Pediatric Sepsis: Diagnosis and Management

Pediatric Sepsis: Diagnosis and Management

Editor: Alonso Egerton

AMERICAN
MEDICAL PUBLISHERS
www.americanmedicalpublishers.com

AMERICAN
MEDICAL PUBLISHERS
www.americanmedicalpublishers.com

Cataloging-in-Publication Data

Pediatric sepsis : diagnosis and management / edited by Alonso Egerton.
p. cm.
Includes bibliographical references and index.
ISBN 979-8-88740-370-0
1. Septicemia in children. 2. Septicemia--Diagnosis. 3. Septicemia--Treatment. 4. Septicemia.
5. Communicable diseases in children. 6. Pediatric hematology. I. Egerton, Alonso.
RJ320.S45 P43 2023
618.920 1--dc23

American Medical Publishers,
41 Flatbush Avenue,
1st Floor, New York,
NY 11217, USA

ISBN 979-8-88740-370-0 (Hardback)

Contents

Preface

In my initial years as a student, I used to run to the library at every possible instance to grab a book and learn something new. Books were my primary source of knowledge and I would not have come such a long way without all that I learnt from them. Thus, when I was approached to edit this book; I became understandably nostalgic. It was an absolute honor to be considered worthy of guiding the current generation as well as those to come. I put all my knowledge and hard work into making this book most beneficial for its readers.

Pediatric sepsis is a medical condition, which involves a severe inflammatory response in the body that can lead to tissue damage and organ failure in children. Premature babies and infants are most susceptible to this condition. The common symptoms include fever, lethargy, nausea, vomiting, dizziness and dehydration. There is no single diagnostic test for sepsis. A combination of tests such as a spinal fluid test, X-ray, or ultrasound may be required for diagnosing sepsis. Urine tests are done to gain information on urinary tract infection and kidney condition. In addition, blood tests are used to detect the presence of elevated or low white blood cells, lactic acid, and C-reactive protein (CRP). Infants and children who have developed sepsis need close monitoring and specialized medical and life-care support systems such as ventilators. Treatment with intravenous fluids, antibiotics, and other medications helps in improving the condition of the patients. Preventive measures such as frequent hand washing, vaccines, and timely medical attention inhibit an infection from developing in the first place. This book contains some path-breaking studies related to pediatric sepsis. It outlines the diagnosis and management of this disease in detail. Those in search of information to further their knowledge will be greatly assisted by this book.

I wish to thank my publisher for supporting me at every step. I would also like to thank all the authors who have contributed their researches in this book. I hope this book will be a valuable contribution to the progress of the field.

Editor

1

Life-Threatening Infectious Complications in Sickle Cell Disease

Dominik Ochocinski[1], Mansi Dalal[2], L. Vandy Black[2], Silvana Carr[3], Judy Lew[3], Kevin Sullivan[1,4] and Niranjan Kissoon[5]*

[1] Department of Anesthesiology, University of Florida, Gainesville, FL, United States, [2] Division of Pediatric Hematology/Oncology, University of Florida, Gainesville, FL, United States, [3] Division of Pediatric Infectious Disease, University of Florida, Gainesville, FL, United States, [4] Congenital Heart Center, University of Florida, Gainesville, FL, United States, [5] Department of Pediatrics, University of British Columbia and BC Children's Hospital, Vancouver, BC, Canada

***Correspondence:**
Kevin Sullivan
ksullivan@anest.ufl.edu

Sickle cell disease (SCD) results in chronic hemolytic anemia, recurrent vascular occlusion, insidious vital organ deterioration, early mortality, and diminished quality of life. Life-threatening acute physiologic crises may occur on a background of progressive diminishing vital organ function. Sickle hemoglobin polymerizes in the deoxygenated state, resulting in erythrocyte membrane deformation, vascular occlusion, and hemolysis. Vascular occlusion and increased blood viscosity results in functional asplenia and immune deficiency in early childhood, resulting in life-long increased susceptibility to serious bacterial infections. Infection remains a main cause of overall mortality in patients with SCD in low- and middle-income countries due to increased exposure to pathogens, increased co-morbidities such as malnutrition, lower vaccination rates, and diminished access to definitive care, including antibiotics and blood. Thus, the greatest gains in preventing infection-associated mortality can be achieved by addressing these factors for SCD patients in austere environments. In contrast, in high-income countries, perinatal diagnosis of SCD, antimicrobial prophylaxis, vaccination, aggressive use of antibiotics for febrile episodes, and the availability of contemporary critical care resources have resulted in a significant reduction in deaths from infection; however, chronic organ injury is problematic. All clinicians, regardless of their discipline, who assume the care of SCD patients must understand the importance of infectious disease as a contributor to death and disability. In this concise narrative review, we summarize the data that describes the importance of infectious diseases as a contributor to death and disability in SCD and discuss pathophysiology, prevalent organisms, prevention, management of acute episodes of critical illness, and ongoing care.

Keywords: sickle cell disease, infection, children, sepsis, prophylaxis, vaccination, critical care

INTRODUCTION

Human hemoglobin is a tetramer comprising two alpha (α) and two non-α globin chains that envelop oxygen-carrying heme moieties. Normal hemoglobin is composed of hemoglobin A (95% of total hemoglobin), which contains two α-chains and two beta (β)-chains, hemoglobin A2, which is composed of two α-chains and two delta (δ)-chains (1–4%), and fetal hemoglobin, which consists

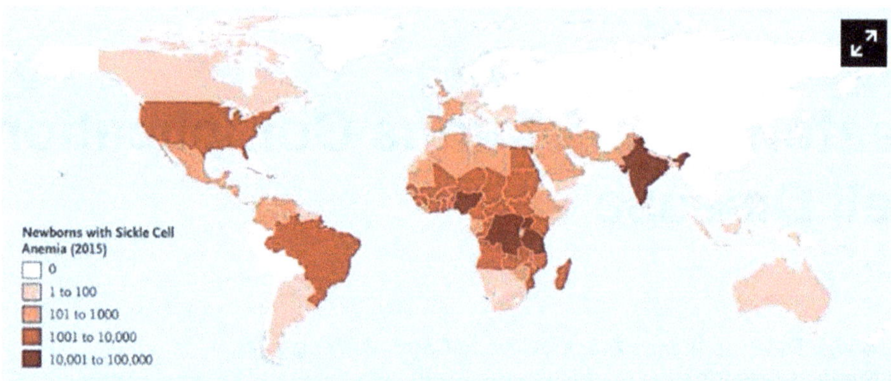

FIGURE 1 | Number of newborns with Sickle Cell Anemia is Each Country in 2015. Data are based on estimates from Piel et al. Alaska is shown separately from the rest of the United States. Used with permission from Piel FB, Steinberg MH, Rees DC. Sickle cell disease. N Engl J Med (2017) 376:1561-1573.

of two α-chains and two gamma (γ)-chains (70–90% at birth, with a subsequent decline through the first 6 months of life).

The sickle cell disease (SCD) phenotype is the result of the substitution of valine for glutamine at the 6th amino acid position of the β-chain. Hemoglobin that incorporates this amino acid substitution is referred to as sickle hemoglobin (HbS). Patients who are heterozygous at this locus have sickle cell trait (HbAS) and are largely asymptomatic, whereas patients homozygous for the sickle β-chain mutation have sickle cell anemia (HbSS). Patients who inherit the sickle β-chain mutation along with other distinct β-chain mutations such as sickle β-thalassemia ($HbS\beta^0$ or $HbS\beta^+$ thalassemia) or hemoglobin C (HbSC disease) also exhibit the SCD phenotype. Patients with HbSS and $HbS\beta^0$ experience severe symptoms, whereas patients with HbSC and $HbS\beta^+$ are generally less affected.

SCD has a worldwide distribution. It is estimated that 300,000 infants are born annually with SCD, most in sub-Saharan Africa (1, 2). In the United States, 1 in 2,500 live births are afflicted with SCD (3), and it is estimated that 100,000 patients with SCD live in the United States (4). However, patients living in high-income countries (HICs) account for only 10% of the world's SCD population (5). The African continent, in particular, bears the burden of SCD, where the United Nations estimates that 12–15 million of the world's 25 million SCD patients live (6). Childhood mortality among SCD patients is highest between 6 months and 3 years of age (5–8), and it is estimated that 75% of all babies born with SCD are born in Africa where the mortality rate for children under 5 is estimated to exceed 50% (5, 9). The worldwide distribution of SCD is illustrated in **Figure 1**.

Immune function in pediatric SCD patients is impaired for a variety of reasons, including deficient splenic clearance of opsonized encapsulated bacteria (10, 11). This results in a propensity to infection by encapsulated bacteria such as *Streptococcus pneumoniae*, *Haemophilus influenzae*, *Salmonella typhi* and *non-typhi*, and *Meningococcal* species. In sub-Saharan Africa, one-half of patients with SCD die from infection before the age of 5, and children with SCD are >50 times more likely to suffer from invasive pneumococcal disease (12–16).

Early childhood SCD mortality has been dramatically reduced in HICs due to neonatal SCD screening, the provision of vaccination and prophylactic antibiotics, the aggressive early use of intravenous antibiotic therapy for febrile episodes, and the availability of contemporary pediatric critical care services. SCD patients in HICs commonly live into the fourth decade and beyond (17–19), during which time they accumulate chronic injury to their cardiovascular, central nervous, renal, pulmonary, and musculoskeletal systems.

SCD is a multisystem disease characterized by disordered hemoglobin structure, aberrant endothelial interactions, systemic inflammation, oxidant stress, and activation of the coagulation system. These derangements result in a tenuous physiology susceptible to infection-mediated acute crises, including splenic sequestration, acute chest syndrome, stroke, aplastic and vaso-occlusive crises, long-term disability, and death.

Herein, we discuss aspects of severe infections in children with SCD, including burden pathophysiology, prevention, therapy, and outcomes.

MATERIALS AND METHODS

The PubMed and Google Scholar databases were queried for English-language original research, literature reviews, systematic reviews, case reports, and meta-analyses relevant to the epidemiology, outcomes, prevention, treatment, and pathophysiology of infectious complications in SCD patients. Search terms included combinations of the following terms; sickle cell disease, sickle, chronic, organ dysfunction, hemoglobinopathy, pathophysiology, bacteria, bacterial, virus, viral, parasitic, malaria, sepsis, pneumococcal, invasive, *Haemophilus*, *Streptococcus*, *Salmonella*, HIV, tuberculosis, infection, complications, pneumonia, osteomyelitis, meningitis, bacteremia, vaccination, spleen, splenic, opsonization, prophylaxis, prevention, guidelines, recommendations, and

Abbreviations: SCD, sickle cell disease; LMIC, low- and middle-income countries; HIC, high-income country.

immunization. Publications identified by the primary search were reviewed, and additional references were retrieved from the bibliographies of the articles identified by the primary search. The publications most appropriate to the pre-selected topics to be covered in this concise review were selected for inclusion.

PREDISPOSITION TO INFECTION

Patients with SCD are prone to infection for a variety of reasons that include splenic dysfunction, defects in opsonization of encapsulated organisms, impaired adaptive immunity, and immune deficiencies associated with malnutrition. The factors that contribute to immune deficiency in patients with SCD are summarized in **Table 1**. Indeed, malnutrition and the onset of splenic dysfunction early in life results in life-long deficiencies in innate, humoral, and cellular immune function.

Splenic Dysfunction

The spleen is primarily responsible for filtering circulating pathogens and promoting innate and adaptive immune functions. Bacterial killing by macrophages is hampered because microbial opsonization with antibodies and/or complement, a prerequisite for the destruction of encapsulated bacteria, is impaired (21, 22, 30). Macrophages also present microbial antigens to T-lymphocytes, which in turn stimulate B-lymphocytes to produce high-affinity antibodies required for opsonization of encapsulated bacteria (31, 32).

Splenic dysfunction, including impaired filtration, deformation, and stagnation of red blood cells, and shunting, begins in infancy and is reflected by the presence of Howell-Jolly bodies in the peripheral blood (33). Chronic vaso-occlusion and ischemia damage the structure and function of the spleen, resulting in auto-splenectomy by 3–5 years of age, but functional asplenia and the resultant susceptibility to serious bacterial infection is present even earlier in childhood (34).

TABLE 1 | Summary of immune system dysfunction and mechanisms leading to increased susceptibility to infections in patients with sickle cell disease.

System	Mechanism
INNATE IMMUNE DYSFUNCTION	
Neutrophil dysfunction (20)	Impaired neutrophil chemotaxis, migration, and killing ability
Splenic dysfunction (21, 22)	Repeated sickling within the spleen leads to compromised splenic filtration of microorganisms
Reduced opsonization (23, 24)	Reduced opsonin production, leading to decreased ability to destroy encapsulated organisms
ADAPTIVE IMMUNE DYSFUNCTION	
Decreased humoral immunity (25)	Loss of splenic marginal zone leads to reduced number of Memory B cells and reduced antigen-specific immunoglobulin M secretion
Impaired virus-directed immunity (26)	Decreased Th1 response with reduced CD4+:CD8 suppressor T Cells
MECHANICAL FACTORS	
Increased susceptibility to osteomyelitis (27)	Bony infarction secondary to sluggish circulation leading to infarcts, which then act a nidus for bacterial proliferation
NUTRITIONAL	
Impaired virus-directed immunity (28, 29)	Zinc deficiency leads to lymphopenia and decreased Th1 response

Opsonization

Splenic opsonization is impaired due to deficient immunoglobulins and impaired production of the opsonins required for bacterial destruction. Efficient opsonization relies on the complement cascade, which is activated by classical and alternative pathways and kills invading microbes by inserting pores into their cell membranes (35, 36). In SCD, the insufficient availability of splenic immunoglobulin (Ig) M results in impaired opsonization and diminished classical pathway activation. Other opsonins, including tuftsin, which are produced in the spleen and needed for the activation of granulocytes, macrophages, and monocytes, are decreased in patients with SCD, suggesting a role for the spleen in their production (23, 24). Similarly, deficient levels of complement factor B, a protease that binds to C3b and amplifies the alternative complement pathway, is deficient, likely due to consumption from clearing sickled erythrocytes (37–39).

Lymphocytes

Children with SCD are also vulnerable to atypical bacteria and viruses, suggesting other defects in immunity. B- and T-cell lymphocyte function are impaired in SCD, resulting in inadequate memory B-cell function and T-cell–independent production of natural anti-polysaccharide antibodies (25, 40, 41). The IgM antibody response to the influenza vaccine is also diminished in SCD patients (41). Circulating CD4+ and CD8+ T-lymphocytes are reduced in patients with SCD, and their differentiation into mature lymphocytes is adversely affected (26). This results in a diminished humoral immune response (referred to as Th2) or a cell-mediated immune response (referred to as a Th1 response) by CD4+ T-lymphocytes. Polarization of naive CD4+ cells away from an effective cell-mediated immunity effector stance may explain the development of severe influenza virus infections in children with SCD (42).

Other Factors

Sluggish blood flow through the bone and bone marrow promotes bone ischemia, necrosis, and increased susceptibility to *Salmonella* osteomyelitis (27). Nutritional deficiencies impair the immune system in children with SCD. Deficiencies of macro- and micronutrients are present in children with SCD due to mechanisms that may include diminished caloric intake, elevated resting metabolic rate, increased red cell synthesis, elevated protein turnover, dysregulated inflammation, and increased myocardial energy demands (43). Micronutrient deficiencies have been implicated in increased susceptibility to infections and increased frequency of SCD-specific complications.

Low serum immunoglobulin levels are a commonly reported immune abnormality in malnourished children. Zinc deficiency develops as a result of poor dietary intake, high protein turnover, and increased losses from the kidneys due to inadequate reabsorption (44). Zinc deficiency has been linked to lymphopenia, reduced IL-2 production (required for adequate development of cell-mediated immunity), and is associated with deficient coordination of the innate and adaptive immune systems (28, 29). Zinc supplementation in SCD children has been demonstrated to improve somatic growth (45, 46), and supplementation of vitamins A, B, and magnesium has been demonstrated to decrease the frequency of infection, painful crisis, and emergency department visits (47, 48).

INFECTIOUS COMPLICATIONS

Infectious pathogens of relevance to patients with SCD include bacteria, viruses, parasites, and mycobacteria. **Table 2** presents a summary of the features of common infections seen in SCD patients. Empiric antibiotic treatment for bacterial infections are summarized in **Table 3** and should be tempered by the local epidemiology and resistance patterns of bacterial pathogens.

Bacterial Pathogens in SCD and Associated Anatomical Sites

Bacteremia and sepsis are commonly detected in SCD patients. In some series, bacteremia accounted for 10–32% of febrile illnesses (49, 52, 69, 70). In Africa, bacteremia was found in 14–32% of children with SCD, a greater incidence than is observed in HICs (49, 69, 70). In contrast, in 165 Jamaican patients, only 6% of the episodes was caused by bacteremia, but 10% of the bacteremic patients died from their infections (71). Mortality from septicemia reaches 35–50% in infants and young children (50).

Prior to the use of augmented vaccination schedules and routine penicillin prophylaxis, *S. pneumoniae* caused the majority of cases of severe sepsis, followed by *Neisseria meningitidis*, *H. influenzae*, and *Escherichia coli* (11, 50, 72, 73). The epidemiology of bacterial infections and sepsis varies with geographic and socioeconomic circumstances, and includes consideration of *Staphylococcus aureus*, Salmonella species, and Bacteroides species, and other Gram-negative enteric bacilli (49, 51). Short- and long-term intravascular catheters are a common risk factor for bacteremia (74, 75).

Studies in several African countries showed Gram-negative bacteria can cause >50% of bacteremic episodes in children with SCD, with *Klebsiella pneumoniae* (25%), Salmonella *species* (12.5%), and other Gram negatives (25%) were detected more often than Gram-positive bacteria such as *S. aureus* (25%) and *S. pneumoniae* (6.3%) in one such study (49, 76, 77). The reasons for differing epidemiologic results in these studies are unclear but may be due to (a) higher carriage of other microorganisms, (b) liberal use of antibiotics before hospital admission, which influences culture results (mainly penicillin derivatives, often available without prescriptions), (c) difficulties of identifying the cause of infection by routine cultures or polymerase chain reaction in resource-limited settings and, (d) early extra-hospital deaths of children with fulminant infections with encapsulated bacteria (49, 76–80).

Taken together, these data suggest that bacteremia is common in SCD patients in all socioeconomic envirnonments. Bacteremia is associated with significant morbidity and mortality. It is essential to treat it with antibiotics that cover *Streptococcal*, *Haemophilus*, and *Salmonella* species, but it is also necessary to consider coverage for *Staphylococcal* species and Gram-negative enteric bacteria, depending on local data.

Meningitis is caused by *S. pneumoniae* (70–75% of cases), *H. influenzae*, and *N. meningitidis*. *Salmonella* species, *E. coli*, and other Gram-negative enteric bacteria also cause meningitis in children with SCD and must be considered in the differential diagnosis. Mortality has been reported as 10–20% for meningitis (11, 52). Meningitis in SCD generally presents and progresses similarly to meningitis in children <5 years of age without SCD (52). However, meningitis in children with SCD may predispose to stroke, a common complication of SCD (52–54).

Pneumonia is commonly due to *S. pneumoniae* in younger children, and *Chlamydia pneumoniae*, *Mycoplasma pneumoniae*, *Mycoplasma hominis*, and *S. aureus* (and to a lesser extent *Legionella* species) in older children and adults (11, 57–59). Pulmonary infection is one of the principal triggers for acute chest syndrome, and it is often difficult to distinguish patients with acute chest syndrome from those with pneumonia or those who have both. Of 670 acute chest syndrome episodes analyzed during a 4-year period, 45.7% had an unknown cause, 29.4% were attributed to infection, 16.1% to infarction, and 8.8% to fat embolism (57). In an analysis of 292 acute chest syndrome episodes in which a cause could be determined, infection was responsible for one-half of the cases, and of these, 25% were caused by a *Chlamydia* species, 22% were caused by *Mycoplasma* species, and 22% were caused by viruses (57).

Osteomyelitis occurs in between 0.5 and 16% in children and adults with SCD (60, 61, 63, 81). *Salmonella* species and *S. aureus* are the most common infectious etiologies of acute osteomyelitis (42–57%) in North America (52, 60). *Salmonella* species are the most common pathogen in West Africa and Saudi Arabia (52, 62). *Salmonella typhi* (the only encapsulated *Salmonella* species), *Salmonella non-typhi* species, Gram-negative enteric bacteria, and *S. aureus* can all cause osteomyelitis (64). It is often challenging to differentiate vaso-occlusive crisis with bone involvement from osteomyelitis on the basis of imaging or laboratory studies. Osteomyelitis commonly affects the diaphysis of the femur, tibia, or humerus. However, any bone can be affected, and it may be multifocal after hematogenous spread (60, 67, 81). The etiologic organism can be identified by blood culture, aspiration of bone lesion, or bone biopsy (67, 72). Septic arthritis may complicate osteomyelitis and osteonecrosis in children with SCD, and the causative bacteria are similar to those of osteomyelitis (65, 67). *Mycobacterial* infection and fastidious pathogens such as *Kingella kingae* (which can be pursued with molecular testing) may be the reason for sterile cultures.

Urinary tract infection (UTI) prevalence in SCD patients ranges from 6 to 26% and is more common in children with SCD than healthy children (82). Vaso-occlusion within the vasa rectae of the inner medulla causes ischemia, renal

TABLE 2 | Most common pathogens in patients with sickle cell disease, including those living in austere environments.

Infection/system	Micro-organism (s)	Complications/chronic organ dysfunction	Treatment
Bacteremia/sepsis	*S. pneumoniae, S. aureus, GNR (Typhi and non-typhi Salmonella, E. coli, Klebsiella* sp., *H. influenzae type B), Bacteroides* sp. (49–51)	Septic shock with multi-organ failure (50, 52)	- *S. pneumoniae,* Gram-negative rods, some Bacteroides: third-generation cephalosporins (Ceftriaxone, Cefotaxime)* - *S. aureus*: oxacillin, nafcillin, or cefazolin (MSSA)*; Vancomycin, clindamycin (MRSA)*
Meningitis/central nervous system infection	*S. pneumoniae*, *H. influenzae*, and *N. meningitides* (11, 52); *Pasteurella multocida* and *Capnocytophaga* sp. (in the presence of dog bite), viruses (Enteroviruses, herpes simplex viruses, mosquito-borne viruses); *Cryptococcus neoformans* and cerebral *Toxoplasma gondii* (especially in the presence of HIV)	Seizures, hemorrhagic stroke, acute ischemic stroke, venous sinus thrombosis, silent cerebral infarction, intra-cranial abscess, cognitive impairment (52–54)	- Third-generation cephalosporins (Ceftriaxone, Cefotaxime)* - *Capnocyphaga* sp.: beta-lactam/beta-lactamase inhibitors and carbapenems (imipenem, meropenem) - *Pasteurella multocida*: penicillin (drug of choice) - *Cryptococcus neoformans*: a. Amphotericin B deoxycholate or liposomal amphotericin B + fluocytosine (induction phase), followed by fluconazole (consolidation therapy). - *Toxoplasma gondii*: pyrimethamine + sulfadiazine + folic acid. Allergy to sulfa: pyrimethamine + folic acid + clindamycin OR atovaquone - Herpes viruses: intravenous acyclovir
Upper and lower respiratory tract infection (sinusitis, epiglottitis, tracheitis, bronchitis, pneumonia)	Viruses (influenza viruses, respiratory syncytial virus, adenovirus, metapneumovirus, rhino-enterovirus, parvovirus B-19, parainfluenza viruses, cytomegalovirus, Epstein-Barr virus, and herpes simplex viruses, etc.) (55, 56); bacteria (*S. pneumoniae*, *H. influenzae*, *Chlamydophila pneumoniae*, *Mycoplasma pneumoniae*, *Legionella* sp., *S. aureus* (methicillin susceptible and resistant) (11, 57–59)	Acute chest syndrome, chronic lung disease/chronic restrictive lung disease, pulmonary hypertension	- Influenza: oseltamivir, inhaled zanamivir, baxtamivir - *S. pneumoniae*, *H. influenza type B*: third-generation cephalosporins (Ceftriaxone, Cefotaxime)*; *S. aureus*: oxacillin, nafcillin, or cefazolin (MSSA)*; Vancomcyin, clindamycin (MRSA)* - Cytomegalovirus: intravenous gancyclovir/oral valganciclovir; Epstein-Barr virus: intravenous ganciclovir; Herpes viruses: intravenous or oral acyclovir, valacyclovir, or famciclovir - *Chlamydophila pneumoniae*, *Mycoplasma pneumoniae*, *Legionella* sp.: macrolides, quinolones
Musculoskeletal (skin and soft tissue infection, septic arthritis, fasciitis, myositis, osteomyelitis)	*Typhi* and *non-typhi Salmonella*, Gram-negative enteric bacteria, other Gram-negative (*Kingella kingae,* especially in the presence of negative cultures); *S. aureus* (methicillin susceptible and resistant), *S. pneumonia* (51, 52, 60–62)	Avascular necrosis, leg ulceration (skin), osteonecrosis (63, 64)	- Third-generation cephalosporins (Ceftriaxone, Cefotaxime)* - *S. aureus*: oxacillin, nafcillin, or cefazolin (MSSA)*; vancomycin, clindamycin (MRSA)* - *Kingella kingae*: ampicillin-sulbactam or a first-, second-, or third-generation cephalosporin
Gastrointestinal (cholelithiasis/ choledocholithiasis, cholecystitis, cholangitis, intussusception), gastroenteritis	Enteric Gram-negative pathogens including *Typhi* and *non-typhi Salmonella*, Enterococci, anaerobic bacteria (65) and *Yersinia enterocolitica* infections (66)	Cholangiopathy (e.g., common biliary duct obstruction, cholestasis), hepatopathy (e.g., hepatic vaso-occlusive crisis, sequestration; hepatic fibrosis secondary to iron overload), mesenteric vaso-occlusion, and bowel infarcts	- Piperacillin-tazobactam or a carbapenem (imipenem, meropenem) - Surgical consult for decompression (stent/drains placement) or open/laparoscopic cholecystectomy - For Yersinia, a third-generation cephalosporin, piperacillin, or trimethoprim-sulfamethoxazole
Urogenital (urinary tract infection, pyelonephritis, renal abscess, urosepsis)	Gram-negative pathogens	Papillary necrosis, hematuria, renal failure, priapism (67)	- Third-generation cephalosporin (Ceftriaxone, Cefotaxime)*

(Continued)

TABLE 2 | Continued

Infection/system	Micro-organism (s)	Complications/chronic organ dysfunction	Treatment
Malaria	*Plasmodium falciparum, Plasmodium vivax, Plasmodium ovale, Plasmodium malariae*, and *P. knowlesi*	Vaso-occlusive crisis and secondary pain crisis, splenic sequestration; acute and chronic severe anemia requiring blood transfusion and causing folate-deficiency anemia; nephrotic syndrome, shock, hypoglycemia, acidosis, thrombocytopenia, and multi-organ failure	- Severe malaria requiring intensive care unit admission: intravenous quinidine until the parasite density <1% and able to tolerate oral therapy; alternative = intravenous artesunate*[2] - Oral therapy: based on the infecting species, possible drug resistance, and severity of disease = Avoid exposure to mosquitoes and avoid areas with outbreaks of mosquito-borne infections.
Tuberculosis (*Mycobacterium tuberculosis*)	*Mycobacterium tuberculosis*	Vaso-occlusive crisis, acute chest syndrome; chronic pulmonary dysfunction, increased hemolysis, sub-optimal reticulocytosis, and anemia; extra-pulmonary tuberculosis (meningeal, lymph nodes, bones, joints, skin, middle ear, mastoid, gastrointestinal, renal)	- Presumed or known drug-susceptible pulmonary tuberculosis (except meningeal disease): a 6-month, 4-drug regimen consisting initially of rifampin, isoniazid, pyrazinamide, and ethambutol for the first 2 months and isoniazid and rifampin for the remaining 4 months - Drug-resistant tuberculosis: an expert in drug-resistant tuberculosis should be consulted for all drug-resistant cases
Human immunodeficiency infection	Human Immunodeficiency Virus (HIV-1 and HIV-2); HIV-2 is mainly prevalent in Western Africa	Increased risk for stroke, splenic dysfunction, avascular necrosis, and pulmonary arterial hypertension; increased risk of sepsis and bacterial infection, mainly pneumococcal infection	Because HIV treatment options and recommendations change with time and vary with occurrence of antiretroviral drug resistance and adverse event profile, consultation with a HIV expert is recommended[¥].
Dengue fever, dengue hemorrhagic fever/dengue shock syndrome	Arbovirus (*Flaviviridae* family; genus *Flavivirus*)	Vaso-occlusive crisis, splenic sequestration, leg ulcers requiring amputation, myocarditis, heart block, shock, plasma leakage and secondary pulmonary and brain edema, ascites, anasarca, hemorrhage, multiorgan failure	- Supportive care: high intake of fluids, soft diet, acetaminophen [avoid salicylate-containing (aspirin) and non-steroidal anti-inflammatory products (ibuprofen)] and tepid sponging for relief of fever, adequate oxygenation, vasopressors, intravenous isotonic crystalloid (0.45% sodium chloride if <6 months of age) and colloids solution (avoid overload), blood products transfusion, diuretics for fluid overload; empirical therapy for bacterial infection pending cultures results. Steroids, anti-viral therapy (chloroquine, balapiravir, celgosivir).
Parasitic infections	Helminths: *Ascaris lumbricoides, Ancylostoma duodenale, Trichuris trichiura, Strongyloides stercoralis*, Schistosomiasis (*S. mansoni, S. haematobium, S. japonicum*), *Toxocara canis*, filariasis (*Onchocerca volvulus*)	- Vaso-occlusive crisis, chronic iron deficiency, chronic eosinophilia - Malnutrition, growth delay, cognitive deficit - Acute intestinal obstruction with intestinal perforation and peritonitis; appendicitis, common bile duct obstruction with secondary biliary colic, cholangitis, or pancreatitis (ascariasis) - Infiltrative eosinophilic pneumonitis syndrome (Ascariasis, Ancylostomiasis, schistosomiasis, filariasis, toxocariasis) with secondary hypoxia and acute chest syndrome	- *lumbricoides, A. duodenale*: albendazole, mebendazole, and pyrantel pamoate - *T. trichiura*: albendazole, mebendazole, and ivermectin - *S. stercoralis*: ivermectin (drug of choice), mebendazole - Schistosomiasis: praziquantel (drug of choice) - *T. canis*: albendazole, mebendazole - Filariasis: ivermectin; alternative = doxycycline (not recommended for children younger than 8 years)

(Continued)

TABLE 2 | Continued

Infection/system	Micro-organism (s)	Complications/chronic organ dysfunction	Treatment
		- Urinary schistosomiasis (*S. haematobium*) causing hematuria and predisposition to bacterial infection - Hepatosplenomegaly, bloody diarrhea, portal hypertension, ascites, esophageal varices, and hematemesis (chronic *S. mansoni* and *S. japonicum* infections) - Visual loss/blindness (filariasis, *T. canis*) - Strongyloides hyperinfection syndrome (in immunocompromised patients); larvae migration to distant organs causing fever, abdominal pain, diffuse pulmonary infiltrates, septicemia, and meningitis caused by enteric Gram-negative bacilli	
	Protozoa (other than malaria): *Entamoeba histolytica*, *Entamoeba coli* and *Giardia lamblia*	Chronic Giardia infection with secondary chronic intestinal malabsorption and failure to thrive - Toxic megacolon, fulminant colitis, ulcerations on colonic mucosa and secondary perforation; hepatic, pleural, lungs, and pericardium abscesses (*E. histolytica*)	- Hand hygiene after defecation, before preparing or eating food, after changing a diaper or caring for someone with diarrhea and after handling an animal or its waste - Sanitary disposal of fecal material - Treatment of drinking water (boiling, chemical disinfection with iodine or chlorine, use of filters) - Sexual transmission: use of condoms and avoidance of sexual practices that may permit fecal-oral transmission (*E. histolytica*). - Refrain from using recreational water venues (e.g., swimming pools, water parks) until asymptomatic and completed treatment

**Antibiotic selection should take into consideration local epidemiology and antibiotic-resistant patterns. For developing countries, also refer to World Health Organization recommendations: https://apps.who.int/medicinedocs/en/d/Js5406e/.*
**[2] Available through the CDC malaria hotline investigational new drug (IND) protocol.*
¥ http://aidsinfo.nih.gov.

infarction, papillary necrosis, and scarring of the renal medulla, which promotes UTI (83). Many episodes of Gram-negative septicemia in SCD are secondary to UTI (82–84). In a recent U.S.-based study, UTI was a common reason for fever in SCD children (70). Thus, screening with urinalysis and urine culture during febrile illnesses is important in SCD children, particularly young children $\leq$2 years of age (70, 84, 85).

Abdominal pain with fever is common among patients with SCD and its prevalence increases with age and severity of hemolysis (83). Abdominal pain, nausea, vomiting, fever, and jaundice are common presenting symptoms of cholecystitis. In a recent cross-sectional, hospital-based study of SCD patients, 92.3% of patients with cholecystitis were older than 5 years (86). The pathogens of concern in cholecystitis include enteric Gram-negative pathogens, *Enterococci*, and anaerobic bacteria. Piperacillin-tazobactam and carbapenem antibiotics are considered first-line therapies. Surgical consultation is needed for decompression (surgical-, percutaneous-, or endoscopic retrograde cholangiopancreatography-placed stent/drains) or open or laparoscopic cholecystectomy. Abdominal pain with fever is also characteristic of infection with *S. typhi* (Typhoid fever), Dengue viruses (Dengue fever), and *Yersinia enterocolitica* (thought to be related to the unusual use of iron by this microorganism). *Y. enterocolitica* has been associated with intussusception in a patient with sickle cell anemia (66).

The oral cavity is a source of infectious and non-infectious complications. Orofacial pain in SCD patients may be due to vaso-occlusion in the facial bones and dental pulp, or osteomyelitis of the facial bones. Osteomyelitis is more likely to occur in the mandible due to the relatively poor blood supply in this area. Pathogens responsible for facial osteomyelitis come from the gastrointestinal tract (cholecystitis or gastroenteritis) by hematogenous spread (87). *Salmonella* is a common etiology for facial osteomyelitis, but mixed flora and *S. aureus* also account for a substantial percentage of cases (87, 88). It is often difficult

TABLE 3 | Prophylaxis for the most common pathogens in patients with sickle cell disease, including those living in austere environments.

Infection/system	Micro-organism(s)	Prophylaxis*+
Bacteremia/sepsis	*S. pneumoniae*, *S. aureus*, GNR (*Typhi* and *non-typhi Salmonella*, *E. coli*, *Klebsiella* sp., *H. influenzae*), *Bacteroides* sp. (49–51)	- Diphtheria/tetanus/pertussis/*H. influenzae type B*/polio/13-valent pneumococcal vaccine at 2, 4, and 6 months (13-valent pneumococcal and *H. influenzae type B* also at 12–15 months); - *S. pneumoniae* 23-valent vaccine (at 2 years of age and 5 years later) at least 2 months after the 13-valent vaccine (68) - Penicillin V prophylaxis; erythromycin if penicillin allergy. Starting at age of 2 months until 5 years or for a history of pneumococcal sepsis or surgical splenectomy and continued lifelong (68) - *Salmonella typhi* vaccine for travel to resource-poor areas
Meningitis/central nervous system	*S. pneumoniae*, *H. influenzae*, and *N. meningitidis* (11, 52); *Pasteurella multocida* and *Capnocytophaga* sp. (in the presence of dog bite), viruses (Enteroviruses, herpes simplex viruses, mosquito-borne viruses); *Cryptococcus neoformans* and cerebral *Toxoplasma gondii* (especially in the presence of HIV)	- Diphtheria/tetanus/pertussis/*H. influenzae type B*/polio/13-valent pneumococcal vaccine/meningococcal vaccine+ at 2, 4, and 6 months (13-valent pneumococcal/*H. influenza type B* also at 12–15 months and meningococcal vaccine+ at 12 months). - *S. pneumoniae* 23-valent vaccine (at 2 years of age and 5 years later) at least 2 months after the 13-valent vaccine (68) - Meningococcal vaccine+2, including travel to resource-poor areas. - Meningococcal B vaccination+3, can start at 10 years of age. - Penicillin V prophylaxis; erythromycin if penicillin allergy. Starting at age of 2 months until 5 years or for a history of pneumococcal sepsis or surgical splenectomy and continued lifelong (68) - Avoid bites, scratches, and have mindful contact with dogs (*Capnocytophaga* sp., *Pasteurella multocida*).
Upper and lower respiratory tract infection (sinusitis, epiglottitis, tracheitis, bronchitis, pneumonia)	Viruses (influenza viruses, respiratory syncytial virus, adenovirus, metapneumovirus, rhino-enterovirus, parvovirus B-19, parainfluenza viruses, cytomegalovirus, Epstein-Barr virus, and herpes simplex viruses, etc.) (55, 56); bacteria (*S. pneumoniae*, *H. influenzae*, *Chlamydophila pneumoniae*, *Mycoplasma pneumoniae*, *Legionella* sp., *S. aureus* (methicillin susceptible and resistant) (11, 57–59)	- Annual influenza vaccine from 6 months. - Diphtheria/tetanus/pertussis/*H. influenzae type B*/polio/13-valent pneumococcal vaccine at 2, 4, and 6 months (13-valent pneumococcal and *H. influenzae type B* also at 12-15 months). - *S. pneumoniae* 23- valent vaccine (at 2 years of age and 5 years later) at least 2 months after the 13-valent vaccine (68) - Penicillin V prophylaxis; erythromycin if penicillin allergy. Starting at age of 2 months until 5 years or for a history of pneumococcal sepsis or surgical splenectomy and continued lifelong (68)
Musculoskeletal (skin and soft tissue infection, septic arthritis, fasciitis, myositis, osteomyelitis)	*Typhi* and *non-typhi Salmonella*, Gram-negative enteric bacteria, other Gram-negative (*Kingella kingae*, especially in the presence of negative cultures), *S. aureus* (methicillin susceptible and resistant), *S. pneumoniae* (51, 52, 60–62) *H. influenzae type B*	- Diphtheria/tetanus/pertussis/*H. influenza type B*/polio/13-valent pneumococcal vaccine at 2, 3, and 4 months (13-valent pneumococcal/H. influenza also at 12–15 months). - *S. pneumoniae* 23-valent vaccine (at 2 years of age and 5 years later) at least 2 months after the 13-valent vaccine (68) - Penicillin V prophylaxis; erythromycin if penicillin allergy. Starting at age of 2 months until 5 years or for a history of pneumococcal sepsis or surgical splenectomy and continued lifelong (68) - *Salmonella typhi* vaccine for travel to resource-poor areas.
Gastrointestinal (cholelithiasis/ choledocholithiasis, cholecystitis, cholangitis, intussusception), gastroenteritis	Enteric Gram-negative pathogens, including *Typhi* and *non-typhi Salmonella*, Enterococci, and anaerobic bacteria (65)	- Prevention of vaso-occlusive crisis: avoid hypoxia, acidosis, hypothermia, infection, hypovolemia, etc.) - Decreased hemolysis/gallstone formation: hydroxyurea, ursodiol, low-fat diet - Prophylactic cholecystectomy? - *Salmonella typhi* vaccine for travel to endemic areas, known exposure to a carrier or laboratorian who works with *S. typhi*.
Urogenital (urinary tract infection, pyelonephritis, renal abscess, urosepsis)	Gram-negative pathogens	Prevention of vaso-occlusive crisis: avoid hypoxia, acidosis, hypothermia, infection, and hypovolemia.
Malaria	*Plasmodium falciparum*, *Plasmodium vivax*, *Plasmodium ovale*, *Plasmodium malariae*, and *P. knowlesi*	- Lifelong antimalarial chemoprophylaxis in patients living in malaria-endemic countries. - Travel to malaria-endemic areas: a. Avoid exposure to mosquitoes and avoid areas with outbreaks of mosquito-borne infections. b. Mosquito barriers: b.1. Wear Permethrin clothing that fully covers arms and legs and closed shoes, especially during early morning and late afternoon. b.2. Bed nets, screens, and nets tucked around strollers and other confined spaces where young children are placed. Insecticide-treated nets. b.3. Use Environmental Protection Agency-registered mosquito repellents. c. Avoid outdoor activities at dawn and dusk in malaria-endemic areas). d. Malaria chemoprophylaxis□

(Continued)

TABLE 3 | Continued

Infection/system	Micro-organism(s)	Prophylaxis*+
Tuberculosis (*Mycobacterium tuberculosis*)	*Mycobacterium tuberculosis*	- Annual tuberculin skin test or interferon-gamma release assay for HIV-infected persons and incarcerated adolescents. - Bacille Calmette-Guerin (BCG) immunization for those living in endemic areas, in U.S.: when risk of exposure is unavoidable and failure or unfeasibility of other control methods. - Latent tuberculosis infection identification and treatment.
Human immunodeficiency infection	Human Immunodeficiency Virus (HIV-1 and HIV-2); HIV-2 is mainly prevalent in Western Africa	- Safe sex practices. - Pre-exposure prophylaxis for men who have sex with men, heterosexual couples, and injection drug users[€]. - Post-exposure prophylaxis (sexual, other non-occupational exposure, occupational exposure)[€]. - Prevention of HIV transmission from infected pregnant mother-to-child[Ω].
Dengue fever, dengue hemorrhagic fever/dengue shock syndrome	Arbovirus (Flaviviridae family; genus Flavivirus)	- Avoid exposure to mosquitoes and avoid areas with outbreaks of mosquito-borne infections. - Eliminate local mosquito breeding sites (elimination/drainage of receptacles for standing water), keep swimming pools, children's wading pools, and bird baths clean; clearing clogged rain gutters. - Mosquito barriers: a. Wear Permethrin clothing that fully covers arms and legs and closed shoes, especially during early morning and late afternoon. b. Bed nets, screens, and nets tucked around strollers and other confined spaces where young children are placed. Insecticide-treated nets. c. Use Environmental Protection Agency- registered mosquito repellents. - Avoid outdoor activities during daylight hours in Dengue-endemic areas. - No chemoprophylaxis available. - In May 2019, Dengvaxia was FDA approved for 9-45 year olds with laboratory-confirmed prior dengue virus infection. Other vaccine candidates are under clinical trials.
Parasitic infections	Helminths: *Ascaris lumbricoides*, *Ancylostoma duodenale*, *Trichuris trichiura*, *Strongyloides stercoralis*, Schistosomiasis (*S. mansoni*, *S. haematobium*, *S. japonicum*), *Toxocara canis*, *T. filariasis* (*Onchocerca volvulus*)	- Sanitary disposal of human feces (all parasitic infections). - Vegetables cultivated in areas where uncomposed human feces are used as fertilizer must be washed thoroughly and cooked before eating (*A. lumbricoides*). - Wear shoes to avoid contact with contaminated soil (*A. duodenale*). - Chemotherapy prophylaxis: albendazole, mebendazole) to pre-school and school-aged children in areas with >20% prevalence of infection (*A. lumbricoides*, *T. trichiura*). - Screening and treatment of high-risk groups (e.g., children, agricultural workers, and immigrants from endemic areas (*A. duodenale*). - *S. stercoralis* serology in all people with unexplained eosinophilia. - Elimination of the intermediate snail host in endemic areas; avoid contact with fresh water streams, rivers, ponds, or lakes in endemic areas (schistosomiasis). - Proper disposal of cats and dog feces, deworming of dogs and cats, covering sandboxes when not in use (*T. canis*). - Repellents and protective clothing (long sleeves and pants) to decrease exposure to black flies' bites during the day; community-wide mass ivermectin treatment: filariasis).
Parasitic infections	Protozoa (other than malaria): *Entamoeba histolytica*, *Entamoeba coli*, and *Giardia lambli*	Protozoa (other than malaria): *Entamoeba histolytica*, *Entamoeba coli*, and *Giardia lamblia* - Chronic Giardia infection with secondary chronic intestinal malabsorption and failure to thrive. - Toxic megacolon, fulminant colitis, ulcerations on colonic mucosa and secondary perforation; hepatic, pleural, lungs, and pericardium abscesses (*E. histolytica*). - *E. histolytica*: a. Asymptomatic cyst excreters (intraluminal infection): paromomycin or diiodohydroxyquinoline/iodoquinol. b. Invasive colitis or extraintestinal disease: metronidazole or tinidazole followed by diiodohydroxyquinoline/iodoquinol or paromomycin. c. Percutaneous or surgical aspiration of large liver abscesses. d. Piperacillin-tazobactam or Meropenem if peritonitis. - Giardiasis: metronidazole, nitazoxanide, or tinidazole. - Hand hygiene after defecation, before preparing or eating food, after changing a diaper or caring someone with diarrhea, and after handling an animal or its waste.

(Continued)

TABLE 3 | Continued

Infection/system	Micro-organism(s)	Prophylaxis*+
		- Sanitary disposal of fecal material. - Treatment of drinking water (boiling, chemical disinfection with iodine or chlorine, use of filters). - Sexual transmission: use of condoms and avoidance of sexual practices that may permit fecal-oral transmission (*E. histolytica*). - Refrain from using recreational water venues (e.g., swimming pools, water parks) until asymptomatic and completed treatment.

*The standard vaccine series of childhood according to the American Academy of Pediatrics and the Advisory Committee on Immunization Practices should also be provided to all patients with sickle cell disease.
+CDC-guided immunization schedule (for 2019) with notes for those with sickle cell disease: https://www.cdc.gov/vaccines/schedules/hcp/imz/child-adolescent.html.
+2Menveo (groups A, C, Y, W-135) or MenHibtix (groups C, Y, and Haemophilus b Tetanus Toxoid conjugate). Menactra not given until child is 2 years old, with two doses given 8 weeks apart unless travel to country with endemic disease—can start at 9–23 months and given 12 (preferred) or 8 weeks apart.
+3Can be given to adolescents 16–23 years of age at clinical discretion. Bexsero: two-dose series at least 1 month apart. Trumenba: three-dose series at 0, 1–2, and 6 months. Bexsero and Trumenba are not interchangeable, and the same product must be given for all doses used in a series.
□www.cdc.gov/malaria/resources/pdf/treatmenttable.pdf.
€www.cdc.gov/hiv/risk/prep/index.html.
Ωhttps://aidsinfo.nih.gov/guidelines/html/3/perinatal/224/whats-new-in-the-guidelines.

to differentiate early bone infarction from osteomyelitis. Blood culture, magnetic resonance imaging, and bone aspiration/biopsy may be diagnostic. Colonization of the oropharynx with *non-albicans Candida* species and unusual fungi has been observed in patients with SCD, suggesting that penicillin may affect the balance of oral flora (89).

Viral Pathogens in SCD

Respiratory viruses (e.g., respiratory syncytial virus, influenza viruses, rhinovirus, human metapneumovirus, parainfluenza viruses) can trigger significant complications in patients with SCD, including acute chest syndrome, bacterial superinfection, aplastic crisis, splenic sequestration, and painful vaso-occlusive crisis (55, 57, 90). Viral respiratory pathogens promote the development of acute chest syndrome by inducing lung inflammation, injury to the microvasculature of the lung, airway hyper-reactivity, mismatch of ventilation and perfusion, and in some instances, secondary bacterial infection (commonly with *S. aureus* or *S. pneumoniae*) (91–93).

Other viruses such as Parvovirus B19, hepatitis B, hepatitis C, Epstein-Barr Virus, influenza, dengue, and human immunodeficiency virus (HIV) cause significant morbidity for SCD patients worldwide (11, 50, 56). Parvovirus B19 causes transient aplastic crisis in 65–80% of infections in SCD patients. It specifically infects erythroid progenitor cells, resulting in a temporary cessation of erythropoiesis and leading to severe anemia (94). Parvovirus B19 has also been associated with the development of acute chest syndrome, splenic and hepatic sequestration, bone marrow necrosis, pain crisis, and stroke (94). Epstein-Barr Virus infection can cause splenic rupture, thrombocytopenia, agranulocytosis, hemolytic anemia, and hemophagocytic lymphohistiocytosis in SCD. SCD individuals are at high risk for complications from influenza infections; they are hospitalized for influenza at a rate 56 times that of children without SCD (56). The liver may be adversely affected by hepatitis B and C, and HIV infections (72). In resource-challenged areas of the world, the blood supply is a major source of these infections, but unsafe injections given by untrained/informal providers and surgical practices such as circumcision and female genital mutilation are additional sources of hepatitis C transmission (95). The worldwide prevalence of hepatitis C and B infections among SCD patients ranges from 2 to 30% (96) and 1.5–18.9%, respectively (96, 97).

The prevalence of HIV seropositivity in SCD patients varies between 0 and 11.5% (98). Few data are available regarding the impact of coexistent HIV infection and SCD but both diseases increase the risk for stroke, splenic dysfunction, avascular necrosis, and pulmonary arterial hypertension (98). SCD patients with HIV may be more susceptible to infection with encapsulated bacteria as well as opportunistic pathogens. In a U.S. hospital-based study, SCD with HIV infection conferred a greater risk for hospitalization for bacterial infection and sepsis but less risk for vaso-occlusive crisis. Inpatient case fatality data for children with SCD and HIV were not different from that of children with SCD alone but fatalities were lower than those of children with HIV infection only (99). SCD may confer protection against HIV infection because of upregulation of inflammation, iron metabolism, and auto-splenectomy, which are not favorable for HIV replication (98).

A final concern emerging among viral pathogens is the significant overlap of the mosquito-borne dengue viruses (DENV 1-4) in geographic areas of the world where SCD is endemic. These include the Caribbean, Central and South America, areas of Africa and the Middle East, Asia, and Oceania (100, 101). Dengue hemorrhagic fever is a viral infection that is characterized by headache, fever, abdominal pain, bleeding, myalgias, and loss of capillary integrity with extensive third-space fluid losses, resulting in hypovolemia and death. Sickle cell patients, because of their intolerance of hypovolemia and proclivity to endothelial cell activation, are at increased risk to die from this viral infection (101, 102).

Parasites

Malaria is caused by a protozoan parasite from the Plasmodium family that is transmitted by the bite of the Anopheles mosquito, a contaminated needle, or a blood transfusion. The sickle cell trait is believed to confer a protective effect against severe, life-threatening malaria because sickled erythrocytes are readily cleared by splenic macrophages (11, 72, 103). The effect of malaria on morbidity and mortality in homozygous SCD patients however is severe, with mortality in the SCD population significantly increased when compared to malaria in persons without SCD (104, 105). Studies in two African nations demonstrated that the incidence of malaria was not increased among patients with SCD, but that the risk of death was much higher in malaria patients with SCD when compared to those without SCD (106–108).

Parasitic infections are a common problem in developing countries, and can increase morbidity in patients with SCD. In a Nigerian study of 100 SCD patients, 27% were found to be infected with intestinal parasites that included four helminths (*Ascaris lumbricoides, Ancylostoma duodenale, Trichuris trichiura,* and *Strongyloides stercoralis*) and three protozoa (*Entamoeba histolytica, Entamoeba coli,* and *Giardia lamblia*) (109). Intestinal parasites increase the severity of anemia and the need for transfusion (109). Finally, urinary schistosomiasis is an endemic disease in rural and urban communities in Africa. Schistosomiasis infection in patients with SCD is associated with increased reticulocyte count and lower hematocrit due to urinary blood loss. In addition, urinary schistosomiasis can promote secondary bacterial UTI (110).

Mycobacteria

M. tuberculosis and SCD are prevalent co-morbidities in austere environments, and features of tuberculosis in children with SCD are comparable to those in the general population with favorable outcomes with standard treatment (111).

INFECTION PROPHYLAXIS

Perhaps the greatest reductions in infectious morbidity and mortality have occurred as a result of advances related to the administration of antibiotic prophylaxis, vaccination, and the prompt administration of parenteral antibiotics during febrile illness. Indeed, the rationale for the perinatal screening of infants for SCD is to facilitate participation in these preventive measures. **Table 3** summarizes the recommended antibiotic prophylaxis and vaccination schedules for the prevention of infections in SCD patients.

Before the advent of penicillin prophylaxis, the incidence of invasive pneumococcal disease was 6 episodes/100 patient years, with a peak in the first 3 years of life. Pneumococcal polysaccharide vaccine markedly reduces the risk of invasive pneumococcal disease in children receiving daily prophylactic penicillin (112). However, whether prophylaxis should be continued throughout adulthood is uncertain. Most pediatric hematologists recommend stopping prophylaxis at 5 years of age (112–114). Similarly, the role of penicillin prophylaxis in patients with HbSC, HbS-β^+ thalassemia, and other compound heterozygotes is controversial. Current evidence-based guidelines from the National Heart, Lung, and Blood Institute (115) recommend oral penicillin prophylaxis [(125 mg for age <3 years and 250 mg for age 3 years and older) twice daily until 5 years of age in all children with homozygous SCD (Hb SS)]. These guidelines endorse the discontinuation of penicillin at 5 years of age if there is no history of invasive pneumococcal disease or surgical splenectomy and pneumococcal vaccination is adequate (115).

The heptavalent pneumococcal conjugate vaccine (PCV7) introduced in 2000 led to a further 70% decrease in the incidence of invasive pneumococcal disease (116), with more recent studies suggesting that the PCV13 vaccine introduced in 2010 has further reduced the incidence of serious pneumococcal disease (117, 118). Current standard practice should include the initiation of daily prophylactic penicillin by 2 months of age and the completion of the pneumococcal vaccine series (both PCV13 and pneumococcal 23-valent vaccine) by 5 years of age before the discontinuation of prophylactic penicillin. Some centers recommend pneumococcal polysaccharide vaccine boosters every 5 years, although this practice has not been endorsed by any set of evidence-based guidelines (68). In addition to standard immunizations recommended by the Advisory Committee on Immunization Practices, children with SCD should also be immunized against meningococcal disease and receive the annual influenza vaccine.

Because of the risk of invasive pneumococcal disease, any fever (typically defined as 38.5°C or higher) is treated as a medical emergency in children with SCD. National Heart, Lung, and Blood Institute Guidelines (115) recommend the urgent evaluation of all febrile episodes, including physical examination, complete blood count, and blood culture. Hospitalization for observation is sometimes necessary but most patients with SCD evaluated for fever without a source who lack certain high-risk features (white blood cell count $>30{,}000/mm^3$ or $<5{,}000/mm^3$, fever >40°C, "ill-appearing") can be managed safely as an outpatient after intravenous administration of an empiric, anti-pneumococcal antibiotic that also provides Gram-negative enteric coverage (e.g., ceftriaxone) as long as other SCD-related complications (such as acute chest syndrome) have been excluded. The average time to positive blood cultures for children with SCD and bacteremia is <24 h (119), thus a single dose of ceftriaxone is probably sufficient in most cases of outpatient management.

In low- to middle-income countries, provision of prophylaxis for endemic infections, including malaria and dengue, should be considered. SCD patients traveling to or living within areas endemic for malaria and dengue fever would benefit from meticulous use of maximal mosquito protection techniques and malaria chemoprophylaxis (101, 105). Additionally, malaria prophylaxis should be considered for patients with SCD visiting endemic regions (105, 120). Long-term malaria chemoprophylaxis has been shown to lower the incidence of crisis and to reduce mortality, but few studies have evaluated its benefit, particularly in SCD (106). A recent Cochrane review reported that malaria prophylaxis reduces the frequency of sickle cell crisis, hospital admission, blood transfusion, and anemia severity but suggested further studies to compare antimalarial prophylaxis medications and to better characterize potential adverse outcomes of long-term prophylaxis (120). It is not known how antimalarial drug resistance affects its efficacy (121).

New consensus guidelines for chemoprophylaxis of SCD remains a priority.

Two *Salmonella typhi* vaccines (oral live-attenuated Ty21a and inactivated Vi capsid polysaccharide for persons >6 and >2 years of age, respectively) are available in the United States typically for travelers to endemic typhoid fever areas. Their efficacy in persons with SCD is unknown (122, 123). Both vaccines are allowed for indication, since for vaccine purposes, persons with SCD are considered to have a medical condition with limited immune deficit (asplenia) (Centers for Disease Control and Prevention: https://wwwnc.cdc.gov/travel/yellowbook/2020/travelers-with-additional-considerations/immunocompromised-travelers). However, if age appropriate, the oral vaccine is recommended over the injectable vaccine, which has more known side effects. A recent phase 3 trial of a typhoid conjugate vaccine in Nepal demonstrated excellent immunogenicity, significantly reduced *Salmonella typhi* bacteremia, and had a similar frequency of adverse events as the group A capsular antigen Meningococcal vaccine that was used as a control vaccine (124).

A summary of considerations for persons with SCD traveling to or living in austere environments is also provided in **Tables 3, 4**. The United States Centers for Disease Control (https://wwwnc.cdc.gov/travel/yellowbook/2020/travelers-with-additional-considerations/immunocompromised-travelers) provides a website and book for travel medicine specialists that offers guidance for vaccination and medical prophylaxis for prevalent and endemic infections based on the location of rural or urban destination, recent outbreaks, length of stay, age and immune competency of the traveler, and other variables.

Vaccination and penicillin prophylaxis are effective. In developed nations where children with SCD are identified by newborn screening programs and receive recommended prophylactic treatment with penicillin and an augmented immunization schedule, rates of bacteremia have been shown to be <1% (127). In resource-challenged socioeconomic environments, the priorities remain: (a) clarification of the spectrum of bacterial pathogens relevant to SCD patients in specific geographic regions, (b) implementation of comprehensive perinatal SCD screening, and (c) implementation of vaccination and antibiotic prophylaxis programs appropriate for the bacterial epidemiology of the region.

TABLE 4 | Recommendation for patients with sickle cell disease traveling to austere countries*.

Issue	Recommendations
Vaccination† (see also **Table 3**)	Ensure all age-appropriate vaccinations in **Table 3**: • *Streptococcus pneumoniae* (within 5 years) • *Neisseria meningitidis* (within previous 3 years) • *Haemophilus influenzae* B (once) • Influenza (annually) Additional vaccinations: • Yellow fever (if traveling to endemic African/American countries) • *Salmonella typhi* vaccination (if traveling to endemic areas)
Mosquito-borne illnesses (malaria/Dengue) (see also **Table 3**)	• Ensure basic preventive methods (mosquito nets, insect repellants, avoiding marshy/wet areas with mosquito habitats) • Chemoprophylaxis (all major prophylactic regimens are acceptable) • Prompt diagnosis and treatment of suspected malaria
Gastroenteritis/enteritis (see also **Table 3**)	• Avoid contaminated food and water • Employing adequate hand washing prior to eating or preparing food, after using bathroom • Carry oral electrolyte replacement solutions to ensure proper hydration and to avoid hypovolemia/vaso-occlusive crisis in the setting of gastroenteritis
Invasive bacterial infection (see also **Table 3**)	• Prophylaxis for duration of travel (amoxicillin 250–500 mg PO BID) • Seek medical advice promptly for management of febrile illness • Standby treatment of febrile illness (amoxicillin 3 g PO vs. fluoroquinolone)

*See Willen et al. (125).
Watson (126).
†The standard vaccine series of childhood according to the American Academy of Pediatrics and the Advisory Committee on Immunization Practices should be provided to all sickle cell patients.

TREATMENT OF LIFE-THREATENING INFECTIONS

Bacteremia presents on a continuum of severity that ranges from indolent to fulminant. The incidence of bacteremia varies from 6 to 25% and progresses to life-threatening disease in 10–25% of children in reports from both HICs and low- to middle-income countries.

These data suggest that bacteremia is not the most common cause of fever in persons with SCD and remains life threatening in a significant percentage of patients despite aggressive treatment. It is reasonable to assume that deficiencies in vaccination, antibiotic prophylaxis, rapid hospital transport, intravenous antibiotics, blood supply, microbiologic diagnostic techniques, and critical care capacity in austere environments serve to increase morbidity and mortality from bacteremia. Indeed, mortality rates of 35–50% from septicemia have been described (50).

Infection and the Pathophysiology of SCD

Deoxygenation of HbS alters the structure of the β-chain of hemoglobin, resulting in reduced solubility, hemoglobin polymerization, and diminished membrane flexibility (128–130). Distortion of globin chains and exposure of intracellular heme iron intensifies intracellular oxidant stress, cell membrane damage, and erythrocyte dehydration (129, 130). Vascular occlusion, tissue ischemia, and a cascade of systemic inflammation activate endothelial cells to interact with erythrocytes, activated leukocytes, the coagulation cascade, and activated platelets (131–143). Potent vasoconstrictors are liberated from the endothelium in response to injury (131–145). These events result in endothelial dysfunction, inflammation, and tissue ischemia, which correlates with SCD symptom severity (146, 147). The clinical presentations of SCD-specific complications and serious infections can overlap. Care of the critically ill SCD patient must address infection while supporting the underlying pathophysiology of the disease to prevent or mitigate SCD-related complications. These interactions are summarized in **Figure 2**.

Chronic endothelial inflammation and dysfunction cause progressive vital organ system deterioration over time. Relevant organ system considerations for critical care management are summarized in **Figure 3**.

SCD produces changes in the **cardiovascular system** of children, including diastolic dysfunction and left and right ventricular dilation, usually with preserved systolic function (148–150). Left ventricular systolic function may be impaired in adulthood in patients with renal disease and longstanding hypertension (151). Pulmonary artery hypertension develops for reasons that are multi-factorial and may reflect the intrinsic elevation of pulmonary vascular resistance or left ventricular dysfunction with normal pulmonary vascular resistance. The development of chronic pulmonary hypertension is an ominous finding associated with the increased occurrence of multi-organ system failure and premature mortality (152–155).

The **pulmonary system** is adversely affected by SCD. Younger patients may have mild restrictive lung disease, whereas adults with SCD can develop a severe form of restrictive lung disease referred to as sickle cell chronic lung disease. Asthma carries great clinical significance in SCD as its presence is associated with more frequent episodes of acute chest syndrome early in life and increased mortality and reduced lifespan in adulthood (156, 157).

The **renal system** suffers repeated ischemic insults in the hypertonic medulla that result in impaired urinary-concentrating ability (158). Dialysis and renal transplantation are sometimes necessary in adulthood. The intensivist managing critically ill SCD patients must be mindful to maintain hydration, intake and output, acid-base balance, and the renal elimination of medications. Continuous renal replacement therapy is often helpful in this regard.

The **central nervous system** is the vital organ system most impaired in childhood. The risk of stroke in SCD is highest in the first decade of life, with an incidence of 1% per year between the ages of 2 and 5 (159). Most strokes in children are ischemic, and hemorrhagic stroke accounts for up to one-third of strokes in adults (160). Increased transcranial Doppler flow velocities in the middle cerebral arteries are predictive of future strokes, and patients with increased transcranial Doppler, prior overt stroke, or silent cerebral infarcts are treated with chronic transfusion therapy to prevent future strokes. Risk factors for the recurrence of stroke include the presence of silent cerebral infarction, non-compliance with chronic transfusion therapy after a first stroke, presence of Moyamoya vasculopathy, acute decrease in hemoglobin concentration, history of transient ischemic attack, recent or recurrent episodes of acute chest syndrome, severity of anemia, and systolic hypertension (159, 161).

Differential Diagnosis of Fever and Infectious Syndromes in SCD

Fever without a source is a common problem in SCD patients and should be regarded as a medical emergency requiring rapid evaluation and initiation of intravenous antibiotics. The presentation of sepsis is similar to children without SCD. The presentation of bacteremia may be subtle, however, and can include sudden fever, few prodromal features with a relatively

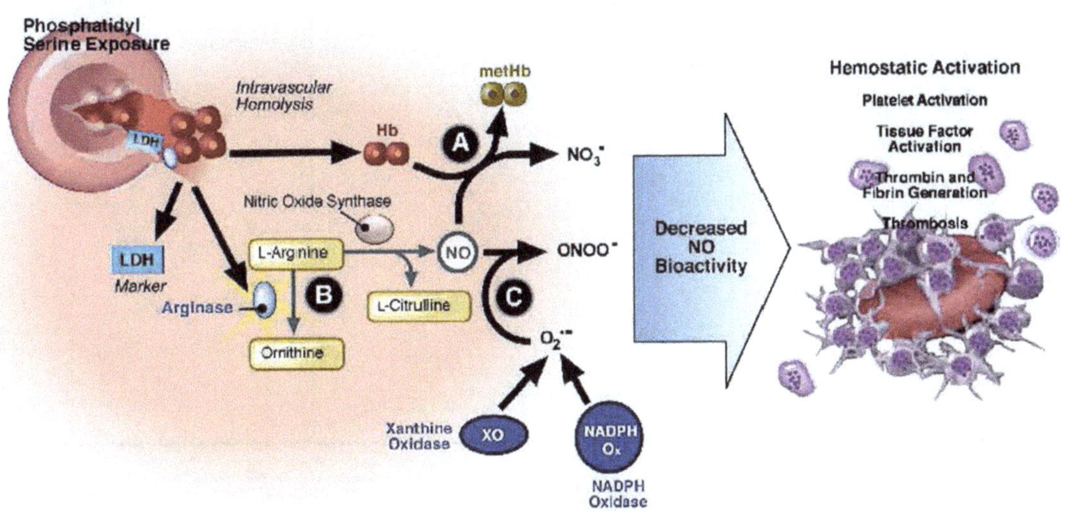

FIGURE 2 | Hemolysis-associated hemostatic activation. Intravascular hemolysis releases hemoglobin into plasma which quenches nitric oxide (NO) and generates reactive oxygen species (directly via fenton chemistry or via induction of xanthine oxidase and NADP oxidase). In addition, arginase I is released from the red blood cell during hemolysis and metabolizes arginine, the substrate for NO synthesis, further impairing NO homeostasis. The depletion of NO is associated with pathological platelet activation and tissue factor expression. Hemolysis and splenectomy are also associated with phosphatidylserine exposure on red cells which can activate tissue factor and form a platform for coagulation. Used with permission from Gladwin MT, Kato GJ. Hemolysis-associated hypercoagulability in sickle cell disease: the plot (and blood) thickens! Haematologica (2008) 93:1-3.

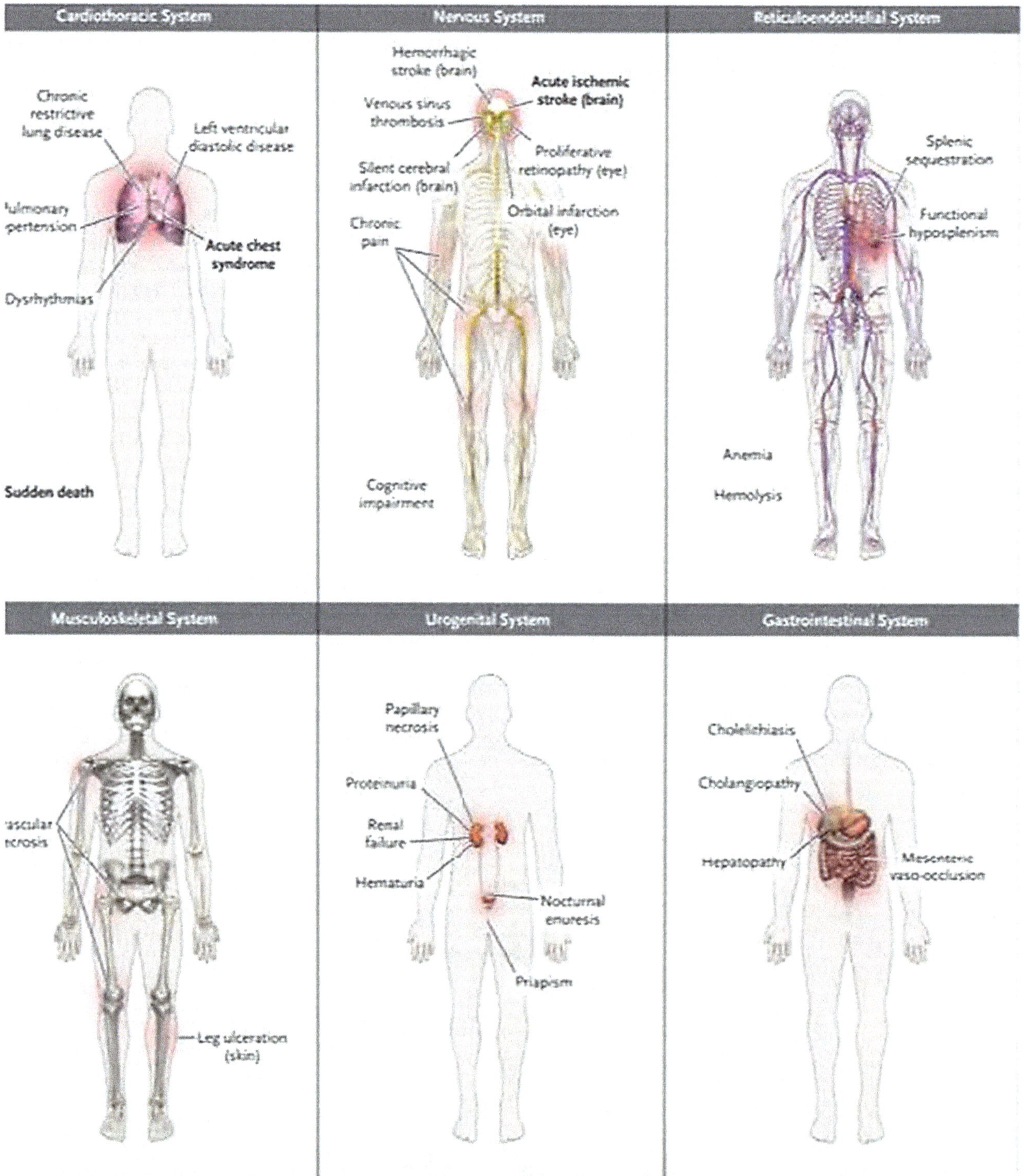

FIGURE 3 | Common clinical complications of sickle cell disease. Data are from Rees et al. and Serjeant. Acute complications are shown in boldface type. Used with permission from Piel FB, Steinberg MH, Rees DC. Sickle cell disease. N Engl J Med (2017) 376:1561-1573.

well appearance, and then rapid deterioration sometimes associated with adrenal hemorrhage, progressive shock, and death (52).

Leukocytes and platelet counts may mimic findings in infections and are similar to children without SCD. An increased hematocrit can signify dehydration due to poor fluid intake or increased fluid losses, whereas decreased hematocrit may result from infection-induced hemolysis, acute chest syndrome, splenic sequestration crisis, malaria, or viral suppression of the bone marrow. Splenomegaly or hepatomegaly may indicate splenic or hepatic sequestration, malaria, or a variety of viral infections.

Diagnostic testing should be guided by the clinical history and physical examination. In the absence of localizing signs or symptoms of infection, blood cultures, urinalysis, and urine culture should be considered (especially in infants and sexually active females). Viral pathogens (i.e., enterovirus, influenza, and others) may also cause severe systemic disease, and molecular diagnostic panels for viral pathogens may also be appropriate. Further infectious testing should be guided by signs and symptoms. Blood cultures, as well as all other clinically indicated culture materials, should be obtained quickly and antibiotic administration should be expedited. Thorough physical examination should seek a focus of infection (indwelling intravascular catheter tunnel sites, facial and long bones, dental sources, and skin/soft tissue infections) that may require source control.

All febrile children should be evaluated for evidence of early focal infection of the respiratory system, central nervous system, abdomen, and musculoskeletal systems as well as SCD-specific complications, including acute chest syndrome, stroke, vaso-occlusive crisis, aplastic crisis, splenic sequestration, and hepatic sequestration.

Fever with respiratory symptoms such as cough, tachypnea, hypoxemia, fever, and chest pain may be due to pneumonia, acute chest syndrome, or both. If intrathoracic infection is suspected, sputum should be sent for bacterial culture, and polymerase chain reaction should be performed for viral detection. Adequate sputum specimens are difficult to obtain from young children who are not intubated but they can be induced from older children or may be obtained by bronchoscopy. Isolation of a predominant bacterial pathogen in the presence of a granulocytic response on Gram stain suggests the bacterial etiology, and the absence of such findings may suggest a mycobacterial infection or non-bacterial cause such as acute chest syndrome. Pleural fluid, if significant, should be sent for cell count, chemistries, pH measurement, bacterial Gram stain, and culture. In the setting of acute chest syndrome and/or pulmonary infection, *Staphylococci, Streptococci*, atypical bacteria, and respiratory viruses (respiratory syncytial virus, human metapneumovirus, rhinovirus, parvovirus, parainfluenza viruses, influenza viruses, cytomegalovirus, Epstein-Barr Virus, and Herpes simplex viruses) comprise a major source of infectious etiologies. Sputum acid-fast staining and Mycobacterial cultures should be considered in the appropriate clinical settings.

Fever with central nervous system symptoms occurs less commonly in SCD and is a medical emergency. Children with a central nervous system infection (meningitis or meningoencephalitis) may present with nuchal rigidity, photophobia, fever, and/or signs of elevated intracranial pressure. Alternatively, they may present with less definitive findings such as seizure, altered sensorium, or headache. Central nervous system differential diagnoses include ischemic or hemorrhagic stroke, seizure, and central nervous system infection. If central nervous system disease is suspected, lumbar puncture should be performed after neuroimaging has excluded the presence of markedly increased intracranial pressure, an alternate diagnosis (hemorrhagic or ischemic stroke), and coagulation status has been confirmed as normal. Administration of antimicrobial therapy should not be delayed for neuroimaging or if lumbar puncture has to be delayed.

Cerebrospinal fluid should be analyzed for cell count, differential, chemistries, and Gram stain, and bacterial culture and molecular diagnostic testing should be performed for bacterial and viral pathogens. Bacterial pathogens likely to be present include *S. pneumoniae, H. influenzae*, or *N. meningitidis*. Gram-negative pathogens occur occasionally and especially in neonates. In the presence of a dog bite, *Capnocytophaga* and *Pasteurella multocida* species should be considered. Bacterial pathogens and viral pathogens may be tested by polymerase chain reaction on cerebrospinal fluid. In the presence of appropriate risk factors, geographic location, and travel history, further testing for tuberculous meningitis, cerebral malaria, HIV and HIV-associated central nervous system infections (HIV, *Cryptococcus neoformans, Toxoplasma gondii*), fungal pathogens, roundworm infections, and amoeba should be considered. Empiric treatment with vancomycin, ceftriaxone, and acyclovir, if clinically indicated, are recommended. Empiric initial antibiotic therapy with vancomycin is recommended when *Staphylococci* or resistant *Streptococci* are in the differential diagnosis. Anti-pseudomonal antibiotics can be considered if nosocomial or neurosurgical infection is considered. Antiviral, antimalarial, and other therapies may be added based on risk factors, lab testing, and infectious disease consultant recommendations.

Regardless of the site of infection, if appropriate risk factors are present (recent hospitalization, inpatient status in a chronic care facility, prolonged broad-spectrum antibiotic or steroid use, or other causes of immune suppression), it may be prudent to consider empiric fungal coverage. Finally, in endemic areas, testing, and treatment for dengue viruses, malaria, tuberculosis, and HIV may be considered. Input from infectious disease and hematology specialists is essential.

Approach to Antimicrobial Coverage

Appropriate initial empiric antibiotic therapy for the most likely pathogens is presented in **Table 2**. Initial antibiotic selection for patients presumed to be bacteremic should be broad and active against encapsulated organisms as well as other common pathogens. Antibiotic selection is further influenced by local epidemiology and antibiotic resistance patterns (162, 163). The empiric use of vancomycin and a third-generation cephalosporin provides coverage against: resistant pneumococci, meningeal penetration, and Staphylococci and enteric Gram-negative pathogens. Antibiotic coverage should be tapered based on culture results to minimize development of bacterial resistance and opportunistic fungal infection. The addition of anti-pseudomonal antibiotics should be considered if hospital-acquired pneumonia is present, and oseltamivir should be administered if influenza is considered likely.

Critical Care Considerations in SCD

An exhaustive discussion of critical care support of sepsis with organ dysfunction is beyond the scope of this review. Critical care support of patients with severe sepsis and organ dysfunction is similar to that provided to patients without SCD with additional considerations specific to persons with SCD.

In this section, we will review the considerations relevant specifically to the management of SCD patients with severe sepsis. We present issues related to (a) hemodynamic assessment and support, (b) respiratory considerations, (c) the role of transfusion therapy in critically ill persons with SCD, and (d) precautions related to granulocyte colony-stimulating factor and coagulation factor replacement.

Initial hemodynamic evaluation and management should consider the patient's pre-morbid SCD-related circulatory system changes. The hemodynamic profile of the SCD patient with infection and shock may vary with respect to contractility and atrial filling pressures. Systemic resistance may be high, low, or normal, and pulmonary vascular resistance may be elevated. Shock states may be caused by systolic and/or diastolic dysfunction of either or both ventricles. The hemodynamic profile can change as infection progresses, necessitating re-evaluation and a willingness to modify treatment. Critically ill SCD patients presenting with presumed infection should undergo thorough echocardiographic examination to determine systolic and diastolic function of both ventricles, the function of cardiac valves, and estimated pulmonary artery pressure.

Circulatory support must be individualized and frequently reassessed. No single inotrope or vasopressor can be recommended, as therapy must be determined on the basis of serial hemodynamic evaluations. Vasoconstrictor medications, though often necessary to maintain vital organ perfusion pressure, should be minimized and weaned whenever possible as they promote sickle hemoglobin polymerization by prolonging transit through the vasculature. Individuals with SCD typically have lower blood pressure than matched African American controls (164), therefore, blood pressure should be viewed in the context of direct and indirect measures of adequate oxygen delivery.

Before permissive hypercapnia and its attendant decrease in pH is adopted, the right ventricle and pulmonary resistance needs to be evaluated, as right heart failure can be precipitated in critically ill patients with SCD. Frequent or continuous assessment of cardiac output, atrial filling pressures, pulmonary artery pressures, and systemic resistance may allow the least harmful ventilatory support to be applied while monitoring for ongoing surveillance of cardiac filling pressures, pulmonary vascular resistance, systemic resistance, and cardiac output. The addition of inhaled nitric oxide may be helpful in supporting right heart function in the face of elevated pulmonary vascular resistance.

Patients with pulmonary artery hypertension are treated with hydroxyurea and chronic transfusion therapy to control the underlying hemolytic state, and oxygen is administered to correct hypoxemia. SCD patients may also be treated with endothelin-1 receptor antagonists (bosentan, ambrisentan) or prostanoids. The use of PDE-5 inhibitors (sildenafil, tadalafil) is not recommended in SCD patients due to frequent hospitalizations for serious adverse events (165).

Respiratory disease in the context of fever can be serious and progress rapidly when associated with pneumonia and/or acute chest syndrome. SCD-specific concerns in the setting of pulmonary infection involve the appreciation for the relationship between severe lung disease, elevated pulmonary vascular resistance, and right ventricular dysfunction or failure, as well as the importance of superimposed reactive airway disease as a contributor to deterioration. Analgesia should be provided to allow the patient to cough and breathe deeply if pleuritic chest pain or vaso-occlusive crisis pain is significant. Inhaled nitric oxide, high-frequency oscillatory ventilation, dexamethasone, and extracorporeal membrane oxygenation support have been used to support SCD patients with severe lung disease (166–169). Reactive airway disease should be sought and treated, as this source of ventilation/perfusion mismatch may promote acute chest syndrome. Finally, pulmonary infection can incite acute chest syndrome with increased hospital morbidity and mortality.

Central nervous system disease in SCD patients with fever has many serious etiologies. Support of patients with a central nervous system infection is similar to other patients with the added concern for proclivity to stroke. Markedly elevated intracranial pressure is treated with sedation, head of the bed elevation, osmolar therapy with hypertonic saline and mannitol, temperature control, normoglycemia, seizure suppression, and appropriate broad-spectrum antibiotics. Neurosurgical consultation for intracranial pressure monitoring, cerebrospinal fluid drainage, and/or surgical evacuation of blood or purulent material should be considered.

Aggressive transfusion therapy can prevent or reverse neurologic injury in patients with SCD (see below). Immediate exchange transfusion to reduce HbS% <30% is protective against stroke, which can be provoked by meningitis, acute chest syndrome, vaso-occlusive crisis, and sepsis. The addition of corticosteroids, which have efficacy in minimizing hearing loss in *H. influenzae* meningitis, but not proven in other forms of meningitis, can be considered as they also have utility in the treatment of acute chest syndrome and reactive airway disease. However, caution is advised, as the use of systemic corticosteroids in SCD is associated with the risk of rebound vaso-occlusive crisis (170).

Aggressive transfusion therapy may be necessary during infection to prevent or treat serious SCD complications, including acute chest syndrome, stroke, acute splenic sequestration, and vaso-occlusive crisis that may occur during or concomitantly with infection and can be life threatening. Simple transfusion (in 10- to 15-mL/kg aliquots) can be administered to optimize oxygen-carrying capacity and minimally changes HbS percentage. Hematocrit should not be increased beyond 30% to avoid an abrupt increase in viscosity that predisposes to stroke. In contrast, exchange transfusion using standard calculations can be performed by automated erythrocytapheresis or manual exchange to quickly decrease the HbS percentage to <30% and increase the hematocrit to approximately 30%. Exchange transfusion can be considered during overwhelming infections to ameliorate and prevent vaso-occlusive crisis, acute chest syndrome, and stroke, and may ameliorate diffuse microvascular occlusion by sickled erythrocytes in patients with multi-organ system failure. Plasma exchange, in addition to red cell exchange, may be helpful for patients with a thrombotic thrombocytopenic purpura-like clinical picture (171).

Although transfusion is regarded as an important therapy to avert serious SCD complications, it is not benign, and repeated transfusions can result in complications such as transfusion-related iron overload, alloimmunization, and delayed hemolytic transfusion reactions, which can result in hyperhemolysis syndrome and death. In many austere environments, the risk of transmission of blood-borne pathogens is prohibitive and precludes transfusion except for the most life-threatening levels of anemia.

The topic of transfusion thresholds frequently arises during the management of persons with SCD who are critically ill. We do not believe that specific thresholds are as helpful as an ongoing evaluation of the risks and benefits of transfusion therapy in the context of the severity of a patient's anemia, adequacy of systemic oxygen delivery, and abundance and safety of the regional blood supply. Simple transfusion of red blood cells should be considered to maintain oxygen-carrying capacity and systemic oxygen delivery and to treat moderate acute chest syndrome. Exchange transfusion should be performed for stroke and severe acute chest syndrome.

Other hematologic considerations relate to the support of coagulation abnormalities in severe infection. Coagulopathy is a common finding in serious infections. Clinical judgment is required to determine how aggressively to replete coagulation factors in a disease that is marked by a propensity to both ischemic and hemorrhagic stroke and diffuse vital organ vascular occlusion. In general, they are used sparingly unless coagulation is severely altered or bleeding is present. It is prudent to correct the platelet count, fibrinogen concentration, and coagulation times sufficiently to stop ongoing bleeding, facilitate invasive procedures, and maintain levels above which spontaneous intracranial hemorrhage is likely to occur.

Finally, granulocyte colony-stimulating factor has been used to treat neutropenia and to increase circulating stem cells in other patient populations with few adverse effects. The use of granulocyte colony-stimulating factor in SCD patients is associated with stimulation of severe vaso-occlusive crisis symptoms, acute chest syndrome, multi-organ system failure, and death (172). Further, symptoms have occurred in the SCD population in previously undiagnosed patients and in SCD patients without an elevated neutrophil count. Granulocyte colony-stimulating factor cannot be recommended for use in SCD with sepsis, as catastrophic illness may result. If it is considered for use in a SCD patient, it should only be done when all other therapies have failed and after a complete disclosure of the risk to the patient and family.

ROADMAP FOR RESEARCH AND IMPLEMENTATION

Therapies designed to interfere with the sickle cascade at many levels of the pathway are ongoing. Such efforts include strategies to reduce hemoglobin polymerization through the stabilization of HbS with medications such as voxelotor and l-glutamine (173, 174), as well as interference with interactions between the cellular elements of the blood and the endothelium with the monoclonal antibody crizanlizumab (158, 175, 176). Molecular strategies designed to nullify the cellular interactions that characterize the pathophysiology of SCD may someday delay or prevent acquired spleen dysfunction, thus allowing the infant's maturing immune system to develop.

In resource-rich environments, morbidity and mortality related to infectious sequelae have been greatly reduced. In such environments, research should include more effective vaccines to more completely immunize SCD children against bacterial and viral pathogens. Likewise, investigation into barriers that prevent 100% compliance with vaccination and antibiotic prophylaxis is necessary to ensure that children capitalize on the availability of optimal nutrition, disease-modifying medications (hydroxyurea), antibiotic prophylaxis, and vaccination participation. Ongoing surveillance into the development of microbial resistance to antibiotics and immunization strains is needed to stay current with effective prophylaxis and immunization.

In austere environments, policy efforts should continue to emphasize the cost-effective therapies already proven effective elsewhere. These include provision of universal neonatal screening for sickle cell disease, enhanced vaccination, and antibiotic prophylaxis. Delineation of pathogens responsible for viral and bacterial disease in SCD patients in austere environments is necessary, as other pathogens may need to be considered for inclusion for vaccination and antibiotic prophylaxis. Hydroxyurea, an oral disease-modifying medication that is generally effective and well-tolerated, should be made available to as many children with SCD as possible. Finally, efforts in the areas of nutrition, safe blood-banking practices, sanitation, and disease control programs for malaria, tuberculosis, and HIV are essential.

STRENGTHS AND LIMITATIONS

The strength of our review is its multidisciplinary approach to the issue of infectious complications that includes the broad perspectives of physicians who specialize in critical care medicine, hematology, and infectious disease.

There are limitations in our review, which include the methodology and the scope of the literature included. This concise review was intended to review pre-determined topics relevant to infectious complications of sickle cell disease. We chose to search the medical literature for case reports, systematic reviews, original research, meta-analyses, narrative reviews, and position/policy statements relevant to SCD and infection. Although we used an extensive combination of terms in our literature search, it is possible that some important references were overlooked. Additionally, we sought only English-language publications, thus limiting our search results.

CONCLUSIONS

SCD confers a high burden and results in morbidity and mortality worldwide. The priorities for the future management of infectious complications in SCD differs by geographic and socioeconomic circumstances. In the resource-rich nations where perinatal screening, antibiotic prophylaxis, and robust vaccination programs exist, mortality from infection is greatly reduced. In these areas of the world, prevention of chronic organ injury and improvement of quality and duration of life have become the principal goals of therapy. Conversely, in resource-poor environments where SCD is more prevalent and lethal, the priorities are more basic. In the face of a serious infection, the basics of excellent critical care, antibiotic therapy, and transfusion therapy still remain the cornerstones for effective treatment.

AUTHOR CONTRIBUTIONS

All authors listed have made a substantial, direct and intellectual contribution to the work, and approved it for publication.

ACKNOWLEDGMENTS

We would like to thank Corey Astrom, ELS, for her editorial expertise and assistance with this manuscript.

REFERENCES

1. Modell B, Darlison M. Global epidemiology of haemoglobin disorders and derived service indicators. *Bull World Health Organ.* (2008) 86:480–7. doi: 10.2471/BLT.06.036673
2. Weatherall DJ. The inherited diseases of hemoglobin are an emerging global health burden. *Blood.* (2010) 115:4331–6. doi: 10.1182/blood-2010-01-251348
3. Therrell BL, Hannon WH. National evaluation of US newborn screening system components. *Ment Retard Dev Disabil Res Rev.* (2006) 12:236–45. doi: 10.1002/mrdd.20124
4. Piel FB, Steinberg MH, Rees DC. Sickle cell disease. *N Engl J Med.* (2017) 377:305. doi: 10.1056/NEJMc1706325
5. Aygun B, Odame, I. A global perspective on sickle cell disease. *Pediatr Blood Cancer.* (2012) 59:386–90. doi: 10.1002/pbc.24175
6. Aliyu ZY, Kato GJ, Taylor JT, Babadoko A, Mamman AI, Gordeuk VR, et al. Sickle cell disease and pulmonary hypertension in Africa: a global perspective and review of epidemiology, pathophysiology, and management. *Am J Hematol.* (2008) 83:63–70. doi: 10.1002/ajh.21057
7. Davies SC, Brozovic M. The presentation, management and prophylaxis of sickle cell disease. *Blood Rev.* (1989) 3:29–44. doi: 10.1016/0268-960X(89)90023-4
8. Adewuyi JO. Morbidity of sickle cell disease in early childhood. *J Trop Pediatr.* (1988) 34:93.
9. Makani J, Cox SE, Soka D, Komba AN, Oruo J, Mwamtemi H, et al. Mortality in sickle cell anemia in Africa: a prospective cohort study in Tanzania. *PLoS ONE.* (2011) 6:e14699. doi: 10.1371/journal.pone.0014699
10. Brousse V, Buffet P, Rees D. The spleen and sickle cell disease: the sick(led) spleen. *Br J Haematol.* (2014) 166:165–76. doi: 10.1111/bjh.12950
11. Booth C, Inusa B, Obaro SK. Infection in sickle cell disease: a review. *Int J Infect Dis.* (2010) 14:e2–12. doi: 10.1016/j.ijid.2009.03.010
12. Davies EG, Riddington C, Lottenberg R, Dower N. Pneumococcal vaccines for sickle cell disease. *Cochrane Database Syst Rev.* (2004) 10:CD003885. doi: 10.1002/14651858.CD003885.pub2
13. Van Beneden C, Whitney C, Levine O. Preventing pneumococcal disease among infants and young children; recommendations of the Advisory Committee on Immunization Practices (ACIP). *MMWR Recomm Rep.* (2000) 49:1–35.
14. Gill FM, Sleeper LA, Weiner SJ, Brown AK, Bellevue R, Grover R, et al. Clinical events in the first decade in a cohort of infants with sickle cell disease. Cooperative Study of Sickle Cell Disease. *Blood.* (1995) 86:776–83. doi: 10.1182/blood.V86.2.776.bloodjournal862776
15. Adamkiewicz TV, Sarnaik S, Buchanan GR, Iyer RV, Miller ST, Pegelow CH, et al. Invasive pneumococcal infections in children with sickle cell disease in the era of penicillin prophylaxis, antibiotic resistance, and 23-valent pneumococcal polysaccharide vaccination. *J Pediatr.* (2003) 143:438–44. doi: 10.1067/S0022-3476(03)00331-7
16. Quinn CT, Rogers ZR, Buchanan GR. Survival of children with sickle cell disease. *Blood.* (2004) 103:4023–7. doi: 10.1182/blood-2003-11-3758
17. Serjeant GR, Ndugwa CM. Sickle cell disease in Uganda: a time for action. *East Afr Med J.* (2003) 80:384–7. doi: 10.4314/eamj.v80i7.8724
18. Hassell KL. Population estimates of sickle cell disease in the U.S. *Am J Prev Med.* (2010) 38:S512–21. doi: 10.1016/j.amepre.2009.12.022
19. Platt OS, Brambilla DJ, Rosse WF, Milner PF, Castro O, Steinberg MH, et al. Mortality in sickle cell disease. Life expectancy and risk factors for early death. *N Engl J Med.* (1994) 330:1639–44. doi: 10.1056/NEJM199406093302303
20. Humbert JR, Winsor EL, Githens JM, Schmitz JB. Neutrophil dysfunctions in sickle celldisease. *Biomed Pharmacother.* (1990) 44:153–8. doi: 10.1016/0753-3322(90)90002-Q
21. Bohnsack JF, Brown EJ. The role of the spleen in resistance to infection. *Annu Rev Med.* (1986) 37:49–59. doi: 10.1146/annurev.me.37.020186.000405
22. William BM, Corazza GR. Hyposplenism: a comprehensive review. Part I: basic concepts and causes. *Hematology.* (2007) 12:1–13. doi: 10.1080/10245330600938422
23. Drew PA, Kiroff GK, Ferrante A, Cohen RC. Alterations in immunoglobulin synthesis by peripheral blood mononuclear cells from splenectomized patients with and without splenic regrowth. *J Immunol.* (1984) 132:191–6.
24. Spirer Z, Weisman Y, Zakuth V, Fridkin M, Bogair N Decreased serum tuftsin concentrations in sickle cell disease. *Arch Dis Child.* (1980) 55:566–7. doi: 10.1136/adc.55.7.566
25. Cameron PU, Jones P, Gorniak M, Dunster K, Paul E, Lewin S, et al. Splenectomy associated changes in IgM memory B cells in an adult spleen registry cohort. *PLoS ONE.* (2011) 6:e23164. doi: 10.1371/journal.pone.0023164
26. Koffi KG, Sawadogo D, Meite M, Nanho DC, Tanoh ES, Attia AK, et al. Reduced levels of T-cell subsets CD4+ and CD8+ in homozygous sickle cell anaemia patients with splenic defects. *Hematol J.* (2003) 4:363–5. doi: 10.1038/sj.thj.6200310
27. Atkins BL, Price EH, Tillyer L, Novelli V, Evans J. Salmonella osteomyelitis in sickle cell disease children in the east end of London. *J Infect.* (1997) 34:133–8. doi: 10.1016/S0163-4453(97)92452-X
28. Hoyjo S, Fukada T. Roles of zinc signaling in the immune system. *J Immunol Res.* (2016) 2016:6762343. doi: 10.1155/2016/6762343
29. Fraker PJ, King LE, Laakko T, Vollmer TL. The dynamic link between the integrity of the immune system and zinc status. *J Nutr.* (2000) 130:1399S–1406S. doi: 10.1093/jn/130.5.1399S
30. Holdsworth RJ, McKenzie H, Parratt D, Irving AD, Cuschieri A. The role of the spleen in the immune response following naturally acquired exposure to encapsulated bacteria. *Int J Exp Pathol.* (1990) 71:835–43.

31. Mebius RE, Kraal G. Structure and function of the spleen. *Nat Rev Immunol.* (2005) 5:606–16. doi: 10.1038/nri1669
32. Hendricks J, Bos NA, Kroese FGM. Heterogeneity of memory marginal zone B cells. *Crit Rev Immunol.* (2018) 38:145–58. doi: 10.1615/CritRevImmunol.2018024985
33. Pearson HA, Spencer RP, Cornelius EA. Functional asplenia in sickle-cell anemia. *N Engl J Med.* (1969) 281:923–6. doi: 10.1056/NEJM196910232811703
34. Brown AK, Sleeper LA, Miller ST, Pegelow CH, Gill FM, Waclawiw MA. Reference values and hematologic changes from birth to 5 years in patients with sickle cell disease. Cooperative Study of Sickle Cell Disease. *Arch Pediatr Adolesc Med.* (1994) 148:796–804. doi: 10.1001/archpedi.1994.02170080026005
35. Janeway CA Jr., Travers P, Walport M, Shlomchik MJ. *Immunobiology: The Immune System in Health and Disease.* 5th ed. New York, NY: Garland Science (2001).
36. Dunkelberger JR, Song WC. Complement and its role in innate and adaptive immune responses. *Cell Res.* (2010) 20:34–50. doi: 10.1038/cr.2009.139
37. Wilson WA, Thomas EJ. Activation of the alternative pathway of human complement by haemoglobin. *Clin Exp Immunol.* (1979) 36:140–4.
38. DeCeulaer K, Wilson WA, Morgan AG, Serjeant GR. Plasma haemoglobin and complement activation in sickle cell disease. *J Clin Lab Immunol.* (1981) 6:57–60.
39. Wilson WA, Hughes GR, Lachmann PJ. Deficiency of factor B of the complement system in sickle cell anaemia. *Br Med J.* (1976) 1:367–9. doi: 10.1136/bmj.1.6006.367
40. Weller S, Braun MC, Tan BK, Rosenwald A, Cordier C, Conley ME, et al. Human blood IgM "memory" B cells are circulating splenic marginal zone B cells harboring a prediversified immunoglobulin repertoire. *Blood.* (2004) 104:3647–54. doi: 10.1182/blood-2004-01-0346
41. Ballester OF, Abdallah JM, Prasad AS. Impaired IgM antibody responses to an influenza virus vaccine in adults with sickle cell anemia. *Am J Hematol.* (1985) 20:409–12. doi: 10.1002/ajh.2830200413
42. Romagnani S. T-cell subsets (Th1 versus Th2). *Ann Allergy Asthma Immunol.* (2000) 85:9–18; quiz 18, 21. doi: 10.1016/S1081-1206(10)62426-X
43. Hibbert JM, Creary MS, Gee BE, Buchanan I, Quarshie A, Hsu LL. Erythropoiesis and myocardial energy requirements contribute to the hypermetabolism of childhood sickle cell anemia. *J Pediatr Gastroenterol Nutr.* (2006) 43:680–7. doi: 10.1097/01.mpg.0000228120.44606.d6
44. Prasad AS, Schoomaker EB, Ortega J, Brewer GJ, Oberleas D, Oelshlegel FJ Jr. Zinc deficiency in sickle cell disease. *Clin Chem.* (1975) 21:582–7. doi: 10.1093/clinchem/21.4.582
45. Prasad AS, Cossack ZT. Zinc supplementation and growth in sickle cell disease. *Ann Intern Med.* (1984) 100:367–71. doi: 10.7326/0003-4819-100-3-367
46. Zemel BS, Kawchak DA, Fung EB, Ohene-Frempong K, Stallings VA. Effect of zinc supplementation on growth and body composition in children with sickle cell disease. *Am J Clin Nutr.* (2002) 75:300–7. doi: 10.1093/ajcn/75.2.300
47. Schall JI, Zemel BS, Kawchak DA, Ohene-Frempong K, Stallings VA. Vitamin A status, hospitalizations, and other outcomes in young children with sickle cell disease. *J Pediatr.* (2004) 145:99–106. doi: 10.1016/j.jpeds.2004.03.051
48. De Franceschi L, Bachir D, Galacteros F, Tchernia G, Cynober T, Neuberg D, et al. Oral magnesium pidolate: effects of long-term administration in patients with sickle cell disease. *Br J Haematol.* (2000) 108:284–9. doi: 10.1046/j.1365-2141.2000.01861.x
49. Brown B, Dada-Adegbola H, Trippe C, Olopade O. Prevalence and etiology of bacteremia in febrile children with sickle cell disease at a Nigeria tertiary hospital. *Mediterr J Hematol Infect Dis.* (2017) 9:e2017039. doi: 10.4084/mjhid.2017.039
50. Cannas G, Merazga S, Virot E. Sickle cell disease and infections in high- and low-income countries. *Mediterr J Hematol Infect Dis.* (2019) 11:e2019042. doi: 10.4084/mjhid.2019.042
51. Richards LH, Howard J, Klein JL. Community-acquired Salmonella bacteraemia in patients with sickle-cell disease 1969–2008: a single centre study. *Scand J Infect Dis.* (2011) 43:89–94. doi: 10.3109/00365548.2010.526958
52. Onwubalili JK. Sickle cell disease and infection. *J Infect.* (1983) 7:2–20. doi: 10.1016/S0163-4453(83)90863-0
53. Seeler RA, Royal JE. Commentary: sickle cell anemia, stroke, and transfusion. *J Pediatr.* (1980) 96:243–4. doi: 10.1016/S0022-3476(80)80811-0
54. Jordan LC, Casella JF, DeBaun MR. Prospects for primary stroke prevention in children with sickle cell anaemia. *Br J Haematol.* (2012) 157:14–25. doi: 10.1111/j.1365-2141.2011.09005.x
55. Sadreameli SC, Reller ME, Bundy DG, Casella JF, Strouse JJ. Respiratory syncytial virus and seasonal influenza cause similar illnesses in children with sickle cell disease. *Pediatr Blood Cancer.* (2014) 61:875–8. doi: 10.1002/pbc.24887
56. Bundy DG, Strouse JJ, Casella JF, Miller MR. Burden of influenza-related hospitalizations among children with sickle cell disease. *Pediatrics.* (2010) 125:234–43. doi: 10.1542/peds.2009-1465
57. Vichinsky EP, Neumayr LD, Earles AN, Williams R, Lennette ET, Dean D, et al. Causes and outcomes of the acute chest syndrome in sickle cell disease. National Acute Chest Syndrome Study Group. *N Engl J Med.* (2000) 342:1855–65. doi: 10.1056/NEJM200006223422502
58. Neumayr L, Lennette E, Kelly D, Earles A, Embury S, Groncy P, et al. Mycoplasma disease and acute chest syndrome in sickle cell disease. *Pediatrics.* (2003) 112:87–95. doi: 10.1542/peds.112.1.87
59. Jain S, Bakshi N, Krishnamurti L. Acute chest syndrome in children with sickle cell disease. *Pediatr Allergy Immunol Pulmonol.* (2017) 30:191–201. doi: 10.1089/ped.2017.0814
60. Chambers JB, Forsythe DA, Bertrand SL, Iwinski HJ, Steflik DE. Retrospective review of osteoarticular infections in a pediatric sickle cell age group. *J Pediatr Orthop.* (2000) 20:682–5. doi: 10.1097/01241398-200009000-00025
61. Neonato MG, Guilloud-Bataille M, Beauvais P, Begue P, Belloy M, Benkerrou M, et al. Acute clinical events in 299 homozygous sickle cell patients living in France. French Study Group on Sickle Cell Disease. *Eur J Haematol.* (2000) 65:155–64. doi: 10.1034/j.1600-0609.2000.90210.x
62. Mallouh A, Talab Y. Bone and joint infection in patients with sickle cell disease. *J Pediatr Orthop.* (1985) 5:158–62. doi: 10.1097/01241398-198505020-00007
63. Bahebeck J, Atangana R, Techa A, Monny-Lobe M, Sosso M, Hoffmeyer P. Relative rates and features of musculoskeletal complications in adult sicklers. *Acta Orthop Belg.* (2004) 70:107–11.
64. Anand AJ, Glatt AE. Salmonella osteomyelitis and arthritis in sickle cell disease. *Semin Arthritis Rheum.* (1994) 24:211–21. doi: 10.1016/0049-0172(94)90076-0
65. Hernigou P, Daltro G, Flouzat-Lachaniette CH, Roussignol X, Poignard A. Septic arthritis in adults with sickle cell disease often is associated with osteomyelitis or osteonecrosis. *Clin Orthop Relat Res.* (2010) 468:1676–81. doi: 10.1007/s11999-009-1149-3
66. Gupta G, Kumar S, Singh R, Shanmugasamy K. Intussusception caused by *Yersinia enterocolitica* Enterocolitis in a patient with sickle cell anemia. *Clin Med Insights Pathol.* (2010) 3:7–11. doi: 10.4137/CPath.S4943
67. Vanderhave KL, Perkins CA, Scannell B, Brighton BK. Orthopaedic manifestations of sickle cell disease. *J Am Acad Orthop Surg.* (2018) 26:94–101. doi: 10.5435/JAAOS-D-16-00255
68. Santoro JD, Myers L, Kanter J. Assessing the immunogenic response of a single center's pneumococcal vaccination protocol in sickle cell disease. *J Pediatr Hematol Oncol.* (2016) 38:e102–6. doi: 10.1097/MPH.0000000000000510
69. Brown BJ, Jacob NE, Lagunju IA, Jarrett OO. Morbidity and mortality pattern in hospitalized children with sickle cell disorders at the University College Hospital, Ibadan, Nigeria. *Nig J Paediatr.* (2013) 40:34–9. doi: 10.4314/njp.v40i1.6
70. Bansil NH, Kim TY, Tieu L, Barcega B. Incidence of serious bacterial infections in febrile children with sickle cell disease. *Clin Pediatr.* (2013) 52:661–6. doi: 10.1177/0009922813488645
71. Wierenga KJ, Hambleton IR, Wilson RM, Alexander H, Serjeant BE, Serjeant GR. Significance of fever in Jamaican patients with homozygous sickle cell disease. *Arch Dis Child.* (2001) 84:156–9. doi: 10.1136/adc.84.2.156
72. Sobota A, Sabharwal V, Fonebi G, Steinberg M. How we prevent and manage infection in sickle cell disease. *Br J Haematol.* (2015) 170:757–67. doi: 10.1111/bjh.13526

73. Zarkowsky HS, Gallagher D, Gill FM, Wang WC, Falletta JM, Lande WM, et al. Bacteremia in sickle hemoglobinopathies. *J Pediatr.* (1986) 109:579–85. doi: 10.1016/S0022-3476(86)80216-5
74. Alkindi S, Matwani S, Al-Maawali A, Al-Maskari B, Pathare A. Complications of PORT-A-CATH(R) in patients with sickle cell disease. *J Infect Public Health.* (2012) 5:57–62. doi: 10.1016/j.jiph.2011.10.004
75. Yeral M, Boga C, Oguzkurt L, Asma S, Kasar M, Kozanoglu I. Short-term central venous catheter complications in patients with sickle cell disease who undergo apheresis. *J Thromb Thrombolysis.* (2014) 37:97–101. doi: 10.1007/s11239-013-0914-z
76. Kizito ME, Mworozi E, Ndugwa C, Serjeant GR. Bacteraemia in homozygous sickle cell disease in Africa: is pneumococcal prophylaxis justified? *Arch Dis Child.* (2007) 92:21–3. doi: 10.1136/adc.2005.088807
77. Musa A, Ogunrinde OG, Mamman AI, Saad YM, Ibrahim A, Yakubu AM. Prevalence and pattern of bacterial isolate in febrile children with sickle cell anemia in a tertiary hospital in Northern Nigeria. *Sub-Saharan Afr J Med.* (2018) 5:80–85. doi: 10.4103/ssajm.ssajm_1_19
78. Bello N, Kudu ATD, Adetokun AB, Taura DW, Jobbi YD, Umar M, et al. Characterization and antimicrobial susceptibility profile of bacteraemia causing pathogens isolated from febrile children with and without sickle cell disease in Kano, Nigeria. *Mediterr J Hematol Infect Dis.* (2018) 10:e2018016. doi: 10.4084/mjhid.2018.016
79. Akuse RM. Variation in the pattern of bacterial infection in patients with sickle cell disease requiring admission. *J Trop Pediatr.* (1996) 42:318–23. doi: 10.1093/tropej/42.6.318
80. Lepage P, Bogaerts J, Van Goethem C, Ntahorutaba M, Nsengumuremyi F, Hitimana DG, et al. Community-acquired bacteraemia in African children. *Lancet.* (1987) 1:1458–61. doi: 10.1016/S0140-6736(87)92207-0
81. Vaishya R, Agarwal AK, Edomwonyi EO, Vijay V. Musculoskeletal manifestations of sickle cell disease: a review. *Cureus.* (2015) 7:e358. doi: 10.7759/cureus.358
82. Tarry WF, Duckett JW Jr., Snyder HM 3rd. Urological complications of sickle cell disease in a pediatric population. *J Urol.* (1987) 138:592–4. doi: 10.1016/S0022-5347(17)43267-8
83. Barrett-Connor E. Bacterial infection and sickle cell anemia. An analysis of 250 infections in 166 patients and a review of the literature. *Medicine.* (1971) 50:97–112. doi: 10.1097/00005792-197103000-00002
84. Yanda ANA, Nansseu JRN, Mbassa Awa HD, Tatah SA, Seung J, Eposse C, et al. Burden and spectrum of bacterial infections among sickle cell disease children living in Cameroon. *BMC Infect Dis.* (2017) 17:211. doi: 10.1186/s12879-017-2317-9
85. Rogers ZR. Management of fever in sickle cell disease. In: *UpToDate.* Available online at https://www.uptodate.com/contents/management-of-fever-in-sickle-cell-disease (2019).
86. Qhalib HA, Zain GH. Hepatobiliary complications of sickle cell disease among children admitted to Al Wahda Teaching Hospital, Aden, Yemen. *Sultan Qaboos Univ Med J.* (2014) 14:e556–60.
87. Chekroun M, Cherifi H, Fournier B, Gaultier F, Sitbon IY, Ferre FC, et al. Oral manifestations of sickle cell disease. *Br Dent J.* (2019) 226:27–31. doi: 10.1038/sj.bdj.2019.4
88. Olaitan AA, Amuda JT, Adekeye EO. Osteomyelitis of the mandible in sickle cell disease. *Br J Oral Maxillofac Surg.* (1997) 35:190–2. doi: 10.1016/S0266-4356(97)90562-3
89. de Matos BM, Ribeiro ZE, Balducci I, Figueiredo MS, Back-Brito GN, Mota AJ, et al. Oral microbial colonization in children with sickle cell anaemia under long-term prophylaxis with penicillin. *Arch Oral Biol.* (2014) 59:1042–7. doi: 10.1016/j.archoralbio.2014.05.014
90. Jacobs JE, Quirolo K, Vichinsky E. Novel influenza A (H1N1) viral infection in pediatric patients with sickle-cell disease. *Pediatr Blood Cancer.* (2011) 56:95–8. doi: 10.1002/pbc.22656
91. Vinekar K, Schaad N, Ber Lucien MA, Leshem E, Oboho IK, Joseph G, et al. Hospitalizations and deaths because of respiratory and diarrheal diseases among Haitian children under five years of age, 2011–2013. *Pediatr Infect Dis J.* (2015) 34:e238–43. doi: 10.1097/INF.0000000000000805
92. Lagare A, Ousmane S, Issa I, Mainassara HB, Mamadou S. Molecular detection of respiratory pathogens among children aged younger than 5 years hospitalized with febrile acute respiratory infections: s prospective hospital based observational study in Niamey, Niger. *Health Sci Rep.* (2019) 2:e137. doi: 10.1002/hsr2.137
93. Nascimento-Carvalho AC, Ruuskanen O, Nascimento-Carvalho CM. Comparison of the frequency of bacterial and viral infections among children with community-acquired pneumonia hospitalized across distinct severity categories: a prospective cross-sectional study. *BMC Pediatr.* (2016) 16:105. doi: 10.1186/s12887-016-0645-3
94. Smith-Whitley K, Zhao H, Hodinka RL, Kwiatkowski J, Cecil R, Cecil T, et al. Epidemiology of human parvovirus B19 in children with sickle cell disease. *Blood.* (2004) 103:422–7. doi: 10.1182/blood-2003-01-0069
95. El Katsha S, Labeeb S, Watts S, Younis A. Informal health providers and the transmission of hepatitis C virus: pilot study in two Egyptian villages. *East Mediterr Health J.* (2006) 12:758–67.
96. Mousa SM, El-Ghamrawy MK, Gouda H, Khorshied M, El-Salam Ahmed DA, Shiba H. Prevalence of hepatitis C among Egyptian children with sickle cell disease and the role of IL28b gene polymorphisms in spontaneous viral clearance. *Mediterr J Hematol Infect Dis.* (2016) 8:e2016007. doi: 10.4084/mjhid.2016.007
97. Bakarey AS, Olaniyan OD. Hepatitis B virus infection among asymptomatic residents of low-income community in Ibadan, Southwest, Nigeria. *J Immunoassay Immunochem.* (2018) 39:377–89. doi: 10.1080/15321819.2018.1467928
98. Owusu ED, Visser BJ, Nagel IM, Mens PF, Grobusch MP. The interaction between sickle cell disease and HIV infection: a systematic review. *Clin Infect Dis.* (2015) 60:612–26. doi: 10.1093/cid/ciu832
99. Kourtis AP, Bansil P, Posner SF, Johnson C, Jamieson DJ. Trends in hospitalizations of HIV-infected children and adolescents in the United States: analysis of data from the 1994–2003 Nationwide Inpatient Sample. *Pediatrics.* (2007) 120:e236–43. doi: 10.1542/peds.2006-3268
100. Jentes ES, Lash RR, Johansson MA, Sharp TM, Henry R, Brady OJ, et al. Evidence-based risk assessment and communication: a new global dengue-risk map for travellers and clinicians. *J Travel Med.* (2016) 23:taw062. doi: 10.1093/jtm/taw062
101. Wilder-Smith A, Leong WY. Risk of severe dengue is higher in patients with sickle cell disease: a scoping review. *J Travel Med.* (2019) 26:937–41. doi: 10.1093/jtm/tay136
102. Rankine-Mullings A, Reid ME, Moo Sang M, Richards-Dawson MA, Knight JM. A retrospective analysis of the significance of Haemoglobin SS and SC in disease outcome in patients with sickle cell disease and Dengue fever. *EBioMedicine.* (2015) 2:937–41. doi: 10.1016/j.ebiom.2015.07.002
103. Makani J, Williams TN, Marsh K. Sickle cell disease in Africa: burden and research priorities. *Ann Trop Med Parasitol.* (2007) 101:3–14. doi: 10.1179/136485907X154638
104. Luzzatto L. Sickle cell anaemia and malaria. *Mediterr J Hematol Infect Dis.* (2012) 4:e2012065. doi: 10.4084/mjhid.2012.065
105. McAuley CF, Webb C, Makani J, Macharia A, Uyoga S, Opi DH, et al. High mortality from *Plasmodium falciparum* malaria in children living with sickle cell anemia on the coast of Kenya. *Blood.* (2010) 116:1663–8. doi: 10.1182/blood-2010-01-265249
106. Aluoch JR. Higher resistance to *Plasmodium falciparum* infection in patients with homozygous sickle cell disease in western Kenya. *Trop Med Int Health.* (1997) 2:568–71. doi: 10.1046/j.1365-3156.1997.d01-322.x
107. Makani J, Komba AN, Cox SE, Oruo J, Mwamtemi K, Kitundu J, et al. Malaria in patients with sickle cell anemia: burden, risk factors, and outcome at the outpatient clinic and during hospitalization. *Blood.* (2010) 115:215–20. doi: 10.1182/blood-2009-07-233528
108. Uyoga S, Macharia AW, Ndila CM, Nyutu G, Shebe M, Awuondo KO, et al. The indirect health effects of malaria estimated from health advantages of the sickle cell trait. *Nat Commun.* (2019) 10:856. doi: 10.1038/s41467-019-08775-0
109. Ahmed SG, Uraka J. Impact of intestinal parasites on haematological parameters of sickle-cell anaemia patients in Nigeria. *East Mediterr Health J.* (2011) 17:710–13. doi: 10.26719/2011.17.9.710
110. Ahmed SG, Ibrahim UA. A compendium of pathophysiologic basis of etiologic risk factors for painful vaso-occlusive crisis in sickle cell disease. *Niger J Basic Clin Sci.* (2017) 14:57–77. doi: 10.4103/njbcs.njbcs_11_17
111. Droz N, De Lauzanne A, Holvoet L, Missud F, Benkerrou M, Brousse V, et al. Tuberculosis in children with sickle cell anaemia: a retrospective

study in French tertiary care centres. *Eur J Pediatr.* (2017) 176:723–9. doi: 10.1007/s00431-017-2905-0

112. Gaston MH, Verter JI, Woods G, Pegelow C, Kelleher J, Presbury G, et al. Prophylaxis with oral penicillin in children with sickle cell anemia. A randomized trial. *N Engl J Med.* (1986) 314:1593–9. doi: 10.1056/NEJM198606193142501
113. Falletta JM, Woods GM, Verter JI, Buchanan GR, Pegelow CH, Iyer RV, et al. Discontinuing penicillin prophylaxis in children with sickle cell anemia. Prophylactic Penicillin Study II. *J Pediatr.* (1995) 127:685–90.
114. McCavit TL, Gilbert M, Buchanan GR. Prophylactic penicillin after 5 years of age in patients with sickle cell disease: a survey of sickle cell disease experts. *Pediatr Blood Cancer.* (2013) 60:935–9. doi: 10.1002/pbc.24395
115. Yawn BP, Buchanan GR, Afenyi-Annan AN, Ballas SK, Hassell KL, James AH, et al. Management of sickle cell disease: summary of the 2014 evidence-based report by expert panel members. *JAMA.* (2014) 312:1033–48. doi: 10.1001/jama.2014.10517
116. Halasa NB, Shankar SM, Talbot TR, Arbogast PG, Mitchel EF, Wang WC, et al. Incidence of invasive pneumococcal disease among individuals with sickle cell disease before and after the introduction of the pneumococcal conjugate vaccine. *Clin Infect Dis.* (2007) 44:1428–33. doi: 10.1086/516781
117. Espsito S, Principi N. Impacts of the 13-valent pneumococcal conjugate vaccine in children. *J Immunol Res.* (2015) 59:1580–6. doi: 10.1155/2015/591580
118. Waight PA, Andrews NJ, Ladhani SN, Sheppard CL, Slack MP, Miller E. Effect of the 13-valet pneumococcal conjugate vaccine on invasive pneumococcal disease in England and Wales 4 years after its introduction: an observational cohort study. *Lancet Infec Dis.* (2015) 15:535–43. doi: 10.1016/S1473-3099(15)70044-7
119. Norris CF, Smith-Whitley K, McGowan KL. Positive blood cultures in sickle cell disease: time to positivity and clinical outcome. *J Pediatr Hematol Oncol.* (2003) 25:390–5. doi: 10.1097/00043426-200305000-00008
120. Oniyangi O, Omari AA. Malaria chemoprophylaxis in sickle cell disease. *Cochrane Database Syst Rev.* (2019) 2019. doi: 10.1002/14651858.CD003489.pub2
121. Aneni EC, Hamer DH, Gill CJ. Systematic review of current and emerging strategies for reducing morbidity from malaria in sickle cell disease. *Trop Med Int Health.* (2013) 18:313–27. doi: 10.1111/tmi.12056
122. Obaro SK, Iroh Tam PY. Preventing infections in sickle cell disease: the unfinished business. *Pediatr Blood Cancer.* (2016) 63:781–5. doi: 10.1002/pbc.25911
123. Odey F, Okomo U, Oyo-Ita A. Vaccines for preventing invasive salmonella infections in people with sickle cell disease. *Cochrane Database Syst Rev.* (2018) 12:CD006975. doi: 10.1002/14651858.CD006975.pub4
124. Shakya M, Colin-Jones R, Theiss-Nyland K, Voysey M, Pant D, Smith N, et al. Phase 3 efficacy analysis of a typhoid conjugate vaccine trial in Nepal. *N Engl J Med.* (2019) 381:2209–18. doi: 10.1056/NEJMoa1905047
125. Willen SM, Thornburg CD, Lantos PM. The traveler with sickle cell disease. *J Travel Med.* (2014) 21:332–9. doi: 10.1111/jtm.12142
126. Watson AR. Pretravel health advice for asplenic individuals. *J Travel Med.* (2003) 10:117–21. doi: 10.2310/7060.2003.31772
127. Baskin MN, Goh XL, Heeney MM, Harper MB. Bacteremia risk and outpatient management of febrile patients with sickle cell disease. *Pediatrics.* (2013) 131:1035–41. doi: 10.1542/peds.2012-2139
128. Eaton WA, Hofrichter J. Hemoglobin S gelation and sickle cell disease. *Blood.* (1987) 70:1245–66. doi: 10.1182/blood.V70.5.1245.bloodjournal7051245
129. Aslan M, Thornley-Brown D, Freeman BA. Reactive species in sickle cell disease. *Ann N Y Acad Sci.* (2000) 899:375–91. doi: 10.1111/j.1749-6632.2000.tb06201.x
130. Hebbel RP, Morgan WT, Eaton JW, Hedlund BE. Accelerated autoxidation and heme loss due to instability of sickle hemoglobin. *Proc Natl Acad Sci USA.* (1988) 85:237–41. doi: 10.1073/pnas.85.1.237
131. Kato GJ, Martyr S, Blackwelder WC, Nichols JS, Coles WA, Hunter LA, et al. Levels of soluble endothelium-derived adhesion molecules in patients with sickle cell disease are associated with pulmonary hypertension, organ dysfunction, and mortality. *Br J Haematol.* (2005) 130:943–53. doi: 10.1111/j.1365-2141.2005.05701.x
132. Strijbos MH, Landburg PP, Nur E, Teerlink T, Leebeek FW, Rijneveld AW, et al. Circulating endothelial cells: a potential parameter of organ damage in sickle cell anemia? *Blood Cells Mol Dis.* (2009) 43:63–7. doi: 10.1016/j.bcmd.2009.02.007
133. Kaul DK, Liu XD, Zhang X, Ma L, Hsia CJ, Nagel RL. Inhibition of sickle red cell adhesion and vasoocclusion in the microcirculation by antioxidants. *Am J Physiol Heart Circ Physiol.* (2006) 291:H167–75. doi: 10.1152/ajpheart.01096.2005
134. Haynes J Jr., Obiako B, King JA, Hester RB, Ofori-Acquah S. Activated neutrophil-mediated sickle red blood cell adhesion to lung vascular endothelium: role of phosphatidylserine-exposed sickle red blood cells. *Am J Physiol Heart Circ Physiol.* (2006) 291:H1679–85. doi: 10.1152/ajpheart.00256.2006
135. Villagra J, Shiva S, Hunter LA, Machado RF, Gladwin MT, Kato GJ. Platelet activation in patients with sickle disease, hemolysis-associated pulmonary hypertension, and nitric oxide scavenging by cell-free hemoglobin. *Blood.* (2007) 110:2166–72. doi: 10.1182/blood-2006-12-061697
136. Singer ST, Ataga KI. Hypercoagulability in sickle cell disease and beta-thalassemia. *Curr Mol Med.* (2008) 8:639–45. doi: 10.2174/156652408786241366
137. Assis A, Conran N, Canalli AA, Lorand-Metze I, Saad ST, Costa FF. Effect of cytokines and chemokines on sickle neutrophil adhesion to fibronectin. *Acta Haematol.* (2005) 113:130–6. doi: 10.1159/000083451
138. Belcher JD, Marker PH, Weber JP, Hebbel RP, Vercellotti GM. Activated monocytes in sickle cell disease: potential role in the activation of vascular endothelium and vaso-occlusion. *Blood.* (2000) 96:2451–9. doi: 10.1182/blood.V96.7.2451.h8002451_2451_2459
139. Zhou Z, Han H, Cruz MA, Lopez JA, Dong JF, Guchhait P. Haemoglobin blocks von Willebrand factor proteolysis by ADAMTS-13: a mechanism associated with sickle cell disease. *Thromb Haemost.* (2009) 101:1070–7. doi: 10.1160/TH08-10-0677
140. Peters M, Plaat BE, Ten Cate H, Wolters HJ, Weening RS, Brandjes DP. Enhanced thrombin generation in children with sickle cell disease. *Thromb Haemost.* (1994) 71:169–72.
141. Liesner R, Mackie I, Cookson J, McDonald S, Chitolie A, Donohoe S, et al. Prothrombotic changes in children with sickle cell disease: relationships to cerebrovascular disease and transfusion. *Br J Haematol.* (1998) 103:1037–44. doi: 10.1046/j.1365-2141.1998.01121.x
142. Hagger D, Wolff S, Owen J, Samson D. Changes in coagulation and fibrinolysis in patients with sickle cell disease compared with healthy black controls. *Blood Coagul Fibrinolysis.* (1995) 6:93–9. doi: 10.1097/00001721-199504000-00001
143. Solovey A, Gui L, Key NS, Hebbel RP. Tissue factor expression by endothelial cells in sickle cell anemia. *J Clin Invest.* (1998) 101:1899–904. doi: 10.1172/JCI1932
144. Graido-Gonzalez E, Doherty JC, Bergreen EW, Organ G, Telfer M, McMillen MA. Plasma endothelin-1, cytokine, and prostaglandin E2 levels in sickle cell disease and acute vaso-occlusive sickle crisis. *Blood.* (1998) 92:2551–5. doi: 10.1182/blood.V92.7.2551.2551_2551_2555
145. Hammerman SI, Kourembanas S, Conca TJ, Tucci M, Brauer M, Farber HW. Endothelin-1 production during the acute chest syndrome in sickle cell disease. *Am J Respir Crit Care Med.* (1997) 156:280–5. doi: 10.1164/ajrccm.156.1.9611085
146. Hebbel RP, Boogaerts MA, Eaton JW, Steinberg MH. Erythrocyte adherence to endothelium in sickle-cell anemia. A possible determinant of disease severity. *N Engl J Med.* (1980) 302:992. doi: 10.1056/NEJM198005013021803
147. Schnog JJ, Kremer Hovinga JA, Krieg S, Akin S, Lammle B, Brandjes DP, et al. ADAMTS13 activity in sickle cell disease. *Am J Hematol.* (2006) 81:492–8. doi: 10.1002/ajh.20653
148. Hankins JS, McCarville MB, Hillenbrand CM, Loeffler RB, Ware RE, Song R, et al. Ventricular diastolic dysfunction in sickle cell anemia is common but not associated with myocardial iron deposition. *Pediatr Blood Cancer.* (2010) 55:495–500. doi: 10.1002/pbc.22587
149. Johnson MC, Kirkham FJ, Redline S, Rosen CL, Yan Y, Roberts I, et al. Left ventricular hypertrophy and diastolic dysfunction in children with sickle cell disease are related to asleep and waking oxygen desaturation. *Blood.* (2010) 116:16–21. doi: 10.1182/blood-2009-06-227447
150. Covitz W, Espeland M, Gallagher D, Hellenbrand W, Leff S, Talner N. The heart in sickle cell anemia. The cooperative study of sickle cell disease (CSSCD). *Chest.* (1995) 108:1214–9. doi: 10.1378/chest.108.5.1214

151. Willens HJ, Lawrence C, Frishman WH, Strom JA. A noninvasive comparison of left ventricular performance in sickle cell anemia and chronic aortic regurgitation. *Clin Cardiol.* (1983) 6:542–8. doi: 10.1002/clc.4960061105
152. Gladwin MT. Cardiovascular complications and risk of death in sickle-cell disease. *Lancet.* (2016) 387:2565–74. doi: 10.1016/S0140-6736(16)00647-4
153. Caldas MC, Meira ZA, Barbosa MM. Evaluation of 107 patients with sickle cell anemia through tissue Doppler and myocardial performance index. *J Am Soc Echocardiogr.* (2008) 21:1163–7. doi: 10.1016/j.echo.2007.06.001
154. Sachdev V, Kato GJ, Gibbs JS, Barst RJ, Machado RF, Nouraie M, et al. Echocardiographic markers of elevated pulmonary pressure and left ventricular diastolic dysfunction are associated with exercise intolerance in adults and adolescents with homozygous sickle cell anemia in the United States and United Kingdom. *Circulation.* (2011) 124:1452–60. doi: 10.1161/CIRCULATIONAHA.111.032920
155. Mekontso Dessap A, Leon R, Habibi A, Nzouakou R, Roudot-Thoraval F, Adnot S, et al. Pulmonary hypertension and cor pulmonale during severe acute chest syndrome in sickle cell disease. *Am J Respir Crit Care Med.* (2008) 177:646–53. doi: 10.1164/rccm.200710-1606OC
156. Boyd JH, Macklin EA, Strunk RC, DeBaun MR. Asthma is associated with acute chest syndrome and pain in children with sickle cell anemia. *Blood.* (2006) 108:2923–7. doi: 10.1182/blood-2006-01-011072
157. Boyd JH, Macklin EA, Strunk RC, DeBaun MR. Asthma is associated with increased mortality in individuals with sickle cell anemia. *Haematologica.* (2007) 92:1115–8. doi: 10.3324/haematol.11213
158. Brewin J, Howard J. Sickle cell disease: an update on management. *Paediatr Child Health.* (2017) 27:506–10. doi: 10.1016/j.paed.2017.07.005
159. Ohene-Frempong K, Weiner SJ, Sleeper LA, Miller ST, Embury S, Moohr JW, et al. Cerebrovascular accidents in sickle cell disease: rates and risk factors. *Blood.* (1998) 91:288–94.
160. Pavlakis SG, Prohovnik I, Piomelli S, DeVivo DC. Neurologic complications of sickle cell disease. *Adv Pediatr.* (1989) 36:247–76.
161. Dobson SR, Holden KR, Nietert PJ, Cure JK, Laver JH, Disco D, et al. Moyamoya syndrome in childhood sickle cell disease: a predictive factor for recurrent cerebrovascular events. *Blood.* (2002) 99:3144–50. doi: 10.1182/blood.V99.9.3144
162. Murphy RA. Preventable deaths in sickle-cell anaemia in African children. *Lancet.* (2010) 375:460–1. doi: 10.1016/S0140-6736(10)60194-8
163. Ramakrishnan M, Moisi JC, Klugman KP, Iglesias JM, Grant LR, Mpoudi-Etame M, et al. Increased risk of invasive bacterial infections in African people with sickle-cell disease: a systematic review and meta-analysis. *Lancet Infect Dis.* (2010) 10:329–37. doi: 10.1016/S1473-3099(10)70055-4
164. Pegelow CH, Colangelo L, Steinberg M, Wright EC, Smith J, Phillips G, et al. Natural history of blood pressure in sickle cell disease: risks for stroke and death associated with relative hypertension in sickle cell anemia. *Am J Med.* (1997) 102:171–7. doi: 10.1016/S0002-9343(96)00407-X
165. Machado RF, Barst RJ, Yovetich NA, Hassell KL, Kato GJ, Gordeuk VR, et al. Hospitalization for pain in patients with sickle cell disease treated with sildenafil for elevated TRV and low exercise capacity. *Blood.* (2011) 118:855–64. doi: 10.1182/blood-2010-09-306167
166. Bernini JC, Rogers ZR, Sandler ES, Reisch JS, Quinn CT, Buchanan GR. Beneficial effect of intravenous dexamethasone in children with mild to moderately severe acute chest syndrome complicating sickle cell disease. *Blood.* (1998) 92:3082–9. doi: 10.1182/blood.V92.9.3082.421k15_3082_3089
167. Atz AM, Wessel DL. Inhaled nitric oxide in sickle cell disease with acute chest syndrome. *Anesthesiology.* (1997) 87:988–90. doi: 10.1097/00000542-199710000-00037
168. Sullivan KJ, Goodwin SR, Evangelist J, Moore RD, Mehta P. Nitric oxide successfully used to treat acute chest syndrome of sickle cell disease in a young adolescent. *Crit Care Med.* (1999) 27:2563–8. doi: 10.1097/00003246-199911000-00039
169. Hoffmann M, Geldner G, Leschke M. Life-threatening acute chest syndrome with hemolytic crisis in sickle cell disease. Treatment using a venovenous extracorporeal membrane oxygenation (ECMO). *Dtsch Med Wochenschr.* (2011) 136:2192–5. doi: 10.1055/s-0031-1292031
170. Black LV, Smith W. Evidence-based mini-review: are systemic corticosteroids an effective treatment for acute pain in sickle cell disease? *Hematology.* (2010) 2010:416–7. doi: 10.1182/asheducation-2010.1.416
171. Novelli EM, Gladwin MT. Crises in sickle cell disease. *Chest.* (2016) 149:1082–93. doi: 10.1016/j.chest.2015.12.016
172. Fitzhugh CD, Hsieh MM, Bolan CD, Saenz C, Tisdale JF. Granulocyte colony-stimulating factor (G-CSF) administration in individuals with sickle cell disease: time for a moratorium? *Cytotherapy.* (2009) 11:464–71. doi: 10.1080/14653240902849788
173. Vichinsky E, Hoppe CC, Ataga KI, Ware RE, Nduba V, El-Beshlawy A, et al. A phase 3 randomized trial of Voxelotor in sickle cell disease. *N Engl J Med.* (2019) 381:509–19. doi: 10.1056/NEJMoa1903212
174. Niihara Y, Miller ST, Kanter J, Lanzkron S, Smith WR, Hsu LL, et al. A phase 3 trial of l-Glutamine in sickle cell disease. *N Engl J Med.* (2018) 379:226–35. doi: 10.1056/NEJMoa1715971
175. Kutlar A, Kanter J, Liles DK, Alvarez OA, Cancado RD, Friedrisch JR, et al. Effect of crizanlizumab on pain crises in subgroups of patients with sickle cell disease: a sustain study analysis. *Am J Hematol.* (2019) 94:55–61. doi: 10.1002/ajh.25308
176. Ataga KI, Kutlar A, Kanter J. Crizanlizumab in sickle cell disease. *N Engl J Med.* (2017) 376:1796. doi: 10.1056/NEJMc1703162

2

Similarities and Differences Between Staphylococcal and Streptococcal Toxic Shock Syndromes in Children: Results from a 30-Case Cohort

Etienne Javouhey[1,2], Pierre-Adrien Bolze[3], Claire Jamen[1], Gerard Lina[4,5,6], Cédric Badiou[6], Claire Poyart[7,8,9,10], Aurelie Portefaix[1,11], Anne Tristan[2,4,5,6], Frédéric Laurent[2,4,5,6], Michèle Bes[4,6], François Vandenesch[2,4,5,6], Yves Gilletand[1,4,6] and Olivier Dauwalder[4,5,6]*

[1] Pediatric Emergency and Critical Care Unit, Hospices Civils de Lyon, Hôpital Femme Mère Enfant, Bron, France, [2] Faculté de Médecine Lyon Est, Université de Lyon, Domaine de la Buire, Lyon, France, [3] Service de Gynécologie et Obstétrique, Hospices Civils de Lyon, Hôpital Femme Mère Enfant, Bron, France, [4] Centre National de Référence des Staphylocoques, Institut des Agents Infectieux, Centre de Biologie et de Pathologie Nord, Hospices Civils de Lyon, Lyon, France, [5] Laboratoire de Bactériologie, Centre de Biologie et de Pathologie Nord, Institut des Agents Infectieux, Hospices Civils de Lyon, Lyon, France, [6] Centre International de Recherche en Infectiologie (CIRI), Inserm U1111, Université Lyon 1, Ecole Normale Supérieure de Lyon, CNRS UMR5308, Lyon, France, [7] Centre National de Références des Streptocoques - Groupe Hospitalier Paris Centre Cochin-Hôtel Dieu-Broca, Assistance Publique Hôpitaux de Paris, Paris, France, [8] Institut Cochin Université Sorbonne Paris Descartes, Paris, France, [9] INSERM 1016, Institut Cochin, Paris, France, [10] CNRS, UMR8104, Institut Cochin, Paris, France, [11] EPICIME-CIC 1407 de Lyon, Inserm, Service de Pharmacotoxicologie, Hospices Civils de Lyon, Bron, France

***Correspondence:**
Etienne Javouhey
etienne.javouhey@chu-lyon.fr

Introduction: Toxic shock syndromes (TSS) are severe shocks due to staphylococcal or streptococcal infection that require specific treatments. The early recognition of these shocks is crucial to improve their outcomes.

Objectives: The primary objective of this study was to compare characteristics and outcomes of staphylococcal and streptococcal TSS in children, in order to identify putative early clinical diagnostic criteria. Secondary objectives were to determine the toxin gene profiles of associated isolated strains and the relevance of measuring Vβ T-cell signatures to confirm the diagnosis.

Study design: We performed a multicenter retrospective evaluation of clinical data, biological results, and treatment outcomes of children with a confirmed or probable case of staphylococcal or streptococcal TSS. Children were consecutively included if they were admitted to the pediatric intensive care units of Lyon (France), between January 2005 and July 2011.

Results: Among the 30 analyzed children, 15 presented staphylococcal TSS and 15 streptococcal TSS. The most frequent origin of staphylococcal and streptococcal TSS was the lower respiratory tract (53%) and the genital tract (47%) respectively. Non-menstrual TSS syndrome cases presented more frequently with neurological alterations, and digestive signs were predominant in menstrual forms. Compared to Staphylococcal TSS, Streptococcal TSS presented with higher organ dysfunction scores (median Pediatric Index of Mortality 2 score 20.9 (4.1–100) vs. 1.7 (1.3–2.3), $p = 0.001$), required respiratory support more frequently (80 vs. 33%, $p = 0.02$), were intubated for a longer time (3 days (0.75–5) vs. 1 day (0–1.5), $p = 0.006$) and had a non-significant trend of higher, case-fatality rate (20 vs. 7%, $p = 0.60$). The lack of antitoxin therapy was associated with higher case-fatality rate (50 vs. 4%, $p = 0.04$). The Vβ repertoire measurements exhibited toxin dependent-alterations in accordance with the toxin gene profiles of isolated strains in both types of toxic shock syndromes. Regarding toxin gene profiles of isolated strains, 10/15 *Staphylococcus aureus* belonged to clonal complex (CC) 30 and 6/12 *Streptococcus pyogenes* were *emm1* type suggesting clonal etiologies for both staphylococcal and streptococcal TSS.

Conclusion: Despite the involvement of functionally similar toxins, staphylococcal and streptococcal TSS differed by their clinical signs, origin of infection and prognosis. The detection of Vβ profiles was useful to confirm the diagnosis of staphylococcal and streptococcal TSS and for the identification of involved toxins.

Keywords: toxic shock syndrome, children, *Staphylococcus aureus, Streptococcus pyogenes*, Vβ T-cell signature, antitoxin therapy

INTRODUCTION

Toxic Shock Syndrome (TSS) is a severe acute illness characterized by high fever, hypotension, rash, multi-organ system dysfunction, and desquamation during convalescence. TSS is caused by toxin-producing strains of *Staphylococcus aureus* or *Streptococcus pyogenes* and occurs in both adult and pediatric patients (1–5). TSS remains a rare but severe disease, with a mortality rate that varies from 4 to 27% for streptococcal (Str) TSS (2–4) and from 0 to 22% for menstrual and non-menstrual staphylococcal (Sta) TSS (1). Studies conducted in pediatric intensive care units (PICU) reported a mortality rate that can reach 25% for Str-TSS (2–6). The outcome of Sta-TSS is more favorable in children than in adults (7, 8). TSSs have a specific pathophysiology linked to superantigen exotoxins. Superantigens (SAg), in contrast with conventional antigens, do not need to be processed by antigen-presenting cells before being presented to T cells. They instead directly stimulate T cells by cross-linking major histocompatibility complex class II molecules on the antigen-presenting cells with the variable portion of the T-cell antigen receptor chain (Vβ TCR), thereby inducing massive polyclonal cell proliferation (9, 10). Due to their structural differences, each SAg links preferentially to one or several Vβ repertoire, thus inducing targeted T cell expansion and the massive pro-inflammatory response (11). A transient depletion of targeted Vβ TCRs may be observed at the early phase of TSS due to the concomitant lymphopenia, to the mobilization/accumulation of T cells from peripheral blood to lymph nodes or to the spleen, and/or from downregulation of TCR molecules binding the toxin targeted Vβ repertoire(s) soon after T cell activation (12).

The diagnosis of TSS is based on the association of standardized clinical signs defined by the Centers for Disease Control (CDC), but some of them may be transient (i.e., hypotension), lacking (i.e., cutaneous rash) or of delayed occurrence (i.e., desquamation), and diagnosis is often difficult during the early stages of the diseases (13, 14). Distinction from septic shock, Kawasaki disease with shock, drug reaction with eosinophilia and systemic symptoms (DRESS) syndrome is sometimes difficult (15). Nevertheless, treatments of these differential diagnoses differ significantly and early recognition of these diseases is a key point for the prognosis. Because SAgs are active at very low concentrations (<1 pg/mL) that are barely detectable *in vivo*, the identification of *ex vivo* specific Vβ TCR alterations could help to diagnose or to confirm TSS (16–26).

Early diagnosis of TSS is required because specific TSS treatments with antitoxin effects must be added (1, 27) to adapted antimicrobial chemotherapy: clindamycin, rifampicin or linezolid to reduce exotoxin synthesis (2, 9, 28, 29), and intravenous immunoglobulin (IVIG) therapy to neutralize the SAg, especially in severe TSS (1–4, 7, 8, 30–36). Because of severity of the disease, the clinical characteristics of Sta- and Str-TSS have been primarily described in adult patients.

The objectives of this pediatric study were to compare the characteristics and the outcome of staphylococcal and streptococcal TSS in children to identify putative early clinical diagnostic criteria; to identify factors associated with case-fatality; to study the toxin gene profiles of associated isolated strains; and to assess the relevance of measuring Vβ T-cell signatures to confirm the diagnosis.

MATERIALS AND METHODS

Patient Selection

Selection of Eligible TSS Cases

The Sta- and Str-TSS cases were retrospectively selected by searching for the keywords “toxic” or “toxin-associated shock syndrome” in the hospital information system, as well as in the medical records and databases of the two PICUs of the Hospices Civils de Lyon, France (Debrousse Hospital and Edouard Herriot Hospital from 2005 to 2008), then the PICU of the “Hôpital Femme Mère Enfant” from 2008 to 2011 grouping those two units when they closed. A supplemental research was performed from the database of the French Staphylococcal and Streptococcal National Reference Centers (NRC) which collects prospectively strains involved in staphylococcal and streptococcal diseases, and notably toxin associated diseases. Appointed by Santé Publique France, an agency of the French Ministry of health, NRC missions include (i) strain expertises (identification, resistance, virulence, and typing), (ii) epidemiological surveillance of infections (i.e., increase of incidence, new virulent factor, etc.), and (iii) advice to public authorities, health agencies, and health professionals.

Included Cases

All records of the cases identified were reviewed by two authors (CJ, EJ) to check if they met the CDC criteria for confirmed and probable TSS cases (13, 14). Sta-TSS patients with all CDC criteria but desquamation were included in the probable Sta-TSS group, as this sign mainly occurred lately in the course of the disease and was therefore lacking in the PICU's medical record.

Collected Data

Clinical and biological data, including pediatric index of mortality (PIM 2), pediatric logistic organ dysfunction (PELOD) scores and 30 days outcomes (length of PICU stay and mortality) were collected anonymously (37, 38).

Ethics Statements

According to the French policies, our study was defined as a non-interventional study as it met the following two criteria: (i) parents of children included in the database have received information about the study and (ii) an non-formalized right of opposition was collected in the clinical records. Regarding this lack of written informed consent, patient records were collected anonymously and de-identified prior to analysis. Thus, this study was approved by an institutional ethics review board ("Comité de Protection des personnes Sud Est IV, DC-2008-176").

Immunological Data

Blood samples were collected in EDTA tubes from 1 to 4 days (D) after PICU admission to measure Vβ CD3+T cell alterations. Due to the initial lymphopenia, the mobilization/accumulation of T cells from peripheral blood to lymph nodes or to the spleen, and/or from downregulation of TCR molecules binding the toxin targeted Vβ repertoire(s) soon after T cell activation, a second measurement was performed between D+3 and D+8 of PICU admission in case of massive decrease of one or association of Vβ repertoires known to be targetet by SAg. These measurements could only be performed 5 days a week (Monday–Friday) which explains that the first determination could range from D+1 to D+4 and the second from D+3 to D+8. The physicians responsible for case coding as well as those responsible for the clinical PICU's databases were not aware of the results of these immunological investigations.

The peripheral blood mononuclear cells were stained with CD3 and 24 TCR Vβ element antibodies (IO Test Beta Mark® kit, Beckman Coulter, Marseille, France) and analyzed with FACScan® flow cytometer (BD, Pont de Claix, France), as previously described (25). Based on our previous data that showed an association between TCR Vβ expansions and involved staphylococcal toxin, we limited the measure of Vβ CD3+T cell alterations to these 24 out of 65 known human Vβ elements.

Microbiological Data

Different anatomical sites were sampled and sent for microbiological analysis (culture and isolation of *S. aureus* or *S. pyogenes*) in order to identify etiology and source of infection. Strains were identified by biochemical tests, such as clumping factor, the coagulase test or Lancefield group agglutination (bioMérieux, Marcy l'Etoile, France), and with Phoenix® strips (BD, Pont de Claix, France) or mass spectrometry (VITEK MS®, BioMérieux, France). Antibiotic susceptibilities were determined using a Phoenix 100® instrument (BD) or by the disc diffusion method (SIRSCAN® I2A, Peyrols, France) following CA-SFM guidelines.

Toxin Gene Profiles of *S. aureus* Strains Determined by the French NRC of Staphylococci

The toxin gene profiles of *S. aureus* isolates were characterized for all patients. Staphylococcal DNA was extracted (Qiagen, Courtaboeuf, France), and the toxin gene profile was determined using Identibac *S. aureus* Genotyping® DNA microarrays (Alere, Jouy en Josas, France), as previously described (39). This Identibac *S. aureus* Genotyping® DNA microarray screened genes for strains identification, virulence factors, resistance and allow for the assignment to a probable clonal complex (CC) (39).

Toxin Gene Profiles and M Protein Typing of *S. pyogenes* Strains Determined by the French NRC of Streptococci

The toxin gene profiles of *S. pyogenes* isolates were characterized for 12/15 patients (three strains were not transmitted to the French NRC for streptococci). As previously described, *S. pyogenes* strains were analyzed to determine their gene profiles of superantigenic toxins and M protein types (*emm*) (8) by PCR.

Statistical Analysis

Data were analyzed with SPSS for Windows version 17.0 (SPSS Inc., Chicago, Illinois, USA). Qualitative variables were compared with a Chi-Square test supplemented by Fisher's exact test for low effective groups ($n < 5$). Quantitative variables are reported as the means and standard deviation or as medians and quartiles 1 and 3 for the variables that had distributions that were not normal. The Kolmogorov-Smirnov test was used to study the normality of the distribution of the continuous variables. The quantitative variables were compared with Student's *t*-test or with a non-parametric Wilcoxon test depending on the normality of their distribution. *P*-values below 0.05 were considered to indicate statistical significance.

RESULTS

Characteristics of the Study Population

Among the 34 patients identified from the cross-analysis of the databases, 30 (11 boys and 19 girls) were finally included in the study. Among them, 15 Str-TSS cases (11 confirmed and 4 probable cases according to the CDC criteria) and 15 Sta-TSS cases, 6 of which were menstrual Sta-TSS and 9 non-menstrual Sta-TSS (4 confirmed cases and 8 probable cases according to the CDC criteria) were included. The four excluded patients were 1

Stevens-Johnson syndrome, 1 Kawasaki syndrome with shock, 1 severe Panton-Valentine staphylococcal infection and 1 patient hospitalized in an intermediate care unit. The median age was 5.2 years (interquartile range: 1.4-12.8, **Table 1**). *S. pyogenes* were isolated in all the patients.

Comparison Between Patients With Staphylococcal and Streptococcal Toxic Shock Syndrome

Children with Str-TSS were significantly younger than children with Sta-TSS [1.7 years (0.7-5.4) vs. 12.8 years (5–15.7), $p = 0.001$]. At day 1, compared to Sta-TSS patients, Str-TSS patients needed ventilation support more often and had longer ventilation duration [3 days (0.75–5) vs. 1 day (0–1.5), $p = 0.006$]; had higher leukocyte counts (22.3 vs. 14.6 G/L, $p = 0.049$) and significantly higher CRP levels (238.8+/– 103.8 vs. 164+/– 82.8 mg/l, $p = 0.04$, respectively) and presented with significantly higher PIM 2 score (median 20.9 (4.1–100) vs. 1.7 (1.3–2.3), $p = 0.001$) Other clinical variable were similar in the two groups.

The primary origin of the Str-TSS was the lower respiratory tract (53% of Str-TSS cases) whereas menstrual and non-menstrual Sta-TSS involved the vagina, and the skin or the upper respiratory tract respectively (**Table 2**).

TABLE 1 | Clinical and biological characteristics of patients with staphylococcal or streptococcal toxic shock syndrome.

		Missing data	Sta-TSS[a] ($n = 15$)	Str-TSS[b] ($n = 15$)	*p*
Demographical characteristics	Male (%[c])	0	4 (27%)	7 (47%)	0.45[d]
	Age (years) median (Q1-Q3[e])	0	12.8 (5–15.7)	1.7 (0.7–5.4)	0.001[f,*]
Hemodynamic characteristics	Hypotension (%)	0	15 (100%)	15 (100%)	1[g]
	Need of amine support (%)	0	10 (67%)	12 (80%)	0.68[g]
	Duration of treatment with amines (days) median (Q1-Q3)	0	1 (0–1.8)	2 (0.8–3)	0.17[f]
Pulmonary signs	$FiO_2^h > 50\%$ (%)	1	5/14 (36%)	13/15 (87%)	0.01[g,*]
	Requirement of mechanical ventilation (%)	0	5 (33%)	12 (80%)	0.02[g,*]
	Duration of intubation median (days) (Q1-Q3)	0	1 (0–1.5)	3 (0.75–5)	0.006[f,*]
	ARDS[i] (%)	2	1/14 (7%)	5/14 (36%)	0.16[d]
Organ dysfunctions	Creatinine, maximum value (μmol/L) mean (SD[j])	0	122.1 (115.8)	68.3 (49.6)	0.11[k]
	Liver alterations[l] (%)	2	10/14 (71%)	8/14 (57%)	0.69[g]
	Number of organ dysfunction[l] median (Q1-Q3)	0	3 (2–4)	4 (3–5)	0.13[f]
Cutaneous signs	Rash (%)	0	15 (100%)	11 (73%)	0.10[g]
	Desquamation (%)	6	5/13 (39%)	3/11 (27%)	0.68[d]
	Digestive signs (%)	0	11 (73%)	7 (47%)	0.26[g]
Inflammatory parameters	Fever ≥ 38.9°C (%)	0	15 (100%)	15 (100%)	1[g]
	Leukocytes, minimum value (G/L)mean (*SD*)	0	8.6 (3.7)	8.5 (6.3)	0.95[k]
	Leukocytes, maximum value (G/L) mean (*SD*)	0	14.6 (6.2)	22.3 (13)	0.049[k,*]
	Lymphocytes, minimum value (G/L) median (Q1-Q3)	2	0.2 (0.1–1.2)	0.6 (0.5–0.9)	0.056[f]
	C-Reactive Protein (mg/L) mean (SD)	2	164 (82.8)	238.8 (103.8)	0.044[k,*]
Hemostasis parameters	Platelets, minimum value (G/L) mean (SD)	0	124.8 (52.5)	140.2 (100.6)	0.61[k]
	Disseminated Intravascular Coagulation	1	8/15 (53%)	8/14 (57%)	1[g]
Severity scores and outcome	PIM2[m] score median (Q1-Q3)	3	1.7 (1.3-2.3)	20.9 (4.1-100)	0.001[f,*]
	PELOD[n] J1 score median (Q1-Q3)	1	11 (11-21)	16.5 (11.8–25)	0.15[f]
	Length of stay in ICU[o] (days) median (Q1-Q3)	0	3 (2-4)	6 (3–9)	0.02[f,*]
	30 day death	0	1 (7%)	3 (20%)	0.60 [d]

[a] *Sta-TSS, Staphylococcal Toxic Shock Syndrome.*
[b] *Str-TSS, Streptococcal Toxic Shock Syndrome.*
[c] *% percent of total population.*
[d] *Statistical analysis performed with Fisher exact test.*
[e] *Q1-Q3, Interquartile range.*
[f] *Statistical analysis performed with Wilcoxon test.*
[g] *Statistical analysis performed with Chi-square test.*
[h] *FiO_2, Fraction of inspired Oxygen.*
[i] *ARDS, Acute Respiratory Distress Syndrome.*
[j] *SD, standard deviation.*
[k] *Statistical analysis performed with Student t-test.*
[l] *Liver alterations and organ dysfunctions were defined in CDC criteria for case definition of toxic shock syndrome (13, 14).*
[m] *PIM2 Pediatric Index of Mortality 2 score.*
[n] *PELOD Pediatric Logistic Organs Dysfunctions score.*
[o] *ICU, Intensive Care Unit.*
[*] *Statistically significant data with the corresponding statistical test.*

TABLE 2 | Infectious source of patients with staphylococcal and streptococcal toxic shock syndrome.

Etiological infectious sites	Staphylococcal TSS[a] (n = 15)	Streptococcal TSS (n = 15)	p^b
Bacteremia	1 (7%)	6 (40%)	0.08
Pleura or lung	1 (7%)	8 (53%)	0.01*
Postoperative TSS	0 (0%)	2 (13%)	0.48
Skin and soft tissues	4 (27%)	3 (20%)	1
Upper respiratory tract	3 (20%)	3 (20%)	1
Vagina	7 (47%)	0 (0%)	0.006*
Varicella superinfection	2 (13%)	3 (20%)	1
Indefinite	0 (0%)	1 (7%)	1

[a]*TSS, Toxic Shock Syndrome;* [b]*Statistical analysis performed with Chi-square test.*
**Statistically significant data (p<0.05) with the corresponding statistical test.*

There was no difference between groups regarding IVIG use (53% for Str-TSS and 47% for Sta-TSS, p=1) or the use of anti-infectious agents with antitoxin effects (clindamycin, linezolid, rifampicin; 93% for Str-TSS and 87% for Sta-TSS, $p = 1$).

Comparison Between Menstrual and Non-menstrual Staphylococcal Toxic Shock Syndrome

The most striking difference between menstrual and non-menstrual Sta-TSS was the constant presence of gastrointestinal signs (i.e., abdominal pain and emesis) in menstrual Sta-TSS (100 vs. 50%, $p = 0.08$) There was also a non-significant trend toward a higher frequency of neurological symptoms (i.e., confusion, impaired consciousness) in non-menstrual Sta-TSS (50 vs. 14%, $p = 0.28$).

Factors Associated With Case-Fatality:

Our retrospective study reported 4/30 deaths (13%) (**Table 3**). The non-survivors significantly presented with more organ dysfunctions, with a higher occurrence of acute respiratory distress syndrome and with a higher PELOD score measured at D+1. The case-fatality rate was not significantly different between the Staphylococcal and Streptococcal TSS groups (7 vs. 20% $p = 0.60$). All the children received adapted antimicrobial therapies for *S. aureus* or *S. pyogenes*, and 27/30 received an antitoxin therapy (clindamycin or clindamycin + IVIG) with a significant association with survival (**Table 3**). Among the 4 non-survivors, three died rapidly (one during the transport to PICU, one 4 h after arrival, one had presented a cardiac arrest just prior to PICU admission), and only one of them received an antitoxin antibiotic.

Microbiological Features

S. aureus strains belonged to the accessory gene regulator (Agr)1 (2/15), Agr2 (2/15) or Agr3 (11/15) genetic backgrounds. According to DNA microarrays assignments, 10/15 belongs to clonal complex (CC) 30, 1/15 to CC5, 1/ 15 to CC45, 1/15 to CC22, and the sole MRSA strain is CC5 and belongs to Geraldine clone. All menstrual Sta-TSS strains contained the TSS toxin gene (*tst)* that encodes TSS toxin −1 (TSST-1), the staphylococcal enterotoxin A gene (*sea)* gene that encodes staphylococcal enterotoxin (SE) A (4/7), the enterotoxin gene clusters (*egc*) that encode SEG, SEI, staphylococcal enterotoxin like (SE*l)* M, SE*l*N and SE*l*O (5/7). The non-menstrual Sta-TSS isolates were characterized by the presence of the *tst* gene encoding TSST-1 (6/8), *seb* (1/8), or *sec* (1/8) in association with other toxin genes; the most frequently found toxin genes were *sea* (4/8) and *egc* (7/8). Only one strain involved in non-menstrual Sta-TSS was resistant to methicillin.

S. pyogenes strains were primarily types *emm*1 (6/12) or *emm*12 (2/12). Toxin gene analysis showed the following 4 different profiles: contained the streptococcal pyrogenic exotoxin A (*spe*A) and *spe*C genes encoding streptococcal pyrogenic exotoxin (SPE) A and SPEC, respectively (2/12), contained only the *spe*A gene (4/12), contained only *spe*C (5/12) or contained neither *spe*A nor *spe*C but did encode *spe*B (1/12). The gene *spe*B was present in all *S. pyogenes* strains included in our study.

Immunological Features: Superantigenic Toxins and Vβ T-Cell Signatures

The Vβ repertoire profile of CD3+ T cells (Vβ profile) was determined at D1-4 after PICU admission in a subset of 18/30 patients that included 12 Sta-TSS and 6 Str-TSS cases (**Tables 4, 5**). Targeted by TSST-1, a significant Vβ2 alteration was observed in all confirmed and probable TSS-Sta cases. Whereas, a Vβ2 increase was measured for 8/12 (67%) Sta-TSS patients, it was delayed for 4 Sta-TSS cases with initially a large decrease of Vβ2 repertoire followed by a large expansion at the second measurement performed between D3 and D5. A correlation between the number of organ dysfunctions and the level of Vβ2 expression on CD3+ T cells between days 3 and 5 post-Sta-TSS onset was found (**Figure 1**). Regarding 6 Str-TSS cases, expansions of some or all Vβ repertoires targeted by SPEA or SPEC were also measured in all confirmed and probable Str-TSS cases at the first determination (**Table 5**).

DISCUSSION

This retrospective analysis of 30 consecutive cases of Staphylococcal and Streptococcal TSS, admitted to the PICUs of the city of Lyon in France, showed differences between groups regarding clinical presentation, origin of infection, and outcome. However, pathophysiological mechanisms involving superantigenic toxins were consistent between groups. We showed that the detection of Vβ profiles could confirm the diagnosis of Staphylococcal and Streptococcal TSS cases, signing a toxin involvement, correlated to the toxin gene profile of the isolated strains.

Clinical Findings

Str-TSS patients were younger than Sta-TSS patients, with 47% of patients younger than 2 years, in agreement with previous studies (2, 4–6). Regarding their clinical signs, TSS associated with para-pneumonic empyema was highly suggestive of a

TABLE 3 | Comparison of clinical characteristics and effects of antitoxin therapies on live vs. dead TSS cases.

	Dead ($n = 4$)	Survivor ($n = 26$)	P
Etiology of toxic shock syndrome			$p = 0.5977$
- Sta-TSS[a] (%)[b]	1 (7%)	14 (93%)	
- Str-TSS[c] (%)	3 (20%)	12 (80%)	
Number of organ dysfunctions (SD[d])	5 (0, 8)	4 (1, 3)	$p = 0.04^*$
ARDS[e] (%)	4/4 (100%)	4/26 (15%)	$p = 0.04^*$
PELOD[f] score at D+1 (SD)	28 (13, 7)	12 (7, 1)	$p = 0.04^*$
Antitoxin therapies (overall)			$p = 0.04^*$
- No treatment (%)	2 (67%)	1 (33%)	
- At least one antitoxin therapies (clindamycin; clindamycin + IVIG[g]) (%)	2 (7%)	25 (93%)	
Antitoxin therapy: clindamycin only			$p = 0.0813$
- No treatment (%)	2 (67%)	1 (33%)	
- Clindamycin only (%)	1 (8%)	11 (92%)	
Antitoxin therapy: clindamycin + IVIG			$p = 0.5977$
- No treatment (%)	3 (20%)	12 (80%)	
- Clindamycin + IVIG (%)	1 (7%)	14 (93%)	
Antitoxin therapy: clindamycin + IVIG			$p = 1.0000$
- Clindamycin only (%)	1 (8%)	11 (92%)	
- Clindamycin + IVIG (%)	1 (7%)	14 (93%)	

[a]Sta-TSS, Staphylococcal Toxic Shock Syndrome.
[b]%, percent of total population.
[c]Str-TSS, Streptococcal Toxic Shock Syndrome.
[d]SD, standard deviation.
[e]ARDS, Acute Respiratory Distress Syndrome.
[f]PELOD, Pediatric Logistic Organs Dysfunctions score.
[g]IVIG, Intravenous Immunoglobulin.
**Statistically significant data with the corresponding statistical test.*

streptococcal origin. Conversely, menstrual Sta-TSS should be suspected in a young adolescent girl with hypotension, rash, gastrointestinal symptoms and fever, whereas non-menstrual Sta-TSS may include a very heterogeneous group of patients in terms of age, gender and comorbidities.

Str-TSS cases had a more severe prognosis than the Sta-TSS cases, including longer PICU stay, higher PIM2 scores, higher number of organ failure with more frequent acute respiratory distress syndrome, and required mechanical ventilation more often and for a longer time, in accordance to UK and Australian studies (5, 6, 40). Although not significant, the case-fatality rate for Str-TSS (20%) was higher than Sta-TSS (7%), that is consistent with the meta-analysis of Chuang et al., who analyzed 27 and 30 studies focused on Sta- and Str-TSS, respectively. They found a 5 to 10% case-fatality rate for Str-TSS, a 3% case-fatality rate for menstrual Sta-TSS and a 5% rate for non-menstrual Sta-TSS (7). Moreover, three later studies that included critically ill children found a case-fatality rate between 20 and 30% for Str-TSS (2, 4, 6); however, that remains below the case-fatality rate (45%) estimated for adults by the French NRC between 2006 and 2010 (1). Recently, Chen et al. reported an absence of death in a large cohort of 62 Staphylococcal and Streptococcal TSS cases (5, 6).

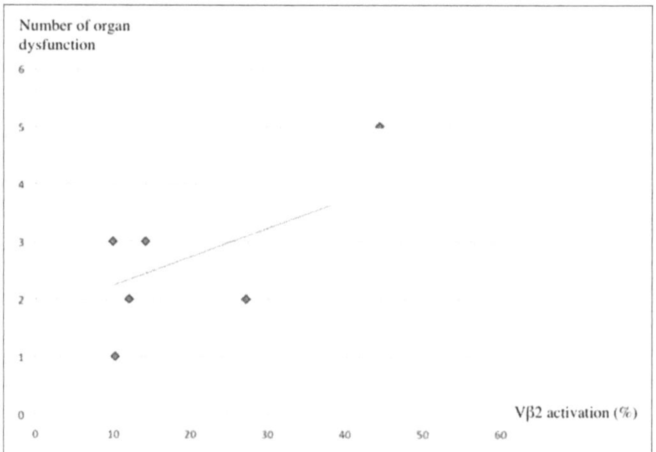

FIGURE 1 | Correlation between organ dysfunctions and Vβ2 expression on CD3+ T cells. Correlation between the number of organ dysfunctions and the Vβ2 expression measured on CD3+ T cells between days 3 and 5 after the onset of staphylococcal toxic shock syndrome. Pearson's correlation (R^2) was used to measure co-linearity between the selected independent variables.

Factors Associated With Case-Fatality

We found a significantly lower case-fatality rate in patients treated with at least one antitoxin therapy (clindamycin or clindamycin + IVIG) (**Table 3**). This result was in line with a recent study on TSS-Str demonstrating that clindamycin treatment substantially reduced mortality rate (41, 42). This effect may be enhanced by concurrent treatment with IVIG,

TABLE 4 | Vβ T cell signatures and *Staphylococcus aureus* toxin gene profiles of patients with staphylococcal toxic shock syndrome.

	Gender	Treatments		Immunological data		Toxin suspected according to Vβ modification profile	Microbiological data				Clonal complexe
		Antitoxin antibiotic	IVIG[a] (Dose)	Vβ alterations of CD3+ T cells (%)[b] Measurement 1 [day post shock onset]	Vβ alterations of CD3+ T cells (%)[b] Measurement 2 [day post shock onset]		Site of isolation – Infection or carriage strain	Methicillin suscepti-bility	Allele of Agr system	Toxin gene profile	
Menstrual staphylococcal toxic shocks	F[c]	Yes	Yes (NA[d])	Vβ2 ↗ (44.4%) [D[e]+4]	ND[f]	TSST-1[g]	Vagina (c)[h]	MSSA[i]	3	*tst*[j]; *sea*[k]; *egc*[l]	CC30
	F	Yes	No	Vβ2 ↘ (1.1%) [D+1]	Vβ2 ↔ (10.2%) [D+5]	TSST-1	Vagina (c)	MSSA	1	*tst; egc*	CC22
	F	Yes	No	Vβ2 ↗ (19%) [D+1]	ND	TSST-1	Vagina (c)	MSSA	3	*tst*	CC30
	F	Yes	No	Vβ2 ↗ (22%) [D+2]	ND	TSST-1	Vagina (c)	MSSA	3	*tst; sea; egc; selu*[m]	CC30
	F	Yes	Yes (1g/kg)	Vβ2 ↘ (5.7%) [D+1]	Vβ2 ↗ (14.1%) [D+3]	TSST-1	Vagina (c)	MSSA	3	*tst; sea; egc; selu*	CC30
	F	Yes	No	Vβ2 ↗ (12%) [D+3]	Vβ2 ↗ (27.2%) [D+5]	TSST-1	Vagina (c)	MSSA	3	*tst*	CC30
	ccF	Yes	Yes (0.5g/kg)	Vβ2 ↗ (29.3%) [D+2]	ND	TSST-1	Vagina (c)	MSSA	3	*tst; sea; egc; selu*	CC30
Non menstrual staphylococcal toxic shocks	M[n]	Yes	Yes (2g/kg)	Vβ2 ↘ (0.9%) [D+1]	Vβ2 ↗ (52.4%) [D+3]	TSST-1	Throat (c)	MSSA	3	*tst; sea; egc*	CC30
	M	Yes	Yes (2g/kg)	Vβ2 ↗ (27.3%) [D+1]	ND	TSST-1	Furuncle (i)[o]	MSSA	3	*tst; egc; selu*	CC30
	F	Yes	Yes (1g/kg)	Vβ2 ↗ (46.5%) [D+4]	ND	TSST-1	Blood (i)	MSSA	3	*tst; sea; egc; selu*	CC30
	M	Yes	No	Vβ2 ↘ (0.6%) [D+2]	Vβ2 ↔ (9.9%) [D+4]	TSST-1	Nose (c)	MSSA	3	*tst; sea; egc; selu*	CC30
	F	Yes	Yes (1g/kg)	Vβ2 ↗ (47.6%) [D+4]	ND	TSST-1	Superficial wound (i)	MSSA	3	*tst; sea; egc; selu*	CC30
	F	Yes	No	ND	ND	ND	Skin (i)	MRSA[p]	2	*tst; sec*[q]; *sed*[r]; *selj*[s]; *sell*[t]; *egc; selu; ser*[u]	CC5
	F	Yes	No	ND	ND	ND	Skin (i)	MSSA	1	*sec; sell; egc; selu*	CC45
	M	No	No	ND	ND	ND	Lung (i)	MSSA	2	*seb; selp*[v]	ND

[a]*IVIG, Intravenous immunoglobulins;*
[b]*Vβ alterations of CD3+ T cells (%), The expression of 24 main Vβ CD3+ T cells was determined by flow cytometry. Since all our staphylococcal toxic shock syndromes were due to toxic shock syndrome toxin-1 (TSST-1), only Vβ2 repertoire was reported according to it's the only Vβ repertoire targeted by TSST-1. Normal adult range for Vβ2 repertoire according to kit manufacturer, 5.84 to 10.76%.*
[c]*F, female.*
[d]*NA, not available.*
[e]*D, day.*
[f]*ND, not determined.*
[g]*TSST-1, toxic shock syndrome toxin−1.*
[h]*(c): carriage strain.*
[i]*MSSA, Methicillin Susceptible Staphylococcus aureus;* [j]*tst: gene encoding staphylococcal toxic shock toxin 1.*
[k]*sea, gene encoding staphylococcal enterotoxin A.*
[l]*egc, enterotoxin gene cluster encoding staphylococcal enterotoxin G, I, M, N, and O.*
[m]*selu, gene encoding staphylococcal enterotoxin like U.*
[n]*M, male;* [o]*(i): infection strain.*
[p]*MRSA, Methicillin Resistant Staphylococcus aureus.*
[q]*sec, gene encoding staphylococcal enterotoxin C.*
[r]*sed, gene encoding staphylococcal enterotoxin D.*
[s]*selj, gene encoding staphylococcal enterotoxin like J.*
[t]*sell, gene encoding staphylococcal enterotoxin like L.*
[u]*ser, gene encoding staphylococcal enterotoxin R.*
[v]*selp, gene encoding staphylococcal enterotoxin like P.*

contrasting with a previous study suggesting that IVIG had no effect (3, 41). Causality of our results cannot be ascertained because of the retrospective study design with no adjustment for disease severity (i.e., the lack of antitoxin therapy could be due to a misdiagnosis). This supports the need for a large randomized prospective trial, especially to test IVIG. Moreover, this difference in survival rates is likely to be due to the impossibility to receive such urgent treatments in time, because of the very high severity of the disease.

Microbiological and Immunological Findings

In accordance with DeVries et al. study which included any positive culture for *S. aureus* (including infection as well as carriage strains) and obtained strain in 72% of the examined cases, we systematically isolated *S. aureus* strains, suggesting a selection bias in our population based on TSS criteria (43). However, in agreement with other studies, bacteremia was rare in Sta-TSS (<5%) and significantly more frequent in the Str-TSS (40 to 60%) (7). Because characterization of the toxin gene profile of isolates was not mandatory for the inclusion analysis, only 90% were characterized: The 15 isolated *S. aureus* strains belonged to 3 different *agr* groups, and 13/15 carried at least *tst*. Eleven of the *S. aureus* strains were Agr3, and among them, 6 exhibited similar toxin gene profile associating *tst*, *sea*, *egc* and *seu*, and belongs to clonal complex 30 (44). These results suggest the presence of a dominant *S. aureus* clone involved in Sta-TSS in France as recently described in United Kingdom. This CC30 MSSA produces more TSST-1 and induces more T-cell proliferation than CC30 MRSA (45). Similarly, Str-TSS were due to a dominant clone of *S. pyogenes* characterized by an *emm*1 gene encoding the M1 protein and *spe*A, in agreement with previous studies (8).

Specific treatments appear most effective when administered early in the development of the disease; thus TSS should be diagnosed as early as possible. However, TSS diagnosis based on the CDC criteria is difficult (43) because some criteria occur lately or rarely, resulting in under-diagnosis of TSS cases (11). Moreover, differential diagnosis with septic shock or Kawasaki syndrome with shock and DRESS syndrome is sometimes challenging because of the association of shock, cutaneous rash and multi organ dysfunctions in these conditions. Parsonnet et al. suggested that the integration of other laboratory criteria such as the isolation of *S. aureus,* the production of TSST 1 (or another superantigen) and the absence of antibodies against superantigen produced by the host could increase the accuracy of TSS diagnosis (46). Based on a biological test measuring functional effects of SAgs on immune system, our study used Vβ profile test to improve TSS diagnosis. As previously described (18), Vβ2 alterations (initial decrease followed by large expansion) correspond to the activation of T cells by TSST-1 and were observed in each of the 12 Sta-TSS cases. Each of the eight Sta-TSS cases, classified as probable according to the CDC criteria and for which Vβ profile was studied, showed a Vβ 2 repertoire expansion similar to other confirmed Sta-TSS cases. Similarly, Vβ expansions corresponded to partial or complete profiles of streptococcal SAgs produced by the clinical isolates were measured in 6/6 patients with Str-TSS. However, in two cases of Str-TSS, the Vβ expansions were difficult to interpret due to partial Vβ profiles when they were compared to the Vβ specificity from the literature (16, 19, 21, 23, 24, 26). These partial profiles may be due to residual neutralizing effects of IVIG infusion before measurement of Vβ repertoire profiles. These discrepancies may also be explained by differences in the methods used to detect Vβ expansions (other sets of antibodies or RT-PCR), the length of the incubation and the use of different cut-off values used to define significant enhancement of Vβ alterations. Ideally, we should determine the Vβ specificity of streptococcal superantigens using a flow cytometric test that has been used for *S. aureus* superantigens (10, 25). Although there is no control group due to the retrospective collection of cases, our study described, for the first time, the use of Vβ profiles to characterize a large pediatric TSS population. This biological test, which was positive in probable as well as confirmed TSS, could identify the toxin involved in the TSS and show alterations at the first measurement, which could help diagnosing or confirming TSS cases. This test may allow for an early (within the first 24–48 h) diagnosis of Sta-TSS, especially in non-menstrual cases, showing a large decrease of Vβ2 associated with severe lymphopenia. Later on (after 48 h), when expansion would confirm the diagnosis whenever the doubt persists; for example when no staphylococcus has been isolated yet.

In contrast, Ferry et al. found no discriminant Vβ signature in septic shock (27), suggesting a high specificity of the Vβ profile for TSS. At least, the Vβ profile might thus constitute a new tool to improve the diagnosis of toxic shock and might also improve the TSS diagnosis criteria of the CDC. However, additional studies are required to evaluate its relevance in partial or doubtful form of TSS cases according to CDC criteria.

Limitations

The retrospective nature of our study did not allow interpreting reliably the impact of antitoxin therapy on survival. The inability to perform Vβ profile for all patients at a same time point may bias the analysis of the performance of this biological diagnosis test. However, these preliminary results are consistent with those found in adults and require a validation by a prospective multicenter study.

The low sample size did not allow for multifactorial analysis that would have strengthened our findings.

CONCLUSION

Sta- and Str-TSS are induced by similar toxins produced by strains with limited diversity which suggests a clonal origin of French strains involved in TSS. However, they differ in their clinical presentations (pulmonary involvement vs. gastrointestinal signs), their source of infection (bacteremia vs. vaginal localization), their severity and their prognosis. The detection of Vβ profiles was helpful for the diagnosis of probable TSS cases and for the identification of toxin involvement but

TABLE 5 | VBeta T cell signatures and *Streptococcus pyogenes* toxin gene profiles of patients with streptococcal toxic shock syndrome.

Gender	Treatments		Immunological data			Microbiological data		
	Antitoxin antibiotic (Clindamycin)	IVIG[a] (Dose)	Vβ alterations of CD3⁺ T cells (%)[b] Measurement 1 [day post shock onset]	Vβ alterations of CD3⁺ T cells (%) Measurement 2 [day post shock onset]	Toxin suspected according to Vβ modification profile	Site(s) of isolation	*emm*-types	Toxin gene profile
F[c]	Yes	Yes (2 g/kg)	Vβ1 ↔ (4.6%); Vβ2 ↔ (5.8%); Vβ5.1 ↔ (5.6%); Vβ12 ↔ (1.5%); Vβ14 ↗ (5.6%) [D[d]+3]	Vβ1 ↗ (5.6%); Vβ2 ↔ (9.22%); Vβ5.1 ↔ (4.24%); Vβ12 ↔ (1.32%); Vβ14 ↗ (5.1%) [D[d]+8]	SPEA[e] or SPEC[f]	Throat	89	*speB*[g], *speC*[h]
M[i]	Yes	No	Vβ1 ↔ (2.2%); Vβ2 ↔ (10.6%); Vβ5.1 ↔ (4.7%); Vβ12 ↗ (5.8%); Vβ14 ↗ (22.1%) [D+4]	ND[j]	SPEA	Pleural effusion	1	*speA*[k] *speB*
F	Yes	Yes (2 g/kg)	Vβ1 ↗ (8.2%); Vβ2 ↗ (11.8%); Vβ5.1 ↔ (3.4%); Vβ12 ↔ (1.9%); Vβ14 ↔ (4.4%) [D+3]	ND	SPEC	Blood	87	*speB*, *speC*
M	Yes	Yes (2 g/kg)	Vβ1 ↔ (2.3%); Vβ2 ↗ (19.1%); Vβ5.1 ↘ (3.3%); Vβ12 ↗ (2.3%); Vβ14 ↗ (15.8%) [D+3]	ND	SPEA	Pleural effusion, blood	1	*speA*, speB
M	Yes	Yes (1 g/kg)	Vβ1 ↔ (2.9%); Vβ2 ↗ (27.6%); Vβ5.1 ↘ (2.5%); Vβ12 ↔ (1.4%); Vβ14 ↗ (6.8%) [D+1]	ND	SPEA or SPEC[j]	Pleural effusion, blood	12	*speB*, *speC*
F	Yes	Yes (NA[l])	Vβ1 ↔ (2.5%); Vβ2 ↗ (15.4%); Vβ5.1 ↘ (3.4%); Vβ12 ↗ (3.6%); Vβ14 ↗ (17.7%) [D+4]	ND	SPEA	Pleural effusion	1	*speA*, speB
F	Yes	Yes (1 g/kg)	ND	ND	ND	Wound	28	*speB*, *speC*
M	Yes	Yes (2 g/kg)	ND	ND	ND	Throat	ND	ND
F	No	No	ND	ND	ND	Blood	ND	ND
F	No	No	ND	ND	ND	Pleural effusion	1	*speA*, *speB*, *speC*
M	Yes	No	ND	ND	ND	Blood	12	*speB*
F	Yes	No	ND	ND	ND	Pleural effusion, blood	1	*speA*, *speB*
M	Yes	No	ND	ND	ND	Tracheal secretions	ND	ND
F	Yes	No	ND	ND	ND	Pleural effusion, tracheal secretions	6	*speB*, *speC*
M	Yes	Yes (2 g/kg)	ND	ND[j]	ND	Pleural effusion	1	*speA*, *speB*, *speC*

[a]*IVIG, Intravenous Immunoglobulin.*

[b]*Vβ, alterations of CD3⁺ T cells (%): The expression of 24 main Vβ CD3+ T cells was determined by flow cytometry. Only the altered expression of Vβ CD3⁺ T cells is showed according the following normal adult ranges provided by the kit manufacturer: Vβ1: 2.18 to 4.88%Vβ2: 5.84 to 10.76%; Vβ5.1: 3.85 to 7.05%; Vβ12: 1.12 to 2.2%; Vβ14: 2.13 to 4.85%.*

[c]*F, Female.*

[d]*D, day.*

[e]*SPEA, streptococcal pyrogenic exotoxin A.*

[f]*SPEC, streptococcal pyrogenic exotoxin C.*

[g]*speB, gene encoding streptococcal pyrogenic exotoxin B.*

[h]*speC, gene encoding streptococcal pyrogenic exotoxin C.*

[i]*M, male.*

[j]*ND, not determined.*

[k]*speA, gene encoding streptococcal pyrogenic exotoxin A.*

[l]*NA, not available.*

No specific other fundings for this study.

future investigations are required to extensively identify the Vβ profiles of streptococcal toxins. However, this test might be added to the TSS diagnosis criteria in the future. Antitoxin therapies (clindamycin and/or IVIG) were associated with a better survival. However, a potential bias related to the discrepancy in the timing of treatment delivery may limit the interpretation of these results. The conduct of a large randomized controlled trial is mandatory to assess IVIG and anti-toxin chemotherapy efficacy.

AUTHOR CONTRIBUTIONS

EJ participated in study design, data analysis and interpretation, critically revised and approved the final manuscript as submitted. P-AB participated in the study design, data analysis, and interpretation and wrote the article as submitted. CJ participated in the study design, acquisition of data, statistical analysis, and interpretation, wrote the article and approved the final manuscript as submitted. GL participated in the study design, critically revised, and approved the final manuscript as submitted. CB performed some immunological analyses and approved the final manuscript as submitted. CP helps to analyze data from streptococcal strains and approved the final manuscript as submitted. AP participated in the study design, acquisition of data, statistical analysis and interpretation, and approved the final manuscript as submitted. AT, FL, and MB analyzes data from staphylococcal strains and approved the final manuscript as submitted. FV and YG revised and approved the final manuscript as submitted. OD participated in the study design, patient recruitment, data analysis and interpretation, wrote the article, and approved the final version of the manuscript as submitted. All authors approved the final manuscript as submitted and agree to be accountable for all aspects of the work.

ACKNOWLEDGMENTS

We are grateful to Christine Courtier, Christine Gardon, Céline Spinelli, Caroline Bouveyron, Virginie Dumoulin and Annie Martra for their technical help.

REFERENCES

1. Descloux E, Perpoint T, Ferry T, Lina G, Bes M, Vandenesch F, et al. One in five mortality in non-menstrual toxic shock syndrome versus no mortality in menstrual cases in a balanced French series of 55 cases. *Eur J Clin Microbiol Infect Dis.* (2008) 27:37–43. doi: 10.1007/s10096-007-0405-2
2. Rodriguez-Nunez A, Dosil-Gallardo S, Jordan I, ad hoc Streptococcal Toxic Shock Syndrome collaborative group of Spanish Society of Pediatric Intensive C. Clinical characteristics of children with group A streptococcal toxic shock syndrome admitted to pediatric intensive care units. *Eur J Pediatr.* (2011) 170:639–44. doi: 10.1007/s00431-010-1337-x
3. Shah SS, Hall M, Srivastava R, Subramony A, Levin JE. Intravenous immunoglobulin in children with streptococcal toxic shock syndrome. *Clin Infect Dis.* (2009) 49:1369–76. doi: 10.1086/606048
4. Timmis A, Parkins K, Kustos I, Riordan FA, Efstratiou A, Carrol ED. Invasive group A streptococcal infections in children presenting to a paediatric intensive care unit in the North West of England. *J Infect.* (2010) 60:183–6. doi: 10.1016/j.jinf.2009.12.001
5. Chen KY, Cheung M, Burgner DP, Curtis N. Toxic shock syndrome in Australian children. *Arch Dis Child.* (2016) 101:736–40. doi: 10.1136/archdischild-2015-310121
6. Adalat S, Dawson T, Hackett SJ, Clark JE, In association with the British Paediatric Surveillance U. Toxic shock syndrome surveillance in UK children. *Arch Dis Child.* (2014) 99:1078–82. doi: 10.1136/archdischild-2013-304741
7. Chuang YY, Huang YC, Lin TY. Toxic shock syndrome in children: epidemiology, pathogenesis, and management. *Paediatr Drugs* (2005) 7:11–25. doi: 10.2165/00148581-200507010-00002
8. Plainvert C, Doloy A, Loubinoux J, Lepoutre A, Collobert G, Touak G, et al. Invasive group A streptococcal infections in adults, France (2006-2010). *Clin Microbiol Infect.* (2012) 18:702–10. doi: 10.1111/j.1469-0691.2011.03624.x
9. Lappin E, Ferguson AJ. Gram-positive toxic shock syndromes. *Lancet Infect Dis.* (2009) 9:281–90. doi: 10.1016/S1473-3099(09)70066-0
10. Thomas D, Chou S, Dauwalder O, Lina G. Diversity in Staphylococcus aureus enterotoxins. *Chem Immunol Allergy* (2007) 93:24–41. doi: 10.1159/000100856
11. Xu SX, McCormick JK. Staphylococcal superantigens in colonization and disease. *Front Cell Infect Microbiol.* (2012) 2:52. doi: 10.3389/fcimb.2012.00052
12. Kato H, Takahashi N, Arimura Y, Imanishi K, Nishida H, Uchiyama T. The percentage of superantigen-reactive T cells in peripheral blood significantly decreases before massively increasing in patients with neonatal TSS-like exanthematous disease in the early acute phase. *J Infect Chemother.* (2002) 8:111–4. doi: 10.1007/s101560200018
13. Prevention. CfDCa. *Streptococcal Toxic-Shock Syndrome (STSS) (Streptococcus pyogenes), 2010 Case Definition.*: National Notifiable Diseases Surveillance System (NNDSS) (2010).
14. Prevention. CfDCa. *Toxic Shock Syndrome (other than Streptococcal) (TSS), 2011 Case Definition.*: National Notifiable Diseases Surveillance System (NNDSS) (2011).
15. Lin YJ, Cheng MC, Lo MH, Chien SJ. Early differentiation of kawasaki disease shock syndrome and toxic shock syndrome in a pediatric intensive care unit. *Pediatr Infect Dis J.* (2015) 34:1163–7. doi: 10.1097/INF.0000000000000852
16. Abe J, Forrester J, Nakahara T, Lafferty JA, Kotzin BL, Leung DY. Selective stimulation of human T cells with streptococcal erythrogenic toxins A and B. *J Immunol.* (1991) 146:3747–50.
17. Adrait A, Lebert D, Trauchessec M, Dupuis A, Louwagie M, Masselon C, et al. Development of a protein standard absolute quantification (PSAQ) assay for the quantification of *Staphylococcus aureus* enterotoxin A in serum. *J Proteomics* (2012) 75:3041–9. doi: 10.1016/j.jprot.2011.11.031
18. Dauwalder O, Venet F, Javouhey E, Badiou C, Gillet Y, Guignant C, et al. Assessment of cellular immune parameters in paediatric toxic shock syndrome: a report of five cases. *FEMS Immunol Med Microbiol.* (2012) 66:116–9. doi: 10.1111/j.1574-695X.2012.00990.x
19. De Marzi MC, Fernandez MM, Sundberg EJ, Molinero L, Zwirner NW, Llera AS, et al. Cloning, expression and interaction of human T-cell receptors with the bacterial superantigen SSA. *Eur J Biochem.* (2004) 271:4075–83. doi: 10.1111/j.1432-1033.2004.04345.x
20. Ferry T, Thomas D, Bouchut JC, Lina G, Vasselon-Raina M, Dauwalder O, et al. Early diagnosis of staphylococcal toxic shock syndrome by detection of the TSST-1 Vbeta signature in peripheral blood of a 12-year-old boy. *Pediatr Infect Dis J.* (2008) 27:274–7. doi: 10.1097/INF.0b013e31815c93a3

21. Kotb M, Fraser J. *Superantigens: Molecular Basis for Their Role in Human Diseases.* Washingto, DC: ASM Press (2007).
22. McCormick JK, Yarwood JM, Schlievert PM. Toxic shock syndrome and bacterial superantigens: an update. *Ann Rev Microbiol.* (2001) 55:77–104. doi: 10.1146/annurev.micro.55.1.77
23. Mollick JA, Miller GG, Musser JM, Cook RG, Grossman D, Rich RR. A novel superantigen isolated from pathogenic strains of Streptococcus pyogenes with aminoterminal homology to staphylococcal enterotoxins B and C. *J Clin Invest.* (1993) 92:710–9. doi: 10.1172/JCI116641
24. Rivera A, Rebollo M, Miro E, Mateo M, Navarro F, Gurgui M, et al. Superantigen gene profile, emm type and antibiotic resistance genes among group A streptococcal isolates from Barcelona, Spain. *J Med Microbiol.* (2006) 55(Pt 8):1115–23. doi: 10.1099/jmm.0.46481-0
25. Thomas D, Dauwalder O, Brun V, Badiou C, Ferry T, Etienne J, et al. Staphylococcus aureus superantigens elicit redundant and extensive human Vbeta patterns. *Infect. Immun.* (2009) 77:2043–50. doi: 10.1128/IAI.01388-08
26. Tomai MA, Schlievert PM, Kotb M. Distinct T-cell receptor V beta gene usage by human T lymphocytes stimulated with the streptococcal pyrogenic exotoxins and pep M5 protein. *Infect Immun.* (1992) 60:701–5.
27. Ferry T, Thomas D, Perpoint T, Lina G, Monneret G, Mohammedi I, et al. Analysis of superantigenic toxin Vbeta T-cell signatures produced during cases of staphylococcal toxic shock syndrome and septic shock. *Clin Microbiol Infect.* (2008) 14:546–54. doi: 10.1111/j.1469-0691.2008.01975.x
28. Coyle EA, Cha R, Rybak MJ. Influences of linezolid, penicillin, and clindamycin, alone and in combination, on streptococcal pyrogenic exotoxin a release. *Antimicrob Agents Chemother.* (2003) 47:1752–5. doi: 10.1128/AAC.47.5.1752-1755.2003
29. Sriskandan S, McKee A, Hall L, Cohen J. Comparative effects of clindamycin and ampicillin on superantigenic activity of *Streptococcus pyogenes. J Antimicrob Chemother.* (1997) 40:275–7.
30. Darenberg J, Ihendyane N, Sjolin J, Aufwerber E, Haidl S, Follin P, et al. Intravenous immunoglobulin G therapy in streptococcal toxic shock syndrome: a European randomized, double-blind, placebo-controlled trial. *Clin Infect Dis.* (2003) 37:333–40. doi: 10.1086/376630
31. Darenberg J, Soderquist B, Normark BH, Norrby-Teglund A. Differences in potency of intravenous polyspecific immunoglobulin G against streptococcal and staphylococcal superantigens: implications for therapy of toxic shock syndrome. *Clin Infect Dis.* (2004) 38:836–42. doi: 10.1086/381979
32. Department of Health UK. *Clinical Guidelines for Immunoglobulin Use, Second Edition*, London (2008).
33. Department of Health UK. *Clinical Guidelines for Immunoglobulin Use, Second Edition Update,* London (2011).
34. Kaul R, McGeer A, Norrby-Teglund A, Kotb M, Schwartz B, O'Rourke K, et al. Intravenous immunoglobulin therapy for streptococcal toxic shock syndrome–a comparative observational study. The Canadian Streptococcal Study Group. *Clin Infect Dis.* (1999) 28:800–7. doi: 10.1086/515199
35. Norrby-Teglund A, Kaul R, Low DE, McGeer A, Newton DW, Andersson J, et al. Plasma from patients with severe invasive group A streptococcal infections treated with normal polyspecific IgG inhibits streptococcal superantigen-induced T cell proliferation and cytokine production. *J Immunol.* (1996) 156:3057–64.
36. Valiquette L, Low DE, McGeer AJ. Assessing the impact of intravenous immunoglobulin in the management of streptococcal toxic shock syndrome: a noble but difficult quest. *Clin Infect Dis.* (2009) 49:1377–9. doi: 10.1086/606049
37. Leteurtre S, Duhamel A, Grandbastien B, Lacroix J, Leclerc F. Paediatric logistic organ dysfunction (PELOD) score. *Lancet* (2006) 367:897; author reply 900–2. doi: 10.1016/S0140-6736(06)68371-2
38. Slater A, Shann F, Pearson G, Paediatric index of mortality study G. PIM2: a revised version of the paediatric index of mortality. *Intens Care Med.* (2003) 29:278–85. doi: 10.1007/s00134-002-1601-2
39. Monecke S, Luedicke C, Slickers P, Ehricht R. Molecular epidemiology of Staphylococcus aureus in asymptomatic carriers. *Eur J Clin Microbiol Infect Dis.* (2009) 28:1159–65. doi: 10.1007/s10096-009-0752-2
40. Lithgow A, Duke T, Steer A, Smeesters PR. Severe group A streptococcal infections in a paediatric intensive care unit. *J Paediatr Child Health* (2014) 50:687–92. doi: 10.1111/jpc.12601
41. Carapetis JR, Jacoby P, Carville K, Ang SJ, Curtis N, Andrews R. Effectiveness of clindamycin and intravenous immunoglobulin, and risk of disease in contacts, in invasive group a streptococcal infections. *Clin Infect Dis.* (2014) 59:358–65. doi: 10.1093/cid/ciu304
42. Linner A, Darenberg J, Sjolin J, Henriques-Normark B, Norrby-Teglund A. Clinical efficacy of polyspecific intravenous immunoglobulin therapy in patients with streptococcal toxic shock syndrome: a comparative observational study. *Clin Infect Dis.* (2014) 59:851–7. doi: 10.1093/cid/ciu449
43. DeVries AS, Lesher L, Schlievert PM, Rogers T, Villaume LG, Danila R, et al. Staphylococcal toxic shock syndrome 2000-2006: epidemiology, clinical features, and molecular characteristics. *PLoS ONE* (2011) 6:e22997. doi: 10.1371/journal.pone.0022997
44. Holtfreter S, Grumann D, Schmudde M, Nguyen HT, Eichler P, Strommenger B, et al. Clonal distribution of superantigen genes in clinical *Staphylococcus aureus* isolates. *J Clin Microbiol.* (2007) 45:2669–80. doi: 10.1128/JCM.00204-07
45. Sharma H, Smith D, Turner CE, Game L, Pichon B, Hope R, et al. Clinical and molecular epidemiology of staphylococcal toxic shock syndrome in the United Kingdom. *Emerg Infect Dis.* (2018) 24:258–66. doi: 10.3201/eid2402.170606
46. Parsonnet J. Case definition of staphylococcal TSS: a proposed revision incorporating laboratory findings. *Int Congr Symp Series* (1998) 1998:15.

3

Fluid Bolus Therapy in Pediatric Sepsis: Current Knowledge and Future Direction

Ben Gelbart [1,2,3]*

[1] Paediatric Intensive Care Unit Royal Children's Hospital, Melbourne, VIC, Australia, [2] Murdoch Childrens Research Institute, Melbourne, VIC, Australia, [3] The University of Melbourne, Melbourne, VIC, Australia

***Correspondence:**
Ben Gelbart
ben.gelbart@rch.org.au

Sepsis is a leading cause of morbidity and mortality in children with a worldwide prevalence in pediatric intensive care units of approximately 8%. Fluid bolus therapy (FBT) is a first line therapy for resuscitation of septic shock and has been a recommendation of international guidelines for nearly two decades. The evidence base supporting these guidelines are based on limited data including animal studies and case control studies. In recent times, evidence suggesting harm from fluid in terms of morbidity and mortality have generated interest in evaluating FBT. In view of this, studies of fluid restrictive strategies in adults and children have emerged. The complexity of studying FBT relates to several points. Firstly, the physiological and haemodynamic response to FBT including magnitude and duration is not well described in children. Secondly, assessment of the circulation is based on non-specific clinical signs and limited haemodynamic monitoring with limited physiological targets. Thirdly, FBT exists in a complex myriad of pathophysiological responses to sepsis and other confounding therapies. Despite this, a greater understanding of the role of FBT in terms of the physiological response and possible harm is warranted. This review outlines current knowledge and future direction for FBT in sepsis.

Keywords: fluid therapy, pediatric, septic shock, sepsis, volume responsiveness

INTRODUCTION

The worldwide burden of sepsis in pediatric intensive care in terms of morbidity and mortality remains high and is a key healthcare priority (1–3). Fluid bolus therapy (FBT) has long been the central component of resuscitation of children with sepsis (4). The role of FBT is to improve the circulating volume, cardiac output and mitigate circulatory dysfunction and organ hypoperfusion. It is the recommended forefront therapy of international pediatric and adult consensus guidelines in high-income and low-income settings (5–8). The emergence of evidence demonstrating harm associated with FBT has led to a re-evaluation of its role in sepsis resuscitation.

Data supporting current pediatric sepsis guidelines are limited. Recommendations in relation to FBT have been based on small case control studies and animal data, mostly from two-three decades ago (9–11). Few randomized controlled studies exist. The most recent 2017 ACCM/PALS guidelines recommend that 20–60 ml/kg should be administered, titrated to clinical signs of shock and discontinued at shock resolution or fluid overload (5). Fluid resuscitation (FR) for refractory shock and assessment of response is recommended within 15 min to which adherence has proven difficult (12, 13). The past two decades has seen large multicentre studies targeting optimal fluid composition (14, 15), goal directed therapy (16–18), fluid restrictive protocols (19–23) as well as a pivotal study of FBT vs. no FBT in African children with sepsis (24); all contributing to the current landscape.

Clinicians aim to identify patterns of circulatory dysfunction in septic shock that include myocardial dysfunction, systemic vasodilatation, and hypovolaemia (25). This generally relies on clinical examination and non-invasive haemodynamic parameters. The challenge of investigating whether interventions that independently, or in combination with others, improve outcomes or cause harm may prove difficult (26). The complexity of assessing one component of a suite of interventions to address a multifaceted pathophysiological process will require carefully designed studies. Yet, in the face of many unanswered questions and associated harm, the imperative to investigate the role of FBT in sepsis exists.

This review outlines the current understanding of the role of FBT in children with sepsis and recent research direction.

EPIDEMIOLOGY OF SEPSIS, PATTERNS OF FLUID RESUSCITATION AND OUTCOMES IN CHILDREN

The global burden of sepsis and septic shock is high in pediatric intensive care units (PICUs) with prevalence studies suggesting mortality rates ranging from 6 to 25% (1, 27). Temporal trends suggest that although prevalence may be increasing, severe sepsis mortality might be declining (2). In PICUs in ANZ, the prevalence of sepsis and septic shock is 2.9 and 2.1% respectively and accounts for over a quarter of PICU deaths (28). In the US, an observational study of septic shock in children indicated that a third of deaths occur early (1–3 days) with a high proportion occurring in previously healthy children (29). The most common causes of death being refractory shock followed by secondary organ dysfunction. In ANZ, Schlapbach et al. demonstrated that 50% of deaths from sepsis occurred within 48 h and that predictors of death unsurprisingly relate to presence of markers of multi-organ dysfunction (30). Pediatric sepsis mortality in low income countries range widely (31) due to definitions of shock, disease specific and population specific factors as well as differences in intensive care resources.

There are very few large scale epidemiological or randomized studies of FBT in pediatric septic shock (32). Several pediatric observational studies of the resuscitation phase of sepsis have mostly been small single center studies and compare survivors and non survivors (33, 34), those with or without shock (12), or protocol adherence (13, 35, 36). Those reporting outcomes with volume or timing of FBT show varying results. Paul et al. for instance, showed that those who received 60 ml/kg of FBT within 60 min in the emergency department had a 57% shorter hospital length of stay than children who did not (13). Whether this relates to early recognition and implementation of a range of interventions such as early appropriate antibiotics or FBT is unclear. An audit of pediatric sepsis management from the United Kingdom showed that the initial median volume of FBT prior to intensive care is 50–60 ml/kg (12) suggesting alignment to current guidelines in the initial phase of sepsis management.

A large US adult study of the interaction between fluid administration on day 1 and mortality from sepsis showed increased severity adjusted mortality and cost for each liter above 5L; in the presence of shock, mechanical ventilation or both (37). Leisman et al. however, showed in an observational cohort study of adults with sepsis that less time to initiation of FBT reduced hospital mortality, ICU admission, mechanical ventilation duration and length of ICU and hospital stay. These were adjusted for measures of organ dysfunction, patient source and antibiotic administration (38). The inherent limitations in this study preclude a causal relationship however of note, no difference in hospital mortality was observed for volume of FBT until >35 ml/kg was administered where mortality was increased. Whether improved survival relates to timely recognition of sepsis, improved bundle delivery remains unclear. There are a paucity of similar pediatric data associating outcomes with fluid resuscitation.

PATHOPHYSIOLOGICAL ASPECTS OF SEPSIS AND RESPONSE TO FBT

The pathophysiology and haemodynamic patterns in septic shock are complex, dynamic and not easily determined clinically. The pathophysiological hallmarks of septic shock are cytokine and nitric oxide mediated inflammation, activation of the coagulation cascade, manifesting as myocardial, endothelial, and organ dysfunction (25). Therapeutic targets in the acute management of septic shock are fundamentally aimed at matching oxygen delivery to demand by improving cardiac output for which the key targets are macrovascular.

Circulatory Markers of Shock

Clinical signs of septic shock such as tachycardia, hypotension, impaired skin perfusion, while readily identifiable and indicative of shock, are difficult to rely upon to indicate hypovolaemia or volume responsiveness. Yet these are commonly the triggers or targets available to clinicians in the first hours of pediatric sepsis management. More advanced tools such as echocardiography or invasive haemodynamic monitoring can assist in deciphering myocardial dysfunction from a hyperdynamic circulation as well as volume responsiveness, however even these, as static measures lack predictive accuracy (39). Their availability are not always available outside of the intensive care environment or during anesthesia. Both dynamic and static measures of volume responsiveness are unreliable in children (40, 41) and volume responsiveness as a concept, is somewhat arbitrary. Respiratory variation in aortic blood flow velocities appear better predictors of volume responsiveness in children (42, 43) more so than systolic pressure and pulse pressure variation (44) but this is in the context of ventilated children.

Blood pressure and heart rate are the most highly rated clinical signs among pediatric intensivists (45), ED physicians (46), adult intensive care physicians (47, 48). Yet blood pressure measured non-invasively are prone to underestimation. A study of over 50,000 concurrent non-invasive and invasive BP measurements showed that NIBP has a poor positive predictive value of 58% for hypotension meaning over treatment of low blood pressure is possible (49). The quality and volume of the peripheral and central pulses are also critical signs that rely on experience to elucidate and interpret accurately.

Capillary refill time (CRT) is a simple bedside test universally regarded as a marker of inadequate perfusion and dehydration in children and a specific adjunct sign of shock (50, 51). In children with septic shock in intensive care it relates weakly to stroke volume index (52) but commonly relied upon to determine the responsiveness to FBT. A study of adults with septic shock suggest good interrater reliability, good correlation with lactate and SOFA score and 14 day mortality (53) and trials of tissue perfusion-guided therapy (including CRT) on outcomes in sepsis, have ensued (54).

Several studies describe the haemodynamic patterns in children with septic shock, often following an initial dose of FBT commonly referred to as "fluid refractory shock." Deep et al. showed distinct patterns of "cold' (predominantly reduced myocardial function, vasoconstricted) and "warm" (predominantly hyperdynamic, vasodilatory) shock amongst 36 children with community acquired and hospital acquired sepsis with early and sustained abnormalities in haemodynamic values (55). An Indian study in two PICUs showed that in 48 children who had received 40 ml/kg of FBT the continued presence of both "warm" and "cold" shock based on clinical and echocardiographic indices, was also accompanied by the transformation or evolution over time indicating the dynamic nature of the circulatory disturbance (56). Others have also defined the clinical and haemodynamic phenotypes using a pulmonary artery catheter (57). Ceneviva et al. showed persistence of shock following FBT (60 ml/kg) in over a third of patients. The distribution of shock patterns were low cardiac index (CI) (58%), high CI/low systemic vascular resistive index (SVRI) (20%) and low CI/low SVRI (20%) (57). Similarly, in another small cohort of children with "fluid refractory shock," non-invasive cardiac output monitoring demonstrated marked differences in physiological patterns between those with catheter related sepsis and community acquired pneumonia (58).

Clearly a spectrum of circulatory phenotypes exists, overlap and evolve in the initial stages of septic shock in children. The ability of clinicians to recognize these entities early and repeatedly on the basis of predominantly clinical signs, commence therapies and use clinical, biochemical, echocardiographic, and perhaps microcirculatory markers to judge response to therapy outlines the complex nature of sepsis resuscitation and teasing out the role of one therapeutic intervention.

Sepsis and the Microcirculation

Imaging of the microcirculation to measure the number of perfused capillaries and capillary density can assess the microvascular response to sepsis and therapy. It is performed in intensive care patients with a sublingual camera using side-stream dark field video-microscopy of the sublingual circulation. Alterations in the microvasculature include reduction in capillary density and microvascular blood flow (59, 60). Microvascular dysregulation that occurs in sepsis include altered rheology of red blood cells, impaired regional vascular autoregulation, activation of coagulation and arteriovenous shunting (60). The microvasculature plays an independent role in tissue perfusion and oxygenation that may not be influenced by macrovascular alterations (61). In an observational study of 18 pediatric sepsis patients, persistent reduction in microcirculatory flow in the first few days of sepsis was associated with mortality (59). In relation to response to FBT, few animal studies using intra-vital microscopy and video imaging of the microcirculation have shown both improvement as well as persistence in microcirculatory dysfunction with FBT (62) whereas a small observational study in adults with sepsis showed that fluid responders (determined by a 5% increment in stroke volume), increased capillary density and flow to FBT compared to non-responders (63). Near-infrared spectroscopy is another non-invasive modality that can assess tissue oxygenation at the bedside and may have a place in assessing the microcirculatory manifestations of septic shock and response to therapy. The clinical utility of measures of the microcirculation in the resuscitation phase of septic shock remains to be seen.

Perhaps, in time, assessment of the phenotypic subtypes of septic shock may extend beyond clinical signs and haemodynamic measured and include genetic markers (64). Until then, the fundamental principles of using a constellation of clinical signs and haemodynamic monitoring in the resuscitation of septic shock with an emphasis on repeated assessments of response to therapy, will remain.

PHYSIOLOGICAL RESPONSES TO FBT

Pharmacodynamics assessment of FBT in post-operative adults show that the maximal effect on cardiac output occurs at 1.2 mins in responders and the effect dissipates at 10 min (65). A systematic review of studies looking at haemodynamic responses also support the findings that increases in cardiac output following FBT is unsustained at 30 min (66). In healthy adult volunteers, rapid IV bolus of 30 ml/kg of 0.9% saline and 4% albumin lead to differences in effects on pulmonary mechanics, inflammation and cardiac preload (67). Specifically, those who received 0.9% saline had increased pulmonary oedema with an inflammatory component whereas those who received 4% albumin did not. In adults in an emergency department setting the 5% changes in HR and BP from baseline measured at 10 min post FBT were not sustained at 1 or 2 h (68). There are limited data on the pharmacodynamic effect of FBT in children. A recent small cohort study however, compared echocardiographic changes in the first 24 h following FBT and rehydration vs. rehydration alone in malnourished African children with gastroenteritis (69). There were heterogeneous effects on echocardiographic markers of stroke volume in the bolus group; more so when compared to the continuous rehydration group. Long et al. in a prospective observational study showed a transient increase in cardiac index (a product of heart rate and echocardiographic derived stroke volume per meter squared of body surface area; L/min/m^2) 5 min following a fluid bolus that had dissipated by 60 min to a lower baseline than pre bolus (70). Observational studies such as these are limited by confounding factors but do reflect the reality in clinical practice. It also suggests that that minutely time intervals may be required to understand physiological effects of FBT in a more granular way. The duration, magnitude and dissipation of effect of FBT in children require further examination.

EVIDENCE BASE AND GUIDELINES FOR FBT IN PEDIATRIC SEPSIS

The two recent editions of the Surviving Sepsis Campaign Guidelines (6, 71) and the ACCM PALS guidelines have not altered their recommendations relating to FBT in sepsis (5, 72). They recommend that 20 ml/kg boluses up to 60 ml/kg be administered in the first 15 min of resuscitation unless signs of fluid overload occur. The World Health Organization report on the management of critically ill children, in 2016 recommended that for the treatment of non-specific shock, 10–20 ml of crystalloid be administered between 30 and 60 min with an emphasis on repeated re-assessments (7). The foundation of these recommendations is largely based on limited human and animal data as well as expert opinion. One of the pivotal observational cohort studies from 1991 investigated the association of fluid administration and mortality in children with septic shock. Thirty four subjects were categorized by administered volumes of FBT in the first hour of septic shock; <20 ml/kg, 20–40 ml/kg and more than 40 ml/kg (9). The study showed that those who received >40 ml/kg of FBT had improved survival compared to those who received <20 ml/kg.

There are few randomized studies of FBT in children with septic shock in the context of intensive care resources. Three studies have compared a range of interventions such as fluid types, early inotrope and goal directed therapy with measured outcomes such as shock reversal, mortality, and intensive care resources (18, 73, 74). These studies included a total of 309 children and when systematically reviewed, there were no discernible difference in patient-centered outcomes (75).

The majority of studies of FBT in children relate to disease specific conditions such as malaria (76, 77), dengue fever (78–80), and meningococcal sepsis (81) limiting their broad applicability. Systematic review and meta-analysis of these studies (excluding the FEAST study) do not provide compelling evidence for a mortality benefit from FBT vs. no FBT or for different types of FBT (82).

FLUID EXPANSION AS SUPPORTIVE THERAPY (FEAST) TRIAL

The FEAST study, a RCT of FBT in over 3,000 Sub-Saharan African children with sepsis and impaired perfusion has been a pivotal study in generating interest in the potential harm from FBT. It showed that boluses of 0.9% saline or 5% albumin compared to maintenance fluid significant increased mortality at 48 h (RR 1.45; 95% CI 1.13-1.86; $p = 0.003$). The results were consistent across all pre-specified subgroups including malaria, anemia (hemoglobin concentration <50 mg/l), coma and lactic acidosis (lactate >5 mmol/l). These results generated much interest and debate surrounding the role of FBT in high-income countries (83–85). The investigators assigned causes of death based on clinical features at presentation and concluded that cardiovascular collapse, as the terminal event, was the largest contributor to excess mortality as opposed to pulmonary or neurological failure (86). Important perspectives regarding this trial have been outlined (84, 87) but increasing interest in examining FBT has followed in both adults and children. The main limitations of these findings have been well articulated by Duke (87). Firstly, despite being a clearly unwell population of children, shock, defined by the WHO (7) as presence of cold peripheries and weak pulse, tachycardia and delayed capillary refill >3 s was not present in around 70% of participants. Secondly, the lack of availability of intensive care interventions limits the ability to respond to complications of fluid therapy and thirdly, the population studied may well have been at risk of adverse consequences of fluid therapy such as the presence of cerebral oedema, hyponatremia or excessive antidiuretic hormone secretion.

FLUIDS AND HARM: FLUID OVERLOAD

Fluid accumulation in critical care is recognized as being associated with respiratory and renal morbidity as well as increased ICU Length of stay (LOS) and mortality. The degree to which FBT contributes to fluid accumulation in children is not well established. The association of fluid overload and harm is consistent in a broad spectrum of critically ill children including those following congenital heart disease surgery (88–90), acute kidney injury (91, 92), acute lung injury (93), children on ECMO (94), in a general PICU (95, 96), children with shock (97), and sepsis (98). However, fluid overload is defined, either by percentage of weight accumulation or percentage increase in daily cumulative fluid balance, the association stands in a dose dependant fashion (99). The downstream effects of FBT on fluid accumulation in children with sepsis is likely to represent one of many aetiological factors including non-resuscitation fluid, impaired clearance mechanisms, physiological responses such as SIADH and endothelial dysfunction. Furthermore, how fluid overload (commonly identified from the medical record by net change in fluid input and output) relates to organ oedema, organ perfusion and function, is not clear. Fluid administration is a key modifiable component of fluid accumulation and the impact on organ oedema and function requires further examination.

FLUID RESTRICTIVE RESUSCITATION STRATEGIES

In response to the concern regarding harm from FBT, studies of restrictive fluid resuscitation have emerged to assess feasibility and safety of early inotrope based resuscitation strategies in adults, in high and low income countries (19, 20, 100). Two pediatric studies exist; one in the UK (23) and one in Canada (22). The UK study randomized 75 children with infections and clinical signs of shock after 20 ml/kg of FBT to either 10 ml/kg or 20 ml/kg per bolus for subsequent boluses. At the end of the 4-h study period the mean difference in FBT volume was −11.2 ml/kg (95% CI −16.6 to −5.8 mL/kg; $p < 0.001$). Roughly two-thirds received only 1 further bolus. There were no differences in hospital or PICU based outcomes. The authors concluded that lower than expected severity of illness precludes conduct of a larger study. The Canadian study aims to determine whether early vasoactive therapy, compared to usual fluid resuscitation practice (up to 60 ml/kg of isotonic fluid) reduces time to shock reversal and organ dysfunction. Adult data have shown that fluid restrictive resuscitation can reduce FBT administration. The CLASSIC study randomized 151 adults with septic shock and showed a significant reduction of resuscitation fluid at 5 days [500 ml (IQR;0–2,500) vs. 2,000 ml (IQR; 1,000–4,100) $p < 0.001$] but no difference in total administered fluid [12,411 ml (IQR; 5,518–17,035) vs. 13,687 (IQR; 7,163–17,082) $p = 0.45$] but a trend toward lower fluid accumulation [−1,148(−2,531–235) $p = 0.06$](19). Fluid restriction also led to less AKI but no changes in rates of CRRT, respiratory support or mortality. A summary of fluid restrictive resuscitation studies in children and adults with sepsis is in **Supplementary Table 1**.

For pediatric studies focusing on fluid restriction it will be important to determine feasibility of implementation of a fluid restriction protocol in terms of recruitment and separation between the groups for dose of FBT. Whether restrictive FBT can present a safe, feasible alternative that positively impacts patient centered outcomes is the challenge for these studies.

CHALLENGES OF STUDYING INTERVENTIONS IN PEDIATRIC SEPSIS: FUTURE DIRECTIONS

The time critical nature of recognizing and initiating management of pediatric septic shock belies the challenges of investigating FBT. Determining triggers and targets for interventions will largely rely on haemodynamic markers of shock as well as markers of impaired tissue perfusion such as hyperlactataemia. Despite the inherent difficulties, alternative interventions may prove to be safe equivalent in reversing shock and may reduce harm in terms of morbidity and mortality related to limiting excessive fluid administration. One such strategy is restrictive fluid resuscitation where early vasoactive therapy is initiated rather than repeated FBT.

Population

Targeting children with septic shock would be necessary despite the challenges in recognizing this group early at presentation. A combination of haemodynamic indicators as well as features of organ dysfunction (altered consciousness state, tachypnoea) and tissue dysoxia (lactate elevation) are key features. A study in ANZ showed that these features are easily identifiable early and can accurately discriminate children at risk of death, albeit once admitted to an intensive care unit (30). Recent international consensus definition of sepsis severity (101) specifically recognize markers of organ dysfunction to identify high risk groups but are not designed for children. The range in age specific normal values will necessitate sophisticated trial infrastructure to ensure protocol adherence and appropriate recruitment.

Intervention

Trials of restrictive fluid therapy will require a clinically significant separation of administered fluid volume. Vasoactive agents such as adrenaline or noradrenaline can be administered peripherally and are suitable alternate interventions. Adrenaline being more inotropic with vasoconstrictor activity would be the optimal agent. In most instances, central venous access would not be readily available and hence dilute peripheral administration would be required. The administration of peripheral adrenaline presents several issues warranting consideration. Initial titration of adrenaline would occur using non-invasive blood pressure monitoring and, in the presence of shock, would require clear pathways and ceiling doses to either enable weaning or mandate early intensive care interventions. The entry point of recruitment would need to occur when initial therapy for reversing shock are insufficient. Otherwise one risks exposing a large group of children to an intervention (or comparison therapy) that may not have been indicated thereby exposing a proportion of children to excessive therapy. The presence of septic shock and administration of 20 ml/kg of FBT and a decision to administer further resuscitation would be an example of suitable inclusion criteria.

Outcomes

Appropriate outcomes for studies of FBT in sepsis will be an important consideration for trial designs. The desired range of outcomes should include mortality, measures of organ dysfunction, need for intensive care resources as well as outcomes specific to fluid therapy. Markers of tissue oxygenation, tissue oedema and endothelial dysfunction have also been included as secondary endpoints in current study designs. The sample size required to show a 5–10% difference in outcomes have been suggested to be up to 1,500 participants (1) which would be feasibly achieved by a multinational collaboration.

CONCLUSIONS

FBT has been the frontline recommended therapy in sepsis management guidelines for several decades without a body of evidence supporting its appropriate use. Increasing attention has now turned to the potential consequences of excessive fluid therapy in the context of evidence suggesting harm. This has made the time ripe to further investigate the role of this long standing, fundamental intervention in pediatric sepsis. Restrictive fluid resuscitation is currently at the forefront of alternative strategies being investigated. Whether this approach is safe, feasible and effective in reducing excessive fluid therapy and can be shown to independently improve meaningful outcomes in children with septic shock remains to be seen.

AUTHOR CONTRIBUTIONS

The author confirms being the sole contributor of this work and has approved it for publication.

REFERENCES

1. Weiss SL, Fitzgerald JC, Pappachan J, Wheeler D, Jaramillo-Bustamante JC, Salloo A, et al. Global epidemiology of pediatric severe sepsis: the sepsis prevalence, outcomes, and therapies study. *Am J Respir Crit Care Med.* (2015) 191:1147–57. doi: 10.1164/rccm.201412-2323OC
2. Ruth A, McCracken CE, Fortenberry JD, Hall M, Simon HK, Hebbar KB. Pediatric severe sepsis: current trends and outcomes from the Pediatric Health Information Systems database. *Pediatr Crit Care Med.* (2014) 15:828–38. doi: 10.1097/pcc.0000000000000254
3. Wolfler A, Silvani P, Musicco M, Antonelli M, Salvo I, Italian Pediatric Sepsis Study g. Incidence of and mortality due to sepsis, severe sepsis and septic shock in Italian Pediatric Intensive Care Units: a prospective national survey. *Intens Care Med.* (2008) 34:1690–7. doi: 10.1007/s00134-008-1148-y
4. Carcillo JA, Fields AI, American College of Critical Care Medicine Task Force Committee M. Clinical practice parameters for hemodynamic support of pediatric and neonatal patients in septic shock. *Crit Care Med.* (2002) 30:1365–78.
5. Davis AL, Carcillo JA, Aneja RK, Deymann AJ, Lin JC, Nguyen TC, et al. American College of critical care medicine clinical practice parameters for hemodynamic support of pediatric and neonatal septic shock.*Crit Care Med.* (2017) 45:1061–93. doi: 10.1097/ccm.0000000000002425
6. Rhodes A, Evans LE, Alhazzani W, Levy MM, Antonelli M, Ferrer R, et al. Surviving sepsis campaign: International Guidelines for Management of Sepsis and Septic Shock: 2016. *Crit Care Med.* (2017) 45:486–552. doi: 10.1007/s00134-017-4683-6
7. *Updated Guideline: Paediatric Emrgency Triage, Assessment and Treatment.* Geneva: World Health Organisation (2016).
8. Levy MM, Evans LE, Rhodes A. The surviving sepsis campaign bundle: 2018 update. *Intens Care Med.* (2018) 44:925–8. doi: 10.1007/s00134-018-5085-0
9. Carcillo JA, Davis AL, Zaritsky A. Role of early fluid resuscitation in pediatric septic shock. *JAMA* (1991) 266:1242–5.
10. Ottosson J, Dawidson I, Brandberg A, Idvall J, Sandor Z. Cardiac output and organ blood flow in experimental septic shock: effect of treatment with antibiotics, corticosteroids, and fluid infusion. *Circ Shock* (1991) 35:14–24.
11. Carroll GC, Snyder JV. Hyperdynamic severe intravascular sepsis depends on fluid administration in cynomolgus monkey. *Am J Physiol.* (1982) 243:R131–41.
12. Inwald DP, Tasker RC, Peters MJ, Nadel S, Paediatric Intensive Care Society Study G. Emergency management of children with severe sepsis in the United Kingdom: the results of the Paediatric Intensive Care Society sepsis audit. *Arch Dis Child.* (2009) 94:348–53. doi: 10.1136/adc.2008.153064
13. Paul R, Neuman MI, Monuteaux MC, Melendez E. Adherence to PALS sepsis guidelines and hospital length of stay. *Pediatrics* (2012) 130:e273–80. doi: 10.1542/peds.2012-0094
14. Investigators TSS. A comparison of albumin and saline for fluid resuscitation in the intensive care unit. *N Engl J Med.* (2004) 350:2247–56. doi: 10.1056/NEJMoa040232
15. Semler MW, Self WH, Wanderer JP, Ehrenfeld JM, Wang L, Byrne DW, et al. Balanced crystalloids versus saline in critically ill adults. *N Engl J Med.* (2018) 378:829–39. doi: 10.1056/NEJMoa1711584
16. Investigators A, Group ACT, Peake SL, Delaney A, Bailey M, Bellomo R, et al. Goal-directed resuscitation for patients with early septic shock. *N Engl J Med.* (2014) 371:1496–506. doi: 10.1056/NEJMoa1404380
17. Pro CI, Yealy DM, Kellum JA, Huang DT, Barnato AE, Weissfeld LA, et al. A randomized trial of protocol-based care for early septic shock. *N Engl J Med.* (2014) 370:1683–93. doi: 10.1056/NEJMoa1401602
18. de Oliveira CF, de Oliveira DS, Gottschald AF, Moura JD, Costa GA, Ventura AC, et al. ACCM/PALS haemodynamic support guidelines for paediatric septic shock: an outcomes comparison with and without monitoring central venous oxygen saturation. *Intens Care Med.* (2008) 34:1065–75. doi: 10.1007/s00134-008-1085-9
19. Hjortrup PB, Haase N, Bundgaard H, Thomsen SL, Winding R, Pettila V, et al. Restricting volumes of resuscitation fluid in adults with septic shock after initial management: the CLASSIC randomised, parallel-group, multicentre feasibility trial. *Intens Care Med.* (2016) 42:1695–705. doi: 10.1007/s00134-016-4500-7
20. Macdonald SPJ, Taylor DM, Keijzers G, Arendts G, Fatovich DM, Kinnear FB, et al. REstricted Fluid REsuscitation in Sepsis-associated Hypotension (REFRESH): study protocol for a pilot randomised controlled trial. *Trials* (2017) 18:399. doi: 10.1186/s13063-017-2137-7
21. O'Hara CB, Canter RR, Mouncey PR, Carter A, Jones N, Nadel S, et al. A qualitative feasibility study to inform a randomised controlled trial of fluid bolus therapy in septic shock. *Arch Dis Childh.* (2018) 103:28–32. doi: 10.1136/archdischild-2016-312515
22. Parker MJ, Thabane L, Fox-Robichaud A, Liaw P, Choong K. A trial to determine whether septic shock-reversal is quicker in pediatric patients randomized to an early goal-directed fluid-sparing strategy versus usual care (SQUEEZE): study protocol for a pilot randomized controlled trial. *Trials* (2016) 17:556. doi: 10.1186/s13063-016-1689-2
23. Inwald DP, Canter R, Woolfall K, Mouncey P, Zenasni Z, O'Hara C, et al. Restricted fluid bolus volume in early septic shock: results of the Fluids in Shock pilot trial. *Arch Dis Childh.* (2018). doi: 10.1136/archdischild-2018-314924
24. Maitland K, Kiguli S, Opoka RO, Engoru C, Olupot-Olupot P, Akech SO, et al. Mortality after fluid bolus in African children with severe infection. N Engl J Med. (2011) 364:2483–95. doi: 10.1056/NEJMoa1101549
25. Greer JR. Pathophysiology of cardiovascular dysfunction in sepsis. *BJA Educ.* (2015) 15:316–21. doi: 10.1093/bjaceaccp/mkv003
26. Lane RD, Funai T, Reeder R, Larsen GY. High reliability pediatric septic shock quality improvement initiative and decreasing mortality. *Pediatrics* (2016) 138:e20154153. doi: 10.1542/peds.2015-4153
27. Boeddha NP, Schlapbach LJ, Driessen GJ, Herberg JA, Rivero-Calle I, Cebey-López M, et al. Mortality and morbidity in community-acquired sepsis in European pediatric intensive care units: a prospective cohort study from the European Childhood Life-threatening Infectious Disease Study (EUCLIDS). *Crit Care* (2018) 22:143. doi: 10.1186/s13054-018-2052-7
28. Schlapbach LJ, Straney L, Alexander J, MacLaren G, Festa M, Schibler A, et al. Mortality related to invasive infections, sepsis, and septic shock in critically ill children in Australia and New Zealand, 2002-13: a multicentre retrospective cohort study. *Lancet Infect Dis.* (2015) 15:46–54. doi: 10.1016/S1473-3099(14)71003-5
29. Weiss SL, Balamuth F, Hensley J, Fitzgerald JC, Bush J, Nadkarni VM, et al. The epidemiology of hospital death following pediatric severe sepsis: when, why, and how children with sepsis die. *Pediatr Crit Care Med.* (2017) 18:823–30. doi: 10.1097/PCC.0000000000001222
30. Schlapbach LJ, MacLaren G, Festa M, Alexander J, Erickson S, Beca J, et al. Prediction of pediatric sepsis mortality within 1 h of intensive care admission. *Intens Care Med.* (2017) 43:1085–96. doi: 10.1007/s00134-017-4701-8
31. Akech S, Ledermann H, Maitland K. Choice of fluids for resuscitation in children with severe infection and shock: systematic review. *BMJ* (2010) 341:c4416. doi: 10.1136/bmj.c4416
32. Opiyo N, Molyneux E, Sinclair D, Garner P, English M. Immediate fluid management of children with severe febrile illness and signs of impaired circulation in low-income settings: a contextualised systematic review. *BMJ Open* (2014) 4:e004934. doi: 10.1136/bmjopen-2014-004934
33. Han YY, Carcillo JA, Dragotta MA, Bills DM, Watson RS, Westerman ME, et al. Early reversal of pediatric-neonatal septic shock by community physicians is associated with improved outcome. *Pediatrics* (2003) 112:793–9.
34. Oliveira CF, Nogueira de Sa FR, Oliveira DS, Gottschald AF, Moura JD, Shibata AR, et al. Time- and fluid-sensitive resuscitation for hemodynamic support of children in septic shock: barriers to the implementation of the American College of Critical Care Medicine/Pediatric Advanced Life Support Guidelines in a pediatric intensive care unit in a developing world. *Pediatr Emerg Care.* (2008) 24:810–5. doi: 10.1097/PEC.0b013e31818e9f3a
35. Larsen GY, Mecham N, Greenberg R. An emergency department septic shock protocol and care guideline for children initiated at triage. *Pediatrics* (2011) 127:e1585–92.
36. Cruz AT, Perry AM, Williams EA, Graf JM, Wuestner ER, Patel B. Implementation of goal-directed therapy for children with suspected sepsis in the emergency department. *Pediatrics* (2011) 127:e758–66. doi: 10.1542/peds.2010-2895

37. Marik PE, Linde-Zwirble WT, Bittner EA, Sahatjian J, Hansell D. Fluid administration in severe sepsis and septic shock, patterns and outcomes: an analysis of a large national database. *Intens Care Med.* (2017) 43:625–32. doi: 10.1007/s00134-016-4675-y
38. Leisman DE, Goldman C, Doerfler ME, Masick KD, Dries S, Hamilton E, et al. Patterns and outcomes associated with timeliness of initial crystalloid resuscitation in a prospective sepsis and septic shock cohort. *Crit Care Med.* (2017) 45:1596–606. doi: 10.1097/ccm.0000000000002574
39. Cecconi M, De Backer D, Antonelli M, Beale R, Bakker J, Hofer C, et al. Consensus on circulatory shock and hemodynamic monitoring. Task force of the European Society of Intensive Care Medicine. *Intens Care Med.* (2014) 40:1795–815. doi: 10.1007/s00134-014-3525-z
40. Gan H, Cannesson M, Chandler JR, Ansermino JM. Predicting fluid responsiveness in children: a systematic review. *Anesth Analges.* (2013) 117:1380–92. doi: 10.1213/ANE.0b013e3182a9557e
41. Saxena R, Durward A, Steeley S, Murdoch IA, Tibby SM. Predicting fluid responsiveness in 100 critically ill children: the effect of baseline contractility. *Intens Care Med.* (2015) 41:2161–9. doi: 10.1007/s00134-015-4075-8
42. Choi DY, Kwak HJ, Park HY, Kim YB, Choi CH, Lee JY. Respiratory variation in aortic blood flow velocity as a predictor of fluid responsiveness in children after repair of ventricular septal defect. *Pediatr Cardiol.* (2010) 31:1166–70. doi: 10.1007/s00246-010-9776-8
43. Desgranges FP, Desebbe O, Pereira de Souza Neto E, Raphael D, Chassard D. Respiratory variation in aortic blood flow peak velocity to predict fluid responsiveness in mechanically ventilated children: a systematic review and meta-analysis. *Paediatr Anaesth.* (2016) 26:37–47. doi: 10.1111/pan.12803
44. Durand P, Chevret L, Essouri S, Haas V, Devictor D. Respiratory variations in aortic blood flow predict fluid responsiveness in ventilated children. *Intens Care Med.* (2008) 34:888–94. doi: 10.1007/s00134-008-1021-z
45. Gelbart B, Schlapbach L, Ganeshalingham A, Ganu S, Erickson S, Oberender F, et al. Fluid bolus therapy in critically ill children: a survey of practice among paediatric intensive care doctors in Australia and New Zealand. *Crit Care Resusc.* (2018) 20:131–8.
46. Long E, Babl F, Dalziel S, Dalton S, Etheridge C, Duke T, et al. Fluid resuscitation for paediatric sepsis: a survey of senior emergency physicians in Australia and New Zealand. *Emerg Med Australas.* (2015) 27:245–50. doi: 10.1111/1742-6723.12400
47. Glassford NJ, Jones SL, Martensson J, Eastwoods GM, Bailey M, Cross AM, et al. Characteristics and expectations of fluid bolus therapy: a bi-national survey of acute care physicians. *Anaesth Intens Care* (2015) 43:750–6.
48. Cecconi M, Hofer C, Teboul JL, Pettila V, Wilkman E, Molnar Z, et al. Fluid challenges in intensive care: the FENICE study : a global inception cohort study. *Intens Care Med.* (2015) 41:1529–37. doi: 10.1007/s00134-015-3850-x
49. Ray S, Rogers L, Noren DP, Dhar R, Nadel S, Peters MJ, et al. Risk of over-diagnosis of hypotension in children: a comparative analysis of over 50,000 blood pressure measurements. *Intensive Care Med.* (2017) 43:1540–1. doi: 10.1007/s00134-017-4843-8
50. Carcillo JA. Capillary refill time is a very useful clinical sign in early recognition and treatment of very sick children. *Pediatr Crit Care Med.* (2012) 13:210–2. doi: 10.1097/PCC.0b013e3182231667
51. Fleming S, Gill P, Jones C, Taylor JA, Van den Bruel A, Heneghan C, et al. The diagnostic value of capillary refill time for detecting serious illness in children: a systematic review and meta-analysis. *PLoS ONE* (2015) 10:e0138155. doi: 10.1371/journal.pone.0138155
52. Tibby SM, Hatherill M, Murdoch IA. Capillary refill and core-peripheral temperature gap as indicators of haemodynamic status in paediatric intensive care patients. *Arch Dis Child.* (1999) 80:163–6.
53. Ait-Oufella H, Bige N, Boelle PY, Pichereau C, Alves M, Bertinchamp R, et al. Capillary refill time exploration during septic shock. *Intens Care Med.* (2014) 40:958–64. doi: 10.1007/s00134-014-3326-4
54. Pettila V, Merz T, Wilkman E, Perner A, Karlsson S, Lange T, et al. Targeted tissue perfusion versus macrocirculation-guided standard care in patients with septic shock (TARTARE-2S): study protocol and statistical analysis plan for a randomized controlled trial. *Trials* (2016) 17:384. doi: 10.1186/s13063-016-1515-x
55. Deep A, Goonasekera CD, Wang Y, Brierley J. Evolution of haemodynamics and outcome of fluid-refractory septic shock in children. *Intens Care Med.* (2013) 39:1602–9. doi: 10.1007/s00134-013-3003-z
56. Ranjit S, Aram G, Kissoon N, Ali MK, Natraj R, Shresti S, et al. Multimodal monitoring for hemodynamic categorization and management of pediatric septic shock: a pilot observational study*. *Pediatr Crit Care Med.* (2014) 15:e17–26. doi: 10.1097/PCC.0b013e3182a5589c
57. Ceneviva G, Paschall JA, Maffei F, Carcillo JA. Hemodynamic support in fluid-refractory pediatric septic shock. *Pediatrics* (1998) 102:e19.
58. Brierley J, Peters MJ. Distinct hemodynamic patterns of septic shock at presentation to pediatric intensive care. *Pediatrics* (2008) 122:752–9. doi: 10.1542/peds.2007-1979
59. Top AP, Ince C, de Meij N, van Dijk M, Tibboel D. Persistent low microcirculatory vessel density in nonsurvivors of sepsis in pediatric intensive care. *Crit Care Med.* (2011) 39:8–13. doi: 10.1097/CCM.0b013e3181fb7994
60. Spronk PE, Zandstra DF, Ince C. Bench-to-bedside review: sepsis is a disease of the microcirculation. *Crit Care* (2004) 8:462–8. doi: 10.1186/cc2894
61. Boerma EC, Ince C. The role of vasoactive agents in the resuscitation of microvascular perfusion and tissue oxygenation in critically ill patients. *Intens Care Med.* (2010) 36:2004–18. doi: 10.1007/s00134-010-1970-x
62. Obonyo NG, Fanning JP, Ng ASY, Pimenta LP, Shekar K, Platts DG, et al. Effects of volume resuscitation on the microcirculation in animal models of lipopolysaccharide sepsis: a systematic review. *Intens Care Med Exp.* (2016) 4:38. doi: 10.1186/s40635-016-0112-3
63. Klijn E, van Velzen MH, Lima AP, Bakker J, van Bommel J, Groeneveld AB. Tissue perfusion and oxygenation to monitor fluid responsiveness in critically ill, septic patients after initial resuscitation: a prospective observational study. *J Clin Monitor Comput.* (2015) 29:707–12. doi: 10.1007/s10877-014-9653-8
64. Wong HR. Genetics and genomics in pediatric septic shock. *Crit Care Med.* (2012) 40:1618–26. doi: 10.1097/CCM.0b013e318246b546
65. Aya HD, Ster IC, Fletcher N, Grounds RM, Rhodes A, Cecconi M. Pharmacodynamic analysis of a fluid challenge. *Crit Care Med.* (2016) 44:880–91. doi: 10.1097/CCM.0000000000001517
66. Glassford NJ, Eastwood GM, Bellomo R. Physiological changes after fluid bolus therapy in sepsis: a systematic review of contemporary data. *Crit Care* (2014) 18:696. doi: 10.1186/s13054-014-0696-5
67. Bihari S, Wiersema UF, Schembri D, De Pasquale CG, Dixon DL, Prakash S, et al. Bolus intravenous 0.9% saline, but not 4% albumin or 5% glucose, causes interstitial pulmonary edema in healthy subjects. *J Appl Physiol.* (2015) 119:783–92. doi: 10.1152/japplphysiol.00356.2015
68. Bihari S, Teubner DJ, Prakash S, Beatty T, Morphett M, Bellomo R, et al. Fluid bolus therapy in emergency department patients: indications and physiological changes. *Emerg Med Aust.* (2016) 28:531–7. doi: 10.1111/1742-6723.12621
69. Obonyo N, Brent B, Olupot-Olupot P, Boele van Hensbroek M, Kuipers I, Wong S, et al. Myocardial and haemodynamic responses to two fluid regimens in African children with severe malnutrition and hypovolaemic shock (AFRIM study). *Crit Care* (2017) 21:103. doi: 10.1186/s13054-017-1679-0
70. Long E, Babl FE, Oakley E, Sheridan B, Duke T, Pediatric Research in Emergency Departments International C. Cardiac index changes with fluid bolus therapy in children with sepsis-an observational study. *Pediatr Crit Care Med.* (2018) 19:513–8. doi: 10.1097/PCC.00000000000 01534
71. Dellinger RP, Levy MM, Rhodes A, Annane D, Gerlach H, Opal SM, et al. Surviving Sepsis Campaign: international guidelines for management of severe sepsis and septic shock, 2012. *Intens Care Med.* (2013) 39:165–228. doi: 10.1007/s00134-012-2769-8
72. Brierley J, Carcillo JA, Choong K, Cornell T, Decaen A, Deymann A, et al. Clinical practice parameters for hemodynamic support of pediatric and neonatal septic shock: 2007 update from the American College of Critical Care Medicine.[Erratum appears in Crit Care Med. 2009 Apr;37:1536 Note: Skache, Sara [corrected to Kache, Saraswati]; Irazusta, Jose [corrected to Irazuzta, Jose]]. *Crit Care Med.* (2009) 37:666–88. doi: 10.1097/CCM.0b013e31819323c6
73. Upadhyay M, Singhi S, Murlidharan J, Kaur N, Majumdar S. Randomized evaluation of fluid resuscitation with crystalloid (saline) and colloid (polymer from degraded gelatin in saline) in pediatric septic shock. *Indian Pediatr.* (2005) 42:223-31.

74. Santhanam I, Sangareddi S, Venkataraman S, Kissoon N, Thiruvengadamudayan V, Kasthuri RK. A prospective randomized controlled study of two fluid regimens in the initial management of septic shock in the emergency department. *Pediatr Emerg Care* (2008) 24:647–55. doi: 10.1097/PEC.0b013e31818844cf
75. Gelbart B, Glassford NJ, Bellomo R. Fluid bolus therapy-based resuscitation for severe sepsis in hospitalized children: a systematic review. *Pediatr Crit Care Med.* (2015) 16:e297–307. doi: 10.1097/PCC.0000000000000507
76. Akech S, Gwer S, Idro R, Fegan G, Eziefula AC, Newton CRJC, et al. Volume expansion with albumin compared to gelofusine in children with severe malaria: results of a controlled trial. *PLOS Clin Trial* (2006) 1:e21. doi: 10.1371/journal.pctr.0010021
77. Maitland K, Pamba A, English M, Peshu N, Marsh K, Newton C, et al. Randomized trial of volume expansion with albumin or saline in children with severe malaria: preliminary evidence of albumin benefit. *Clin Infect Dis.* (2005) 40:538–45. doi: 10.1086/427505
78. Dung NM, Day NP, Tam DT, Loan HT, Chau HT, Minh LN, et al. Fluid replacement in dengue shock syndrome: a randomized, double-blind comparison of four intravenous-fluid regimens. *Clin Infect Dis.* (1999) 29:787–94.
79. Ngo NT, Cao XT, Kneen R, Wills B, Nguyen VM, Nguyen TQ, et al. Acute management of dengue shock syndrome: a randomized double-blind comparison of 4 intravenous fluid regimens in the first hour. *Clin Infect Dis.* (2001) 32:204–13. doi: 10.1086/318479
80. Wills BA, Nguyen MD, Ha TL, Dong TH, Tran TN, Le TT, et al. Comparison of three fluid solutions for resuscitation in dengue shock syndrome. *N Engl J Med.* (2005) 353:877–89. doi: 10.1056/NEJMoa044057
81. Booy R, Habibi P, Nadel S, de Munter C, Britto J, Morrison A, et al. Reduction in case fatality rate from meningococcal disease associated with improved healthcare delivery. *Arch Dis Child.* (2001) 85:386–90. doi: 10.1136/adc.85.5.386
82. Ford N, Hargreaves S, Shanks L. Mortality after fluid bolus in children with shock due to sepsis or severe infection: a systematic review and meta-analysis. *PLoS ONE* (2012) 7:e43953. doi: 10.1371/journal.pone.0043953
83. Hilton AK, Bellomo R. A critique of fluid bolus resuscitation in severe sepsis. *Crit Care* (2012) 16:302. doi: 10.1186/cc11154
84. Brewster D. African fluid bolus study: implications for practice. *J Paediatr Child Health* (2012) 48:548–50. doi: 10.1111/j.1440-1754.2012.02431.x
85. Myburgh J, Finfer S. Causes of death after fluid bolus resuscitation: new insights from FEAST. *BMC Med.* (2013) 11:67. doi: 10.1186/1741-7015-11-67
86. Maitland K, George EC, Evans JA, Kiguli S, Olupot-Olupot P, Akech SO, et al. Exploring mechanisms of excess mortality with early fluid resuscitation: insights from the FEAST trial. *BMC Med.* (2013) 11:68. doi: 10.1186/1741-7015-11-68
87. Duke T. What the African fluid-bolus trial means. *Lancet* (2011) 378:1685–7. doi: 10.1016/S0140-6736%2811%2960881-7
88. Hazle MA, Gajarski RJ, Yu S, Donohue J, Blatt NB. Fluid overload in infants following congenital heart surgery. *Pediatric Crit Care Med.*. (2013) 14:44–9. doi: 10.1097/PCC.0b013e3182712799
89. Piggott KD, Soni M, Decampli WM, Ramirez JA, Holbein D, Fakioglu H, et al. Acute kidney injury and fluid overload in neonates following surgery for congenital heart disease. *World J Pediatric Congen Heart Surg.* (2015) 6:401–6. doi: 10.1177/2150135115586814
90. Stein A, de Souza L, Belettini C, Menegazzo W, Viegas J, Costa Pereira E. Fluid overload and changes in serum creatinine after cardiac surgery: predictors of mortality and longer intensive care stay. A prospective cohort study. *Crit Care* (2012) 16:R99. doi: 10.1186/cc11368
91. Foland J, Fortenberry J, Warshaw B, Pettignano R, Merritt R, Heard M. Fluid overload before continuous hemofiltration and survival in critically ill children: a retrospective analysis. *Crit Care Med.* (2004) 32:1771–6. doi: 10.1097/01.CCM.0000132897.52737.49
92. Li Y, Wang J, Bai Z, Chen J, Wang X, Pan J, et al. Early fluid overload is associated with acute kidney injury and PICU mortality in critically ill children. *Eur J Pediatr.* (2016) 175:39–48. doi: 10.1007/s00431-015-2592-7
93. Valentine SL, Sapru A, Higgerson RA, Spinella PC, Flori HR, Graham DA, et al. Fluid balance in critically ill children with acute lung injury. *Crit Care Med.* (2012) 40:2883–9. doi: 10.1097/CCM.0b013e31825bc54d
94. Selewski DT, Askenazi DJ, Bridges BC, Cooper DS, Fleming GM, Paden ML, et al. The impact of fluid overload on outcomes in children treated with extracorporeal membrane oxygenation: a multicenter retrospective cohort study*. *Pediatric Crit Care Med.* (2017) 18:1126–35. doi: 10.1097/pcc.0000000000001349
95. Arikan AA, Zappitelli M, Goldstein SL, Naipaul A, Jefferson LS, Loftis LL. Fluid overload is associated with impaired oxygenation and morbidity in critically ill children. *Pediatric Crit Care Med.* (2012) 13:253–8. doi: 10.1097/PCC.0b013e31822882a3
96. Sinitsky L, Walls D, Nadel S, Inwald DP. Fluid overload at 48 hours is associated with respiratory morbidity but not mortality in a general PICU: retrospective cohort study*. *Pediatric Crit Care Med.* (2015) 16:205–9. doi: 10.1097/pcc.0000000000000318
97. Bhaskar P, Dhar AV, Thompson M, Quigley R, Modem V. Early fluid accumulation in children with shock and ICU mortality: a matched case–control study. *Intens Care Med.* (2015) 41:1445–53. doi: 10.1007/s00134-015-3851-9
98. Chen J, Li X, Bai Z, Fang F, Hua J, Li Y, et al. Association of fluid accumulation with clinical outcomes in critically ill children with severe sepsis. *PLoS ONE* (2016) 11:e0160093. doi: 10.1371/journal.pone.0160093
99. Alobaidi R, Morgan C, Basu RK, Stenson E, Featherstone R, Majumdar SR, et al. Association between fluid balance and outcomes in critically ill children: A systematic review and meta-analysis. *JAMA Pediatr.* (2018) 172:257–68. doi: 10.1001/jamapediatrics.2017.4540
100. Andrews B, Semler MW, Muchemwa L, Kelly P, Lakhi S, Heimburger DC, et al. Effect of an early resuscitation protocol on in-hospital mortality among adults with sepsis and hypotension: a randomized clinical trial. *JAMA* (2017) 318:1233–40. doi: 10.1001/jama.2017.10913
101. Singer M, Deutschman CS, Seymour CW, Shankar-Hari M, Annane D, Bauer M, et al. The third international consensus definitions for sepsis and septic shock (sepsis-3). *JAMA* (2016) 315:801–10. doi: 10.1001/jama.2016.0287

4

Culture-Negative Early-Onset Neonatal Sepsis — At the Crossroad Between Efficient Sepsis Care and Antimicrobial Stewardship

Claus Klingenberg[1,2]*, *René F. Kornelisse*[3], *Giuseppe Buonocore*[4], *Rolf F. Maier*[5] *and Martin Stocker*[6]

[1] Pediatric Research Group, Faculty of Health Sciences, University of Tromsø-Arctic University of Norway, Tromsø, Norway, [2] Department of Pediatrics and Adolescence Medicine, University Hospital of North Norway, Tromsø, Norway, [3] Division of Neonatology, Department of Pediatrics, Erasmus MC-Sophia Children's Hospital, Erasmus University Medical Center, Rotterdam, Netherlands, [4] Department of Molecular and Developmental Medicine, University of Siena, Siena, Italy, [5] Children's Hospital, University Hospital, Philipps University of Marburg, Marburg, Germany, [6] Neonatal and Pediatric Intensive Care Unit, Children's Hospital, Lucerne, Switzerland

***Correspondence:**
Claus Klingenberg
claus.klingenberg@unn.no

Sepsis is a leading cause of mortality and morbidity in neonates. Presenting clinical symptoms are unspecific. Sensitivity and positive predictive value of biomarkers at onset of symptoms are suboptimal. Clinical suspicion therefore frequently leads to empirical antibiotic therapy in uninfected infants. The incidence of culture confirmed early-onset sepsis is rather low, around 0.4–0.8/1000 term infants in high-income countries. Six to 16 times more infants receive therapy for culture-negative sepsis in the absence of a positive blood culture. Thus, culture-negative sepsis contributes to high antibiotic consumption in neonatal units. Antibiotics may be life-saving for the few infants who are truly infected. However, overuse of broad-spectrum antibiotics increases colonization with antibiotic resistant bacteria. Antibiotic therapy also induces perturbations of the non-resilient early life microbiota with potentially long lasting negative impact on the individual's own health. Currently there is no uniform consensus definition for neonatal sepsis. This leads to variations in management. Two factors may reduce the number of culture-negative sepsis cases. First, obtaining adequate blood cultures (0.5–1 mL) at symptom onset is mandatory. Unless there is a strong clinical or biochemical indication to prolong antibiotics physician need to trust the culture results and to stop antibiotics for suspected sepsis within 36–48 h. Secondly, an international robust and pragmatic neonatal sepsis definition is urgently needed. Neonatal sepsis is a dynamic condition. Rigorous evaluation of clinical symptoms ("organ dysfunction") over 36–48 h in combination with appropriately selected biomarkers ("dysregulated host response") may be used to support or refute a sepsis diagnosis.

Keywords: neonate, sepsis, blood culture, C-reactive protein, procalcitonin

INTRODUCTION

Neonatal sepsis is a clinical manifestation of a systemic infection during the first 28 days of life, usually classified as early-onset (<48–72 h) and late-onset sepsis (>48–72 h), depending on the age at onset of the sepsis episode (1). The inability to isolate a microbial pathogen does not exclude sepsis (2, 3). The 2016 consensus definition of sepsis in adults (Sepsis-3) states that sepsis is "a life-threatening condition caused by a dysregulated host response to infection and organ dysfunction" (3). There are also ongoing discussions regarding an adapted definition of pediatric sepsis beyond the neonatal period, similar to the Sepsis-3 definition (4, 5). However, there is unfortunately no uniform consensus definition for neonatal sepsis (2, 6, 7). Many neonates are therefore diagnosed with a "probable or possible" sepsis or a "presumed symptomatic infection but no bacterial cause identified" (8); conditions often referred to as "culture-negative sepsis"(9).

Most publications on neonatal sepsis from high-income countries only include culture-confirmed cases. The large number of neonates treated with antibiotics for a culture-negative sepsis are largely ignored in epidemiological studies. Thus, there is a paucity of data on the latter condition. However, neonates with culture-negative sepsis contribute to the high antibiotic consumption seen in neonatal units (10, 11). Moreover, there is a wide variation in antibiotic use between neonatal intensive care units (NICUs) and countries, with no difference in infection-attributable morbidity and mortality (10, 12). This indicates probable overuse of antibiotics in some NICUs, which again may have important adverse short- and long-term consequences for the infant's individual health (13–15). On the other hand, delayed antibiotic therapy in truly infected neonates may result in increased mortality and morbidity (16). Therefore, culture-negative neonatal sepsis is at the crossroad between efficient sepsis care and antimicrobial stewardship programs.

The main objective of this paper is to critically review the controversial term culture-negative neonatal sepsis (9, 17), with a focus on early-onset neonatal sepsis (EONS). We discuss how we can combine efficient sepsis care with antimicrobial stewardship during first days and weeks of life. Finally, we will discuss possible strategies for defining EONS in the absence of a positive blood culture.

EFFICIENT SEPSIS CARE—BASIC ELEMENTS

Epidemiology

In most high-income countries, the incidence of culture-confirmed EONS has decreased or remained relatively stable around 0.4–0.8 cases per 1000 live-born term infants over the last decade (10, 18–21). Although the incidence of EONS is substantially higher in preterm infants, the majority of patients with EONS are delivered at term (22). Robust epidemiological data on culture-negative sepsis are limited. A number of different studies published since 2012 report that infants receiving systemic antibiotic therapy for culture-negative sepsis outnumber infants receiving therapy for culture-confirmed sepsis by a factor of six to 16 (**Table 1**). The reason for the high number of culture-negative cases is not clear, and diagnostic criteria used in the different publications vary substantially (10, 11, 23, 24, 26, 27). Low levels of bacteremia or only small volumes of blood obtained from sick infants may be one explanation for the high number of culture-negative sepsis cases. Also maternal antibiotic treatment before or during delivery may theoretically in some cases mask detection of bacteremia in the newborn. However, one must also question whether over-diagnosis of sepsis among non-infected infants is an alternative explanation.

Survivors of neonatal sepsis may suffer short- and long-term consequences (28, 29). Delayed recognition and therapy of sepsis increase the risk of morbidity and mortality and early antibiotic treatment of suspected sepsis is a corner stone of every sepsis care bundle (30). Therefore, clinicians have a low threshold to suspect neonatal EONS and to start empirical antibiotic therapy. Most probably due to a lack of a clear definition and a robust gold standard of the diagnosis neonatal sepsis, started therapy is often continued for 5–7 days, even in the absence of a positive blood culture, to minimize the risk of "partial treatment" of a potential true infection (11).

Risk Factors for EONS

Maternal group B streptococcal (GBS) colonization in the current pregnancy, GBS bacteriuria, a previous infant with invasive GBS disease, prolonged rupture of membranes (PROM; ≥18 h) and maternal fever (temperature ≥38°C; often interpreted as a sign of chorioamnionitis) are the risk factors most commonly associated with EONS. These risk factors are additive; the presence of more than one factor increases the likelihood of EONS (31, 32). EONS prevention strategies using a risk factor based approach suggest starting empiric antibiotics based on the presence of one or more risk factors. These strategies decrease the incidence of GBS-EONS (33, 34), but have poor predictive ability, leading to high number of mothers and infants being treated with antibiotics. A quantitative model assessing the indication for empiric therapy including degree of maternal fever, duration of PROM and degree of prematurity seem to perform better, and may reduce the number of infants receiving antibiotics (35).

Reports and guidelines differ in their recommendations on how to act on risk factor based strategies (36). The NICE-guidelines do not specify whether the use of intrapartum antibiotic prophylaxis alter the subsequent EONS risk assessment and infant evaluation (8). In contrast, an EONS sepsis calculator developed by Escobar and co-workers incorporates that intrapartum antibiotic given >2–4 h prior to delivery ameliorates the clinical recommendations regarding EONS risk, and subsequent infant management (37). A recent international survey regarding neonatal sepsis showed a broad variability in management of neonates with only risk factors, whereas a newborn with risk factors in combination with clinical signs were uniformly started on antibiotic therapy (36).

Clinical Signs of EONS

EONS generally presents itself with respiratory distress, apnea, lethargy or irritability, temperature instability, and feeding difficulties. These symptoms are unspecific as many non-infected

TABLE 1 | Reported cases of culture-confirmed vs. culture-negative neonatal sepsis in selected studies published after 2012.

Population and country	Ratio culture-confirmed vs. culture-negative sepsis cases	Definition culture-negative sepsis
Term infants admitted to neonatal units in Norway over a 3 year period (*n* = 10 175) (10)	91: 1447 (1:16)	• Physician assigned ICD-10 diagnosis P36.9 • Clinical symptoms • Antibiotics ≥5 days
Term and preterm infants admitted to one neonatal unit in Norway and one in Denmark over a 3 year period (*n* = 2927) (23)	35: 203 (1:6)	• Physician assigned ICD-10 diagnosis P36.9 • Clinical symptoms • CRP > 10 mg/L • Antibiotics ≥3 days
Term and preterm infants admitted within first 24 h of life to a single neonatal unit in Austria (*n* = 851) (24)	31[x]: 209 (1:7)	• Clinical symptoms • Maternal risk factor or at least one abnormal laboratory marker (incl. CRP > 8 mg/L)
Term and preterm infants evaluated for sepsis in one neonatal unit in Canada (*n* = 1202) (25)	16: 107 (1:7)	• Born to mothers receiving intrapartum antibiotics. • Antibiotics started on the day of birth and continued for > 72 h despite negative culture.
Infants born after 34 weeks gestation with suspected EONS requiring antibiotics. A multi-center study in Europe and Canada. (*n* = 1710) (26)	27: 161 (1:6)	Based on a risk classification scheme including: • Maternal risk factors • Clinical symptoms • Laboratory findings (WBC < 5 x 10^9/mL and/or CRP > 10 mg/L)
Infants born after 34 weeks gestation at a single institution in Switzerland over a 5-year period (*n* = 11 503) (27)	4: 48 (1:12)	• ≥2 clinical signs of sepsis within the first 7 days of life (temperature instability, irritability, or lethargy, feeding difficulties, capillary refill >2 s, apnea, tachycardia and/or tachypnea) • CRP > 20 mg/L • Antibiotics ≥7 days

[x]11 cases of positive tracheal cultures indicating invasive infections were reported in the original paper, but excluded here.
WBC, white blood cells; CRP, C-reactive protein; ICD-10, International Classification of Diseases, 10th revision.

neonates display similar symptoms. During the first days of life, there is a dynamic adaption of different organ systems to extra-uterine life. A single-point, clinical assessment to diagnose EONS therefore seems impossible. Some guidelines suggest that a respiratory rate > 50 or 60/min may be suggestive of an infection (**Table 2**). However, in healthy infants the 95th percentile for the respiratory rate is 65/min at 2 h of age (41). Moreover, non-infected early term infants (37–38 weeks gestation) born by cesarean section have high rates of transient tachypnea (42). Feeding difficulties are also notoriously difficult to assess during the first 1–2 days of life. A capillary refill time > 2 s is included as a sign of EONS in some sepsis criteria (27, 43), while observational studies indicate that the normal refill time in neonates is at least 3 s (44, 45). These examples clearly show the limitations with single-point assessments of clinical signs. In preterm infants, symptoms from respiratory distress syndrome or clinical instability may be impossible to differentiate from sepsis. However, a number of preterm infants are delivered by cesarean section, before rupture of membranes and with no maternal signs of infection. Among these there is a very low risk for EONS (46). Recognizing a "low-risk situation" may provide the opportunity to limit routine empiric antibiotics for preterm infants even when there is some degree of respiratory distress. Nevertheless, there is a broad consensus to start antibiotic therapy in newborns with clinical signs suggestive of possible EONS (36)—the major challenge is when to diagnose this as sepsis or to discard a sepsis diagnosis and stop therapy!

Sensitivity and Positive Predictive Value of Inflammatory Markers

In this paragraph we will focus on inflammatory markers that are commonly used and commercially available today, namely the complete blood cell (CBC) count, the C-reactive protein (CRP), procalcitonin (PCT), and to some extent interleukins (e.g., interleukin [IL]-6 and IL-8). It is not possible within the scope of this article to review all biomarkers used for diagnostics, and we refer to recent reviews on this topic (47). In the future, rapid bedside point-of care tests using e.g., microarray chips to quantify multiple cytokines and acute phase reactants and other "multi-omic" approaches may become excellent and improved diagnostic tools (47, 48).

The diagnostic value of the CBC-count and differential with regard to neonatal sepsis has been extensively evaluated (7, 49, 50). In general, CBC components are neither very sensitive nor specific for EONS (49, 50). The white blood cell (WBC) and the absolute neutrophil counts (ANC) are most informative when very low (49, 50). There is a very wide range between the lower and upper normal limits for WBC and ANC. Increased band form neutrophils, represented by high immature-to-total neutrophil ratio (IT-ratio), is often suggested to indicate sepsis. However, large intra- and inter-laboratory variation in interpretation limits its use (49, 51). Early onset thrombocytopenia is commonly associated with feto-maternal conditions and not very predictive for an infection (52). In the setting of an EONS evaluation, a low platelet count has a low

TABLE 2 | Selected examples of suggested neonatal sepsis definition from experts or societies.

Authors or society	Criteria	Comment
International pediatric sepsis consensus conference: Definitions for sepsis and organ dysfunction in pediatrics–2005 (38)	**Systemic inflammatory response syndrome (SIRS) criteria–1st week of life** • Heart rate < 180/min or < 100/min • Respiratory rate > 50/min • WBC > 34 × 10^9/mL • Core temperature of > 38.5°C or < 36°C Sepsis; SIRS in the presence of suspected or proven infection	Evidence of infection vaguely described
European Medicines Agency definition from 2010 (39)	**Criteria for inclusion in a neonatal sepsis clinical trial** Clinical sign (temperature instability, cardiovascular instability, skin symptoms, respiratory instability, gastrointestinal symptoms, non-specific symptoms) Laboratory signs: Low/high WBCs, I/T-ratio > 0.2, Platelet count < 100, CRP > 15 mg/L or PCT > 2 ng/mL, glucose intolerance and metabolic acidosis	Laboratory signs unspecific and cut-offs with poor predictive ability and not age adapted (PCT)
Wynn and Polin –2018 (2)	**Hypothetical neonatal sequential organ failure assessment (nSOFA) score** Including the following 6 items with scores from 0 to 3: Respiratory status, cardiovascular status, platelet counts, absolute neutrophil count, renal function, and CNS function	Inclusion of WBC indices with poor predictive values.
Hakonsson–2017 (40)	**Definition of a clinical, culture-negative GBS sepsis (in retrospect)** • Relevant symptoms and/or a CRP ≥ 25 mg/L • GBS in the maternal vaginal/rectal swabs or superficial infant cultures • The initiation of antibiotic therapy in the infant	Clinical signs not specified
Norwegian Neonatal Society (10)	**Definition of a culture-negative sepsis (in retrospect)** • Clinical symptoms • CRP > 30 mg/L • Other known clinical reasons for increased CRP excluded • Received antibiotics ≥ 5 days	Clinical signs not specified. Duration of antibiotics as a criteria not useful prospectively

CRP, C-reactive protein; GBS, group B streptococci; CNS, central nervous system; WBC, white blood cells; PCT, procalcitonin, I/T ratio-immature to total neutrophil ratio.

sensitivity and a low positive predictive value (49, 53). Thus, CBC components used alone are inaccurate to define neonatal sepsis in the absence of a positive blood culture (7).

CRP is the most extensively studied acute-phase reactant in neonates. It is widely available and its determination is simple, fast, and cost-effective (54, 55). The mean CRP level in healthy term infants undergoes a physiological rise from ~1 mg/L at 12 h of age to ~4 mg/L at 48 h of life (55). Preterm infants have a less pronounced CRP response compared to term infants (56). A CRP cut-off value at 10 mg/L is often suggested as the upper normal limit (54). However, the 95th percentile of CRP in healthy infants at 48 h of age is 12–14 mg/L (55, 57, 58). Moreover, non-infected infants may have CRP values up to at least 40–50 mg/L, in particular after vaginal delivery (58, 59). Thus, a substantial number of healthy infants will have CRP values > 10 mg/L. CRP levels at the time of initial EONS-evaluation have a low sensitivity (25), because EONS usually originates during labor or at delivery and it then takes 12–24 h for CRP to rise (54). The positive predictive value of an elevated CRP value > 10 mg/L for possible or proven EONS has also consistently been low. This is mainly because there are multiple non-infectious conditions associated with an inflammatory reaction in the perinatal period, including a complicated labor and delivery, meconium aspiration, intraventricular hemorrhage, and tissue injury (25, 54, 60).

Over the last decade, PCT has emerged as a promising and increasingly used sepsis biomarker in neonates. PCT, like CRP, does not cross the placenta; hence is not affected by maternal fever in labor (61). PCT levels start to rise 2 h after start of a septic insult and peak by 12 h (62). The earlier rise after onset of the infectious stimulus makes PCT an attractive alternative to CRP (63). However, there has been few high-quality studies reporting data on the clinical usefulness of PCT at disease onset in "ruling in" EONS (63). Moreover, the interpretation of PCT values is challenging due to a strong physiological rise and fall during the first 72 h of life. Other perinatal factors, such as chorioamnionitis, hypoxemia, perinatal asphyxia, and maternal preeclampsia, can also cause PCT to increase (64). Dynamic reference values of PCT in neonates with and without EONS have been published (57, 65, 66).

Interleukins, predominantly IL-6 and IL-8, are used routinely in some countries and are considered as sensitive "early warning biomarkers" (47, 67, 68). The advantage of using interleukins is the early spike after an infectious insult that may add in early diagnosis. However, due to their short half-life one may not catch the peak level and this may limit sensitivity. Thus, when used they should always be combined with a "later marker" e.g., CRP (67).

In summary, the positive predictive values of the above-mentioned inflammatory markers are relatively low. The reason for this is mainly due to perinatal inflammatory reactions triggered by factors during delivery or in the early postnatal period. Still, many clinicians use abnormal inflammatory markers at disease onset as one reason to prolong antibiotic therapy in infants with a negative blood culture (36).

ANTIMICROBIAL STEWARDSHIP IN THE NEONATAL UNIT

Prolonged Antibiotic Therapy in the Neonatal Period and Associated Risks

The duration of antimicrobial therapy in infants with negative blood cultures is controversial, and there is little evidence to inform practice (8, 31). In the SCOUT-study researchers assessed antibiotic consumption for different conditions among 2500 term and preterm infants (11). Culture-proven infection and necrotizing enterocolitis (NEC) accounted for only 6.9% of antibiotic use. In contrast, prolonged (≥ 5 days) antibiotic therapy for pneumonia or culture-negative sepsis accounted for 26% of total antibiotic use and therapy was continued for median (range) seven (5–14) days for these conditions. The UK NICE-guidelines states that the usual duration of antibiotic treatment for babies with a positive blood culture, and for those with a negative blood culture but in whom there has been strong suspicion of sepsis, should be 7 days (8). In observational studies, infants with culture-negative sepsis are commonly treated for 5–7 days and mortality is very low (10, 11, 23). However, due to variable sepsis definitions it is not possible to assess "safety" vs. a clear possibility of harm due to overtreatment (69). A recent study from India compared the efficacy of 7 vs. 10 days duration of intravenous antibiotics for culture-proven septic neonates and found no difference (70).

There is growing evidence that prolonged antibiotic therapy in preterm infants without proven infection increases the risk of mortality, bronchopulmonary dysplasia, NEC, retinopathy, and periventricular white matter damage (13, 71). The question if antibiotic therapy is a perpetrator or an innocent bystander is still not completely clear, but we must seriously consider that the "administration of antibiotics itself may contribute to mortality and morbidity among preterm infants" (72). It has also been known for decades that overuse of antibiotics paves the way for development of multi-resistant bacteria and there is an urgent call for rational use of antibiotics (73). Unfortunately, the cost of antibiotic resistance for the community compared to the potential risk of delayed or insufficient treated infection is a weak argument for the clinician at the bedside. With the growing knowledge of antibiotic use and the cost on the individual's own health via the collateral damage on their microbiota, this may change (74). Recent data indicate that the perturbations of the non-resilient microbiota in early life may influence both the immune system and stem cell populations with potential negative impact on future health (75–77). Therefore, pediatricians and neonatologists need to measure risk and benefits of every dose of antibiotics for culture-negative situations. The hospitals and lead clinicians in neonatal units have an independent responsibility to educate and keep staff updated about current knowledge of the harmful effects of unnecessary antibiotic use in the neonatal period (78). Recent publications reporting results from antimicrobial stewardship programs in NICUs highlight both the potential for improving antibiotic prescription practice, but also challenges when trying to reduce broad-spectrum antibiotic therapy in vulnerable very preterm infants (79, 80).

Appropriate Blood Culture Diagnostics

A positive microbial culture from a normally sterile site (blood) is frequently used as the gold standard to define neonatal sepsis (2). In the UK, around 50% of all blood cultures obtained in the neonatal period were taken on the day of birth, but only 0.8% of these were positive (81). Thus, the majority of blood cultures are negative in neonates who are evaluated with risk factors or clinical signs of EONS. What is the sensitivity of blood cultures in neonates? Schelonka analyzed, in a laboratory-based study, a range of blood volumes containing known concentrations of common neonatal pathogens injected into pediatric blood culture bottles. If organisms were present at very low densities [< 4 colony forming units (cfu)/mL] a blood culture volume of 1.0 mL was needed to detect bacteremia. Otherwise, blood culture volumes down to 0.5 mL were sufficient to detect most bacteremia's. In a similar *in-vitro* study, placental blood seeded with more than 10 cfu/mL of *E. coli* or GBS required only 0.25 mL blood to be consistently detected (82). Thus, blood cultures with a volume of 1.0 mL have excellent sensitivity even when the infant has low very levels of bacteremia, and blood culture volumes down to as little as 0.5 mL may be sufficient to detect moderate and high grade bacteremia (83). Some authorities recommend obtaining at least two cultures (aerobic and anaerobic) before commencing antibiotics, but there are no neonatal data to support this, and usual practice is to take only one aerobic blood culture bottle before starting antibiotic treatment (84).

Quantitative blood culture methodology (cfu/mL) is not routinely used. However, blood culture time to positivity (TTP) correlates to level of bacterial density as TTP is inversely proportional to the inoculated bacterial concentration. Using modern continuous monitoring blood culture system, median TTP of blood cultures in neonatal sepsis is 9–18 h for true pathogenic bacteria (85–89). For GBS and *E. coli* around 96–100% are positive by 36 h (85, 86, 89), whereas coagulase negative staphylococci may take up to 48 h to be detected. Maternal intrapartum antibiotic therapy does not seem to delay TTP (85, 90). Thus, considering TTP aids in clinical interpretation of blood culture results and is the reason why central guidelines suggest stopping antibiotics if culture results are negative at 36–48 h (8, 31). Ensuring a sufficient blood culture volume (minimum 0.5 mL) and adequate routines for 24/7 immediate entry of blood culture bottles into the blood culture system are essential elements in this diagnostic algorithm (84, 87, 91).

Modern molecular methods may potentially represent more rapid, sensitive, and specific ways of identifying bacteria. These methods include conventional and real-time polymerase chain reaction (PCR) assays targeted at universal and specific gene sites. A systematic review from 2017 concluded that molecular assays have the advantage of producing rapid results and may perform well as "add-on" tests, but cannot replace microbial cultures in the diagnosis of neonatal sepsis (92, 93). This may change in the future. A recent publication reports promising results using multiplex real-time PCR in late-onset neonatal sepsis with results potentially available within 4 h of blood sampling and good concordance with blood culture results (94).

Negative Predictive Value of Inflammatory Markers

In contrast to the low positive predictive value, the negative predictive value of some inflammatory markers like CRP and PCT, and in combination with ILs, are good (26, 54, 67). Available evidence indicates that PCT may have the highest negative predictive value for severe, invasive bacterial infections in neonates (95, 96). Some high-quality intervention studies also show superiority of biomarker-guided duration of antibiotic therapy in neonatal (early- or late-onset) sepsis compared to a standard protocol (26, 67, 68, 97). The NICE-guideline states that if continuing antibiotics for longer than 36 h despite negative blood cultures, one should review the baby at least once every 24 h. Each day one should consider whether it is appropriate to stop antibiotic treatment, taking account of the level of initial clinical suspicion of infection, the baby's clinical progress and current condition, and whether there are "reassuring" levels and trends of CRP (8). One potential weakness with this high-quality guideline is the lack of discussion around which CRP values that can be interpreted as "reassuring." After implementing the NICE guidelines recommending measuring CRP 18–24 h after commencing antibiotics, one report in fact showed that this led to more investigations and longer duration of antibiotic treatment (98).

A recent large randomized trial showed that PCT-guided decision-making was superior to standard care in reducing antibiotic therapy in neonates with suspected EONS. Clinicians may still "struggle" to become familiar with postnatal age specific PCT cut-off values over the first few 72 h of life which may confound the interpretation of a negative and a positive PCT value for the diagnosis of EONS. Therefore, a web-based guide for PCT-guided decision-making will hopefully be published in 2018-2019 (personal communication). A survey performed in 2011-2012 in Europe, North-America and Australia showed that PCT at that time was not as widely used as CRP to diagnose EONS (36). However, like for CRP, PCT seems to be an excellent additional tool to rule out EONS as long as age specific values are taken into account.

FUTURE DEFINITION OF NEONATAL SEPSIS

The International Classification of Diseases, 10th Revision (ICD-10), defines different subtypes of bacterial sepsis in the newborn (P36). When specific pathogens are identified in the blood culture, the codes P36.0-8 are applied. For all other cases, e.g., when the clinician "believes" the newborn has sepsis the code P36.9 "unspecified bacterial sepsis" is applied. Regional differences in the use of P36.9 clearly exemplifies the need for a uniform sepsis definition (10). Both the US and the UK EONS-guidelines present the typical clinical symptoms that may indicate EONS, but do not specify clinical criteria defining sepsis in the absence of a positive blood culture (8, 31). Examples of some suggested neonatal sepsis criteria are presented in **Table 2**.

How can we define sepsis in neonates with a negative blood culture? Current adult sepsis definition is a "dysregulated host response to infection and organ dysfunction." An adoption of this definition for neonatal sepsis may be possible, but the terms "dysregulated host response," "infection," and "organ dysfunction" need to be defined for the neonatal population. Interestingly, there are no risk factors included in the new adult Sepsis-3 definition, although risk factors also exist for sepsis in the adult population. Risk factors for EONS are well anchored in the sepsis framework for pediatricians and neonatologists. Clinical symptoms of sepsis may overlap with non-inflammatory conditions and we suggest that parameters reflecting a host inflammatory response ("dysregulated host response") need to be included in order to establish a sepsis diagnosis in the absence of growth in a blood culture. Moreover, the biochemical picture of neonatal sepsis changes over the first days after antibiotics has been commenced for a suspected sepsis episode, and the kinetics of inflammatory biomarkers could also be included in a future sepsis definition. Finally, there is an urgent need for an international definition of organ dysfunction in neonates, which for the first days of life require a dynamic evaluation. Wynn and Polin recently called for a consensus definition of neonatal sepsis (5). As a group of European authors on neonatal sepsis we strongly agree with this call for action.

FUTURE STRATEGIES FOR EFFICIENT MANAGEMENT OF CULTURE-NEGATIVE SEPSIS

Two important factors may substantially reduce the number of cases coined as culture-negative sepsis.

First, available evidence indicate that blood cultures in neonates are highly sensitive, at least down to volumes of 0.5–1.0 mL. In neonatal units with available equipment and resources for obtaining blood cultures this diagnostic procedure must always be performed prior to commencing antibiotic therapy, with adequate aseptic technique and drawing a sufficient volume, preferably 1 mL and minimum 0.5 mL (9). We suggest to clearly record in the patient chart the blood culture volume taken. Automated 24-h electronic systems for reporting negative or positive (i.e., growth detected) blood culture results at 36–48 h incubation should be implemented in each hospital to support clinical decision-making of stopping antibiotics. Unless there is a strong clinical or biochemical indication to prolong antibiotics physician need to trust the culture results when an adequate volume is obtained and to stop antibiotics for suspected sepsis within 36–48 h. Our recommendations are in line with a recently published perspective article entitled "ending the culture of culture-negative sepsis in the neonatal ICU" where the authors urgently ask clinicians to trust negative cultures (9).

Second, a robust and pragmatic neonatal sepsis definition may reduce subjective variations in antibiotic use and support clinicians providing "appropriate" antibiotic therapy to those infants who need antibiotics. EONS is a dynamic and complex condition. A static definition of clinical symptoms reflecting organ dysfunction at a single point (disease onset) is most likely too unspecific to define EONS and guide antibiotic therapy.

A combination of risk factors, symptoms at disease onset combined with development of symptoms upon evaluation after 36–48 h is an alternative approach. This would concomitantly be in line with clinical guidelines strongly suggesting reviewing the infant and deciding whether one should stop treatment of suspected EONS after 36–48 h. Escobar and co-workers developed an electronic sepsis calculator applicable for newborns ≥34 weeks' gestation including both quantitative maternal risk factors and clinical symptoms after birth. Implementation of this calculator in routine clinical care has been associated with a substantial and concomitantly and probably safe reduction in the number of infants commenced on antibiotics for suspected EONS in several countries (35, 99, 100). We believe a similar strategy for diagnosing EONS; including development of clinical symptoms over 36–48 h combined with a biomarker-guided approach may further reduce the unnecessary prolonged duration of antibiotic treatment. CRP and PCT, optionally combined with interleukin 6 or 8, are currently the most attractive biomarkers for this purpose.

In conclusion, there is a need to align the road toward efficient sepsis care with the road toward antimicrobial stewardship in the neonatal unit. Early antibiotic therapy for truly infected newborns is crucial for an optimal outcome. On the other hand, prolonged antibiotic therapy for non-infected newborns is harmful for their microbiota, for their future health and for the community.

AUTHOR CONTRIBUTIONS

CK wrote the first draft of the manuscript. RK, GB, RM, and MS critically revised the manuscript for important intellectual content. All authors read and approved the final manuscript.

REFERENCES

1. Shane AL, Sanchez PJ, Stoll BJ. Neonatal sepsis. *Lancet* (2017) 390:1770–80. doi: 10.1016/S0140-6736(17)31002-4
2. Wynn JL, Polin RA. Progress in the management of neonatal sepsis: the importance of a consensus definition. *Pediatr Res.* (2018) 83:13–5. doi: 10.1038/pr.2017.224
3. Singer M, Deutschman CS, Seymour CW, Shankar-Hari M, Annane D, Bauer M, et al. The third international consensus definitions for sepsis and septic shock (Sepsis-3). *JAMA* (2016) 315:801–10. doi: 10.1001/jama.2016.0287
4. Schlapbach LJ, Kissoon N. Defining pediatric sepsis. *JAMA Pediatr.* (2018) 172:312–4. doi: 10.1001/jamapediatrics.2017.5208
5. Schlapbach LJ. Time for sepsis-3 in children? *Pediatr Crit Care Med.* (2017) 18:805–6. doi: 10.1097/PCC.0000000000001203
6. Haque KN. Definitions of bloodstream infection in the newborn. *Pediatr Crit Care Med.* (2005) 6(3 Suppl.):S45–9. doi: 10.1097/01.PCC.0000161946.73305.0A
7. Wynn JL, Wong HR, Shanley TP, Bizzarro MJ, Saiman L, Polin RA. Time for a neonatal-specific consensus definition for sepsis. *Pediatr Crit Care Med.* (2014) 15:523–8. doi: 10.1097/PCC.0000000000000157
8. National Institute for Health and Care Excellence (NICE). *Antibiotics for Early-onset Neonatal Infection: Antibiotics for the Prevention and Treatment of Early-Onset Neonatal Infection.* London: Clinical guideline [CG149] (2012). Available online at: https://www.nice.org.uk/guidance/cg149
9. Cantey JB, Baird SD. Ending the culture of culture-negative sepsis in the neonatal ICU. *Pediatrics* (2017) 140:e20170044. doi: 10.1542/peds.2017-0044
10. Fjalstad JW, Stensvold HJ, Bergseng H, Simonsen GS, Salvesen B, Ronnestad AE, et al. Early-onset sepsis and antibiotic exposure in term infants: a nationwide population-based study in Norway. *Pediatr Infect Dis J.* (2016) 35:1–6. doi: 10.1097/INF.0000000000000906
11. Cantey JB, Wozniak PS, Pruszynski JE, Sanchez PJ. Reducing unnecessary antibiotic use in the neonatal intensive care unit (SCOUT): a prospective interrupted time-series study. *Lancet Infect Dis.* (2016) 16:1178–84. doi: 10.1016/S1473-3099(16)30205-5
12. Schulman J, Dimand RJ, Lee HC, Duenas GV, Bennett MV, Gould JB. Neonatal intensive care unit antibiotic use. *Pediatrics* (2015) 135:826–33. doi: 10.1542/peds.2014-3409
13. Esaiassen E, Fjalstad JW, Juvet LK, van den Anker JN, Klingenberg C. Antibiotic exposure in neonates and early adverse outcomes: a systematic review and meta-analysis. *J Antimicrob Chemother.* (2017) 72:1858–70. doi: 10.1093/jac/dkx088
14. Mitre E, Susi A, Kropp LE, Schwartz DJ, Gorman GH, Nylund CM. Association between use of acid-suppressive medications and antibiotics during infancy and allergic diseases in early childhood. *JAMA Pediatr.* (2018) 172:e180315. doi: 10.1001/jamapediatrics.2018.2513
15. Rasmussen SH, Shrestha S, Bjerregaard LG, Angquist LH, Baker JL, Jess T, et al. Antibiotic exposure in early life and childhood overweight and obesity: a systematic review and meta-analysis. *Diabetes Obes Metab.* (2018) 20:1508–14. doi: 10.1111/dom.13230
16. Cordery RJ, Roberts CH, Cooper SJ, Bellinghan G, Shetty N. Evaluation of risk factors for the acquisition of bloodstream infections with extended-spectrum beta-lactamase-producing *Escherichia coli* and Klebsiella species in the intensive care unit; antibiotic management and clinical outcome. *J Hosp Infect.* (2008) 68:108–15. doi: 10.1016/j.jhin.2007.10.011
17. Cantey JB, Sanchez PJ. Prolonged antibiotic therapy for "culture-negative" sepsis in preterm infants: it's time to stop! *J Pediatr.* (2011) 159:707–8. doi: 10.1016/j.jpeds.2011.07.032
18. Stoll BJ, Hansen NI, Sanchez PJ, Faix RG, Poindexter BB, Van Meurs KP, et al. Early onset neonatal sepsis: the burden of group *B Streptococcal* and *E. coli* disease continues. *Pediatrics* (2011) 127:817–26. doi: 10.1542/peds.2010-2217
19. Singh T, Barnes EH, Isaacs D. Early-onset neonatal infections in Australia and New Zealand, 2002-2012. *Arch Dis Child Fetal Neonatal Ed.* (2018). doi: 10.1136/archdischild-2017-314671. [Epub ahead of print].
20. Schrag SJ, Farley MM, Petit S, Reingold A, Weston EJ, Pondo T, et al. Epidemiology of invasive early-onset neonatal sepsis, 2005 to 2014. *Pediatrics* (2016) 138:e20162013. doi: 10.1542/peds.2016-2013
21. Bekker V, Bijlsma MW, van de Beek D, Kuijpers TW, van der Ende A. Incidence of invasive group B streptococcal disease and pathogen genotype distribution in newborn babies in the Netherlands over 25 years: a nationwide surveillance study. *Lancet Infect Dis.* (2014) 14:1083–9. doi: 10.1016/S1473-3099(14)70919-3
22. Cailes B, Kortsalioudaki C, Buttery J, Pattnayak S, Greenough A, Matthes J, et al. Epidemiology of UK neonatal infections: the neonIN infection surveillance network. *Arch Dis Child Fetal Neonatal Ed.* (2017). doi: 10.1136/archdischild-2017-313203. [Epub ahead of print].
23. Drageset M, Fjalstad JW, Mortensen S, Klingenberg C. Management of early-onset neonatal sepsis differs in the north and south of Scandinavia. *Acta Paediatr.* (2017) 106:375–81. doi: 10.1111/apa.13698
24. Hofer N, Muller W, Resch B. Neonates presenting with temperature symptoms: role in the diagnosis of early onset sepsis. *Pediatr Int.* (2012) 54:486–90. doi: 10.1111/j.1442-200X.2012.03570.x
25. Lacaze-Masmonteil T, Rosychuk RJ, Robinson JL. Value of a single C-reactive protein measurement at 18 h of age. *Arch Dis Child Fetal Neonatal Ed.* (2014) 99:F76–9. doi: 10.1136/archdischild-2013-303984
26. Stocker M, van Herk W, El Helou S, Dutta S, Fontana MS, Schuerman FABA, et al. Procalcitonin-guided decision making for duration of antibiotic therapy in neonates with suspected early-onset sepsis: a multicentre, randomized controlled trial (NeoPIns). *Lancet* (2017) 390:871–81. doi: 10.1016/S0140-6736(17)31444-7

27. Duvoisin G, Fischer C, Maucort-Boulch D, Giannoni E. Reduction in the use of diagnostic tests in infants with risk factors for early-onset neonatal sepsis does not delay antibiotic treatment. *Swiss Med Wkly.* (2014) 144:w13981. doi: 10.4414/smw.2014.13981
28. Bakhuizen SE, de Haan TR, Teune MJ, van Wassenaer-Leemhuis AG, van der Heyden JL, van der Ham DP, et al. Meta-analysis shows that infants who have suffered neonatal sepsis face an increased risk of mortality and severe complications. *Acta Paediatr.* (2014) 103:1211–8. doi: 10.1111/apa.12764
29. Schlapbach LJ, Aebischer M, Adams M, Natalucci G, Bonhoeffer J, Latzin P, et al. Impact of sepsis on neurodevelopmental outcome in a Swiss National Cohort of extremely premature infants. *Pediatrics* (2011) 128:e348–57. doi: 10.1542/peds.2010-3338
30. Weiss SL, Fitzgerald JC, Balamuth F, Alpern ER, Lavelle J, Chilutti M, et al. Delayed antimicrobial therapy increases mortality and organ dysfunction duration in pediatric sepsis. *Crit Care Med.* (2014) 42:2409–17. doi: 10.1097/CCM.0000000000000509
31. Polin RA. Management of neonates with suspected or proven early-onset bacterial sepsis. *Pediatrics* (2012) 129:1006–15. doi: 10.1542/peds.2012-0541
32. Jefferies AL. Management of term infants at increased risk for early-onset bacterial sepsis. *Paediatr Child Health* (2017) 22:223–8. doi: 10.1093/pch/pxx023
33. Trijbels-Smeulders M, de Jonge GA, Pasker-de Jong PC, Gerards LJ, Adriaanse AH, van Lingen RA, et al. Epidemiology of neonatal group B streptococcal disease in the Netherlands before and after introduction of guidelines for prevention. *Arch Dis Child Fetal Neonatal Ed.* (2007) 92:F271–6. doi: 10.1136/adc.2005.088799
34. Schrag SJ, Zell ER, Lynfield R, Roome A, Arnold KE, Craig AS, et al. A population-based comparison of strategies to prevent early-onset group B streptococcal disease in neonates. *N Engl J Med.* (2002) 347:233–9. doi: 10.1056/NEJMoa020205
35. Kuzniewicz MW, Puopolo KM, Fischer A, Walsh EM, Li S, Newman TB, et al. A quantitative, risk-based approach to the management of neonatal early-onset sepsis. *JAMA Pediatr.* (2017) 171:365–71. doi: 10.1001/jamapediatrics.2016.4678
36. van Herk W, el Helou S, Janota J, Hagmann C, Klingenberg C, Staub E, et al. Variation in current management of term and late-preterm neonates at risk for early-onset sepsis: an international survey and review of guidelines. *Pediatr Infect Dis J.* (2016) 35:494–500. doi: 10.1097/INF.0000000000001063
37. Puopolo KM, Draper D, Wi S, Newman TB, Zupancic J, Lieberman E, et al. Estimating the probability of neonatal early-onset infection on the basis of maternal risk factors. *Pediatrics* (2011) 128:e1155–63. doi: 10.1542/peds.2010-3464
38. Goldstein B, Giroir B, Randolph A. International pediatric sepsis consensus conference: definitions for sepsis and organ dysfunction in pediatrics. *Pediatr Crit Care Med.* (2005) 6:2–8. doi: 10.1097/00130478-200501000-00049
39. Oeser C, Lutsar I, Metsvaht T, Turner MA, Heath PT, Sharland M. Clinical trials in neonatal sepsis. *J Antimicrob Chemother.* (2013) 68:2733–45. doi: 10.1093/jac/dkt297
40. Hakansson S, Lilja M, Jacobsson B, Kallen K. Reduced incidence of neonatal early-onset group B streptococcal infection after promulgation of guidelines for risk-based intrapartum antibiotic prophylaxis in Sweden: analysis of a national population-based cohort. *Acta Obstet Gynecol Scand.* (2017) 96:1475–83. doi: 10.1111/aogs.13211
41. Tveiten L, Diep LM, Halvorsen T, Markestad T. Respiratory rate during the first 24 hours of life in healthy term infants. *Pediatrics* (2016) 137:e20152326. doi: 10.1542/peds.2015-2326
42. Doan E, Gibbons K, Tudehope D. The timing of elective caesarean deliveries and early neonatal outcomes in singleton infants born 37-41 weeks' gestation. *Aust N Z J Obstet Gynaecol.* (2014) 54:340–7. doi: 10.1111/ajo.12220
43. Koch L, Bosk A, Sasse M, Ruef P, Poeschl J. Managing neonatal severe sepsis in Germany: a preliminary survey of current practices. *Klin Padiatr.* (2015) 227:23–7. doi: 10.1055/s-0034-1389975
44. Raju NV, Maisels MJ, Kring E, Schwarz-Warner L. Capillary refill time in the hands and feet of normal newborn infants. *Clin Pediatr.* (1999) 38:139–44. doi: 10.1177/000992289903800303
45. Strozik KS, Pieper CH, Roller J. Capillary refilling time in newborn babies: normal values. *Arch Dis Child Fetal Neonatal Ed.* (1997) 76:F193–6. doi: 10.1136/fn.76.3.F193
46. Puopolo KM, Mukhopadhyay S, Hansen NI, Cotten CM, Stoll BJ, Sanchez PJ, et al. Identification of extremely premature infants at low risk for early-onset sepsis. *Pediatrics* (2017) 140:e20170925. doi: 10.1542/peds.2017-0925
47. Ng PC, Ma TP, Lam HS. The use of laboratory biomarkers for surveillance, diagnosis and prediction of clinical outcomes in neonatal sepsis and necrotising enterocolitis. *Arch Dis Child Fetal Neonatal Ed.* (2015) 100:F448–52. doi: 10.1136/archdischild-2014-307656
48. Ng S, Strunk T, Jiang P, Muk T, Sangild PT, Currie A. Precision medicine for neonatal sepsis. *Front Mol Biosci.* (2018) 5:70. doi: 10.3389/fmolb.2018.00070
49. Hornik CP, Benjamin DK, Becker KC, Benjamin DK Jr, Li J, Clark RH, et al. Use of the complete blood cell count in early-onset neonatal sepsis. *Pediatr Infect Dis J.* (2012) 31:799–802. doi: 10.1097/INF.0b013e318256905c
50. Newman TB, Puopolo KM, Wi S, Draper D, Escobar GJ. Interpreting complete blood counts soon after birth in newborns at risk for sepsis. *Pediatrics* (2010) 126:903–9. doi: 10.1542/peds.2010-0935
51. van der Meer W, van Gelder W, de Keijzer R, Willems H. Does the band cell survive the 21st century? *Eur J Haematol.* (2006) 76:251–4. doi: 10.1111/j.1600-0609.2005.00597.x
52. Del Vecchio A. Evaluation and management of thrombocytopenic neonates in the intensive care unit. *Early Hum Dev.* (2014) 90(Suppl. 2):S51–5. doi: 10.1016/S0378-3782(14)50014-X
53. Spector SA, Ticknor W, Grossman M. Study of the usefulness of clinical and hematologic findings in the diagnosis of neonatal bacterial infections. *Clin Pediatr.* (1981) 20:385–92. doi: 10.1177/000992288102000602
54. Hofer N, Zacharias E, Muller W, Resch B. An update on the use of C-reactive protein in early-onset neonatal sepsis: current insights and new tasks. *Neonatology* (2012) 102:25–36. doi: 10.1159/000336629
55. Perrone S, Lotti F, Longini M, Rossetti A, Bindi I, Bazzini F, et al. C reactive protein in healthy term newborns during the first 48 hours of life. *Arch Dis Child Fetal Neonatal Ed.* (2018) 103:F163–6. doi: 10.1136/archdischild-2016-312506
56. Turner MA, Power S, Emmerson AJ. Gestational age and the C reactive protein response. *Arch Dis Child Fetal Neonatal Ed.* (2004) 89:F272–3. doi: 10.1136/adc.2002.011288
57. Chiesa C, Natale F, Pascone R, Osborn JF, Pacifico L, Bonci E, et al. C reactive protein and procalcitonin: reference intervals for preterm and term newborns during the early neonatal period. *Clin Chim Acta* (2011) 412:1053–9. doi: 10.1016/j.cca.2011.02.020
58. Chiesa C, Signore F, Assumma M, Buffone E, Tramontozzi P, Osborn JF, et al. Serial measurements of C-reactive protein and interleukin-6 in the immediate postnatal period: reference intervals and analysis of maternal and perinatal confounders. *Clin Chem.* (2001) 47:1016–22.
59. Ishibashi M, Takemura Y, Ishida H, Watanabe K, Kawai T. C-reactive protein kinetics in newborns: application of a high-sensitivity analytic method in its determination. *Clin Chem.* (2002) 48:1103–6.
60. Hofer N, Muller W, Resch B. Non-infectious conditions and gestational age influence C-reactive protein values in newborns during the first 3 days of life. *Clin Chem Lab Med.* (2011) 49:297–302. doi: 10.1515/CCLM.2011.048
61. Robinson P, De SK. How to use. Procalcitonin. *Arch Dis Child Educ Pract Ed.* (2018) 103:257–62. doi: 10.1136/archdischild-2017-313699
62. Dandona P, Nix D, Wilson MF, Aljada A, Love J, Assicot M, et al. Procalcitonin increase after endotoxin injection in normal subjects. *J Clin Endocrinol Metab.* (1994) 79:1605–8.
63. Chiesa C, Pacifico L, Osborn JF, Bonci E, Hofer N, Resch B. Early-onset neonatal sepsis: still room for improvement in procalcitonin diagnostic accuracy studies. *Medicine* (2015) 94:e1230. doi: 10.1097/MD.0000000000001230
64. Chiesa C, Pellegrini G, Panero A, Osborn JF, Signore F, Assumma M, et al. C-reactive protein, interleukin-6, and procalcitonin in the immediate postnatal period: influence of illness severity, risk status, antenatal and perinatal complications, and infection. *Clin Chem.* (2003) 49:60–8. doi: 10.1373/49.1.60
65. Stocker M, Fontana M, El HS, Wegscheider K, Berger TM. Use of procalcitonin-guided decision-making to shorten antibiotic therapy in suspected neonatal early-onset sepsis: prospective randomized intervention trial. *Neonatology* (2010) 97:165–74. doi: 10.1159/000241296
66. Chiesa C, Panero A, Rossi N, Stegagno M, De GM, Osborn JF, et al. Reliability of procalcitonin concentrations for the diagnosis of sepsis in

critically ill neonates. *Clin Infect Dis.* (1998) 26:664–72. doi: 10.1086/514576
67. Franz AR, Steinbach G, Kron M, Pohlandt F. Reduction of unnecessary antibiotic therapy in newborn infants using interleukin-8 and C-reactive protein as markers of bacterial infections. *Pediatrics* (1999) 104(3 Pt 1):447–53.
68. Franz AR, Steinbach G, Kron M, Pohlandt F. Interleukin-8: a valuable tool to restrict antibiotic therapy in newborn infants. *Acta Paediatr.* (2001) 90:1025–32. doi: 10.1111/j.1651-2227.2001.tb01359.x
69. Fjalstad JW, Esaiassen E, Juvet LK, van den Anker JN, Klingenberg C. Antibiotic therapy in neonates and impact on gut microbiota and antibiotic resistance development: a systematic review. *J Antimicrob Chemother.* (2017) 73:569–80. doi: 10.1093/jac/dkx426
70. Rohatgi S, Dewan P, Faridi MMA, Kumar A, Malhotra RK, Batra P. Seven versus 10 days antibiotic therapy for culture-proven neonatal sepsis: a randomized controlled trial. *J Paediatr Child Health* (2017) 53:556–62. doi: 10.1111/jpc.13518
71. Ting JY, Synnes A, Roberts A, Deshpandey A, Dow K, Yoon EW, et al. Association between antibiotic use and neonatal mortality and morbidities in very low-birth-weight infants without culture-proven sepsis or necrotizing enterocolitis. *JAMA Pediatr.* (2016) 170:1181–7. doi: 10.1001/jamapediatrics.2016.2132
72. Mukhopadhyay S, Puopolo KM. Antibiotic use and mortality among premature infants without confirmed infection-perpetrator or innocent bystander? *JAMA Pediatr.* (2016) 170:1144–6. doi: 10.1001/jamapediatrics.2016.2836
73. Laxminarayan R, Duse A, Wattal C, Zaidi AK, Wertheim HF, Sumpradit N, et al. Antibiotic resistance-the need for global solutions. *Lancet Infect Dis.* (2013) 13:1057–98. doi: 10.1016/S1473-3099(13)70318-9
74. Blaser MJ. Antibiotic use and its consequences for the normal microbiome. *Science* (2016) 352:544–5. doi: 10.1126/science.aad9358
75. Gensollen T, Iyer SS, Kasper DL, Blumberg RS. How colonization by microbiota in early life shapes the immune system. *Science* (2016) 352:539–44. doi: 10.1126/science.aad9378
76. Gohir W, Ratcliffe EM, Sloboda DM. Of the bugs that shape us: maternal obesity, the gut microbiome, and long-term disease risk. *Pediatr Res.* (2015) 77:196–204. doi: 10.1038/pr.2014.169
77. Schulfer A, Blaser MJ. Risks of antibiotic exposures early in life on the developing microbiome. *PLoS Pathog.* (2015) 11:e1004903. doi: 10.1371/journal.ppat.1004903
78. Goff DA, Kullar R, Bauer KA, File TM Jr. Eight habits of highly effective antimicrobial stewardship programs to meet the joint commission standards for hospitals. *Clin Infect Dis.* (2017) 64:1134–9. doi: 10.1093/cid/cix065
79. Nzegwu NI, Rychalsky MR, Nallu LA, Song X, Deng Y, Natusch AM, et al. Implementation of an antimicrobial stewardship program in a neonatal intensive care unit. *Infect Control Hosp Epidemiol.* (2017) 38:1137–43. doi: 10.1017/ice.2017.151
80. Ting JY, Paquette V, Ng K, Lisonkova S, Hait V, Shivanada S, et al. Reduction of inappropriate antimicrobial prescriptions in a tertiary neonatal intensive care unit following antimicrobial stewardship care bundle implementation. *Pediatr Infect Dis J.* (2018). doi: 10.1097/INF.0000000000002039. [Epub ahead of print].
81. Blackburn RM, Muller-Pebody B, Planche T, Johnson A, Hopkins S, Sharland M, et al. Neonatal sepsis–many blood samples, few positive cultures: implications for improving antibiotic prescribing. *Arch Dis Child Fetal Neonatal Ed.* (2012) 97:F487–8. doi: 10.1136/archdischild-2012-302261
82. Brown DR, Kutler D, Rai B, Chan T, Cohen M. Bacterial concentration and blood volume required for a positive blood culture. *J Perinatol.* (1995) 15:157–9.
83. Buttery JP. Blood cultures in newborns and children: optimizing an everyday test. *Arch Dis Child Fetal Neonatal Ed.* (2002) 87:F25–8. doi: 10.1136/fn.87.1.F25
84. Paul SP, Caplan EM, Morgan HA, Turner PC. Barriers to implementing the NICE guidelines for early-onset neonatal infection: cross-sectional survey of neonatal blood culture reporting by laboratories in the UK. *J Hosp Infect.* (2018) 98:425–8. doi: 10.1016/j.jhin.2017.12.015
85. Garcia-Prats JA, Cooper TR, Schneider VF, Stager CE, Hansen TN. Rapid detection of microorganisms in blood cultures of newborn infants utilizing an automated blood culture system. *Pediatrics* (2000) 105(3 Pt 1): 523–7.
86. Jardine L, Davies MW, Faoagali J. Incubation time required for neonatal blood cultures to become positive. *J Paediatr Child Health* (2006) 42:797–802. doi: 10.1111/j.1440-1754.2006.00980.x
87. Jardine MA, Kumar Y, Kausalya S, Harigopal S, Wong J, Shivaram A, et al. Reducing antibiotic use on the neonatal unit by improving communication of blood culture results: a completed audit cycle. *Arch Dis Child Fetal Neonatal Ed.* (2003) 88:F255. doi: 10.1136/fn.88.3.F255-a
88. Vamsi SR, Bhat RY, Lewis LE, Vandana KE. Time to positivity of blood cultures in neonates. *Pediatr Infect Dis J.* (2014) 33:212–4. doi: 10.1097/INF.0000000000000018
89. Giannoni E, Agyeman PKA, Stocker M, Posfay-Barbe KM, Heininger U, Spycher BD, et al. Neonatal sepsis of early onset, and hospital-acquired and community-acquired late onset: a prospective population-based cohort study. *J Pediatr.* (2018) 201:106–14.e4. doi: 10.1016/j.jpeds.2018.05.048
90. Sarkar SS, Bhagat I, Bhatt-Mehta V, Sarkar S. Does maternal intrapartum antibiotic treatment prolong the incubation time required for blood cultures to become positive for infants with early-onset sepsis? *Am J Perinatol.* (2015) 32:357–62. doi: 10.1055/s-0034-1387933
91. Jardine LA, Sturgess BR, Inglis GD, Davies MW. Neonatal blood cultures: effect of delayed entry into the blood culture machine and bacterial concentration on the time to positive growth in a simulated model. *J Paediatr Child Health* (2009) 45:210–4. doi: 10.1111/j.1440-1754.2008.01455.x
92. Pammi M, Flores A, Leeflang M, Versalovic J. Molecular assays in the diagnosis of neonatal sepsis: a systematic review and meta-analysis. *Pediatrics* (2011) 128:e973–85. doi: 10.1542/peds.2011-1208
93. Pammi M, Flores A, Versalovic J, Leeflang MM. Molecular assays for the diagnosis of sepsis in neonates. *Cochrane Database Syst Rev.* (2017) 2:CD011926. doi: 10.1002/14651858.CD011926.pub2
94. van den Brand M, van den Dungen FAM, Bos MP, van Weissenbruch MM, van Furth AM, de LA, et al. Evaluation of a real-time PCR assay for detection and quantification of bacterial DNA directly in blood of preterm neonates with suspected late-onset sepsis. *Crit Care* (2018) 22:105. doi: 10.1186/s13054-018-2010-4
95. van Rossum AM, Wulkan RW, Oudesluys-Murphy AM. Procalcitonin as an early marker of infection in neonates and children. *Lancet Infect Dis.* (2004) 4:620–30. doi: 10.1016/S1473-3099(04)01146-6
96. Vouloumanou EK, Plessa E, Karageorgopoulos DE, Mantadakis E, Falagas ME. Serum procalcitonin as a diagnostic marker for neonatal sepsis: a systematic review and meta-analysis. *Intensive Care Med.* (2011) 37:747–62. doi: 10.1007/s00134-011-2174-8
97. Ehl S, Gering B, Bartmann P, Hogel J, Pohlandt F. C-reactive protein is a useful marker for guiding duration of antibiotic therapy in suspected neonatal bacterial infection. *Pediatrics* (1997) 99:216–21. doi: 10.1542/peds.99.2.216
98. Mukherjee A, Davidson L, Anguvaa L, Duffy DA, Kennea N. NICE neonatal early onset sepsis guidance: greater consistency, but more investigations, and greater length of stay. *Arch Dis Child Fetal Neonatal Ed.* (2015) 100:F248–9. doi: 10.1136/archdischild-2014-306349
99. Achten NB, Dorigo-Zetsma JW, van der Linden PD, van BM, Plotz FB. Sepsis calculator implementation reduces empiric antibiotics for suspected early-onset sepsis. *Eur J Pediatr.* (2018) 177:741–6. doi: 10.1007/s00431-018-3113-2
100. Strunk T, Buchiboyina A, Sharp M, Nathan E, Doherty D, Patole S. Implementation of the neonatal sepsis calculator in an Australian tertiary perinatal center. *Neonatology* (2018) 113:379–82. doi: 10.1159/000487298

5

Immunomodulation to Prevent or Treat Neonatal Sepsis: Past, Present and Future

Simone S. Schüller[1,2,3*], *Boris W. Kramer*[4,5], *Eduardo Villamor*[4,5], *Andreas Spittler*[6], *Angelika Berger*[1] *and Ofer Levy*[2,3,7*]

[1] *Division of Neonatology, Pediatric Intensive Care & Neuropediatrics, Department of Pediatrics and Adolescent Medicine, Medical University of Vienna, Vienna, Austria,* [2] *Precision Vaccines Program, Division of Infectious Diseases, Department of Medicine, Boston Children's Hospital, Boston, MA, United States,* [3] *Harvard Medical School, Boston, MA, United States,* [4] *Department of Pediatrics, Maastricht University Medical Centre (MUMC+), Maastricht, Netherlands,* [5] *School for Oncology and Developmental Biology (GROW), Maastricht University, Maastricht, Netherlands,* [6] *Department of Surgery, Research Labs & Core Facility Flow Cytometry, Medical University of Vienna, Vienna, Austria,* [7] *Broad Institute of MIT and Harvard, Boston, MA, United States*

***Correspondence:**
Simone S. Schüller
simone.schueller@meduniwien.ac.at
Ofer Levy
ofer.levy@childrens.harvard.edu

Despite continued advances in neonatal medicine, sepsis remains a leading cause of death worldwide in neonatal intensive care units. The clinical presentation of sepsis in neonates varies markedly from that in older children and adults, and distinct acute inflammatory responses results in age-specific inflammatory and protective immune response to infection. This review first provides an overview of the neonatal immune system, then covers current mainstream, and experimental preventive and adjuvant therapies in neonatal sepsis. We also discuss how the distinct physiology of the perinatal period shapes early life immune responses and review strategies to reduce neonatal sepsis-related morbidity and mortality. A summary of studies that characterize immune ontogeny and neonatal sepsis is presented, followed by discussion of clinical trials assessing interventions such as breast milk, lactoferrin, probiotics, and pentoxifylline. Finally, we critically appraise future treatment options such as stem cell therapy, other antimicrobial protein and peptides, and targeting of pattern recognition receptors in an effort to prevent and/or treat sepsis in this highly vulnerable neonatal population.

Keywords: neonatal sepsis, preterm infant, adjuvant sepsis therapy, immunomodulation, pentoxifylline, lactoferrin, probiotics, human milk

INTRODUCTION

Despite advances in neonatal care leading to improved survival rates and reduced complications in preterm infants (1), there has been little improvement in the prophylaxis, treatment, and adverse neurodevelopmental outcomes associated with neonatal sepsis over the last three decades (2–5). The incidence of neonatal sepsis is inversely correlated with gestational age (GA) and birth weight (BW). While ~20% of very low BW (<1,500 g; VLBW) infants suffer from one or more systemic infections during their hospital stay (6, 7), the rate may reach up to 60% in the most immature infants (8). Inflammatory conditions such as neonatal sepsis and necrotizing enterocolitis (NEC) are associated with persistently high morbidity and mortality rates in these infants (9, 10).

DEFINITION AND CLINICAL COURSE OF NEONATAL SEPSIS

While a consensus definition of pediatric sepsis exists, defined as a systemic inflammatory response syndrome (SIRS) in the presence of suspected or proven infection (11), no such consensus definition has yet been published for neonatal sepsis (12). Although a positive blood culture defines bacteremia and has been included in some proposed definitions of neonatal sepsis, such an approach does not take into account that in most cases of neonatal sepsis clinical signs are not associated with positive blood cultures (13). Recent studies included a combination of laboratory tests, clinical findings and/or the duration of antimicrobial treatment (≥5 days), reflecting complexity and heterogeneity in neonatal sepsis (3). Thus, in clinical practice, diagnosis of neonatal sepsis is complicated by the absence of a consensus definition, non-specific symptoms, and low sensitivity of the low volume bacterial blood cultures typically obtained (12). Furthermore, established diagnostic tests to predict severity and to guide treatment are lacking (3). Complete blood counts, including immature to total neutrophil ratios, C-reactive protein (CRP), interleukin (IL)-6 or CXCL-8 (IL-8), and procalcitonin (PCT) have some clinical utility (14). Cell surface markers on circulating cells, such as soluble CD14, CD64, and HLA-DR, offer some diagnostic value (15–17). However, much remains to be learned regarding optimal diagnostics and research in this area, including the application of systems biology approaches for biomarker discovery (18).

Early empiric treatment with antibiotics is essential for neonatal bacterial sepsis. Rapid clinical deterioration, however, may still ensue even if antibiotic treatment is started promptly. Possible life-threatening complications include the development of disseminated intra-vascular coagulation, pulmonary hypertension, congestive heart failure and shock (19). These complications can result from phases of excessive inflammation as well as immunosuppression (20–22). Until recently, the immunological basis of sepsis was thought to be a biphasic process with an initial hyperinflammatory phase followed by a later anti-inflammatory phase manifesting as functional immune suppression (23). However, genome-wide transcription profiling in human sepsis of term neonates, children, and adults demonstrates that phases of pro- and anti-inflammatory mechanisms occur during variable times over a sepsis episode and that patients may cycle through each phase multiple times during the course of sepsis (22, 24–28).

IMMUNOLOGICAL RISK FACTORS FOR NEONATAL SEPSIS

Little is known regarding the sepsis phases in preterm human neonates, but recent findings indicate that both gestational and postnatal age are significant factors affecting immune responses during the critical window of immune adaptation (20, 29, 30). During this window, pathogen-associated molecular patterns (PAMPs) and damage-associated molecular patterns (DAMPs) are potent inducers of inflammation and might shape immune responses early in life (31). Stimulation of pattern recognition receptors (PRRs) in human preterm blood by exogenous PAMPs induces T helper (Th) and anti-inflammatory profiles with impaired Th1 and pro-inflammatory cytokines (32). In this context, innate immunity in newborns has often been alluded to as "impaired," "defective," or "immature." However, it is more accurately described as "distinct" since the fetus/preterm neonate is well-equipped for life *in utero* and the term newborn immune system appropriately mediates the transition from *in utero* to *ex utero* life. For maintenance of tolerance to maternal antigens and to avoid inflammation-triggered preterm delivery, neonatal immune responses are in general T helper (Th)-2 and Th-17 cell biased (33). However, such polarization also corresponds to GA-dependent susceptibility to invasive infections (32, 34). In addition, decreased complement-mediated/phagocytic activity (35, 36), reduced absolute neutrophil counts and functions (37), as well as altered phenotype and function of professional antigen-presenting cells (APCs) (38–40) in response to most Toll-like-receptor agonists (TLRAs) have been described. Moreover, the distinct composition of neonatal plasma, including high concentrations of adenosine (41–44), prostaglandins (45), placental hormones such as cortisol (46), estradiol, and progesterone (47), inhibits the production of Th1 cytokines. In addition, adenosine may also contribute to impaired neutrophil responses by inhibiting neutrophil-endothelial adhesion molecules (48). In contrast, high perinatal levels of cytokines such as the migration inhibitory factor (MIF) (49) and d-dopachrome tautomerase (DDT, also known as MIF-2) (50) counter regulate the activity of adenosine and prostaglandin E2 and together with interleukin-18 (51) further shape immune responses early in life. Taken together, a tightly regulated distinct balance of pro- and anti-inflammatory mediators in neonates shapes early life innate immune responses.

Of note, with respect to human *in vitro* assays, whereas responses to most pure TLRAs are reduced in early life, live organisms such as Group B *streptococcus* (GBS) may signal robust inflammatory responses including TNF production (52). GBS signals in part via TLR8 (53), a TLR pathway that recognizes microbial viability (54). GBS in human newborn blood potentially acts via vita-PAMPs, that is a subset of PAMPs expressed specifically by live microorganism (55), and TLR8 that detects bacterial RNA (52, 54, 56) and might therefore contribute to an exaggerated inflammation in bacterial neonatal sepsis *in vivo* (20). In addition, pro-inflammatory IL-1β responses are impaired in cord blood of preterm infants, but are restored to adult levels during the neonatal period, indicating rapid maturation of these responses after birth (57). Systemic inflammation characterized by high concentrations of proinflammatory cytokines are associated with poor long-term outcomes, and preterm infants are especially vulnerable to inflammatory injuries (10).

A non-inflammatory profile with mature immunoregulatory capacities is acquired in an age—dependent manner and a delayed adjustment of regulatory signaling pathways might in part explain the preterm infants' susceptibility to inflammatory conditions. Neonatal cord blood of term neonates contains extremely high concentrations of alarmins that act as endogenous DAMPs (58). *In utero*, alarmins induce an "endotoxin-like state" by altering MyD88-dependent pro-inflammatory gene programs with corresponding low Th1 responses (30). After birth, alarmin-levels decrease and regulatory TIR-domain-containing adapter-inducing interferon-β (TRIF)-dependent genes gradually increase (30, 58). A disruption of this critical sequence of transient alarmin programming and subsequent reprogramming of regulatory pathways, as occurs in preterm birth, increase the risk of hyperinflammation and neonatal sepsis (30). Of note, alarmins are increased in intra-amniotic infection/inflammation (59) and histologic chorioamnionitis correlates with a decreased risk of LOS (60) indicating that perinatal inflammation may enhance the immunoregulatory and/or functional maturation of the preterm immune system.

Other counter-inflammatory mechanisms, such as increased numbers of regulatory T cells (61, 62), and myeloid-derived suppressor cells (63, 64), as well as impaired phagocytosis-induced cell death (65, 66) might further affect the outcome of neonatal sepsis. However, the role of these mechanisms in neonatal sepsis has not yet been fully delineated, mostly because of limited access to neonatal peripheral blood samples and difficulties in performing longitudinal studies to investigate neonatal immune ontogeny.

EPIDEMIOLOGICAL RISK FACTORS OF NEONATAL SEPSIS

In addition to GA-specific immunological characteristics, sex (67), genetic predisposition (68, 69), the evolving microbiome/microbial colonization (70), and underlying medical conditions shape immune responses and impact the risk of developing neonatal sepsis (4, 71). Given the number of cellular and molecular factors involved, emerging systems biology offer new avenues to monitor functional immune development in the near future (72–74).

The high susceptibility of preterm infants to invasive infections and associated poor long-term outcomes, have prompted the exploration of alternative therapies for neonatal sepsis. A number of interventions have been evaluated, and some such as oral lactoferrin have demonstrated promise (75), but beyond antibiotics and supportive care, there is presently no approved drug for the treatment or prevention of sepsis in preterm or term neonates (25, 76). This review summarizes past and present immunomodulatory concepts and outlines novel potential targets for the prevention and treatment of neonatal sepsis. A literature search for published meta-analyses, randomized controlled trials (RCTs), systematic reviews, individual clinical studies and emerging work from animal models was performed. A list of current approaches discussed in this article is presented in **Table 1** (treatment) and **Table 2** (prevention); the corresponding literature search strategy is outlined in Supplementary Figure 1.

PRIOR STUDIES THAT HAVE NOT DEMONSTRATED CLINICAL BENEFIT

Immunoglobulins

Preterm neonates born prior to 32 weeks gestation have low levels of passively acquired antibodies, and endogenous immunoglobulin (Ig) synthesis does not begin until 24 weeks of life (93, 94). Immunoglobulins provide opsonic activity, activate complement, and promote antibody-dependent cytotoxicity (95). Given these biological effects and the observation of decreased Ig levels in severe sepsis, several clinical studies have investigated the use of intravenous immunoglobulins (IVIG) to prevent and treat neonatal sepsis (78, 96–98).

A 2015 Cochrane Review, evaluating 9 IVIG studies and including a total of 3,973 infants showed no reduction of in-hospital mortality or in the combined outcome of death or major disability at 2 years of age in preterm infants with suspected or proven infection (**Table 1**) (78). Additionally, IgM-enriched IVIG preparations, which may provide higher opsonization activity and complement activation compared to IgG, did not significantly reduce mortality during hospital stay in infants with suspected sepsis ($n = 66$) (78). Based on these findings, routine administration of IVIG or IgM-enriched IVIG to prevent mortality in infants with suspected or proven neonatal infection cannot be recommended.

Given that >50% of cases of late-onset sepsis (LOS) in VLBW are caused by *Staphylococcus* spp., various type-specific antibodies targeted at different antigenic markers of *Staphylococcus* have been developed and studied in RCTs (82, 83). A 2009 Cochrane Review evaluated the effects of two anti-staphylococcal immunoglobulins, INH-A21 (pooled generic anti-staphylococcal immunoglobulin) and Altastaph (human polyclonal immunoglobulin against capsular polysaccharide antigens type 5 and 8), on the prevention of LOS in infants ≤32 weeks (82). No significant reduction in the risk of infection or mortality was identified (**Table 2**). A third anti-staphylococcal immunoglobulin, pagibaximab (anti-lipoteichoic acid monoclonal antibody) was studied, but again no significant reduction in sepsis or mortality was found (83, 84)(**Table 2**).

The reasons for these failed trials have not yet been elucidated but one might speculate that distinct immune responses in the preterm infant such as reduced complement or leukocyte activity may play a role or that the correct type or combination of antibodies has not yet been found (83). Future studies need to identify antibodies that (i) target optimal epitopes, (ii) have optimal bioactivity and/or (iii) can be targeted to carefully defined populations that are most likely to benefit from them. Studies of protective neutralizing antibodies against neonatal pathogens are ongoing (99). Prior to human studies, such investigations should evaluate the activity of potential immunomodulating products in an age-specific manner including in age-specific human *in vitro* platforms as well as in preterm animal models.

Glutamine

Endogenous glutamine, a conditionally essential amino acid, is insufficiently biosynthesized in states of metabolic stress.

TABLE 1 | Meta-analyses on adjunctive therapy for neonatal sepsis.

Intervention	Population	Outcome	RR (95% CI)	RCTs/infants	References
Pentoxifylline	All infants with confirmed or suspected sepsis	All-cause mortality to discharge	**0.57 (0.35–0.93)**	6/416	(77)
	All Infants with confirmed sepsis	All-cause mortality to discharge	**0.37 (0.19–0.73)**	4/235	(77)
	Preterm infants with confirmed or suspected sepsis	All-cause mortality to discharge	**0.38 (0.20–0.71)**	4/277	(77)
IVIG (polyvalent or IgM-enriched)	All infants with suspected infection	All-cause mortality to discharge	0.95 (0.80–1.13)	9/2527	(78)
IVIG (IgM-enriched)	All infants with suspected infection	All-cause mortality to discharge	0.68 (0.39–1.20)	4/267	(78)
GM-CSF or G-CSF	All infants with confirmed or suspected sepsis	All-cause mortality to 14 days	0.71 (0.38–1.33)	7/257	(79)
	All infants with confirmed or suspected sepsis	All-cause mortality to discharge	0.53 (0.25–1.16)	5/178	(79)
	Neutropenic infants with confirmed or suspected sepsis	All-cause mortality to discharge	0.38 (0.16–0.95)	3/97	(79)
Granulocyte transfusion	Neutropenic infants with confirmed or suspected sepsis	All-cause mortality to discharge	0.89 (0.43–1.86)	3/44	(80)
	Neutropenic preterm infants with confirmed or suspected sepsis	All-cause mortality to discharge	0.94 (0.39–2.24)	2/33	(80)

Cochrane reviews or the most updated meta-analysis on the topic were selected for inclusion in the table. Outcomes were selected based on relevance. Statistically significant results are marked in bold. CI, confidence interval; GM-CSF, granulocyte-macrophage colony stimulating factor; G-CSF, granulocyte colony stimulating factor; IVIG, intravenous immunoglobulin; RCT, randomized controlled trial; RR, risk ratio.

Accordingly the supplementation with glutamine improved clinical outcomes in critically ill adults (100). Glutamine is abundant in human milk, but levels in formula are much lower and it is not routinely supplemented in parenteral nutrition solutions for neonates.

Despite its potential role in metabolic stress, a systematic review of 12 RCTs including 2,877 VLBW did not find any effect of preventive glutamine supplementation on mortality or major neonatal morbidities (**Table 1**) (91). It remains unknown, whether glutamine supplementation may be beneficial in the recovery of critically ill infants, in particular, after gastrointestinal inflammatory processes such as NEC.

Antioxidants: Selenium, Melatonin, and Vitamin A

Preterm neonates are at increased risk of oxidative stress due to lower basal levels of plasma antioxidants and metal-binding proteins (ceruloplasmin, transferrin), reduced activity of antioxidant enzymes, and higher potential for exposure to reactive oxygen species (101–103). A 2003 Cochrane review including 297 preterm neonates (<32 weeks of gestation and/or BW $\leq$ 2,000 g) showed a significant reduction of sepsis episodes associated with prophylactic selenium supplementation but no difference in survival (**Table 2**) (92). A more recent RCT confirmed these findings (104); an updated meta-analysis is pending. Thus, selenium supplementation in preterm infants might reduce the incidence of sepsis, but does not affect overall mortality.

Melatonin has antioxidant, anti-inflammatory and anti-apoptotic properties that may improve neonatal sepsis outcome, in particular in mitochondrial injury (105). Three small single-center studies investigated the use of melatonin as adjuvant therapy in neonatal sepsis and results indicate a beneficial effect of melatonin (106–108). However, so far no follow-up RCTs have been conducted, thus, firm conclusions here are precluded.

No reduction of neonatal sepsis in vitamin A-treated patients has been demonstrated so far (109), and a recent meta-analysis could not demonstrate a significant reduction of mortality in term neonates, who were supplemented with vitamin A (110). Further results of on-going clinical trials investigating the effect of vitamin A for the treatment of sepsis and NEC are still pending (111).

Granulocyte and Granulocyte-Macrophage Colony Stimulating Factors

Myeloid colony stimulating factors (CSFs), including granulocyte-macrophage CSF (GM-CSF; CSF-2) and granulocyte CSF (G-CSF; CSF-3), stimulate innate immune function, improve myelopoiesis, and limit apoptosis. (112). The clearance of apoptotic cells is essential for the resolution of inflammation and phagocytosis of apoptotic granulocytes is diminished in neonates compared to adults (113). Neonates rapidly deplete their small neutrophil pool when septic, resulting in neutropenia and Gram negative sepsis was partially reversed by administration of G-CSF in preterm infants (114, 115). Thus, a number of clinical trials investigated the effect of G-CSF and GM-SCF in the prevention and treatment of neonatal sepsis over the last decades. A 2003 Cochrane Review of seven treatment and three prophylaxis studies however, demonstrated no significant survival advantage at 14 days from the start of therapy (79) (**Table 1**). Of note, a subgroup analysis of 97 infants, who in addition to systemic infection, had clinically significant neutropenia at trial entry, did show a significant reduction in mortality (79). Three prophylactic studies, on the other hand,

TABLE 2 | Meta-analyses on preventive strategies for sepsis in preterm infants.

Intervention	Outcome	RR (95% CI)	RCTs/infants	References
IVIG	All-cause mortality	0.89 (0.75–1.05)	15/4125	(81)
	Mortality (infectious)	0.83 (0.56–1.22)	10/1690	(81)
	Late-onset sepsis	**0.85 (0.74–0.98)**	10/3795	(81)
INH-A21	All-cause mortality	0.80 (0.59–1.08)	2/2488	(82)
	Staphylococcal infection	1.07 (0.94–1.22)	2/2488	(82)
Altastaph	All-cause mortality	1.31 (0.30–5.70)	1/206	(82)
	Staphylococcal infection	0.86 (0.32–2.28)	1/206	(82)
Pagibaximab	All-cause mortality	1.16 (0.82–1.64)[a]	2/1669	(83, 84)
	Staphylococcal infection	1.17 (0.90–1.50)[a]	2/1669	(83, 84)
GM-CSF	All-cause mortality	1.05 (0.64–1.72)	4/639	(79, 85)
	Late-onset sepsis	1.05 (0.84–1.30)	3/564	(79, 85)
Donor human milk vs. formula	All-cause mortality	0.75 (0.44–1.27)	4/721	(86)
	Invasive infection	0.89 (0.67–1.19)	2/219	(86)
	Necrotizing enterocolitis	**0.36 (0.18–0.71)**	6/431	(86)
Probiotics (single or multiple strains)	All-cause mortality	**0.77 (0.65–0.92)**	27/8056	(87)
	Late-onset sepsis	**0.86 (0.78–0.94)**	37/9416	(88)
	Invasive fungal infection	**0.48 (0.33–0.71)**	6/916	(89)
Probiotics (single strains)	All-cause mortality	0.95 (0.72–1.26)	11/3424	(90)
	Late-onset sepsis	**0.86 (0.76–0.97)**	14/3455	(88)
Probiotics (multiple strains)	All-cause mortality	**0.67 (0.50–0.89)**	10/2867	(90)
	Late-onset sepsis	**0.85 (0.74–0.97)**	23/5691	(88)
Oral lactoferrin	All-cause mortality	0.65 (0.37–1.11)	6/1041	(75)
	Late-onset sepsis	**0.59 (0.40–0.87)**	6/886	(75)
Oral lactoferrin + probiotics	All-cause mortality	0.54 (0.25–1.18)	1/496	(75)
	Late-onset sepsis	**0.27 (0.12–0.60)**	1/319	(75)
Glutamine	All-cause mortality	0.97 (0.80–1.17)	12/2877	(91)
	Late-onset sepsis	0.94 (0.86–1.04)	11/2815	(91)
Selenium supplementation	All-cause mortality	0.92 (0.48–1.75)	2/549	(92)
	Late-onset sepsis	**0.73 (0.57–0.93)**	3/583	(92)

Cochrane reviews or the most updated meta-analysis on the topic were selected for inclusion in the table. Outcomes were selected based on relevance. Statistically significant results are marked in bold. Altastaph, antibody against capsular polysaccharide antigen type 5 and 8; CI, confidence interval; GM-CSF, granulocyte-macrophage colony stimulating factor; INH-A21, pooled generic antistaphylococcal immunoglobulin; IVIG, intravenous immunoglobulin; Pagibaximab, anti-lipoteichoic acid monoclonal antibody; RCT, randomized controlled trial; RR, risk ratio. [a]No complete meta-analysis has been conducted. RR, calculated from preliminary results.

did not demonstrate significantly reduced mortality in neonates receiving GM-CSF (79). The authors concluded that due to the small sample size, there was insufficient evidence to support the introduction of either G-CSF or GM-CSF into neonatal practice, either as treatment of established systemic infection to reduce resulting mortality, or as prophylaxis to prevent systemic infection in high-risk neonates (79).

A study from 2009 investigating 280 neonates ≤31 weeks' gestation demonstrated that even higher doses of postnatal prophylactic GM-CSF (10 μg/kg per day administrated subcutaneously on 5 consecutive days) did not reduce sepsis or improve survival or short-term outcomes (85). When this study was pooled with the three previously published small RCTs, no significant effects of prophylactic GM-CSF on mortality or sepsis incidence were observed (79, 85) (**Table 2**).

In summary, available data do not support the use of G- or GM-CSF for prophylaxis of infections in neonates. This might in part be explained by a hyporesponsiveness of neonatal granulocytes to G- or GM-CSF induced anti-apoptotic effects compared to adults (116). Preterm neonates with moderate (<1,700/μL) or severe (<500/μL) neutropenia and systemic infection, however, might benefit from adjuvant treatment with G-CSF or GM-CSF, respectively (117). Optimal timing of administration and monitoring of G- or GM-CSF levels will be crucial to maximize the beneficial aspects of these cytokines in these infants.

Granulocyte Transfusions

Granulocytes of term and preterm neonates exhibit quantitative and qualitative differences compared to those of adults, which may contribute to the neonates' higher risk for developing bacterial infections (114). Treatment of neonatal sepsis with granulocyte transfusions was thus investigated to determine whether it might enhance quality and quantity of neutrophils thereby leading to improved outcome. However, no significant difference in mortality was found in infants with sepsis and neutropenia who received granulocyte transfusions when compared to placebo (**Table 1**) (80). Of importance, potentially severe side effects have been reported: fluid overload, transmission of blood-borne infection, graft-vs.-host disease, pulmonary complications secondary to leukocyte aggregation and sequestration and sensitization to donor erythrocyte and leukocytes (80, 101). Thus, the application of granulocyte transfusions cannot be recommended due to insufficient evidence of safety and efficacy in preterm infants.

Exchange Transfusions

Exchange transfusion may remove toxic bacterial products and potentially harmful circulating inflammatory mediators, including cytokines, in an effort to improve perfusion and tissue oxygenation, replace clotting factors, and enhance humoral immune responses.

One retrospective and one prospective single center study investigated the effect of exchange transfusions in a cohort of 101 and 83 preterm infants, respectively. In these cohorts of preterm infants with severe sepsis/septic shock no significant reduction in mortality rates was found (118, 119). Nevertheless, a trend in mortality reduction was reported (119) and another study found a statistically significant protective effect, after controlling for potential confounding factors significantly associated with death (GA, serum lactate, inotropic drugs, oligo/anuria) (118). Although hypoglycemia, electrolyte disturbances, hemodynamic instability, and thrombosis are potential complications of exchange transfusion, the authors reported no side effects (120). Thus, based on the current evidence and safety data, no firm conclusion on the recommendation of exchange transfusions for the treatment of neonatal sepsis can be made.

Recombinant Activated Human Protein C

Recombinant human activated protein C (rhAPC) possesses a broad spectrum of activity including modulation of coagulation, inflammation, and apoptosis (121). However, results among adults and children demonstrated lack of efficacy and an increased risk of bleeding associated with higher mortality rates (122, 123). Consequently, rhAPC was withdrawn from the market before any randomized trials were performed in preterm neonates, and in 2012 a clear recommendation against the treatment with rhAPC for neonatal sepsis was proclaimed (124).

CURRENT INTERVENTIONS WITH CLINICAL EVIDENCE OF BENEFIT

Human Milk

Human milk contains multiple distinct bioactive molecules, including antimicrobial proteins and peptides (APPs), that protect against infection and contribute to immune maturation, and healthy microbial colonization (**Figure 1C**) (140). Ethical limitations preclude RCTs on the topic but feeding preterm infants with their own mother's milk (MOM) offers an impressive array of benefits, including decreased rates of LOS, NEC and retinopathy of prematurity, lower rates of re-hospitalizations in the first year of life, and improved neurodevelopmental outcomes (141–144).

The term "human milk feeding" is frequently used to encompass both MOM and donor human milk (DHM), implying that the multiple beneficial outcomes attributed to MOM can be generalized to DHM (145, 146). This assumption, however, may only be partially correct due to differences in milk composition and processing. Preterm mothers' milk shows great variation in total protein levels and inverse correlation with lactation and daily milk volume (147). This demand-adapted regulation of protein intake, including APPs is hampered in DHM, because GA of donors' infants and infants receiving their milk might be mismatched or DHM might be pooled. More importantly, pasteurization of DHM destroys or significantly decreases the concentration of many of the protective elements in human milk, including lysozymes, secretory IgA, growth factors, lactoferrin, antioxidants, and microbiota (145, 146, 148–150). Nevertheless, improved outcomes of infants fed DHM may be primarily to avoiding potentially injurious effects of formula feeding (145, 146, 151). A meta-analysis showed that feeding with formula compared with DHM results in a higher risk of developing NEC (86). However, feeding DHM instead of formula did not significantly affect mortality or rate of invasive infection (**Table 2**) (86).

Prebiotics

A wide range of prebiotic components (substrates that are selectively utilized by host microorganisms conferring a health benefit) and antimicrobial and anti-inflammatory factors are delivered by breast milk (141–143). These provide passive protection to the neonate and stimulate maturation of host intestinal defenses, which are particularly relevant for premature infants (144). Prebiotic components of human milk promote the growth of a physiologic, probiotic flora including *Bifidobacteria* spp. and *Lactobacilli* spp. in the colon. Although there is currently no evidence regarding the effectiveness of the isolated application of prebiotics in preventing nosocomial sepsis in preterm infants (152), combinations of probiotics and synbiotics, i.e., a synergistic combination of probiotics and prebiotics, may be beneficial for prevention of LOS, as described below (153).

Probiotics

In healthy term infants the gut is colonized with maternal probiotic bacteria including *Lactobacilla* spp. and *Bifidobacteria* spp., which upregulate local and systemic immunity, increase anti-inflammatory cytokines, and decrease the permeability of the gut to bacteria and toxins (**Figure 1B**). Treatment with antibiotics and delayed enteral feeding are common in preterm infants and contribute to the development of sepsis and NEC (154). Probiotics, live non-pathogenic microorganisms, might confer a benefit to neonatal host immunity. By altering host epithelial and immunological responses (155), they may reduce several neonatal inflammatory conditions (156).

A 2014 Cochrane review of 24 randomized or quasi-RCTs evaluated the effect of probiotics in the prevention of NEC and LOS in preterm infants <37 weeks GA or <2,500 g birth weight, or both (157). Enteral probiotic supplementation significantly

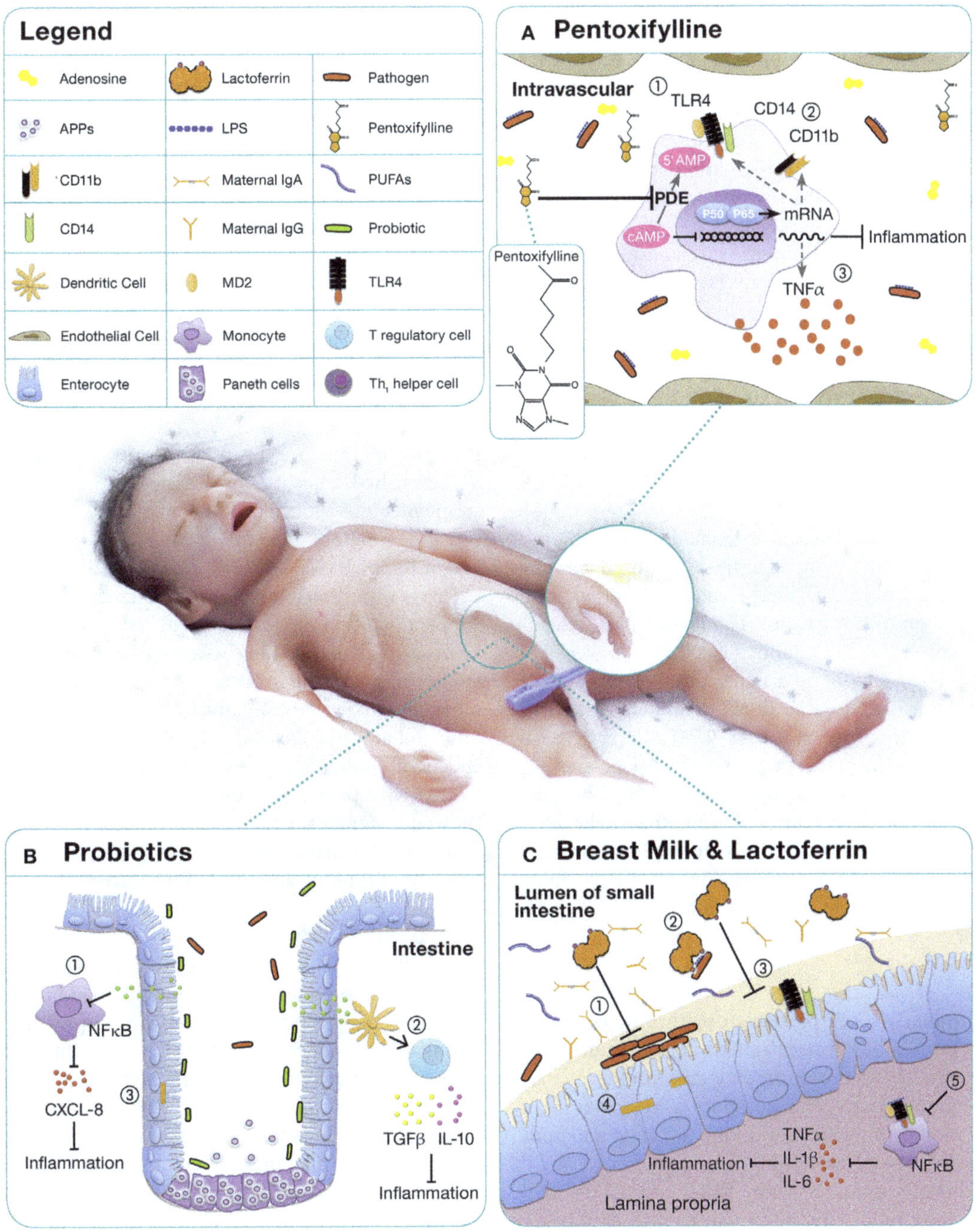

FIGURE 1 | Immunomodulatory approaches for the treatment and prevention of neonatal sepsis. **(A)** PTX, a phosphodiesterase inhibitor, mediates most of its functions by enhanced cyclic AMP (cAMP) due to a reduced degradation of cAMP (125, 126). Relatively high concentrations of adenosine are present in neonatal blood plasma and neonatal mononuclear cells demonstrate increased sensitivity to the cAMP-mediated inhibitory effects of adenosine (127, 128). As immunomodulatory properties of PTX are mediated via adenosine-dependent pathways, adenosine and PTX in combination, lead to a profound inhibitory effect on pro-inflammatory cytokine production (129). On neonatal APCs, PTX demonstrates anti-inflammatory properties by (1) down-regulating TLR4 expression and signaling, (2) downregulation of surface molecules such as CD14 and CD11b, and (3) inhibition of inflammatory cytokine production (70). **(B)** The microbiome of premature infants has a smaller proportion of beneficial bacteria and higher numbers of pathogenic bacteria compared to term infants, likely owing to higher frequencies of cesarean sections, antibiotic use, exposure to the hospital environment, and artificial feeding (130). The administration of probiotics up-regulates local and systemic immunity by (1) decreasing proinflammatory cytokines, (2) increasing the production of anti-inflammatory cytokines, and (3) decreasing the permeability of the gut to bacteria and toxins (131). **(C)** Human milk contains a range of distinct bioactive molecules that protect against infection and inflammation including immunoglobulins, long-chain PUFAs, and LF. Among them, the antimicrobial and immunomodulatory effects of lactoferrin are best studied: (1) Inhibition of bacterial adhesion and biofilm formation (132–134), (2) binding of endotoxins from intestinal pathogens (135), (3) blocking of receptors essential for epithelial invasion of microbes (136) thereby (4) prevention of bacterial translocation (137), (5) promotion of anergic/anti-inflammatory effects in LPS or LTA stimulated macrophages by TLR expression and pathway interference (138, 139).

reduced the incidence of severe NEC ≥ stage II and mortality but initially, no evidence of significant reduction of LOS was found (157). Recent meta-analyses, including 37 RCTs ($n = 9{,}416$) have demonstrated a significant protective effect of probiotics against LOS and all cause mortality (87, 88, 158) (**Table 2**). The optimal composition of probiotics remains to be determined, but there is evidence that probiotics consisting of multiple strains are more effective than single-strain probiotics in preventing mortality and NEC (90).

Side effects of probiotic treatment are rare and most clinical studies did not report significant adverse effects. However, occasional cases of sepsis caused by administered probiotic species have been reported (159).

In summary, growing evidence suggests that the preventive use of probiotics reduces the risk for neonatal sepsis in preterm infants. Further studies are necessary to optimize formulation, composition, standardization and optimal dosing of probiotics.

Synbiotics

The potential benefit of synbiotics, a combination of probiotics and prebiotics is currently being investigated and so far one large RCT has been published. This recent RCT of an oral synbiotics preparation (*Lactobacillus plantarum* plus fructo-oligosaccharide) enrolled 4,556 infants >2,000 g or 35 weeks of gestation, in rural India and found a significant reduction of the primary outcome sepsis and death in the treatment arm (risk ratio 0.60, 95% confidence interval 0.48–0.74) (160). Preterm infants represent a major challenge in resource-poor settings where NEC and sepsis carry greater risks of death (161). The risk–benefit ratio of prophylactic probiotics or synbiotics might differ between healthcare settings. Results indicate an equal or even more pronounced beneficial effect in neonates from developing countries and support further RCTs in both, high and low resource settings.

Lactoferrin

Lactoferrin is the major whey protein in mature human milk and is present in even higher concentrations in colostrum (153). This multifunctional, 80 kDa iron-binding glycoprotein is part of the innate immune system and possesses a broad range of antimicrobial, immunostimulatory, anti-inflammatory, and anti-apoptotic properties (**Figure 1C**) (162).

Lactoferrin directly interacts with TLR4 and CD14 and demonstrates bacteriostatic activity through its high affinity for iron its ability to directly bind LPS (163, 164). In addition to its function as an antimicrobial protein, lactoferrin has also demonstrated immunoregulatory properties *in vitro* and *in vivo* (131, 165, 166). These studies indicate a potential role of lactoferrin as an immune-sensor to maintain immune homeostasis with an immunosuppressive effect on inflammatory monocytes/macrophages of preterm neonates (30, 131, 167).

Bovine lactoferrin (bLF) is only 69% homologous to human lactoferrin (hLF), but both serve similar biological functions (168). In RCTs the oral supplementation with bLF was associated with a decreased incidence of LOS caused by bacteria and invasive fungal infections in preterm infants (169). A recent Cochrane Review including six RCTs demonstrated that oral bLF supplementation with or without probiotics decreased LOS and NEC stage II or III but not mortality (**Table 2**) (75). Of note, to date no adverse effects regarding the use of bLF in human infants have been reported (75). Talactoferrin, a recombinant hLF, has been tested in a phase I study in preterm neonates (170). In contrast to bLF, talactoferrin does not need to be pasteurized and might therefore differ in function and effectiveness. Studies comparing talactoferrin and bLF remain to be done. Given the common use of probiotics, potential interactions between oral probiotics and bLF/talactoferrin should be tested (171).

Thus, optimum dosing regimens, type of lactoferrin (human or bovine), and effects on long-term outcomes still need to be defined, but lactoferrin might prove to be an effective agent in helping to prevent LOS in very preterm infants.

Zinc

Preterm infants are born with low zinc (Zn) stores and a diminished capacity for Zn absorption and retention. Zn supplementation decreases oxidative stress markers and limits pro-inflammatory cytokine production by targeting Nuclear Factor Kappa B (NF-κB) (172, 173). A RCT in 352 infants aged 7–120 days with probable serious bacterial infection showed that Zn supplementation significantly reduced treatment failure, defined as need to change antibiotics, need for intensive care, or death (174). In a RCT high doses of Zn (9.7–10.7 mg/day) reduced mortality in preterm infants (24–32 weeks) without signs of infection at initial inclusion (175). Two RCTs have evaluated the effects of enteral Zn supplementation in preterm infants (≥32 weeks) with suspected sepsis (176, 177) and one of them (177) showed a significant reduction in mortality (178). A Cochrane review of the effects of enteral Zn supplementation in preterm neonates morbidity and mortality is currently pending (179).

Pentoxifylline

Pentoxifylline (PTX), a non-specific phosphodiesterase inhibitor with immunomodulatory properties (**Figure 1A**), may be beneficial in preterm neonates with sepsis and NEC. PTX inhibits the production of TLR—and inflammasome-mediated inflammatory cytokines and the expression of LPS-stimulated surface markers *in vitro* (127, 128). PTX's effects are more pronounced in neonatal immune cells than in adults and it suppresses pro-inflammatory cytokines to a greater degree than anti-inflammatory cytokines (127, 128). This corresponds to the observation of limited clinical benefit in adult sepsis, but promising results from RCTs in neonates. Moreover, PTX's anti-inflammatory effects on PRR signaling are distinct from those of other anti-inflammatory agents such as dexamethasone and azithromycin with which PTX can act in synergy (180).

A meta-analysis of six RCTs encompassing 416 infants concluded that PTX, when used as an adjunct therapy to antibiotics in neonatal sepsis, might decrease mortality (**Table 1**) (77). Statistical subgroup analyses of four of these studies revealed lower mortality in preterm infants, infants with confirmed sepsis, and infants with Gram-negative sepsis. However, according to the authors, the overall quality of evidence was low (77). A recent double-blind RCT of 120 preterm infants with LOS demonstrated several beneficial adjuvant effects of PTX including a reduced length of hospital stay ($p = 0.04$), duration of respiratory support ($p = 0.02$) and less need for vasopressors ($p = 0.01$) but was not powered for clinical outcomes (181). Of note, no adverse effects of PTX were reported. Further *in vivo* studies, both in animal sepsis models and in human clinical trials, may help to define the optimal timing and dosing of PTX as well as its efficacy in improving short—and long-term outcomes following neonatal inflammation. Initiated in 2016, a randomized, placebo controlled multi-center study with a cohort size of 900 very preterm infants with LOS or NEC, is currently investigating PTX's effect on disability-free survival (Australian New Zealand Clinical Trials Registry 12616000405415).

FUTURE CONCEPTS WITH POTENTIAL BENEFITS

Although certain measures have indicated benefit, there remains an urgent and unmet need for novel, safe and efficacious strategies to reduce the huge burden of sepsis-related morbidity in the preterm population. We herein discuss new approaches with potential future applications that have not yet been tested beyond phase 1 clinical trials.

Maternal Immunization

Maternal immunization boosts the concentration of vaccine-specific IgG antibodies in the mother and increases antibody concentration in the infant at birth. Currently three vaccines have specific recommendations for routine use in pregnancy: tetanus, influenza and pertussis (182). Future prospects include potential development of maternal vaccines against GBS (183), cytomegalovirus (CMV) (184) and respiratory syncytial virus (RSV) (185).

In term infants, maternal vaccination may provide protection until the period of maximum susceptibility or risk has passed or until the infant has completed the routine immunizations. This benefit may be reduced in preterm infants due to reduced transplacental antibody transport before the third trimester with resulting lower antibody-concentrations compared to term infants (186). While much remains to be learned regarding the optimal timing, safety and efficacy of maternal vaccines as well as their potential effect on subsequent infant responses to vaccines (187), maternal immunization is an important strategy to substantially reduce morbidity and mortality from infectious diseases after birth.

Antimicrobial Proteins and Peptides (APPs)

Both *in vitro* and *in vivo* data support the hypothesis that APPs are important contributors to intrinsic mucosal immunity. Alterations in the level of APP expression or biologic activity can predispose the organism to microbial infection (188). Primarily released by neutrophils, monocytes, and macrophages, APPs are also produced within the skin and at mucosal surfaces by epithelial cells and thus are present within body fluids, including saliva, airway surface liquid, and breast milk (189). Circulating and intracellular levels of APPs are relatively low in early life, especially in preterm infants, potentially lessening protective immunity (190). APPs expressed in neonates include α- and β-defensins, cathelicidins, bactericidal/permeability-increasing protein (BPI), and lactoferrin (191). While some studies argue for lactoferrin in the prevention of LOS in VLBW infants (192), preclinical data also support antibacterial and anti-endotoxin properties of therapeutic APPs. For example, the recombinant bactericidal/permeability-increasing protein ($rBPI_{21}$) has demonstrated beneficial effects in children with severe meningococcal sepsis (193, 194). Further research on APPs for prevention and treatment of neonatal sepsis is ongoing and has recently been reviewed in detail (190). Synthetic peptides with combined antimicrobial and immunomodulatory properties, such as clavanin-MO, an adenosine monophosphate (AMP) isolated from *Styela clava*, and Innate defense regulator (IDR)-1018, derived from bovine bactenecin, represent a promising approach to treat invasive infections of various bacterial strains, including multidrug-resistant hospital isolates (195, 196). Of the APPs lactoferrin (Lf) has demonstrated benefit as oral agent in the prevention of neonatal sepsis (75). Regarding other APPs, although the results of preclinical studies are encouraging, to our knowledge neonatal clinical trials have not yet been conducted.

Innate Immune Stimulants

Exposure to non-pathogenic components that augment the innate immune responses to prevent neonatal sepsis is promising, but has not yet been thoroughly investigated. Possible candidates are PRR- agonists; among them TLRAs are most extensively studied. In newborn mice, pre-treatment with TLRAs was associated with increased cytokine responses to subsequent polymicrobial infection, induced via intraperitoneal injection of a cecal slurry, with enhanced recruitment of phagocytes and reduced mortality (197). Although Th1-polarizing TLR-responses are diminished in preterm neonates compared to term neonates and adults (38, 39, 198), Th1 cytokine responses to TLR7/8 agonists such as R848 reach adult levels (37, 199). Whether any benefits confer to human neonates from TLRAs currently used as stand-alone agents (e.g., imiquimod cream, TLR7A) or as components of adjuvanted vaccines in clinical and preclinical trials in adults (200) needs to be carefully investigated in preclinical studies.

Most recently a beneficial effect of subcutaneously administered aluminum salts (alum) in the prevention of neonatal polymicrobial sepsis in mice was demonstrated (201). Alum, the most widely used adjuvant in human vaccines, does not activate TLRs but, rather, promotes caspase-1 activation and IL-1β production via the NACHT, LRR and PYD domains-containing protein 3 (NLRP3)-inflammasome (202).

Live attenuated vaccines such as Bacille Calmette–Guérin (BCG) provide inherent PRR-activating activity that may contribute to enhanced immune responses and a decreased susceptibility to invasive non-TB infections in developing countries, where BCG is routinely administered (54, 203). BCG may exert its beneficial potential through heterologous, "non-specific" effects. This heterologous innate immune protection may be due to "trained immunity," the phenomenon whereby innate activation results in a heightened state of innate responses to a broad range of pathogens and thus broad protection, via innate memory as has been reviewed elsewhere

(204). Of note, the combined administration of BCG plus the alum-adjuvanted hepatitis B vaccine (HBV) demonstrates age-dependent synergistic enhancement of IL-1ß, production potentially enhancing both innate and adaptive immune responses (205).

Thus, results from animal and human *in vitro* studies are indicative for a beneficial effect of innate immune stimulants in the prevention of neonatal sepsis and should be further investigated.

Stem Cells

Mesenchymal stromal cells (MSCs) are non-hematopoietic, multipotent stromal precursor cells that can be isolated from the placenta, cord blood, and Wharton's Jelly (206, 207). MSCs are capable of modulating immune responses (208) by both cell-to-cell contact and through the release of soluble paracrine factors including nitric oxide, indoleamine 2,3-dioxygenase, PGE_2, TGF-β, and IL-10 (209, 210). MSCs may improve bacterial clearance by various mechanisms, including enhancement of phagocytic activity of APCs and up-regulation of TLR-2 and TLR-4, and β-defensin 2 secretion (211, 212). A comprehensive review of 18 preclinical studies published between 2009 and 2015 demonstrated that MSC therapy in animal models of sepsis significantly reduced the overall odds of death (OR 0.27, 95% CI 0.18–0.40) (213). A clinical trial of infusion of MSCs to adults demonstrated a significant increase in survival rate (214, 215). Further adult clinical trials are on-going, but to our knowledge neonatal sepsis trials have not yet been conducted (216). However, several studies currently investigate the use of umbilical cord blood derived-MSCs for the prevention and treatment of bronchopulmonary dysplasia (BPD) in human preterm infants at risk, after phase 1 trials showed an acceptable safety profile (217).

Of note, the abundance of hematopoietic stem and progenitor cells (HSPCs) in preterm compared to term cord blood, may contribute to the beneficial effects of delayed cord clamping in very preterm infants (218, 219). A recent systemic review of 2,834 preterm infants found high-quality evidence for reduced hospital mortality, but no clear evidence for a reduction of LOS in infants with delayed cord clamping (220).

Inflammasome Inhibitors

The inflammasome is a newly identified group of PRRs and specific blockage of these by small-molecule inflammasome inhibitors is a promising approach in different inflammatory conditions, including microbe-induced inflammation (221, 222). Numerous inflammasomes have been described so far; among them the (NLRP3) has been best characterized. Interactions among the three proteins of the NLRP3 inflammasome (NLRP3 protein, adapter protein apoptosis-associated speck-like protein (ASC) and procaspase-1) tightly regulate inflammasome function to ensure immune activity only when appropriate. *In vivo* neutralization of the NLRP3 inflammasome with an orally available small molecule inhibitor decreased inflammasome dependent cytokine secretion (IL-1β /IL-18) in a murine *Staph. aureus* infection, and improved the bacterial clearance through improved acidification of the phagosome (223). Newborn neonatal caspase-1/11 knockout mice, showed improved survival following septic challenge compared with wild-type mice (224). This effect was independent of NLRP3 activation (224). Despite promising results from clinical trials in adults treated with inflammasome inhibitors for inflammatory diseases other than sepsis (225, 226), more information is needed regarding the mode of inflammasome action in neonates to inform potential targeted therapeutic inhibition in this distinct age group.

Antibiotics With Anti-inflammatory Properties

Inflammation in sepsis is usually triggered by microbial components, hypoxia, arterial hypotension, and reperfusion. Some antimicrobial agents, such as β-lactam antibiotics, may exacerbate inflammation through the lysis of bacteria (227).

In contrast to proinflammatory effects of certain antibiotics that lyse bacteria, several protein synthesis inhibiting antibiotics exhibit anti-inflammatory activities. Macrolides, rifampicin, and tetracycline demonstrate anti-inflammatory and immunomodulatory properties with a potential application in systemic inflammation (228–231). Rifampicin and tetracycline are contraindicated in the neonatal period; the use of macrolides for other indications, namely, *Ureaplasma spp.* infection and the prevention of BPD in preterm neonates, however, has been studied (232, 233). Prophylactic azithromycin significantly reduced BPD and the composite outcome of BPD/death in preterm infants (232).

The macrolide azithromycin, specifically inhibits IL-1α and IL-1β secretion and non-canonical inflammasome activation upon TLR agonist, including LPS, stimulation *in vitro* (180) and *in vivo* (234). A decrease in IL-1β-mediated inflammation has been attributed to destabilizing mRNA levels for NALP3, a key inflammasome component (235). In a murine sepsis model, mortality was lower along with decreased sepsis scores when mice were treated with a combination of ampicillin and azithromycin instead of ampicillin alone (236). In adults, azithromycin was associated with more ICU-free days in severe sepsis patients with and without pneumonia (237), however questions on the applicability of these results in neonates remain including the consideration of side effects (238–240).

None of these new approaches has been tested in human neonates thus far and the potential *in vitro* and *in vivo* effects of new therapies need to be fully explored before any clinical studies in neonates can be performed. In addition to possibly beneficial single agent such as PTX, future studies will evaluate if a multimodal approach including a combination of immunomodulatory agents may prevent or mitigate neonatal sepsis and associated long term- morbidities in preterm infants.

CONCLUSION

Administration of human milk is a key approach in preventing neonatal sepsis. The use of probiotics and lactoferrin might be effective but more evidence is needed to confirm preliminary observations and to optimize formulation, composition, and dosing of these agents. In certain settings/populations, vaccination with BCG is associated with a reduction in neonatal sepsis via heterologous ("non-specific") effects possibly related to trained immunity. With respect to treatment of neonatal sepsis, PTX holds promise, but larger studies with long-term outcome data are still pending. Several other immunotherapies evaluated for the prophylaxis of neonatal sepsis including IVIG, myeloid CSFs and granulocyte transfusions have failed to demonstrate benefit. As we look to the future, APPs, PRR-agonists, stem cell therapy and inhibitors of the inflammasome might offer new therapeutic or preventive avenues in neonatal sepsis with preclinical and clinical studies yet to be done.

The successful development of new prophylactic and treatment options should take into account age-specific immune responses. Timing of therapy and dosage may determine whether immunomodulatory agents induce a protective immune response or whether the same approach causes potentially harmful interference with the developing immune system.

AUTHOR CONTRIBUTIONS

SS conducted the literature review and drafted the paper. EV designed the tables and assisted in drafting. BK, AS, OL, and AB contributed to critical revision of the article, assisted in drafting, and suggested additional references for inclusion in the final version. OL edited the final manuscript. All authors approved the final manuscript as submitted.

ACKNOWLEDGMENTS

We thank Tobias Strunk, Ludwig Gortner, and David Dowling for helpful discussions and suggestions. We thank Scott Lapinski for professional assistance with the literature research, Karen Pepper for proof reading and Jens-Christian Schwindt for providing a picture of a premature baby simulator. The graphical support by Sheila Ehm is gratefully appreciated. SS thanks the Max Kade Foundation for supporting her fellowship at Boston Children's Hospital.

REFERENCES

1. Soll RF. Progress in the care of extremely preterm infants. *JAMA* (2015) 314:1007–8. doi: 10.1001/jama.2015.10911
2. Stoll BJ, Hansen NI, Adams-Chapman I, Fanaroff AA, Hintz SR, Vohr B, Higgins RD. National Institute of child health and human development neonatal research network. neurodevelopmental and growth impairment among extremely low-birth-weight infants with neonatal infection. *JAMA* (2004) 292:2357. doi: 10.1001/jama.292.19.2357
3. Wynn JL, Wong HR, Shanley TP, Bizzarro MJ, Saiman L, Polin RA. Time for a neonatal-specific consensus definition for sepsis. *Pediatr Crit Care Med.* (2014) 15:523–8. doi: 10.1097/PCC.0000000000000157
4. Camacho-Gonzalez A, Spearman PW, Stoll BJ. Neonatal infectious diseases: evaluation of neonatal sepsis. *Pediatr Clin North Am.* (2013) 60:367–89. doi: 10.1016/j.pcl.2012.12.003
5. Hornik CP, Fort P, Clark RH, Watt K, Benjamin DK, Smith PB, et al. Early and late onset sepsis in very-low-birth-weight infants from a large group of neonatal intensive care units. *Early Hum Dev.* (2012) 88 (Suppl. 2):S69–74. doi: 10.1016/S0378-3782(12)70019-1
6. Stoll BJ, Hansen N, Fanaroff AA, Wright LL, Carlo WA, Ehrenkranz RA, et al. Late-onset sepsis in very low birth weight neonates: the experience of the NICHD Neonatal Research Network. *Pediatrics* (2002) 110:285–91. doi: 10.1542/peds.110.2.285
7. Stoll BJ, Hansen NI, Higgins RD, Fanaroff AA, Duara S, Goldberg R. Very low birth weight preterm infants with early onset neonatal sepsis: the predominance of gram-negative infections continues in the National Institute of Child Health and Human Development Neonatal Research Network, 2002-2003. *Pediatr Infect Dis J.* (2005) 24:635–9. doi: 10.1097/01.inf.0000168749.82105.64
8. Stoll BJ, Hansen NI, Bell EF, Shankaran S, Laptook AR, Walsh MC, et al. Neonatal Outcomes of Extremely Preterm Infants From the NICHD Neonatal Research Network. *Pediatrics* (2010) 126:443–56. doi: 10.1542/peds.2009-2959
9. Adams-Chapman I, Stoll BJ. Neonatal infection and long-term neurodevelopmental outcome in the preterm infant. *Curr Opin Infect Dis.* (2006) 19:290–7. doi: 10.1097/01.qco.0000224825.57976.87
10. Strunk T, Inder T, Wang X, Burgner D, Mallard C, Levy O. Infection-induced inflammation and cerebral injury in preterm infants. *Lancet Infect Dis.* (2014) 14:751–62. doi: 10.1016/S1473-3099(14)70710-8
11. Goldstein B, Giroir B, Randolph A, International Consensus Conference on Pediatric Sepsis. International pediatric sepsis consensus conference: definitions for sepsis and organ dysfunction in pediatrics*. *Pediatr Crit Care Med.* (2005) 6:2–8. doi: 10.1097/01.PCC.0000149131.72248.E6
12. Wynn JL. Defining neonatal sepsis. *Curr Opin Pediatr.* (2016) 28:135–40. doi: 10.1097/MOP.0000000000000315
13. Fanaroff AA, Korones SB, Wright LL, Verter J, Poland RL, Bauer CR, et al. Incidence, presenting features, risk factors and significance of late onset septicemia in very low birth weight infants. The National Institute of Child Health and Human Development Neonatal Research Network. *Pediatr Infect Dis J.* (1998) 17:593–8.

14. Shane AL, Sánchez PJ, Stoll BJ. Neonatal sepsis. *Lancet* (2017) 390:1770–80. doi: 10.1016/S0140-6736(17)31002-4
15. Gilfillan M, Bhandari V. Biomarkers for the diagnosis of neonatal sepsis and necrotizing enterocolitis: Clinical practice guidelines. *Early Hum Dev.* (2017) 105:25–33. doi: 10.1016/j.earlhumdev.2016.12.002
16. Juskewitch JE, Abraham RS, League SC, Jenkins SM, Smith CY, Enders FT, et al. Monocyte HLA-DR expression and neutrophil CD64 expression as biomarkers of infection in critically ill neonates and infants. *Pediatr Res.* (2015) 78:683–90. doi: 10.1038/pr.2015.164
17. Topcuoglu S, Arslanbuga C, Gursoy T, Aktas A, Karatekin G, Uluhan R, et al. Role of presepsin in the diagnosis of late-onset neonatal sepsis in preterm infants. *J Matern Neonatal Med.* (2015) 29:1–6. doi: 10.3109/14767058.2015.1064885
18. Dickinson P, Smith CL, Forster T, Craigon M, Ross AJ, Khondoker MR, et al. Whole blood gene expression profiling of neonates with confirmed bacterial sepsis. *Genomics data* (2015) 3:41–8. doi: 10.1016/j.gdata.2014.11.003
19. Wynn JL, Wong HR. Pathophysiology and treatment of septic shock in neonates. *Clin Perinatol.* (2010) 37:439–79. doi: 10.1016/j.clp.2010.04.002
20. Zhao J, Kim KD, Yang X, Auh S, Fu Y-X, Tang H. Hyper innate responses in neonates lead to increased morbidity and mortality after infection. *Proc Natl Acad Sci USA.* (2008) 105:7528–33. doi: 10.1073/pnas.0800152105
21. Boomer JS, To K, Chang KC, Takasu O, Osborne DF, Walton AH, et al. Immunosuppression in patients who die of sepsis and multiple organ failure. *JAMA* (2011) 306:2594–605. doi: 10.1001/jama.2011.1829
22. Raymond SL, López MC, Baker HV, Larson SD, Efron PA, Sweeney TE, et al. Unique transcriptomic response to sepsis is observed among patients of different age groups. *PLoS ONE* (2017) 12:e0184159. doi: 10.1371/journal.pone.0184159
23. Tang BMP, McLean AS, Dawes IW, Huang SJ, Lin RCY. Gene-expression profiling of peripheral blood mononuclear cells in sepsis*. *Crit Care Med.* (2009) 37:882–8. doi: 10.1097/CCM.0b013e31819b52fd
24. Wynn JL, Cvijanovich NZ, Allen GL, Thomas NJ, Freishtat RJ, Anas N, et al. The influence of developmental age on the early transcriptomic response of children with septic shock. *Mol Med.* (2011) 17:1146–56. doi: 10.2119/molmed.2011.00169
25. Boomer JS, Green JM, Hotchkiss RS. The changing immune system in sepsis: is individualized immuno-modulatory therapy the answer? *Virulence* (2014) 5:45–56. doi: 10.4161/viru.26516
26. Maslove DM, Wong HR. Gene expression profiling in sepsis: timing, tissue, and translational considerations. *Trends Mol Med.* (2014) 20:204–13. doi: 10.1016/j.molmed.2014.01.006
27. Hotchkiss RS, Monneret G, Payen D. Immunosuppression in sepsis: a novel understanding of the disorder and a new therapeutic approach. *Lancet Infect Dis.* (2013) 13:260–8. doi: 10.1016/S1473-3099(13)70001-X
28. Tang BM, Huang SJ, McLean AS. Genome-wide transcription profiling of human sepsis: a systematic review. *Crit Care* (2010) 14:R237. doi: 10.1186/cc9392
29. Wynn JL, Guthrie SO, Wong HR, Lahni P, Ungaro R, Lopez MC, et al. Postnatal age is a critical determinant of the neonatal host response to sepsis. *Mol Med.* (2015) 21:496–504. doi: 10.2119/molmed.2015.00064
30. Ulas T, Pirr S, Fehlhaber B, Bickes MS, Loof TG, Vogl T, et al. S100-alarmin-induced innate immune programming protects newborn infants from sepsis. *Nat Immunol.* (2017) 18:622–32. doi: 10.1038/ni.3745
31. Bianchi ME. DAMPs, PAMPs and alarmins: all we need to know about danger. *J Leukoc Biol.* (2006) 81:1–5. doi: 10.1189/jlb.0306164
32. Kollmann TR, Levy O, Montgomery RR, Goriely S. Innate immune function by Toll-like receptors: distinct responses in newborns and the elderly. *Immunity* (2012) 37:771–83. doi: 10.1016/j.immuni.2012.10.014
33. van Well GTJ, Daalderop LA, Wolfs T, Kramer BW. Human perinatal immunity in physiological conditions and during infection. *Mol Cell Pediatr.* (2017) 4:4. doi: 10.1186/s40348-017-0070-1
34. Dowling DJ, Levy O. Ontogeny of early life immunity. *Trends Immunol.* (2014) 35:299–310. doi: 10.1016/j.it.2014.04.007
35. Zilow EP, Hauck W, Linderkamp O, Zilow G. Alternative pathway activation of the complement system in preterm infants with early onset infection. *Pediatr Res.* (1997) 41:334–9. doi: 10.1203/00006450-199703000-00005
36. Bektas S, Goetze B, Speer CP. Decreased adherence, chemotaxis and phagocytic activities of neutrophils from preterm neonates. *Acta Paediatr Scand.* (1990) 79:1031–8.
37. Levy O. Innate immunity of the newborn: basic mechanisms and clinical correlates. *Nat Rev Immunol.* (2007) 7:379–90. doi: 10.1038/nri2075
38. Förster-Waldl E, Sadeghi K, Tamandl D, Gerhold B, Hallwirth U, Rohrmeister K, et al. Monocyte toll-like receptor 4 expression and LPS-induced cytokine production increase during gestational aging. *Pediatr Res.* (2005) 58:121–4. doi: 10.1203/01.PDR.0000163397.53466.0F
39. Schüller SS, Sadeghi K, Wisgrill L, Dangl A, Diesner SC, Prusa AR, et al. Preterm neonates display altered plasmacytoid dendritic cell function and morphology. *J Leukoc Biol.* (2013) 93:781–8. doi: 10.1189/jlb.1011525
40. Burl S, Townend J, Njie-Jobe J, Cox M, Adetifa UJ, Touray E, et al. Age-dependent maturation of Toll-like receptor-mediated cytokine responses in Gambian infants. *PLoS ONE* (2011) 6:e18185. doi: 10.1371/journal.pone.0018185
41. Belderbos ME, Levy O, Meyaard L, Bont L. Plasma-mediated immune suppression: a neonatal perspective. *Pediatr Allergy Immunol.* (2013) 24:102–13. doi: 10.1111/pai.12023
42. Power Coombs MR, Belderbos ME, Gallington LC, Bont L, Levy O. Adenosine modulates Toll-like receptor function: basic mechanisms and translational opportunities. *Expert Rev Anti Infect Ther.* (2011) 9:261–9. doi: 10.1586/eri.10.158
43. Haskó G, Kuhel DG, Chen JF, Schwarzschild MA, Deitch EA, Mabley JG, et al. Adenosine inhibits IL-12 and TNF-[alpha] production via adenosine A2a receptor-dependent and independent mechanisms. *FASEB J.* (2000) 14:2065–74. doi: 10.1096/fj.99-0508com
44. Haskó G, Cronstein BN. Adenosine: an endogenous regulator of innate immunity. *Trends Immunol.* (2004) 25:33–9. doi: 10.1016/j.it.2003.11.003
45. Mitchell MD, Lucas A, Etches PC, Brunt JD, Turnbull AC. Plasma prostaglandin levels during early neonatal life following term and pre-term delivery. *Prostaglandins* (1978) 16:319–26.
46. Kauppila A, Koivisto M, Pukka M, Tuimala R. Umbilical cord and neonatal cortisol levels. Effect of gestational and neonatal factors. *Obstet Gynecol.* (1978) 52:666–72.
47. Giannoni E, Guignard L, Knaup Reymond M, Perreau M, Roth-Kleiner M, Calandra T, et al. Estradiol and progesterone strongly inhibit the innate immune response of mononuclear cells in newborns. *Infect Immun.* (2011) 79:2690–8. doi: 10.1128/IAI.00076-11
48. Pettengill M, Robson S, Tresenriter M, Millán JL, Usheva A, Bingham T, et al. Soluble ecto-5′-nucleotidase (5′-NT), alkaline phosphatase, and adenosine deaminase (ADA1) activities in neonatal blood favor elevated extracellular adenosine. *J Biol Chem.* (2013) 288:27315–26. doi: 10.1074/jbc.M113.484212
49. Roger T, Schneider A, Weier M, Sweep FCGJ, Le Roy D, Bernhagen J, et al. High expression levels of macrophage migration inhibitory factor sustain the innate immune responses of neonates. *Proc Natl Acad Sci USA.* (2016) 113:E997–1005. doi: 10.1073/pnas.1514018113
50. Roger T, Schlapbach LJ, Schneider A, Weier M, Wellmann S, Marquis P, et al. Plasma Levels of macrophage migration inhibitory factor and d-dopachrome tautomerase show a highly specific profile in early life. *Front Immunol.* (2017) 8:26. doi: 10.3389/fimmu.2017.00026
51. Wynn JL, Wilson CS, Hawiger J, Scumpia PO, Marshall AF, Liu J-H, et al. Targeting IL-17A attenuates neonatal sepsis mortality induced by IL-18. *Proc Natl Acad Sci USA.* (2016) 113:E2627–35. doi: 10.1073/pnas.1515793113
52. Levy O, Jean-Jacques RM, Cywes C, Sisson RB, Zarember KA, Godowski PJ, et al. Critical role of the complement system in group B streptococcus-induced tumor necrosis factor alpha release. *Infect Immun.* (2003) 71:6344–53. doi: 10.1128/iai.71.11.6344-6353.2003
53. Ehrnström B, Beckwith KS, Yurchenko M, Moen SH, Kojen JF, Lentini G, et al. Toll-Like receptor 8 is a major sensor of group bstreptococcusbut notescherichia coliin human primary monocytes and macrophages. *Front Immunol.* (2017) 8:1243. doi: 10.3389/fimmu.2017.01243
54. Ugolini M, Gerhard J, Burkert S, Jensen KJ, Georg P, Ebner F, et al. Recognition of microbial viability via TLR8 drives TFH cell differentiation and vaccine responses. *Nat Immunol.* (2018) 19:386–96. doi: 10.1038/s41590-018-0068-4

55. Moretti J, Blander JM. Detection of a vita-PAMP STINGs cells into reticulophagy. *Autophagy* (2018). doi: 10.1080/15548627.2018.1441471. [Epub ahead of print].
56. Blander JM, Sander LE. Beyond pattern recognition: five immune checkpoints for scaling the microbial threat. *Nat Rev Immunol.* (2012) 12:215–25. doi: 10.1038/nri3167
57. Sharma AA, Jen R, Kan B, Sharma A, Marchant E, Tang A, et al. Impaired NLRP3 inflammasome activity during fetal development regulates IL-1β production in human monocytes. *Eur J Immunol.* (2015) 45:238–49. doi: 10.1002/eji.201444707
58. Austermann J, Friesenhagen J, Fassl SK, Petersen B, Ortkras T, Burgmann J, et al. Alarmins MRP8 and MRP14 induce stress tolerance in phagocytes under sterile inflammatory conditions. *Cell Rep.* (2014) 9:2112–23. doi: 10.1016/j.celrep.2014.11.020
59. Romero R, Chaiworapongsa T, Alpay Savasan Z, Xu Y, Hussein Y, Dong Z, et al. Damage-associated molecular patterns (DAMPs) in preterm labor with intact membranes and preterm PROM: a study of the alarmin HMGB1. *J Matern Neonatal Med.* (2011) 24:1444–55. doi: 10.3109/14767058.2011.591460
60. Strunk T, Doherty D, Jacques MBiostat A, Simmer K, Richmond P, Kohan R, et al. Histologic chorioamnionitis is associated with reduced risk of late-onset sepsis in preterm infants. *Pediatrics* (2012) 129:e134–41. doi: 10.1542/peds.2010-3493
61. Scheible KM, Emo J, Yang H, Holden-Wiltse J, Straw A, Huyck H, et al. Developmentally determined reduction in CD31 during gestation is associated with CD8+ T cell effector differentiation in preterm infants. *Clin Immunol.* (2015) 161:65–74. doi: 10.1016/j.clim.2015.07.003
62. Luciano AA, Arbona-Ramirez IM, Ruiz R, Llorens-Bonilla BJ, Martinez-Lopez DG, Funderburg N, et al. Alterations in regulatory t cell subpopulations seen in preterm infants. *PLoS ONE* (2014) 9:e95867. doi: 10.1371/journal.pone.0095867
63. Gervassi A, Lejarcegui N, Dross S, Jacobson A, Itaya G, Kidzeru E, et al. Myeloid derived suppressor cells are present at high frequency in neonates and suppress in vitro t cell responses. *PLoS ONE* (2014) 9:e107816. doi: 10.1371/journal.pone.0107816
64. Rieber N, Gille C, Köstlin N, Schäfer I, Spring B, Ost M, et al. Neutrophilic myeloid-derived suppressor cells in cord blood modulate innate and adaptive immune responses. *Clin Exp Immunol.* (2013) 174:45–52. doi: 10.1111/cei.12143
65. Dreschers S, Saupp P, Hornef M, Prehn A, Platen C, Morschhäuser J, et al. Reduced PICD in monocytes mounts altered neonate immune response to *Candida albicans*. *PLoS ONE* (2016) 11:e0166648. doi: 10.1371/journal.pone.0166648
66. Gille C, Leiber A, Spring B, Kempf VAJ, Loeffler J, Poets CF, et al. Diminished Phagocytosis-Induced Cell Death (PICD) in Neonatal Monocytes upon Infection with *Escherichia coli*. *Pediatr Res.* (2008) 63:33–8. doi: 10.1203/PDR.0b013e31815b8e9f
67. O'Driscoll DN, Greene CM, Molloy EJ. Immune function? A missing link in the gender disparity in preterm neonatal outcomes. *Expert Rev Clin Immunol.* (2017) 13:1061–71. doi: 10.1080/1744666X.2017.1386555
68. Sampath V, Mulrooney N, Patel AL, Cohen J, Zhang L, Garland J, et al. A potential role for the NOD1 Variant (rs6958571) in Gram-positive blood stream infection in ELBW infants. *Neonatology* (2017) 112:354–8. doi: 10.1159/000477433
69. Esposito S, Zampiero A, Pugni L, Tabano S, Pelucchi C, Ghirardi B, et al. Genetic polymorphisms and sepsis in premature neonates. *PLoS ONE* (2014) 9:e101248. doi: 10.1371/journal.pone.0101248
70. Amenyogbe N, Kollmann TR, Ben-Othman R. Early-life host–microbiome interphase: the key frontier for immune development. *Front Pediatr.* (2017) 5:111. doi: 10.3389/fped.2017.00111
71. Gerdes JS. Diagnosis and management of bacterial infections in the neonate. *Pediatr Clin North Am.* (2004) 51:939–59. doi: 10.1016/j.pcl.2004.03.009
72. Smith CL, Dickinson P, Forster T, Craigon M, Ross A, Khondoker MR, et al. Identification of a human neonatal immune-metabolic network associated with bacterial infection. *Nat Commun.* (2014) 5:4649. doi: 10.1038/ncomms5649
73. Fragiadakis GK, Baca QJ, Gherardini PF, Ganio EA, Gaudilliere DK, Tingle M, et al. Mapping the fetomaternal peripheral immune system at term pregnancy. *J Immunol.* (2016) 197:4482–92. doi: 10.4049/jimmunol.1601195
74. Amenyogbe N, Levy O, Kollmann TR. Systems vaccinology: a promise for the young and the poor. *Philos Trans R Soc Lond B Biol Sci.* (2015) 370:20140340. doi: 10.1098/rstb.2014.0340
75. Pammi M, Suresh G. Enteral lactoferrin supplementation for prevention of sepsis and necrotizing enterocolitis in preterm infants. *Cochrane Database Syst Rev.* (2017) 6:CD007137. doi: 10.1002/14651858.CD007137.pub5
76. EMA. *Report on the Expert Meeting on Neonatal and Paediatric Sepsis, 8 June 2010.* (2010)
77. Pammi M, Haque KN. Pentoxifylline for treatment of sepsis and necrotizing enterocolitis in neonates. *Cochrane Database Syst Rev.* (2015) 3:CD004205. doi: 10.1002/14651858.CD004205.pub3
78. Ohlsson A, Lacy JB. Intravenous immunoglobulin for suspected or proven infection in neonates. *Cochrane Database Syst Rev.* (2015) 3:CD001239. doi: 10.1002/14651858.CD001239.pub5
79. Carr R, Modi N, Doré C. G-CSF and GM-CSF for treating or preventing neonatal infections. *Cochrane database Syst Rev.* (2003) CD003066. doi: 10.1002/14651858.CD003066
80. Pammi M, Brocklehurst P. Granulocyte transfusions for neonates with confirmed or suspected sepsis and neutropenia. *Cochrane Database Syst Rev.* (2011) CD003956. doi: 10.1002/14651858.CD003956.pub2
81. Ohlsson A, Lacy JB. Intravenous immunoglobulin for preventing infection in preterm and/or low birth weight infants. In: Ohlsson A, editor. *Cochrane Database of Systematic Reviews* (Chichester: John Wiley & Sons, Ltd), (2013) CD000361. doi: 10.1002/14651858.CD000361.pub2
82. Shah PS, Kaufman DA. Antistaphylococcal immunoglobulins to prevent staphylococcal infection in very low birth weight infants. *Cochrane Database Syst Rev.* (2009) CD006449. doi: 10.1002/14651858.CD006449.pub2
83. Patel M, Kaufman DA. Anti-lipoteichoic acid monoclonal antibody (pagibaximab) studies for the prevention of staphylococcal bloodstream infections in preterm infants. *Expert Opin Biol Ther.* (2015) 15:595–600. doi: 10.1517/14712598.2015.1019857
84. Weisman LE, Thackray HM, Steinhorn RH, Walsh WF, Lassiter HA, Dhanireddy R, et al. A randomized study of a monoclonal antibody (pagibaximab) to prevent staphylococcal sepsis. *Pediatrics* (2011) 128:271–9. doi: 10.1542/peds.2010-3081
85. Carr R, Brocklehurst P, Doré CJ, Modi N. Granulocyte-macrophage colony stimulating factor administered as prophylaxis for reduction of sepsis in extremely preterm, small for gestational age neonates (the PROGRAMS trial): a single-blind, multicentre, randomised controlled trial. *Lancet* (2009) 373:226–33. doi: 10.1016/S0140-6736(09)60071-4
86. Quigley M, McGuire W. Formula versus donor breast milk for feeding preterm or low birth weight infants. *Coch Database Syst Rev.* (2014) CD002971. doi: 10.1002/14651858.CD002971.pub3
87. Dermyshi E, Wang Y, Yan C, Hong W, Qiu G, Gong X, et al. The "Golden Age" of probiotics: a systematic review and meta-analysis of randomized and observational studies in preterm infants. *Neonatology* (2017) 112:9–23. doi: 10.1159/000454668
88. Rao SC, Athalye-Jape GK, Deshpande GC, Simmer KN, Patole SK. Probiotic supplementation and late-onset sepsis in preterm infants: a meta-analysis. *Pediatrics* (2016) 137:e20153684. doi: 10.1542/peds.2015-3684
89. Agrawal S, Rao S, Patole S. Probiotic supplementation for preventing invasive fungal infections in preterm neonates–a systematic review and meta-analysis. *Mycoses* (2015) 58:642–51. doi: 10.1111/myc.12368
90. Chang H-Y, Chen J-H, Chang J-H, Lin H-C, Lin C-Y, Peng C-C. Multiple strains probiotics appear to be the most effective probiotics in the prevention of necrotizing enterocolitis and mortality: an updated meta-analysis. *PLoS ONE* (2017) 12:e0171579. doi: 10.1371/journal.pone.0171579
91. Moe-Byrne T, Brown JV, McGuire W. Glutamine supplementation to prevent morbidity and mortality in preterm infants. *Cochrane Database Syst Rev.* (2016) 4:CD001457. doi: 10.1002/14651858.CD001457.pub6
92. Darlow BA, Austin NC. Selenium supplementation to prevent short-term morbidity in preterm neonates. *Cochrane Database Syst Rev.* (2003) CD003312. doi: 10.1002/14651858.CD003312
93. Kaufman D, Fairchild KD. Clinical microbiology of bacterial and fungal sepsis in very-low-birth-weight infants. *Clin Microbiol Rev.* (2004) 17:638–80. doi: 10.1128/CMR.17.3.638-680.2004

94. van den Berg JP, Westerbeek EAM, van der Klis FRM, Berbers GAM, van Elburg RM. Transplacental transport of IgG antibodies to preterm infants: a review of the literature. *Early Hum Dev.* (2011) 87:67–72. doi: 10.1016/j.earlhumdev.2010.11.003
95. Shankar-Hari M, Spencer J, Sewell WA, Rowan KM, Singer M. Bench-to-bedside review: Immunoglobulin therapy for sepsis - biological plausibility from a critical care perspective. *Crit Care* (2012) 16:206. doi: 10.1186/cc10597
96. Benjamin DK, Schelonka R, White R, Holley HP, Bifano E, Cummings J,et al. A blinded, randomized, multicenter study of an intravenous *Staphylococcus aureus* immune globulin. *J Perinatol.* (2006) 26:290–5. doi: 10.1038/sj.jp.7211496
97. Baker CJ, Melish ME, Hall RT, Casto DT, Vasan U, Givner LB. Intravenous immune globulin for the prevention of nosocomial infection in low-birth-weight neonates. *N Engl J Med.* (1992) 327:213–9. doi: 10.1056/NEJM199207233270401
98. INIS Collaborative Group, Brocklehurst P, Farrell B, King A, Juszczak E, Darlow B, Haque K, et al. Treatment of neonatal sepsis with intravenous immune globulin. *N Engl J Med.* (2011) 365:1201–11. doi: 10.1056/NEJMoa1100441
99. Sause WE, Buckley PT, Strohl WR, Lynch AS, Torres VJ. Antibody-based biologics and their promise to combat *Staphylococcus aureus* infections. *Trends Pharmacol Sci.* (2016) 37:231–41. doi: 10.1016/j.tips.2015.11.008
100. Tao K-M, Li X-Q, Yang L-Q, Yu W-F, Lu Z-J, Sun Y-M, et al. Glutamine supplementation for critically ill adults. *Cochrane Database Syst Rev.* (2014) CD010050. doi: 10.1002/14651858.CD010050.pub2
101. Tarnow-Mordi W, Isaacs D, Dutta S. Adjunctive immunologic interventions in neonatal sepsis. *Clin Perinatol.* (2010) 37:481–99. doi: 10.1016/j.clp.2009.12.002
102. Saugstad OD. Oxidative stress in the newborn–a 30-year perspective. *Biol Neonate* (2005) 88:228–36. doi: 10.1159/000087586
103. Belik J, González-Luis GE, Perez-Vizcaino F, Villamor E. Isoprostanes in fetal and neonatal health and disease. *Free Radic Biol Med.* (2010) 48:177–88. doi: 10.1016/j.freeradbiomed.2009.10.043
104. Aggarwal R, Gathwala G, Yadav S, Kumar P. Selenium supplementation for prevention of late-onset sepsis in very low birth weight preterm neonates. *J Trop Pediatr.* (2016) 62:185–93. doi: 10.1093/tropej/fmv096
105. D'Angelo G, Marseglia L, Reiter RJ, Buonocore G, Gitto E. Melatonin and neonatal sepsis: a promising antioxidant adjuvant agent. *Am J Perinatol.* (2017) 34:1382–8. doi: 10.1055/s-0037-1604244
106. El Frargy M, El-sharkawy HM, Attia GF. Use of melatonin as an adjuvant therapy in neonatal sepsis. *J Neonatal Perinatal Med.* (2015) 8:227–32. doi: 10.3233/NPM-15814072
107. Gitto E, Karbownik M, Reiter RJ, Tan DX, Cuzzocrea S, Chiurazzi P, et al. Effects of melatonin treatment in septic newborns. *Pediatr Res.* (2001) 50:756–60. doi: 10.1203/00006450-200112000-00021
108. El-Gendy FM, El-Hawy MA, Hassan MG. Beneficial effect of melatonin in the treatment of neonatal sepsis. *J Matern Fetal Neonatal Med.* (2017) 31:2299-303. doi: 10.1080/14767058.2017.1342794
109. Uberos J, Miras-Baldo M, Jerez-Calero A, Narbona-López E. Effectiveness of vitamin a in the prevention of complications of prematurity. *Pediatr Neonatol.* (2014) 55:358–62. doi: 10.1016/j.pedneo.2013.12.002
110. Haider BA, Sharma R, Bhutta ZA. Neonatal vitamin A supplementation for the prevention of mortality and morbidity in term neonates in low and middle income countries. *Cochrane Database Syst Rev.* (2017) 2:CD006980. doi: 10.1002/14651858.CD006980.pub3
111. *Effect of Vitamin A in the Treatment of Neonatal Sepsis and Necrotizing Enterocolitis - Full Text View - ClinicalTrials.gov.* Available online at: https://clinicaltrials.gov/ct2/show/NCT00707785 [Accessed April 4, 2017]
112. Mathias B, Szpila BE, Moore FA, Efron PA, Moldawer LL. A review of GM-CSF Therapy in Sepsis. *Medicine (Baltimore)* (2015) 94:e2044. doi: 10.1097/MD.0000000000002044
113. Gille C, Steffen F, Lauber K, Keppeler H, Leiber A, Spring B, et al. Clearance of apoptotic neutrophils is diminished in cord blood monocytes and does not lead to reduced il-8 production. *Pediatr Res.* (2009) 66:507–12. doi: 10.1203/PDR.0b013e3181b9b470
114. Melvan JN, Bagby GJ, Welsh DA, Nelson S, Zhang P. Neonatal sepsis and neutrophil insufficiencies. *Int Rev Immunol.* (2010) 29:315–48. doi: 10.3109/08830181003792803
115. Christensen RD, Rothstein G. Exhaustion of mature marrow neutrophils in neonates with sepsis. *J Pediatr.* (1980) 96:316–8.
116. Molloy EJ, O'Neill AJ, Grantham JJ, Sheridan-Pereira M, Fitzpatrick JM, Webb DW, et al. Granulocyte colony-stimulating factor and granulocyte-macrophage colony-stimulating factor have differential effects on neonatal and adult neutrophil survival and function. *Pediatr Res.* (2005) 57:806–12. doi: 10.1203/01.PDR.0000156500.13600.B5
117. Castagnola E, Dufour C. Role of G-CSF GM-CSF in the management of infections in preterm newborns: an update. *Early Hum Dev.* (2014) 90:S15–17. doi: 10.1016/S0378-3782(14)50005-9
118. Pugni L, Ronchi A, Bizzarri B, Consonni D, Pietrasanta C, Ghirardi B, et al. Exchange transfusion in the treatment of neonatal septic shock: a ten-year experience in a neonatal intensive care unit. *Int J Mol Sci.* (2016) 17:695. doi: 10.3390/ijms17050695
119. Aradhya AS, Sundaram V, Kumar P, Ganapathy SM, Jain A, Rawat A. Double volume exchange transfusion in severe neonatal sepsis. *Indian J Pediatr.* (2016) 83:107–13. doi: 10.1007/s12098-015-1841-0
120. Jackson JC. Adverse events associated with exchange transfusion in healthy and ill newborns. *Pediatrics* (1997) 99:E7.
121. Sarangi PP, Lee H, Kim M. Activated protein C action in inflammation. *Br J Haematol.* (2010) 148:817–33. doi: 10.1111/j.1365-2141.2009.08020.x
122. Thachil J, Toh CH, Levi M, Watson HG. The withdrawal of Activated Protein C from the use in patients with severe sepsis and DIC [Amendment to the BCSH guideline on disseminated intravascular coagulation]. *Br J Haematol.* (2012) 157:493–4. doi: 10.1111/j.1365-2141.2011.09019.x
123. Nadel S, Goldstein B, Williams MD, Dalton H, Peters M, Macias WL, et al. Drotrecogin alfa (activated) in children with severe sepsis: a multicentre phase III randomised controlled trial. *Lancet* (2007) 369:836–43. doi: 10.1016/S0140-6736(07)60411-5
124. Kylat RI, Ohlsson A. Recombinant human activated protein C for severe sepsis in neonates. In: Kylat RI editor. *Cochrane Database of Systematic Reviews* (Chichester: John Wiley & Sons, Ltd), (2012) CD005385. doi: 10.1002/14651858.CD005385.pub3
125. Caccavo D, Pellegrino NM, Altamura M, Rigon A, Amati L, Amoroso A, et al. Antimicrobial and immunoregulatory functions of lactoferrin and its potential therapeutic application. *J Endotoxin Res.* (2002) 8:403–17. doi: 10.1179/096805102125001000
126. Elass E, Masson M, Mazurier J, Legrand D. Lactoferrin inhibits the lipopolysaccharide-induced expression and proteoglycan-binding ability of interleukin-8 in human endothelial cells. *Infect Immun.* (2002) 70:1860–6. doi: 10.1128/iai.70.4.1860-1866.2002
127. Schüller SS, Wisgrill L, Herndl E, Spittler A, Förster-Waldl E, Sadeghi K, et al. Pentoxifylline modulates LPS-induced hyperinflammation in monocytes of preterm infants *in vitro*. *Pediatr Res.* (2017) 82:215–25. doi: 10.1038/pr.2017.41
128. Speer EM, Dowling DJ, Ozog LS, Xu J, Yang J, Kennady G, et al. Pentoxifylline inhibits TLR- and inflammasome-mediated in vitro inflammatory cytokine production in human blood with greater efficacy and potency in newborns. *Pediatr Res.* (2017) 81:806–16. doi: 10.1038/pr.2017.6
129. Anaya JM, Espinoza LR. Phosphodiesterase inhibitor pentoxifylline: an antiinflammatory/immunomodulatory drug potentially useful in some rheumatic diseases. *J Rheumatol.* (1995) 22:595–9.
130. Sherman MP. New concepts of microbial translocation in the neonatal intestine: mechanisms and prevention. *Clin Perinatol.* (2010) 37:565–79. doi: 10.1016/j.clp.2010.05.006
131. Wisgrill L, Wessely I, Spittler A, Förster-Waldl E, Berger A, Sadeghi K. Human lactoferrin attenuates the proinflammatory response of neonatal monocyte-derived macrophages. *Clin Exp Immunol.* (2018) 192:315–24. doi: 10.1111/cei.13108
132. Kallapur SG, Nitsos I, Moss TJM, Polglase GR, Pillow JJ, Cheah F-C, et al. IL-1 mediates pulmonary and systemic inflammatory responses to chorioamnionitis induced by lipopolysaccharide. *Am J Respir Crit Care Med.* (2009) 179:955–61. doi: 10.1164/rccm.200811-1728OC
133. Nold MF, Mangan NE, Rudloff I, Cho SX, Shariatian N, Samarasinghe TD, et al. Interleukin-1 receptor antagonist prevents murine bronchopulmonary dysplasia induced by perinatal inflammation and hyperoxia. *Proc Natl Acad Sci USA.* (2013) 110:14384–9. doi: 10.1073/pnas.1306859110

134. Rudloff I, Cho SX, Bui CB, McLean C, Veldman A, Berger PJ, et al. Refining anti-inflammatory therapy strategies for bronchopulmonary dysplasia. *J Cell Mol Med.* (2017) 21:1128–38. doi: 10.1111/jcmm.13044
135. Liao J, Kapadia VS, Brown LS, Cheong N, Longoria C, Mija D, et al. The NLRP3 inflammasome is critically involved in the development of bronchopulmonary dysplasia. *Nat Commun.* (2015) 6:8977. doi: 10.1038/ncomms9977
136. Singh PK, Parsek MR, Greenberg EP, Welsh MJ. A component of innate immunity prevents bacterial biofilm development. *Nature* (2002) 417:552–5. doi: 10.1038/417552a
137. Elass-Rochard E, Legrand D, Salmon V, Roseanu A, Trif M, Tobias PS, et al. Lactoferrin inhibits the endotoxin interaction with CD14 by competition with the lipopolysaccharide-binding protein. *Infect Immun* (1998) 66:486–91.
138. Kawasaki Y, Tazume S, Shimizu K, Matsuzawa H, Dosako S, Isoda H, et al. Inhibitory effects of bovine lactoferrin on the adherence of enterotoxigenic *Escherichia coli* to host cells. *Biosci Biotechnol Biochem.* (2000) 64:348–54.
139. Ochoa TJ, Noguera-Obenza M, Ebel F, Guzman CA, Gomez HF, Cleary TG. Lactoferrin impairs type III secretory system function in enteropathogenic *Escherichia coli. Infect Immun.* (2003) 71:5149–55.
140. Ballard O, Morrow AL. Human milk composition: nutrients and bioactive factors. *Pediatr Clin North Am.* (2013) 60:49–74. doi: 10.1016/j.pcl.2012.10.002
141. Schanler RJ, Shulman RJ, Lau C. Feeding strategies for premature infants: beneficial outcomes of feeding fortified human milk versus preterm formula. *Pediatrics* (1999) 103:1150–7.
142. de Silva A, Jones PW, Spencer SA. Does human milk reduce infection rates in preterm infants? A systematic review. *Arch Dis Child* (2004) 89:F509–13. doi: 10.1136/adc.2003.045682
143. Cacho NT, Lawrence RM. Innate immunity and breast milk. *Front Immunol.* (2017) 8:584. doi: 10.3389/fimmu.2017.00584
144. Underwood MA. Human milk for the premature infant. *Pediatr Clin North Am.* (2013) 60:189–207. doi: 10.1016/j.pcl.2012.09.008
145. Cacho NT, Parker LA, Neu J. Necrotizing enterocolitis and human milk feeding: a systematic review. *Clin Perinatol.* (2017) 44:49–67. doi: 10.1016/j.clp.2016.11.009
146. Meier P, Patel A, Esquerra-Zwiers A. Donor human milk update: evidence, mechanisms, and priorities for research and practice. *J Pediatr.* (2017) 180:15–21. doi: 10.1016/j.jpeds.2016.09.027
147. Kreissl A, Zwiauer V, Repa A, Binder C, Thanhaeuser M, Jilma B, et al. Human milk analyser shows that the lactation period affects protein levels in preterm breastmilk. *Acta Paediatr.* (2016) 105:635–40. doi: 10.1111/apa.13348
148. Gormaz M, Torres-Cuevas I, Cernada M, Kuligowski J, Cubells E, Escobar J, et al. Role of human milk in oxidative stress associated with prematurity. *J Pediatr Biochem.* (2013) 3:169–77. doi: 10.3233/JPB-130090
149. Peila C, Moro GE, Bertino E, Cavallarin L, Giribaldi M, Giuliani F, et al. The effect of holder pasteurization on nutrients and biologically-active components in donor human milk: a review. *Nutrients* (2016) 8:477. doi: 10.3390/nu8080477
150. Daniels B, Schmidt S, King T, Israel-Ballard K, Amundson Mansen K, Coutsoudis A. The effect of simulated flash-heat pasteurization on immune components of human milk. *Nutrients* (2017) 9:178. doi: 10.3390/nu9020178
151. Villamor-Martínez E, Pierro M, Cavallaro G, Mosca F, Kramer BW, Villamor E. Donor human milk protects against bronchopulmonary dysplasia: a systematic review and meta-analysis. *Nutrients* (2018) 10:238. doi: 10.3390/nu10020238
152. Gibson GR, Hutkins R, Sanders ME, Prescott SL, Reimer RA, Salminen SJ, et al. Expert consensus document: the international scientific association for probiotics and prebiotics (ISAPP) consensus statement on the definition and scope of prebiotics. *Nat Rev Gastroenterol Hepatol.* (2017) 14:491–502. doi: 10.1038/nrgastro.2017.75
153. Jakaitis BM, Denning PW. Human breast milk and the gastrointestinal innate immune system. *Clin Perinatol.* (2014) 41:423–35. doi: 10.1016/j.clp.2014.02.011
154. Nair V, Soraisham AS. Probiotics and prebiotics: role in prevention of nosocomial sepsis in preterm infants. *Int J Pediatr.* (2013) 2013:874726. doi: 10.1155/2013/874726
155. Sanders ME, Guarner F, Guerrant R, Holt PR, Quigley EM, Sartor RB, et al. An update on the use and investigation of probiotics in health and disease. *Gut* (2013) 62:787–96. doi: 10.1136/gutjnl-2012-302504
156. Madan JC, Salari RC, Saxena D, Davidson L, O'Toole GA, Moore JH, Sogin ML, et al. Gut microbial colonisation in premature neonates predicts neonatal sepsis. *Arch Dis Child Fetal Neonatal Ed.* (2012) 97:F456–62. doi: 10.1136/fetalneonatal-2011-301373
157. AlFaleh K, Anabrees J. Probiotics for prevention of necrotizing enterocolitis in preterm infants. *Cochrane Database Syst Rev.* (2014) CD005496. doi: 10.1002/14651858.CD005496.pub4
158. Deshpande G, Jape G, Rao S, Patole S. Benefits of probiotics in preterm neonates in low-income and medium-income countries: a systematic review of randomised controlled trials. *BMJ Open* (2017) 7:e017638. doi: 10.1136/bmjopen-2017-017638
159. Dani C, Coviello C C, Corsini I I, Arena F, Antonelli A, Rossolini GM. Lactobacillus sepsis and probiotic therapy in newborns: two new cases and literature review. *AJP Rep.* (2016) 6:e25–9. doi: 10.1055/s-0035-1566312
160. Panigrahi P, Parida S, Nanda NC, Satpathy R, Pradhan L, Chandel DS, et al. A randomized synbiotic trial to prevent sepsis among infants in rural India. *Nature* (2017) 548:407–12. doi: 10.1038/nature23480
161. Embleton ND, Zalewski S, Berrington JE. Probiotics for prevention of necrotizing enterocolitis and sepsis in preterm infants. *Curr Opin Infect Dis.* (2016) 29:256–61. doi: 10.1097/QCO.0000000000000269
162. Kruzel ML, Zimecki M, Actor JK. Lactoferrin in a context of inflammation-induced pathology. *Front Immunol.* (2017) 8:1438. doi: 10.3389/fimmu.2017.01438
163. Elass-Rochard E, Roseanu A, Legrand D, Trif M, Salmon V, Motas C, et al. Lactoferrin-lipopolysaccharide interaction: involvement of the 28-34 loop region of human lactoferrin in the high-affinity binding to *Escherichia coli* 055B5 lipopolysaccharide. *Biochem J.* (1995) 312 (Pt 3):839–45.
164. Curran CS, Demick KP, Mansfield JM. Lactoferrin activates macrophages via TLR4-dependent and -independent signaling pathways. *Cell Immunol.* (2006) 242:23–30. doi: 10.1016/j.cellimm.2006.08.006
165. Zimecki M, Właszczyk A, Zagulski T, Kübler A. Lactoferrin lowers serum interleukin 6 and tumor necrosis factor alpha levels in mice subjected to surgery. *Arch Immunol Ther Exp. (Warsz)* (1998) 46:97–104.
166. Zimecki M, Właszczyk A, Wojciechowski R, Dawiskiba J, Kruzel M. Lactoferrin regulates the immune responses in post-surgical patients. *Arch Immunol Ther Exp. (Warsz)* (2001) 49:325–33.
167. Kruzel ML, Actor JK, Boldogh I, Zimecki M. Lactoferrin in health and disease. *Postepy Hig Med Dosw (Online)* (2007) 61:261–7.
168. Pierce A, Colavizza D, Benaissa M, Maes P, Tartar A, Montreuil J, et al. Molecular cloning and sequence analysis of bovine lactotransferrin. *Eur J Biochem.* (1991) 196:177–84.
169. Manzoni P, Rinaldi M, Cattani S, Pugni L, Romeo MG, Messner H, et al. Bovine lactoferrin supplementation for prevention of late-onset sepsis in very low-birth-weight neonates<subtitle>a randomized trial</subtitle> *JAMA* (2009) 302:1421. doi: 10.1001/jama.2009.1403
170. Sherman MP, Adamkin DH, Niklas V, Radmacher P, Sherman J, Wertheimer F, et al. Randomized controlled trial of talactoferrin oral solution in preterm infants. *J Pediatr.* (2016) 175:68–73.e3. doi: 10.1016/j.jpeds.2016.04.084
171. Strunk T, Hibbert J, Doherty D, Granland C, Trend S, Simmer K, et al. Probiotics and antimicrobial protein and peptide levels in preterm infants. *Acta Paediatr.* (2017) 106:1747–53. doi: 10.1111/apa.13826
172. Gammoh NZ, Rink L. Zinc in Infection and Inflammation. *Nutrients* (2017) 9:624. doi: 10.3390/nu9060624
173. Prasad AS. Zinc: mechanisms of host defense. *J Nutr.* (2007) 137:1345–9. doi: 10.1093/jn/137.5.1345
174. Bhatnagar S, Wadhwa N, Aneja S, Lodha R, Kabra SK, Natchu UCM, et al. Zinc as adjunct treatment in infants aged between 7 and 120 days with probable serious bacterial infection: a randomised, double-blind, placebo-controlled trial. *Lancet* (2012) 379:2072–8. doi: 10.1016/S0140-6736(12)60477-2
175. Terrin G, Berni Canani R, Passariello A, Messina F, Conti MG, Caoci S, Smaldore A, et al. Zinc supplementation reduces morbidity and mortality in very-low-birth-weight preterm neonates: a hospital-based randomized, placebo-controlled trial in an industrialized country. *Am J Clin Nutr.* (2013) 98:1468–74. doi: 10.3945/ajcn.112.054478

176. Mehta K, Bhatta NK, Majhi S, Shrivastava MK, Singh RR. Oral zinc supplementation for reducing mortality in probable neonatal sepsis: a double blind randomized placebo controlled trial. *Indian Pediatr.* (2013) 50:390–3. doi: 10.1007/s13312-013-0120-2
177. Banupriya N, Bhat BV, Benet BD, Catherine C, Sridhar MG, Parija SC. Short term oral zinc supplementation among babies with neonatal sepsis for reducing mortality and improving outcome - a double-blind randomized controlled trial. *Indian J Pediatr.* (2018) 85:5–9. doi: 10.1007/s12098-017-2444-8
178. Tang Z, Wei Z, Wen F, Wu Y. Efficacy of zinc supplementation for neonatal sepsis: a systematic review and meta-analysis. *J Matern Fetal Neonatal Med.* (2017). doi: 10.1080/14767058.2017.1402001. [Epub ahead of print].
179. Staub E, Evers K, Askie LM. Enteral zinc supplementation for prevention of morbidity and mortality in preterm neonates (Protocol). *Coch Database Syst Rev.* (2017) CD012797. doi: 10.1002/14651858.CD012797
180. Speer EM, Dowling DJ, Xu J, Ozog LS, Mathew JA, Chander A, et al. Pentoxifylline, dexamethasone and azithromycin demonstrate distinct age-dependent and synergistic inhibition of TLR- and inflammasome-mediated cytokine production in human newborn and adult blood in vitro. *PLoS ONE* (2018) 13:e0196352. doi: 10.1371/journal.pone.0196352
181. Shabaan AE, Nasef N, Shouman B, Nour I, Mesbah A, Abdel-Hady H. Pentoxifylline therapy for late-onset sepsis in preterm infants: a randomized controlled trial. *Pediatr Infect Dis J.* (2015) 34:e143-8. doi: 10.1097/INF.0000000000000698
182. Jones CE, Calvert A, Le Doare K. Vaccination in pregnancy—recent developments. *Pediatr Infect Dis J.* (2018) 37:191–3. doi: 10.1097/INF.0000000000001822
183. Heath PT, Culley FJ, Jones CE, Kampmann B, Le Doare K, Nunes MC, et al. Group B streptococcus and respiratory syncytial virus immunisation during pregnancy: a landscape analysis. *Lancet Infect Dis.* (2017) 17:e223–4. doi: 10.1016/S1473-3099(17)30232-3
184. Krause PR, Bialek SR, Boppana SB, Griffiths PD, Laughlin CA, Ljungman P, et al. Priorities for CMV vaccine development. *Vaccine* (2013) 32:4–10. doi: 10.1016/j.vaccine.2013.09.042
185. Munoz FM, Piedra PA, Glezen WP. Safety and immunogenicity of respiratory syncytial virus purified fusion protein-2 vaccine in pregnant women. *Vaccine* (2003) 21:3465–7. doi: 10.1016/s0264-410x(03)00352-9
186. van den Berg JP, Westerbeek EAM, Smits GP, van der Klis FRM, Berbers GAM, van Elburg RM. Lower transplacental antibody transport for measles, mumps, rubella and varicella zoster in very preterm infants. *PLoS ONE* (2014) 9:e94714. doi: 10.1371/journal.pone.0094714
187. Marchant A, Sadarangani M, Garand M, Dauby N, Verhasselt V, Pereira L, et al. Maternal immunisation: collaborating with mother nature. *Lancet Infect Dis.* (2017) 17:e197–208. doi: 10.1016/S1473-3099(17)30229-3
188. Martin L, van Meegern A, Doemming S, Schuerholz T. Antimicrobial peptides in human sepsis. *Front Immunol.* (2015) 6:404. doi: 10.3389/fimmu.2015.00404
189. Huttner KM, Bevins CL. Antimicrobial peptides as mediators of epithelial host defense. *Pediatr Res.* (1999) 45:785–94. doi: 10.1203/00006450-199906000-00001
190. Battersby AJ, Khara J, Wright VJ, Levy O, Kampmann B. Antimicrobial proteins and peptides in early life: ontogeny and translational opportunities. *Front Immunol.* (2016) 7:309. doi: 10.3389/fimmu.2016.00309
191. Kai-Larsen Y, Gudmundsson GH, Agerberth B. A review of the innate immune defence of the human foetus and newborn, with the emphasis on antimicrobial peptides. *Acta Paediatr.* (2014) 103:1000–8. doi: 10.1111/apa.12700
192. Pammi M, Abrams SA. Oral lactoferrin for the prevention of sepsis and necrotizing enterocolitis in preterm infants. In: Pammi M editor. *Cochrane Database of Systematic Reviews* (Chichester: John Wiley & Sons, Ltd) (2015) CD007137. doi: 10.1002/14651858.CD007137.pub4
193. Levin M, Quint PA, Goldstein B, Barton P, Bradley JS, Shemie SD, et al. Recombinant bactericidal/permeability-increasing protein (rBPI21) as adjunctive treatment for children with severe meningococcal sepsis: a randomised trial. rBPI21 Meningococcal Sepsis Study Group. *Lancet* (2000) 356:961–7. doi: 10.1016/s0140-6736(00)02712-4
194. Giroir BP, Scannon PJ, Levin M. Bactericidal/permeability-increasing protein–lessons learned from the phase III, randomized, clinical trial of rBPI21 for adjunctive treatment of children with severe meningococcemia. *Crit Care Med.* (2001) 29:S130–5. doi: 10.1097/00003246-200107001-00039
195. Silva ON, de la Fuente-Núñez C, Haney EF, Fensterseifer ICM, Ribeiro SM, Porto WF, et al. An anti-infective synthetic peptide with dual antimicrobial and immunomodulatory activities. *Sci Rep.* (2016) 6:35465. doi: 10.1038/srep35465
196. Mansour SC, de la Fuente-Núñez C, Hancock REW. Peptide IDR-1018: modulating the immune system and targeting bacterial biofilms to treat antibiotic-resistant bacterial infections. *J Pept Sci.* (2015) 21:323–9. doi: 10.1002/psc.2708
197. Wynn JL, Scumpia PO, Winfield RD, Delano MJ, Kelly-Scumpia K, Barker T, et al. Defective innate immunity predisposes murine neonates to poor sepsis outcome but is reversed by TLR agonists. *Blood* (2008) 112:1750–8. doi: 10.1182/blood-2008-01-130500
198. Sharma AA, Jen R, Brant R, Ladd M, Huang Q, Skoll A, et al. Hierarchical maturation of innate immune defences in very preterm neonates. *Neonatology* (2014) 106:1–9. doi: 10.1159/000358550
199. Schüller S, Wisgrill L, Sadeghi K, Gindl E, Helmer H, Husslein P, et al. The TLR-specific Adjuvants R-848 and CpG-B endorse the immunological reaction of neonatal antigen presenting cells. *Pediatr Res.* (2016) 80:311–8. doi: 10.1038/pr.2016.71
200. Savva A, Roger T. Targeting toll-like receptors: promising therapeutic strategies for the management of sepsis-associated pathology and infectious diseases. *Front Immunol.* (2013) 4:387. doi: 10.3389/fimmu.2013.00387
201. Rincon JC, Cuenca AL, Raymond SL, Mathias B, Nacionales DC, Ungaro R, et al. Adjuvant pretreatment with alum protects neonatal mice in sepsis through myeloid cell activation. *Clin Exp Immunol.* (2017) 191:268–78. doi: 10.1111/cei.13072
202. Li H, Willingham SB, Ting JP-Y, Re F. Cutting edge: inflammasome activation by alum and alum's adjuvant effect are mediated by NLRP3. *J Immunol.* (2008) 181:17–21. doi: 10.4049/jimmunol.181.1.17
203. Aaby P, Roth A, Ravn H, Napirna BM, Rodrigues A, Lisse IM, et al. Randomized trial of BCG vaccination at birth to low-birth-weight children: beneficial nonspecific effects in the neonatal period? *J Infect Dis.* (2011) 204:245–52. doi: 10.1093/infdis/jir240
204. Levy O, Netea MG. Innate immune memory: implications for development of pediatric immunomodulatory agents and adjuvanted vaccines. *Pediatr Res.* (2014) 75:184–8. doi: 10.1038/pr.2013.214
205. Scheid A, Borriello F, Pietrasanta C, Christou H, Diray-Arce J, Pettengill MA, et al. Adjuvant effect of bacille calmette-guérin on hepatitis b vaccine immunogenicity in the preterm and term newborn. *Front Immunol.* (2018) 9:29. doi: 10.3389/fimmu.2018.00029
206. Chamberlain G, Fox J, Ashton B, Middleton J. Concise review: mesenchymal stem cells: their phenotype, differentiation capacity, immunological features, and potential for homing. *Stem Cells* (2007) 25:2739–49. doi: 10.1634/stemcells.2007-0197
207. Cóndor JM, Rodrigues CE, Sousa Moreira R de, Canale D, Volpini RA, Shimizu MHM, et al. Treatment with human wharton's jelly-derived mesenchymal stem cells attenuates sepsis-induced kidney injury, liver injury, and endothelial dysfunction. *Stem Cells Transl Med.* (2016) 5:1048–57. doi: 10.5966/sctm.2015-0138
208. Le Blanc K, Tammik L, Sundberg B, Haynesworth SE, Ringdén O. Mesenchymal stem cells inhibit and stimulate mixed lymphocyte cultures and mitogenic responses independently of the major histocompatibility complex. *Scand J Immunol.* (2003) 57:11–20. doi: 10.1046/j.1365-3083.2003.01176.x
209. Ren G, Zhang L, Zhao X, Xu G, Zhang Y, Roberts AI, et al. Mesenchymal stem cell-mediated immunosuppression occurs via concerted action of chemokines and nitric oxide. *Cell Stem Cell* (2008) 2:141–50. doi: 10.1016/j.stem.2007.11.014
210. English K, Ryan JM, Tobin L, Murphy MJ, Barry FP, Mahon BP. Cell contact, prostaglandin E(2) and transforming growth factor beta 1 play non-redundant roles in human mesenchymal stem cell induction of CD4+CD25(High) forkhead box P3+ regulatory T cells. *Clin Exp Immunol.* (2009) 156:149–60. doi: 10.1111/j.1365-2249.2009.03874.x
211. Krasnodembskaya A, Samarani G, Song Y, Zhuo H, Su X, Lee J-W, et al. Human mesenchymal stem cells reduce mortality and bacteremia in gram-negative sepsis in mice in part by enhancing the phagocytic activity of

blood monocytes. *Am J Physiol Lung Cell Mol Physiol.* (2012) 302:L1003–13. doi: 10.1152/ajplung.00180.2011

212. Sung DK, Chang YS, Sung SI, Yoo HS, Ahn SY, Park WS. Antibacterial effect of mesenchymal stem cells against *Escherichia coli* is mediated by secretion of beta- defensin- 2 via toll- like receptor 4 signalling. *Cell Microbiol.* (2016) 18:424–36. doi: 10.1111/cmi.12522
213. Lalu MM, Sullivan KJ, Mei SH, Moher D, Straus A, Fergusson DA, et al. Evaluating mesenchymal stem cell therapy for sepsis with preclinical meta-analyses prior to initiating a first-in-human trial. *Elife* (2016) 5:e17850. doi: 10.7554/eLife.17850
214. Johnson CL, Soeder Y, Dahlke MH. Concise review: mesenchymal stromal cell-based approaches for the treatment of acute respiratory distress and sepsis syndromes. *Stem Cells Transl Med.* (2017) 6:1141–51. doi: 10.1002/sctm.16-0415
215. Galstian GM, Parovichnikova EN, Makarova PM, Kuzmina LA, Troitskaya VV. Gemdzhian E, et al. The results of the russian clinical trial of mesenchymal stromal cells (MSCs) in severe neutropenic patients (pts) with septic shock (SS) (RUMCESS trial). *Blood* (2015) 126:2220.
216. *Cellular Immunotherapy for Septic Shock: A Phase I Trial - Full Text View - ClinicalTrials.gov.* Available online at: https://clinicaltrials.gov/ct2/show/NCT02421484 [Accessed April 17, 2017]
217. Chang YS, Ahn SY, Yoo HS, Sung SI, Choi SJ, Oh W Il, et al. Mesenchymal stem cells for bronchopulmonary dysplasia: phase 1 dose-escalation clinical trial. *J Pediatr.* (2014) 164:966–72.e6. doi: 10.1016/j.jpeds.2013.12.011
218. Mercer JS, Vohr BR, McGrath MM, Padbury JF, Wallach M, Oh W. Delayed cord clamping in very preterm infants reduces the incidence of intraventricular hemorrhage and late-onset sepsis: a randomized, controlled trial. *Pediatrics* (2006) 117:1235–42. doi: 10.1542/peds.2005-1706
219. Wisgrill L, Schüller S, Bammer M, Berger A, Pollak A, Radke TF, et al. Hematopoietic stem cells in neonates: any differences between very preterm and term neonates? *PLoS ONE* (2014) 9:e106717. doi: 10.1371/journal.pone.0106717
220. Fogarty M, Osborn DA, Askie L, Seidler AL, Hunter K, Lui K, et al. Delayed vs early umbilical cord clamping for preterm infants: a systematic review and meta-analysis. *Am J Obstet Gynecol.* (2018) 218:1–18. doi: 10.1016/j.ajog.2017.10.231
221. Coll RC, Robertson AAB, Chae JJ, Higgins SC, Muñoz-Planillo R, Inserra MC, et al. A small-molecule inhibitor of the NLRP3 inflammasome for the treatment of inflammatory diseases. *Nat Med.* (2015) 21:248–55. doi: 10.1038/nm.3806
222. Shao B-Z, Xu Z-Q, Han B-Z, Su D-F, Liu C. NLRP3 inflammasome and its inhibitors: a review. *Front Pharmacol.* (2015) 6:262. doi: 10.3389/fphar.2015.00262
223. Cohen TS, Boland ML, Boland BB, Takahashi V, Tovchigrechko A, Lee Y, et al. *S. aureus* evades macrophage killing through NLRP3-dependent effects on mitochondrial trafficking. *Cell Rep.* (2018) 22:2431–41. doi: 10.1016/j.celrep.2018.02.027
224. Gentile LF, Cuenca AL, Cuenca AG, Nacionales DC, Ungaro R, Efron PA, et al. Improved emergency myelopoiesis and survival in neonatal sepsis by caspase-1/11 ablation. *Immunology* (2015) 145:300–11. doi: 10.1111/imm.12450
225. Fenini G, Contassot E, French LE. Potential of IL-1, IL-18 and Inflammasome Inhibition for the Treatment of Inflammatory Skin Diseases. *Front Pharmacol.* (2017) 8:278. doi: 10.3389/fphar.2017.00278
226. Ridker PM, Everett BM, Thuren T, MacFadyen JG, Chang WH, Ballantyne C, et al. Antiinflammatory therapy with canakinumab for atherosclerotic disease. *N Engl J Med.* (2017) 377:1119–31. doi: 10.1056/NEJMoa1707914
227. Orman KL, English BK. Effects of antibiotic class on the macrophage inflammatory response to *Streptococcus pneumoniae*. *J Infect Dis.* (2000) 182:1561–5. doi: 10.1086/315861
228. von Seth M, Sjölin J, Larsson A, Eriksson M, Hillered L, Lipcsey M. Effects of tigecycline and doxycycline on inflammation and hemodynamics in porcine endotoxemia. *Shock* (2015) 43:604–11. doi: 10.1097/SHK.0000000000000351
229. Krakauer T, Buckley M. Doxycycline is anti-inflammatory and inhibits staphylococcal exotoxin-induced cytokines and chemokines. *Antimicrob Agents Chemother* (2003) 47:3630–3. doi: 10.1128/aac.47.11.3630-3633.2003
230. Bi W, Zhu L, Jing X, Zeng Z, Liang Y, Xu A, et al. Rifampicin improves neuronal apoptosis in LPS-stimulated co-cultured BV2 cells through inhibition of the TLR-4 pathway. *Mol Med Rep.* (2014) 10:1793–9. doi: 10.3892/mmr.2014.2480
231. Altenburg J, de Graaff CS, van der Werf TS, Boersma WG. Immunomodulatory effects of macrolide antibiotics - part 1: biological mechanisms. *Respiration* (2011) 81:67–74. doi: 10.1159/000320319
232. Nair V, Loganathan P, Soraisham AS. Azithromycin and other macrolides for prevention of bronchopulmonary dysplasia: a systematic review and meta-analysis. *Neonatology* (2014) 106:337–47. doi: 10.1159/000363493
233. Kallapur SG, Kramer BW, Jobe AH. Ureaplasma and BPD. *Semin Perinatol.* (2013) 37:94–101. doi: 10.1053/j.semperi.2013.01.005
234. Gualdoni GA, Lingscheid T, Schmetterer KG, Hennig A, Steinberger P, Zlabinger GJ. Azithromycin inhibits IL-1 secretion and non-canonical inflammasome activation. *Sci Rep.* (2015) 5:12016. doi: 10.1038/srep12016
235. Lendermon EA, Coon TA, Bednash JS, Weathington NM, McDyer JF, Mallampalli RK. Azithromycin decreases NALP3 mRNA stability in monocytes to limit inflammasome-dependent inflammation. *Respir Res.* (2017) 18:131. doi: 10.1186/s12931-017-0608-8
236. Upadhyay K, Hiregoudar B, Meals E, English BK, Talati AJ. Combination therapy with ampicillin and azithromycin improved outcomes in a mouse model of group B streptococcal sepsis. *PLoS ONE* (2017) 12:e0182023. doi: 10.1371/journal.pone.0182023
237. Afshar M, Foster CL, Layden JE, Burnham EL. Azithromycin use and outcomes in severe sepsis patients with and without pneumonia. *J Crit Care* (2016) 32:120–5. doi: 10.1016/j.jcrc.2015.12.010
238. Ruiz VE, Battaglia T, Kurtz ZD, Bijnens L, Ou A, Engstrand I, et al. A single early-in-life macrolide course has lasting effects on murine microbial network topology and immunity. *Nat Commun.* (2017) 8:518. doi: 10.1038/s41467-017-00531-6
239. Murchison L, De Coppi P, Eaton S. Post-natal erythromycin exposure and risk of infantile hypertrophic pyloric stenosis: a systematic review and meta-analysis. *Pediatr Surg Int.* (2016) 32:1147–52. doi: 10.1007/s00383-016-3971-5
240. Eberly MD, Eide MB, Thompson JL, Nylund CM. Azithromycin in Early Infancy and Pyloric Stenosis. *Pediatrics* (2015) 135:483–8. doi: 10.1542/peds.2014-2026

6

Etiology and Clinical Features of Full-Term Neonatal Bacterial Meningitis

Min Xu[1†], *Lan Hu*[2†], *Heyu Huang*[3], *Liping Wang*[1], *Jintong Tan*[1], *Yongjun Zhang*[1], *Chao Chen*[2*], *Xi Zhang*[4*] *and Lisu Huang*[3*]

[1] Department of Neonatology, Xinhua Hospital, Shanghai Jiaotong University School of Medicine, Shanghai, China, [2] Department of Neonatology, Children Hospital of Fudan University, Shanghai, China, [3] Department of Pediatric Infectious Diseases, Xinhua Hospital, Shanghai Jiaotong University School of Medicine, Shanghai, China, [4] Clinical Research Unit, Xinhua Hospital, Shanghai Jiaotong University School of Medicine, Shanghai, China

***Correspondence:**
Chao Chen
chen6010@163.com
Xi Zhang
zhangxi@xinhuamed.com.cn
Lisu Huang
huanglisu@xinhuamed.com.cn

† These authors have contributed equally to this work and are first authors

Objective: Neonatal bacterial meningitis is a severe infectious disease with a high risk of neurodevelopmental sequelae. The causative pathogens may be related to specific clinical features of the disease. Therefore, this study aimed at determining the pathogen-specific and clinical features of bacterial meningitis in full-term neonates.

Methods: We enrolled neonates from the Shanghai Neonate Meningitis Cohort (2005–2017), which is a multicenter retrospective cohort that recruits almost all full-term neonates in Shanghai who underwent lumbar puncture. Patient history and clinical examination results were extracted from the computer-documented information systems of four hospitals. The trends of pathogen distribution were analyzed and differences in the clinical manifestations, treatment, and clinical outcomes at discharge were compared according to the causative pathogen. Logistic regression was used to evaluate the pathogen-specific risk of neurological complications.

Results: In total, 518 cases of neonatal meningitis, including 189 proven cases, were included. *Group B Streptococcus* (GBS) and *Escherichia coli* (*E. coli*) were the leading pathogens in proven cases of early-onset and late-onset neonatal meningitis, respectively. The proportion of early-onset and late-onset GBS and late-onset *E. coli* meningitis cases increased gradually. GBS meningitis had the highest risk of neurological complications, whereas the overall incidence of hydrocephalus and brain abscess in *E. coli* was higher than that in GBS.

Conclusions: Rates of neonatal GBS and *E. coli* meningitis were high in 2005–2017 in Shanghai, and the risk of neurological complications was also high. Therefore, active prevention, rational use of antibiotics, and continuous monitoring of GBS and *E. coli* in neonates should be initiated in Shanghai.

Keywords: pathogens, clinical features, neonatal bacterial meningitis, *Group B Streptococcus*, *Escherichia coli*, neurological complications

INTRODUCTION

Despite advances in infant intensive care, neonatal meningitis remains a devastating disease. In some developed countries, *Group B Streptococcus* (GBS) and *Escherichia coli* (*E. coli*) were reported as the main pathogens of bacterial meningitis in young infants (1–4). However, in the developing world, the microbiology of bacterial meningitis in neonates varies geographically. A World Health Organization-supported study in four African countries showed that *Klebsiella pneumoniae* and *E. coli* were the most-prevalent causative pathogens in cases of neonatal meningitis (5). Reports from the central and western provinces of China showed that *E. coli* was a commonly isolated bacterium in cases of neonatal meningitis; other pathogens included *Staphylococcus epidermidis*, *K. pneumonia,* and GBS (6, 7). However, no large-scale study has examined the etiology of neonatal bacterial meningitis in the eastern regions of China.

The morbidity rate of neonatal meningitis, especially the incidence of neurological sequelae, is currently high worldwide (8, 9), and the clinical severity and prognosis of neonatal bacterial meningitis may be associated with the type of invading pathogen. Most studies have focused on the clinical features of a single pathogen. For instance, both hyper-, and hypothermia were reported as being the most frequent clinical signs of *E. coli* meningitis at admission (10). Further, GBS meningitis, an isolated illness caused by a gram-positive pathogen, was found to be characterized by the presence of specific signs of meningitis, such as lethargy and seizure (2, 11). Symptomatically, gram-negative pathogens are more likely to cause seizures as the initial manifestation of meningitis and are associated with higher cerebrospinal fluid (CSF) white blood cell counts than gram-positive pathogens (12). However, studies on the systematic identification of the clinical features of different pathogens are lacking. Selection bias in such comparative studies can only be reduced by simultaneously comparing the clinical differences of different pathogens in the same study.

Understanding the differences in the clinical manifestations of these pathogens is important for early identification of pathogens and the rational use of antibiotics. In addition, the lack of studies examining the etiology of neonatal bacterial meningitis in the eastern regions of China impedes the development of strategies for the prevention of neonatal bacterial meningitis in these regions. Therefore, this large-scale study aimed to identify the trends in bacterial infection among cases of meningitis in full-term neonates in Shanghai and explore the pathogen-specific and clinical features of bacterial meningitis among full-term neonates.

MATERIALS AND METHODS

The Shanghai Neonate Meningitis Cohort is a multicenter retrospective cohort, including almost all full-term neonates who underwent lumbar puncture in Shanghai (2005–2017). It was conducted at neonatal wards of four tertiary class A pediatric hospitals in Shanghai that examined approximately 95% of the neonates with bacterial meningitis in Shanghai (Xinhua Hospital, affiliated to Shanghai Jiaotong University School of Medicine; Shanghai Children's Medical Center, affiliated to Shanghai Jiaotong University School of Medicine; Children's Hospital of Shanghai Jiaotong University, and Children Hospital of Fudan University).

The history and clinical examination results for all neonates were abstracted from the computer-documented hospital information systems. Approval for the study and sharing data with the coordinating institution was granted by Xinhua Hospital affiliated to Shanghai Jiaotong University School of Medicine and was consented by the other hospitals (No. XHEC-C-2017-084).

In this study, the inclusion criteria for neonatal bacterial meningitis included one or more of the following: (a) isolation of a bacterial pathogen from CSF culture; (b) isolation of the same bacterial pathogen from blood drawn simultaneously at two different sites, with CSF pleocytosis ($\geq$20 cells/mm^3) (13–15); and (c) no pathogen isolated from either CSF or blood, with clinical symptoms and CSF pleocytosis ($\geq$20 cells/mm^3). Proven meningitis was defined in patients with either inclusion criterion (a) or (b). Clinically diagnosed meningitis was defined in patients with inclusion criterion (c). Exclusion criteria were as follows: (a) gestational age $<$37 weeks, (b) onset of bacterial meningitis after $>$28 days of life, (c) history of severe neurological disease or ventricular drain, or (d) receipt of traumatic lumbar puncture ($\geq$10,000 $\times$ 10^6/L red blood cells in CSF) (16) with negative CSF culture result.

Coagulase-negative staphylococci (CoNS), considered as being potential contaminants were further evaluated as follows: Three neonatologists gathered clinical data from the hospital's computerized information system, and pathogens were assessed to determine their clinical significance.

The following data were retrieved from the computer-documented hospital information systems: bacterial species, antimicrobial susceptibility testing, demographic information, clinical signs and symptoms, first laboratory examination of CSF, cranial magnetic resonance imaging (MRI) results during treatment, and clinical outcomes at discharge. Three independent neonatologists performed the data input and checked to avoid data mis-recording as much as possible.

The threshold for early-onset and late-onset diseases was seven days after birth (17, 18). Neonates presenting with symptoms of fever, lethargy, poor feeding, vomiting, cyanosis, and apnea were considered to have nonspecific symptoms. Neonates presenting with symptoms of seizures, dystonia, irritability, abnormal primitive reflexes, bulging fontanelle, and screaming were considered to have neurological symptoms. Neonates presenting with complications including omphalitis, pneumonia, skin infection, diarrhea, and urinary infection were considered to have non-neurological complications. Neurological complications were limited to abnormal cranial MRI results including ventriculitis, intracranial hemorrhage, subdural effusion, hydrocephalus, and brain abscess, which were confirmed by MRI experts. The clinical prognosis at discharge

Abbreviations: CoNS, Coagulase-negative staphylococci; *E. coli*, *Escherichia coli;* ESBL, extended spectrum beta-lactamase; GBS, *Group B Streptococcus;* GOS, Glasgow Outcome Scale; IAP, intrapartum antibiotic prophylaxis; CSF, cerebrospinal fluid.

was evaluated using the Glasgow Outcome Scale (GOS) (1, death; 2, persistent vegetative state; 3, severe disability; 4, moderate disability; 5, good recovery). Moderate or severe disability was defined as any of the following conditions: spasticity, muscle weakness, and immobility in one or more limbs; microcephaly; hydrocephalus; seizure disorder; hearing loss. A GOS score of ≤4 was defined as poor prognosis (19). During the antibiotic treatment, some families decided to withdraw treatment. These neonates had been using antibiotics during hospitalization and did not complete antibiotic treatment before the families withdrew treatment. Once the families withdrew treatment, these neonates were discharged immediately. There were two reasons why the families withdrew treatment: (a) they can no longer afford hospitalization expenses; (b) the neonates had complications during treatment, or parents felt that the prognosis will be poor, and they lost confidence in the recovery of the neonates.

We calculated the median and interquartile range for continuous variables (as most data were not normally distributed), and frequency for categorical variables. Continuous variables were compared using nonparametric methods (Mann-Whitney U-test). Categorical variables were compared using the chi-square test or Fisher's exact test, where appropriate. Considering the multiple comparisons, we used the Bonferroni

TABLE 1 | Pathogen distribution of 189 full-term neonatal cases with proven meningitis.

Pathogen	Total	CSF& Blood	CSF only	Blood only
GBS	55 (29.1)	22 (43.1)	10 (21.7)	23 (25.0)
E. coli	55 (29.1)	20 (39.2)	13 (28.3)	22 (23.9)
CoNS	42 (22.2)	4 (7.9)	7 (15.3)	31 (33.8)
Staphylococcus epidermidis	21 (11.1)	1 (2.0)	1 (2.2)	19 (20.7)
Staphylococcus haemolyticus	3 (1.6)	0 (0.0)	1 (2.2)	2 (2.2)
Staphylococcus hominis	3 (1.6)	1 (2.0)	0 (0.0)	2 (2.2)
Staphylococcus saprophyticus	2 (1.1)	0 (0.0)	1 (2.2)	1 (1.1)
Staphylococcus warneri	1 (0.5)	0 (0.0)	1 (2.2)	0 (0.0)
Staphylococcus lentus	1 (0.5)	0 (0.0)	0 (0.0)	1 (1.1)
Staphylococcus cohnii	1 (0.5)	0 (0.0)	1 (2.2)	0 (0.0)
Other types	10 (5.3)	2 (3.9)	2 (4.3)	6 (6.5)
Enterobacteriaceae (except *E. coli*)	11 (5.8)	1 (2.0)	5 (10.9)	5 (5.4)
Klebsiella pneumoniae	7 (3.7)	1 (2.0)	2 (4.3)	4 (4.3)
Enterobacter cloacae	1 (0.5)	0 (0.0)	1 (2.2)	0 (0.0)
Proteus species	1 (0.5)	0 (0.0)	1 (2.2)	0 (0.0)
Klebsiella oxytoca	1 (0.5)	0 (0.0)	1 (2.2)	0 (0.0)
Plesiomonas shigelloides	1 (0.5)	0 (0.0)	0 (0.0)	1 (1.1)
Enterococcus	10 (5.3)	1 (2.0)	4 (8.7)	5 (5.4)
Enterococcus faecium	8 (4.2)	1 (2.0)	3 (6.5)	4 (4.3)
Enterococcus faecalis	1 (0.5)	0 (0.0)	1 (2.2)	0 (0.0)
Enterococcus gallinarum	1 (0.5)	0 (0.0)	0 (0.0)	1 (1.1)
Staphylococcus aureus	3 (1.6)	1 (2.0)	0 (0.0)	2 (2.2)
Chryseobacterium meningosepticum	3 (1.6)	1 (2.0)	2 (4.3)	0 (0.0)
Listeria monocytogenes	3 (1.6)	0 (0.0)	3 (6.5)	0 (0.0)
Stenotrophomonas maltophilia	2 (1.1)	0 (0.0)	1 (2.2)	1 (1.1)
Acinetobacter bauman	1 (0.5)	0 (0.0)	1 (2.2)	0 (0.0)
Haemophilus influenzae	1 (0.5)	0 (0.0)	0 (0.0)	1 (1.1)
Bacillus subtilis	1 (0.5)	1 (2.0)	0 (0.0)	0 (0.0)
Streptococcus gallolyticus	1 (0.5)	0 (0.0)	0 (0.0)	1 (1.1)
Micrococcus luteus	1 (0.5)	0 (0.0)	0 (0.0)	1 (1.1)
Total	189 (100.0)	51 (100.0)	46 (100.0)	92 (100.0)

Numbers are presented as n (%). "CSF & Blood," "CSF only," and "Blood only" represent pathogens detected in both the CSF and blood cultures; CSF culture only; and blood culture only, respectively. E. coli, Escherichia coli; GBS, Group B Streptococcus; CSF, cerebrospinal fluid.

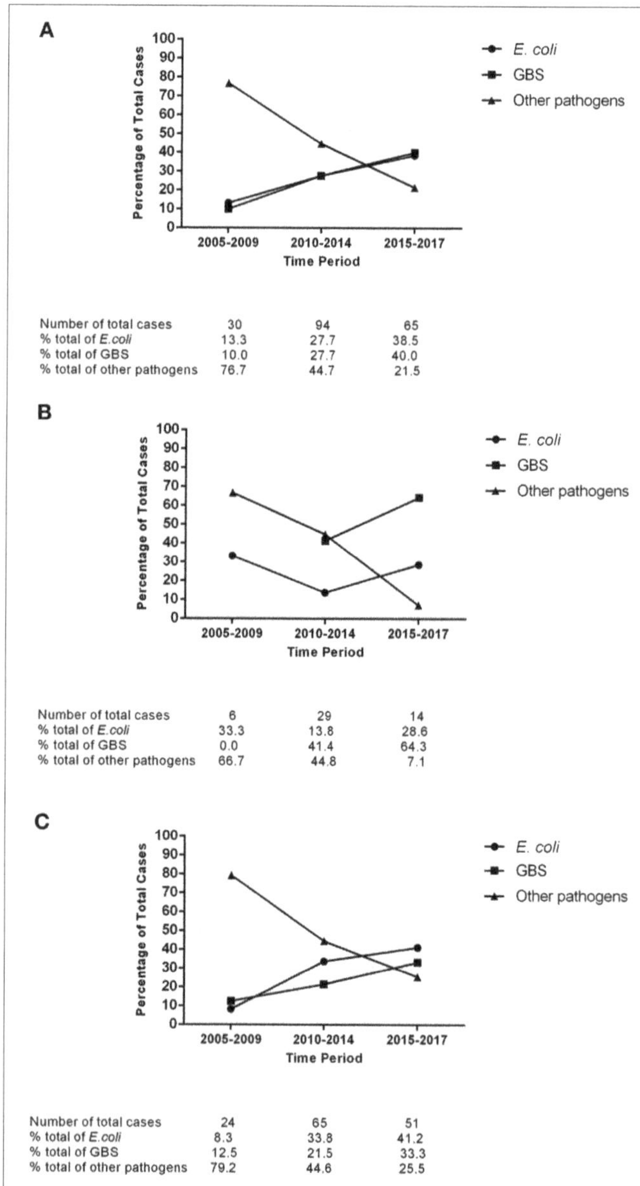

FIGURE 1 | Trends in the pathogen distribution of full-term neonatal meningitis in Shanghai, 2005–2017. **(A)** All meningitis cases; **(B)** Early-onset meningitis cases; **(C)** Late-onset meningitis cases. *E. coli*, *Escherichia coli*; GBS, Group *B Streptococcus*.

method to adjust for the type I error rate. Multivariate logistic regression models were used to evaluate risk factors for poor prognosis and neurological complications. All statistical analyses were performed using SPSS 17.0 (SPSS Inc, Chicago, IL, USA). The figures were produced using GraphPad Prism 6.0 (GraphPad Software, La Jolla, CA, USA).

RESULTS

Pathogen Distribution

We identified 518 cases of neonatal meningitis, including 189 proven cases and 329 clinically diagnosed cases. In the proven cases, gram-positive pathogens accounted for 116 cases (61.4%), and gram-negative pathogens accounted for the remaining 73 cases (38.6%). GBS ($n =$ 55, 29.1%) and *E. coli* ($n = 55$, 29.1%) were the leading pathogens in the proven cases of neonatal meningitis. Other pathogens involved in <5 cases included CoNS ($n = 42$, 22.2%), *Enterobacteriaceae* (except *E. coli*) ($n = 11$, 5.8%), and *Enterococcus* ($n = 10$, 5.3%) (**Table 1**).

Trends in Pathogen Distribution

Early-onset bacterial meningitis accounted for 31.2% of the proven cases among full-term neonates in Shanghai during 2005–2017. There was an upward trend in the proportions of both early-onset and late-onset GBS meningitis (**Figure 1**). Over the study duration, GBS was the leading pathogen in early-onset meningitis (21/49, 42.9%). The proportion of late-onset *E. coli* meningitis cases increased gradually, and *E. coli* was the most-common pathogen in cases of late-onset meningitis (45/140, 32.1%). The proportion of all other pathogens decreased gradually in cases of both early-onset and late-onset meningitis.

Antibiotic Susceptibility

All GBS strains were sensitive to gentamicin, ampicillin, vancomycin, and linezolid while only 16.2% of GBS cases were sensitive to clindamycin (**Table 2**). Only one strain was resistant to penicillin. *E. coli* showed a high sensitivity to cefepime (88.6%) and meropenem (100.0%), a varying resistance to ampicillin, gentamicin, cefotaxime, and ceftriaxone (71.4, 36.8, 50.0, and 43.3%, respectively), and a high proportion of extended spectrum beta-lactamase (ESBL)-producing isolates (41.2%).

Demographic Information and Clinical Symptoms

Of the 518 neonates, 307 (59.3%) were boys, 15 (2.9%) had low birth weights (<2,500 g), and 344 (66.4%) were born by cesarean section. Fever was the predominant symptom in all cases, regardless of the etiology, and 197 cases (38.0%) showed neurological symptoms. Seizures ($n = 83$, 16.0%) were the leading presentation of neurological symptoms. Poor feeding, seizures, and irritability occurred more frequently in GBS cases than in the clinically diagnosed cases ($P < 0.05$). Incidence rates of the other symptoms did not differ among the clinically diagnosed, GBS and *E. coli* cases (**Table 3**).

CSF Findings

Lumbar puncture was performed in all 518 cases. The GBS and *E. coli* cases showed higher CSF white blood cell counts, protein levels, and lower glucose levels than the clinically diagnosed cases ($P < 0.05$). There were no significant differences in CFS findings between the GBS and *E. coli* cases.

Clinical Outcomes at Discharge

A total of 3 neonates died in hospital, and 140 neonates (27.0%) had poor prognosis (GOS score $\leq$4) at discharge. Seventy-six neonates (14.7%) were discharged after families chose to withdraw treatment, in which 25 neonates received >2 weeks of treatment. The rates of in-hospital deaths and treatment withdrawal did not differ significantly between the clinically diagnosed, GBS, and *E. coli* meningitis cases. There was also no difference between the clinically diagnosed group and each proven group in terms of the incidence of poor prognosis. However, the rate of poor prognosis was significantly higher in *E. coli* cases than in GBS cases ($P < 0.05$), and this difference was consistent when we further adjusted for gender, birth weight, and early or late-onset pattern in the multivariate analyses (**Supplementary Table 1**).

Most neonates (501/518, 96.7%) underwent cranial MRI during treatment, and the results of 146 neonates (29.1%) were abnormal, including ventriculitis (21/501, 4.2%), intracranial hemorrhage (88/501, 17.6%), subdural effusion (41/501, 8.2%), hydrocephalus (33/501, 6.6%), and brain abscess (17/501, 3.4%). Neonates with GBS meningitis had a much higher risk of total neurological complications, especially subdural effusion and brain abscess, than clinically diagnosed cases (total neurological complications: odds ratio [OR], 2.3; 95% confidence interval [CI], 1.3–4.1; subdural effusion: OR, 5.0; 95% CI, 2.2–11.3; and brain abscess: OR, 6.3; 95% CI, 1.8–22.8). Neonates with *E. coli* meningitis had a relatively higher risk of total neurological complications, subdural effusion, hydrocephalus, and brain abscess than the clinically diagnosed cases (total neurological complications: OR, 2.0; 95% CI, 1.1–3.6; subdural effusion: OR, 3.5; 95% CI, 1.5–8.4; hydrocephalus: OR, 4.0; 95% CI, 1.7–9.3; and brain abscess: OR, 6.3; 95% CI, 1.8–22.8). Compared to neonates with GBS meningitis, those with *E. coli* meningitis showed a higher overall incidence of hydrocephalus and brain abscess.

Multivariate analysis of the neurological complications showed that neonates with GBS and *E. coli* meningitis had a significantly higher risk of neurological complications than those with clinically diagnosed meningitis (GBS: OR, 2.3; 95% CI, 1.3–4.3; *E. coli*: OR, 2.0; 95% CI, 1.1–3.6). There was no significant difference in the risk of neurological complications between the clinically diagnosed cases and the cases of the other pathogens (**Table 4**).

DISCUSSION

To the best of our knowledge, this is the first long-term study of full-term neonatal meningitis with a large sample size in Shanghai, China. We found that GBS and *E. coli* were the leading pathogens in proven cases of neonatal meningitis,

TABLE 2 | *In vitro* antimicrobial susceptibility testing of common pathogens from full-term neonatal cases with proven meningitis.

Organism	PEN	AMP	GEN	CLI	VAN	LNZ	CTX	CRO	FEP	MEM	ESBL (+)
GBS	42/43 (97.7)	25/25 (100.0)	–	6/37 (16.2)	43/43 (100.0)	40/40 (100.0)	11/11 (100.0)	41/43 (95.3)	–	10/10 (100.0)	–
E. coli	–	10/35 (28.6)	24/38 (63.2)	–	–	–	19/38 (50.0)	17/30 (56.7)	31/35 (88.6)	25/25 (100.0)	7/17 (41.2)
CoNS	3/32 (9.4)	–	19/30 (63.3)	18/32 (56.3)	32/32 (100.0)	31/31 (100.0)	–	–	–	–	–
Enterobacteriaceae (except *E. coli*)	–	0/8 (0.0)	6/8 (75.0)	–	–	–	3/8 (37.5)	2/2 (100.0)	4/7 (57.1)	6/6 (100.0)	–
Enterococcus	2/4 (50.0)	4/6 (66.7)	5/6 (83.3)	–	7/7 (100.0)	6/6 (100.0)	–	–	–	–	–

Numbers represent susceptible pathogens/pathogens tested (% susceptible). PEN, penicillin; AMP, ampicillin; GEN, gentamicin; CLI, clindamycin; VAN, vancomycin; LNZ, linezolid; CTX: cefotaxime; CRO, ceftriaxone; FEP, cefepime; MEM, meropenem; ESBL (+), extended spectrum beta-lactamase (+).

which was similar with that of the developed countries. GBS and *E. coli* were the most-common pathogens in early-onset and late-onset neonatal meningitis, respectively, both of which showed an increasing trend and had a high risk of neurological complications.

In some developed countries and regions, GBS is the most-prevalent pathogen causing meningitis in young infants, and is confined to this population (1, 2, 4). In the USA, approximately 16.7–22.7% of pregnant women showed GBS colonization (20). GBS prevention activities increased since the 1990s, and the first recommendation for universal screening was issued in 2002. This resulted in an estimated 80% decrease in early-onset GBS infection in the USA (21). In China, GBS infection occurs in 7.1–10.4% of pregnant women, a lower prevalence than that of the USA (22, 23). However, in our study, GBS was the leading pathogen in early-onset meningitis, and the prevalence of both early-onset and late-onset GBS meningitis has shown an increasing trend in recent years. Regarding antimicrobial susceptibility, neonates with GBS meningitis showed high sensitivity to penicillin and ampicillin, which remain the agents of choice for intrapartum antibiotic prophylaxis (IAP) (24, 25). These results may be partially related to the non-wide implementation of IAP in China.

In this study, neonates with GBS meningitis had a significantly higher incidence of poor feeding, seizures, and irritability than neonates with clinically diagnosed meningitis. In addition, the incidence of nonspecific and neurological symptoms of GBS and *E. coli* meningitis was both slightly higher than those of clinically diagnosed meningitis (although not significantly). As for the CSF findings, GBS and *E. coli* meningitis were significantly more serious than clinically diagnosed meningitis. Based on these, if a newborn presents with several clinical symptoms combined with severe CSF findings, we should be wary of GBS or *E. coli* meningitis.

The fact that neonatal GBS meningitis had the highest risk of neurological complications may be related to the virulence of GBS and the severe damage to the brain caused by its infection. *In vitro* and clinical studies have found that GBS can promote blood-brain barrier penetration (26–28) and may cause severe cerebrovascular diseases (29). Abnormal findings on full-term neonatal MRI were associated with a poor neurodevelopmental outcome (30). A meta-analysis on neurodevelopmental impairment after GBS disease in infants aged <90 days showed that GBS meningitis was an important risk factor for moderate-to-severe neurodevelopmental impairment, affecting approximately 20% of survivors (31). Therefore, it is important to conduct brain imaging on neonates with GBS meningitis and to follow-up for long-term neurological sequelae. In addition, the implementation of IAP may be associated with a low mortality in cases of early-onset GBS disease, and mild late-onset GBS disease (32, 33). Currently, in China, only a few hospitals perform IAP by strictly following a risk-based strategy. Hence, IAP should be promoted and continuous monitoring of GBS should be initiated in China.

Similar to GBS, we also found that *E. coli* meningitis had a significantly higher risk of neurological complications than those of clinically diagnosed meningitis, especially subdural effusion, hydrocephalus, and brain abscess. As reported in other studies, neonatal *E. coli* meningitis may cause learning and memory impairments in adulthood (34), which may be related to the high incidence of *E. coli* neurological complications. Although *E. coli* meningitis had a similar incidence of neurological complications to GBS, the overall incidence of hydrocephalus and brain abscess was higher than the latter. As serious neurological complications, hydrocephalus and brain abscess were associated with significant long-term morbidity and mortality (35, 36). We further speculate that the high proportion of ESBL-producing isolates in *E. coli* cases increases the risk of serious neurological complications. The high proportion of ESBL-producing isolates in *E. coli* cases is similar to that reported in a large multicenter study in China, which may be related to the universal antibiotic overuse or misuse in China (37). At present, there is no national guideline for the treatment of neonatal meningitis in China, so the choice and course of antimicrobial treatment may vary in different hospitals. Therefore, a consensus guideline for treatment of neonatal meningitis should be established and better monitoring of drug-resistant bacteria should be encouraged.

To our knowledge, this is the first large-scale study of neonatal meningitis in Shanghai investigating pathogen trends in the past 13 years, and its results have furthered the understanding of the

TABLE 3 | Characteristics of full-term neonatal meningitis cases caused by the three most commonly cultured pathogens.

Characteristics	Clinically diagnosed cases ($n = 329$)	GBS cases ($n = 55$)	*E. coli* cases ($n = 55$)
Men, *n* (%)	203 (61.7)	28 (50.9)	27 (49.1)
Gestational age (weeks), median (IQR)	39.1 (38.2–40.0)	39.0 (38.0–40.0)	39.0 (38.0–40.1)
Birth weight (kg), median (IQR)	3.4 (3.1–3.6)	3.3 (3.1–3.5)	3.2 (3.0–3.6)
Early-onset, *n* (%)	108 (32.8)	21 (38.2)	10 (18.2)
Cesarean delivery, *n* (%)	213 (64.7)	42 (76.4)	35 (63.6)
Course of treatment (days), median (IQR)	25 (19–33)	36 (29–51)[†‡]	28 (22–40)
Nonspecific symptoms, *n* (%)[a]	294 (89.4)	54 (98.2)	52 (94.5)
Fever	253 (76.9)	50 (90.9)	49 (89.1)
Lethargy	95 (28.9)	24 (43.6)	22 (40.0)
Poor feeding	82 (24.9)	24 (43.6)[†]	20 (36.4)
Vomit	23 (7.0)	4 (7.3)	2 (3.6)
Cyanosis	19 (5.8)	2 (3.6)	2 (3.6)
Apnea	7 (2.1)	2 (3.6)	1 (1.8)
Neurological symptoms, *n* (%)[b]	122 (37.1)	27 (49.1)	23 (41.8)
Seizures	47 (14.3)	15 (27.3)[†]	9 (16.4)
Dystonia	36 (10.9)	12 (21.8)	9 (16.4)
Irritability	18 (5.5)	10 (18.2)[†]	6 (10.9)
Abnormal primitive reflexes	56 (17.0)	4 (7.3)	9 (16.4)
Bulging fontanelle	14 (4.3)	3 (5.5)	4 (7.3)
Screaming	1 (0.3)	1 (1.8)	2 (3.6)
CSF findings, median (IQR)			
WBC count ($\times 10^6$/L)	102 (37–420)	1111 (114–3,920)[†]	491 (79–3,248)*
Protein, g/L	1.3 (0.9–2.0)	2.9 (1.6–4.7)[†]	2.0 (1.5–3.3)*
Glucose, mmol/L	2.0 (1.1–2.4)	1.0 (0.8–2.0)[†]	1.6 (0.1–2.0)*
Non-neurological complications, *n* (%)[c]	176 (53.5)	27 (49.1)	21 (38.2)
Omphalitis	20 (6.1)	2 (3.6)	5 (9.1)
Pneumonia	131 (39.8)	21 (38.2)	14 (25.5)
Skin infection	5 (1.5)	0 (0.0)	2 (3.6)
Diarrhea	49 (14.9)	7 (12.7)	3 (5.5)
Urinary infection	6 (1.8)	0 (0.0)	0 (0.0)
Neurological complications, *n* (%)[d]	82 (25.9)	24 (44.4)[†]	22 (40.7)*
Ventriculitis	13 (4.1)	2 (3.7)	3 (5.6)
Intracranial hemorrhage	59 (18.7)	12 (22.2)	7 (13.0)
Subdural effusion	17 (5.4)	12 (22.2)[†]	9 (16.7)*
Hydrocephalus	17 (5.4)	2 (3.7)[‡]	10 (18.5)*
Brain abscess	5 (1.6)	5 (9.3)[†]	5 (9.3)*
Poor prognosis, *n* (%)[e]	88 (26.7)	10 (18.2)	21 (38.2)
Death, *n* (%)	2 (0.6)	0 (0.0)	0 (0.0)
Withdrew treatment, *n* (%)[f]	47 (14.3)	5 (9.1)	12 (21.8)

[a]Any one or more of the symptoms including fever, lethargy, poor feeding, vomit, cyanosis, and apnea were defined as the presence of nonspecific symptoms.
[b]Any one or more of the symptoms including seizure, dystonia, irritability, abnormal primitive reflexes, bulging fontanelle, and screaming were defined as the presence of neurological symptoms.
[c]Any one or more of the complications including omphalitis, pneumonia, skin infection, diarrhea, and urinary infection were defined as the presence of non-neurological complications.
[d]Any one or more of the neurological complications including ventriculitis, intracranial hemorrhage, subdural effusion, hydrocephalus and brain abscess confirmed by cranial magnetic resonance imaging were defined as the presence of neurological complications.
[e]Glasgow Outcome Scale score of ≤ 4 is defined as poor prognosis.
[f]Families withdrew treatment due to economic difficulties and/or poor prognosis.
**Comparison between clinically diagnosed cases and E. coli cases (adjusted $P < 0.05$ by the Bonferroni method).*
[†]Comparison between clinically diagnosed cases and GBS cases (adjusted $P < 0.05$ by the Bonferroni method).
[‡]Comparison between E. coli cases and GBS cases (adjusted $P < 0.05$ by the Bonferroni method).
IQR, interquartile range; CSF, cerebrospinal fluid; WBC, white blood cell; GBS, Group B Streptococcus; E. coli, Escherichia coli.

TABLE 4 | Univariate and multivariate analyses of risk factors for neurological complications in full-term neonatal meningitis cases.

Variables	Univariate analysis		Multivariate analysis	
	OR (95% CI)	*P*	OR (95% CI)	*P*
Men vs. women	1.1 (0.8–1.7)	0.55	1.2 (0.8–1.8)	0.43
Birth weight <2,500 g vs. ≥2,500 g	0.7 (0.2–2.6)	0.60	0.7 (0.2–2.7)	0.61
Early-onset vs. Late-onset	1.1 (0.7–1.7)	0.62	1.1 (0.7–1.7)	0.75
PATHOGEN				
Clinically diagnosed cases	Reference		Reference	
E. coli cases	2.0 (1.1–3.6)	0.03	2.0 (1.1–3.6)	0.03
GBS cases	2.3 (1.3–4.1)	0.006	2.3 (1.3–4.3)	0.005
Cases of other pathogens	0.9 (0.5–1.6)	0.64	0.9 (0.5–1.6)	0.74

GBS, Group B Streptococcus; E. coli, Escherichia coli; OR, odds ratio; CI, confidence interval.

pathogen-specific and clinical features of bacterial meningitis in full-term neonates. However, there are some limitations. First, the meningitis cases in our study were diagnosed based on CSF pleocytosis, but the interpretation of CSF pleocytosis parameters are not yet standardized (38). This, together with the exclusion of infants who received traumatic lumbar punctures, may have led to underdiagnoses of meningitis in some cases and overdiagnoses in others, limiting this study's ability to estimate of overall burden of neonatal meningitis in Shanghai. Second, viral studies were not routinely considered without significant clinical signs and symptoms in neonates. However, CSF leukocytosis may also occur in neonatal viral meningitis. For example, a proportion of neonatal enteroviral meningitis can cause CSF leukocytosis (39, 40), thus the incidence of neonatal viral meningitis has likely been underestimated. Further, intracranial hemorrhage might also lead to CSF leukocytosis and be confused with clinically diagnosed cases. Third, although CoNS is sometimes a contaminant, it has increasingly been recognized as a cause of clinically significant nosocomial bloodstream infections, particularly in neonates (41). As a result, we did not rule out CoNS cases, which might introduce misdiagnosis; we only included cases with typical meningitis symptoms and signs, in addition to those with positive CSF culture or positive blood culture from blood drawn simultaneously at two different sites. Fourth, some families withdrew treatment, which increased the lost to follow-up rate. This might have introduced bias to the results, such as the incidence of neurological complications. To follow-up on this hospital-based retrospective survey, we plan to address these limitations by conducting a more detailed prospective study on neonatal meningitis in the future.

Rates of neonatal GBS and *E. coli* meningitis were high in 2005–2017 in Shanghai, and the risk of neurological complications was also high. Therefore, active prevention, rational use of antibiotics and continuous monitoring of GBS and *E. coli* in neonates should be initiated in Shanghai.

AUTHOR CONTRIBUTIONS

MX, LaH, YZ, CC, XZ, and LiH conceptualized and designed the study. HH, LW, and JT collected the data. MX, YZ, XZ, and LiH analyzed the data. MX drafted the initial manuscript. All authors contributed to the interpretation of the data and contributed to the final draft of the manuscript.

REFERENCES

1. Okike IO, Johnson AP, Henderson KL, Blackburn RM, Muller-Pebody B, Ladhani SN, et al. Incidence, etiology, and outcome of bacterial meningitis in infants aged <90 days in the United kingdom and Republic of Ireland: prospective, enhanced, national population-based surveillance. *Clin Infect Dis.* (2014) 59:e150–7. doi: 10.1093/cid/ciu514
2. Gaschignard J, Levy C, Romain O, Cohen R, Bingen E, Aujard Y, et al. Neonatal bacterial meningitis: 444 cases in 7 years. *Pediatr Infect Dis J* (2011) 30:212–7. doi: 10.1097/INF.0b013e3181fab1e7
3. Ouchenir L, Renaud C, Khan S, Bitnun A, Boisvert AA, McDonald J, et al. The epidemiology, management, and outcomes of bacterial meningitis in infants. *Pediatrics* (2017) 140:e20170476. doi: 10.1542/peds.2017-0476
4. Thigpen MC, Whitney CG, Messonnier NE, Zell ER, Lynfield R, Hadler JL, et al. Bacterial meningitis in the United States, 1998-2007. *N Engl J Med.* (2011) 364:2016–25. doi: 10.1056/NEJMoa1005384
5. Furyk JS, Swann O, Molyneux E. Systematic review: neonatal meningitis in the developing world. *Trop Med Int Health* (2011) 16:672–9. doi: 10.1111/j.1365-3156.2011.02750.x
6. The Collaborative Group For Neonatal Meningitis Study TC, Liu CQ. Epidemiology of neonatal purulent meningitis in Hebei Province, China: a multicenter study. *Zhongguo Dang Dai Er Ke Za Zhi* (2015) 17:419–24. doi: 10.7499/j.issn.1008-8830.2015.05.001

7. Jiang H, Su M, Kui L, Huang H, Qiu L, Li L, et al. Prevalence and antibiotic resistance profiles of cerebrospinal fluid pathogens in children with acute bacterial meningitis in Yunnan province, China, 2012-2015. *PloS ONE* (2017) 12:e0180161. doi: 10.1371/journal.pone.0180161
8. Harvey D, Holt DE, Bedford H. Bacterial meningitis in the newborn: a prospective study of mortality and morbidity. *Semin Perinatol.* (1999) 23:218–25. doi: 10.1016/S0146-0005(99)80066-4
9. Stevens JP, Eames M, Kent A, Halket S, Holt D, Harvey D. Long term outcome of neonatal meningitis. *Arch Dis Child Fetal Neonatal Ed.* (2003) 88:F179–84. doi: 10.1136/fn.88.3.F179
10. Houdouin V, Bonacorsi S, Bidet P, de La Rocque F, Cohen R, Aujard Y, et al. Clinical outcome and bacterial characteristics of 99 Escherichia coli meningitis in young infants. *Arch Pediatr.* (2008) 15(Suppl. 3):S138–47. doi: 10.1016/S0929-693X(08)75497-6
11. Baud O, Aujard Y. Neonatal bacterial meningitis. *Handb Clin Neurol.* (2013) 112:1109–13. doi: 10.1016/B978-0-444-52910-7.00030-1
12. Smith PB, Cotten CM, Garges HP, Tiffany KF, Lenfestey RW, Moody MA, et al. A comparison of neonatal Gram-negative rod and Gram-positive cocci meningitis. *J Perinatol.* (2006) 26:111–4. doi: 10.1038/sj.jp.7211438
13. Garges HP, Moody MA, Cotten CM, Smith PB, Tiffany KF, Lenfestey R, et al. Neonatal meningitis: what is the correlation among cerebrospinal fluid cultures, blood cultures, and cerebrospinal fluid parameters? *Pediatrics* (2006) 117:1094–100. doi: 10.1542/peds.2005-1132
14. Byington CL, Kendrick J, Sheng X. Normative cerebrospinal fluid profiles in febrile infants. *J Pediatr.* (2011) 158:130–4. doi: 10.1016/j.jpeds.2010.07.022
15. Kestenbaum LA, Ebberson J, Zorc JJ, Hodinka RL, Shah SS. Defining cerebrospinal fluid white blood cell count reference values in neonates and young infants. *Pediatrics* (2010) 125:257–64. doi: 10.1542/peds.2009-1181
16. Lyons TW, Cruz AT, Freedman SB, Neuman MI, Balamuth F, Mistry RD, et al. Interpretation of cerebrospinal fluid white blood cell counts in young infants with a traumatic lumbar puncture. *Ann Emerg Med.* (2017) 69:622–31. doi: 10.1016/j.annemergmed.2016.10.008
17. May M, Daley AJ, Donath S, Isaacs D. Australasian study group for neonatal infections. Early onset neonatal meningitis in Australia and New Zealand, 1992-2002. *Arch Dis Child Fetal Neonatal Ed.* (2005) 90:F324–7. doi: 10.1136/adc.2004.066134
18. Heath PT, Nik Yusoff NK, Baker CJ. Neonatal meningitis. *Arch Dis Child Fetal Neonatal Ed.* (2003) 88:F173–8. doi: 10.1136/fn.88.3.F173
19. Tan J, Kan J, Qiu G, Zhao D, Ren F, Luo Z, et al. Clinical prognosis in neonatal bacterial meningitis: the role of cerebrospinal fluid protein. *PLoS ONE* (2015) 10:e0141620. doi: 10.1371/journal.pone.0141620
20. Kwatra G, Cunnington MC, Merrall E, Kwatra G, Cunnington MC, Merrall E, et al. Prevalence of maternal colonisation with group B streptococcus: a systematic review and meta-analysis. *Lancet Infect Dis.* (2016) 16:1076–84. doi: 10.1016/S1473-3099(16)30055-X
21. Phares CR, Lynfield R, Farley MM, Mohle-Boetani J, Harrison LH, Petit S, et al. Epidemiology of invasive group B streptococcal disease in the United States, 1999-2005. *JAMA* (2008) 299:2056–65. doi: 10.1001/jama.299.17.2056
22. Lu B, Li D, Cui Y, Sui W, Huang L, Lu X. Epidemiology of Group B streptococcus isolated from pregnant women in Beijing, China. *Clin Microbiol Infect.* (2014) 20:O370–3. doi: 10.1111/1469-0691.12416
23. Tsui MH, Ip M, Ng PC, Sahota DS, Leung TN, Lau TK. Change in prevalence of group B Streptococcus maternal colonisation in Hong Kong. *Hong Kong Med J.* (2009) 15:414–9.
24. Verani JR, McGee L, Schrag SJ. Prevention of perinatal group B streptococcal disease–revised guidelines from CDC, 2010. MMWR *Recomm Rep.* (2010) 59:1–36.
25. Tunkel AR, Hartman BJ, Kaplan SL, Kaufman BA, Roos KL, Scheld WM, et al. Practice guidelines for the management of bacterial meningitis. *Clin Infect Dis.* (2004) 39:1267–84. doi: 10.1086/425368
26. Magalhaes V, Andrade EB, Alves J, Ribeiro A, Kim KS, Lima M, et al. Group B Streptococcus hijacks the host plasminogen system to promote brain endothelial cell invasion. *PLoS ONE* (2013) 8:e63244. doi: 10.1371/journal.pone.0063244
27. van Sorge NM, Quach D, Gurney MA, Sullam PM, Nizet V, Doran KS. The group B streptococcal serine-rich repeat 1 glycoprotein mediates penetration of the blood-brain barrier. *J Infect Dis.* (2009) 199:1479–87. doi: 10.1086/598217
28. Cutting AS, Del Rosario Y, Mu R, Rodriguez A, Till A, Subramani S, et al. The role of autophagy during group B Streptococcus infection of blood-brain barrier endothelium. *J Biol Chem.* (2014) 289:35711–23. doi: 10.1074/jbc.M114.588657
29. Tibussek D, Sinclair A, Yau I, Teatero S, Fittipaldi N, Richardson SE, et al. Late-onset group B streptococcal meningitis has cerebrovascular complications. *J Pediatr.* (2015) 166:1187–92.e1. doi: 10.1016/j.jpeds.2015.02.014
30. Massaro AN. MRI for neurodevelopmental prognostication in the high-risk term infant. *Semin Perinatol.* (2015) 39:159–67. doi: 10.1053/j.semperi.2015.01.009
31. Kohli-Lynch M, Russell NJ, Seale AC, Dangor Z, Tann CJ, Baker CJ, et al. Neurodevelopmental impairment in children after group B streptococcal disease worldwide: systematic review and meta-analyses. *Clin Infect Dis.* (2017) 65:S190–9. doi: 10.1093/cid/cix663
32. Edmond KM, Kortsalioudaki C, Scott S, Schrag SJ, Zaidi AK, Cousens S, et al. Group B streptococcal disease in infants aged younger than 3 months: systematic review and meta-analysis. *Lancet* (2012) 379:547–56. doi: 10.1016/S0140-6736(11)61651-6
33. Berardi A, Rossi C, Lugli L, Creti R, Bacchi Reggiani ML, Lanari M, et al. Group B streptococcus late-onset disease: 2003-2010. *Pediatrics* (2013) 131:e361–8. doi: 10.1542/peds.2012-1231
34. Barichello T, Dagostim VS, Generoso JS, Simoes LR, Dominguini D, Silvestre C, et al. Neonatal *Escherichia coli* K1 meningitis causes learning and memory impairments in adulthood. *J Neuroimmunol.* (2014) 272:35–41. doi: 10.1016/j.jneuroim.2014.05.003
35. Tully HM, Dobyns WB. Infantile hydrocephalus: a review of epidemiology, classification and causes. *Eur J Med Genet.* (2014) 57:359–68. doi: 10.1016/j.ejmg.2014.06.002
36. Felsenstein S, Williams B, Shingadia D, Coxon L, Riordan A, Demetriades AK, et al. Clinical and microbiologic features guiding treatment recommendations for brain abscesses in children. *Pediatr Infect Dis J.* (2013) 32:129–35. doi: 10.1097/INF.0b013e3182748d6e
37. Quan J, Zhao D, Liu L, Chen Y, Zhou J, Jiang Y, et al. High prevalence of ESBL-producing Escherichia coli and Klebsiella pneumoniae in community-onset bloodstream infections in China. *J Antimicrob Chemother.* (2017) 72:273–80. doi: 10.1093/jac/dkw372
38. Srinivasan L, Harris MC, Shah SS. Lumbar puncture in the neonate: challenges in decision making and interpretation. *Semin Perinatol.* (2012) 36:445–53. doi: 10.1053/j.semperi.2012.06.007
39. Seiden JA, Zorc JJ, Hodinka RL, Shah SS. Lack of cerebrospinal fluid pleocytosis in young infants with enterovirus infections of the central nervous system. *Pediatr Emerg Care* (2010) 26:77–81. doi: 10.1097/PEC.0b013e3181ce2fad
40. Tan NW, Lee EY, Khoo GM, Tee NW, Krishnamoorthy S, Choong CT. Cerebrospinal fluid white cell count: discriminatory or otherwise for enteroviral meningitis in infants and young children? *J Neurovirol.* (2016) 22:213–7. doi: 10.1007/s13365-015-0387-2
41. von Eiff C, Jansen B, Kohnen W, Becker K. Infections associated with medical devices: pathogenesis, management and prophylaxis. *Drugs* (2005) 65:179–214. doi: 10.2165/00003495-200565020-00003

7

Early Inflammatory Markers for the Diagnosis of Late-Onset Sepsis in Neonates: The Nosodiag Study

Laurence Dillenseger[1], Claire Langlet[1], Silvia Iacobelli[2], Thomas Lavaux[3], Charline Ratomponirina[3], Marc Labenne[4], Dominique Astruc[1], François Severac[5], Jean Bernard Gouyon[2] and Pierre Kuhn[1]*

[1] Service de Pédiatrie II, Hôpital de Hautepierre, Strasbourg, France, [2] Service de Réanimation Néonatale et Pédiatrique, Néonatologie, CHU La Réunion, Saint Pierre, France, [3] Laboratoire de Biochimie et de Biologie Moléculaire, Hôpital de Hautepierre, Strasbourg, France, [4] Service de Réanimation Pédiatrique, Hôpital Timone 2, Marseille, France, [5] Service de Santé Publique, Nouvel Hôpital Civil, Strasbourg, France

***Correspondence:**
Pierre Kuhn
pierre.kuhn@chru-strasbourg.fr*

Background: Early diagnosis is essential to improve the treatment and prognosis of newborn infants with nosocomial bacterial infections. Although cytokines and procalcitonin (PCT) have been evaluated as early inflammatory markers, their diagnostic properties have rarely been compared.

Objectives: This study evaluated and compared the ability of individual inflammatory markers available for clinician (PCT, semi-quantitative determination of IL-8) and of combinations of markers (CRP_i plus IL-6 or quantitative or semi-quantitative determination of IL-8) to diagnose bacterial nosocomial infections in neonates.

Methods: This prospective two-center study included neonates suspected of nosocomial infections from September 2008 to January 2012. Inflammatory markers were measured initially upon suspicion of nosocomial infection, and CRP was again measured 12–24 h later. Newborns were retrospectively classified into two groups: those who were infected (certainly or probably) and uninfected (certainly or probably).

Results: The study included 130 infants of median gestational age 28 weeks (range, 24–41 weeks). Of these, 34 were classified as infected and 96 as uninfected. The sensitivity, specificity, positive and negative predictive values (PPV and NPV), and positive and negative likelihood ratios (LR+ and LR-) for PCT were 59.3% (95% confidence interval [CI], 38.8–77.6%), 78.5% (95% CI, 67.8–86.9%), 48.5% (95% CI, 30.8–66.5%), 84.9% (95% CI, 74.6–92.2%), 2.7 (95% CI, 1.6–4.9), and 0.5 (95% CI, 0.3–0.8), respectively. Semi-quantitative IL-8 had the highest specificity (92.19%; 95% CI, 82.70–97.41%), PPV (72.22%; 95% CI, 46.52–90.30%) and LR+ (6.17, 95% CI, 2.67–28.44), but had low specificity (48.15%; 95% CI, 28.67–68.05%). Of all markers tested, the combination of IL-6 and CRP_i had the highest sensitivity (78.12%; 95% CI, 60.03–90.72%), NPV (91.3%; 95% CI, 82.38–96.32%) and LR- (0.29; 95% CI, 0.12–0.49). The combination of IL-6 and CRP_i had a higher area under the curve than PCT, but with borderline significance (p = 0.055).

Conclusions: The combination of IL-6 and CRP_i was superior to other methods, including PCT, for the early diagnosis of nosocomial infection in neonates, but was not sufficient for sole use. The semi-quantitative determination of IL-8 had good diagnostic properties but its sensitivity was too low for use in clinical practice.

Keywords: Late-onset neonatal sepsis, newborn infant, C-reactive protein, Procalcitonin, Interleukin 6, Interleukin 8

INTRODUCTION

Nosocomial bacterial infection (NBI) increases mortality and morbidity in neonates, especially in very low birth weight or extremely preterm newborn infants. NBI-associated complications have been observed in one-quarter of these infants, lengthening their hospital stay. These infections have been associated with poor neurodevelopment and growth and with altered lung development (1, 2). A rapid diagnosis of NBI is difficult because of the low sensitivity and the lack of specificity of clinical signs as well as the delayed increase in C-reactive protein (CRP) levels and the time required to obtain full bacteriological results. Due to the lack of a perfect gold standard, the best references for the diagnosis of NBI are positive bacteriological results. However, blood cultures have inherent limitations. The number of blood samples that can be safely obtained is limited. The quality of these samples and the amount of blood available for cultures are also challenging. Insufficient sampling can yield false negative results, whereas sample contamination can yield false positive results. Owing to the possible severity of NBI, antibiotic treatment is frequently initiated immediately in neonates with a suspected diagnosis of NBI. This strategy, however, results in the exposure of a large number of newborn infants to needless antibiotic administration, carries a potential risk for the selection in these patients of multiple drug-resistant bacteria and increases health care costs. Several cytokines increasing early during inflammatory cascades, including interleukin IL-6, IL-8 and procalcitonin (PCT) have been evaluated as early inflammatory markers of NBI in neonates. Although studies have shown that these proteins have diagnostic value, they have often led to conflicting results (3–5). Recommendations of the Evidence Based Medicine Working Group (6) have attempted to standardize the methodology of studies evaluating diagnostic markers. These include the need for blinded comparisons; the inclusion in the study population of patients to whom these tests are applicable in clinical practice; and the reporting of the diagnostic properties of these markers as likelihood ratios to assess at best their clinical value.

Studies have also assessed the diagnostic properties of combinations of CRP with IL-6 and IL-8 (7–9), with these combinations clinically used in some neonatal care units. These assays required a minimum time of 85 min to obtain the results, an amount of time compatible with clinical decision making but which should be shortened. Several studies have evaluated the ability of PCT to diagnose NBI in neonates (5, 10–12), with the minimum time required by the Kryptor™ (Brahms™) assay of only 40 min. A semi-quantitative method of measuring IL-8 (Quickline™; Milenia™) has been reported to detect minimum concentrations beyond the threshold of 50 $ng.L^{-1}$, with the results available in 20 min using a densitometer and available at the bedside. Although, all of these methods are faster and/or less expensive than the commonly used assays, their diagnostic properties have rarely been compared.

The main objectives of this study were to evaluate and compare the ability of individual inflammatory markers (PCT, CRP, quantitative and semi-quantitative determination of IL-8) and of combinations of markers (CRP plus IL-6 or quantitative or semi-quantitative determination of IL-8) to diagnose NBI in neonates.

MATERIALS AND METHODS

This prospective two-center study was undertaken in the neonatal intensive care units (NICU) of the University Hospitals of Strasbourg and Dijon between September 2008 and January 2012. This trial was registered in June 2008 on the U.S. National Institutes of Health ClinicalTrials.gov website under identification number NCT00701948.

Study Population

The study included all infants aged >72 h hospitalized in the NICU with a clinical suspicion of nosocomial sepsis, based on the presence of at least three clinical criteria and at least one risk factor reported in **Table 1** (13).

Newborn infants were excluded if they were in early postoperative phase (<48 h after surgery), had major congenital anomalies, had necrotizing enterocolitis with radiological signs, had previously been included in this study for an earlier episode of suspected NBI, or had been treated with antibiotics during the 24 h prior to being suspected of NBI.

Timing and Methods of Determination

Inflammatory markers were measured initially upon suspicion of nosocomial infection. Semi-quantitative IL-8 and PCT were measured at the time of measurement of IL-6 and/or quantitative IL-8 and initial CRP (CRP_i). assays usually performed in patients with suspected infection at each center. The total volume of blood required was 1.6 ml (1.1 ml for semi-quantitative IL-8 and PCT and 0.5 ml for CRP_i and IL-6). If the volume of blood required for semi-quantitative IL-8 and PCT measurements was insufficient, no additional puncture was performed. An additional sample for measurement of CRP was taken from each patient 12–24 h after the first sample. The times required to obtain results were 20 min for CRP (RxL™; Dade Behring™), 85 min for quantitative IL-8 (Immulite™; DPC™), 85 min for IL-6 (Immulite™; DPC™),

TABLE 1 | Criteria and clinical risk factors for nosocomial bacterial infection.

Systems	Clinical signs and risk factors
Respiratory	- Tachypnea - Dyspnea - Increased need of ventilatory supports or oxygen requirements - Apnea
Hemodynamics	- Gray color - Paleness or CRT> 3s - Tachycardia (HR> 180 beats / min) - Bradycardia (HR <100 beats / min) - High blood pressure, or need for inotropic therapy
Digestive	- Vomiting - Abdominal distension - Increased gastric residuals - Hepatomegaly
Neurological	- Lethargy - Hypotonia or hypertonia - Irritability
Thermoregulation	- Hypothermia - Hyperthermia
Metabolic - biological -	- Hyperglycemia - Metabolic acidosis - Leukopenia (<5,000 cells /mm^3) or leukocytosis (> 20,000 cells/mm^3) - Thrombocytopenia
Risk factors	- Endotracheal tube - Central venous catheter - Parenteral nutrition - Presence of a nasogastric tube - Presence of a urinary catheter - Presence of ventricular derivation catheters - Postnatal corticosteroids - Pre-surgery

40 min for PCT (Kryptor™; Brahms™), and 20 min for semi-quantitative IL-8 (Quickline™; Milenia™).

Microbiological Analyses

Blood samples (1 ml) for culture were systematically collected before the initiation of any treatment. Samples were incubated for 72 h, based on recommendations regarding the time to positivity of neonatal cultures (14). Cultures of other samples were based on the clinical signs exhibited by the newborn infant. Cerebrospinal fluid samples were obtained by lumbar puncture of newborns with neurological signs or blood cultures positive for particular pathogens. Tracheal aspirates were obtained through sterile maneuvers. Urine was obtained non-invasively using urine collection pads after rigorous disinfection of the perineal area or invasively using a catheter if a bladder sondage was present.

Antibiotic Treatment

The decision to start antibiotic treatment was made by the clinician in charge of each infant according to the standard protocol of each unit and based on a combination of clinical signs and inflammatory markers results. Those with life-threatening conditions or with hemodynamic clinical signs were started on antibiotics immediately. Those with moderate clinical signs were started on antibiotics only in case of elevated inflammatory markers (IL-6 or CRP_i in center A and quantitative IL-8 or CRP_i in center B) or in case of persistence. The choice of antibiotics was specific to each center. Treatments were started prior to knowledge of the semi-quantitative IL-8 and PCT assays.

Classification

Newborn infants were retrospectively classified into two groups—infected infants (certainly or probably) and uninfected infants (certainly or probably)—by independent physicians who did not participate in the care of the children and who had no knowledge of the results of the marker assays, except for maximum CRP concentration during the episode. Infants were classified based on bacteriological, clinical, and biological criteria.

A newborn with bacteriologically proven sepsis was considered certainly infected. Septicemia was defined by the presence of a positive blood culture. Newborns were considered certainly infected with typical skin contaminants, including such as *coagulase-negative staphylococci, bacilli, propionibacteria* and yeast, if they had positive blood cultures with clinical signs of infection and a CRP concentration >10 mg/l within 12–60 h after the initial assessment of infection (7–9, 13). Meningitis was defined as positive results on lumbar puncture (>10 cells/mL). Pneumonia required the presence of pathogenic bacteria in bronchoalveolar lavage fluid ($>10^4$ bacteria/mL) or in protected tracheal aspiration, with chest radiographs showing new or progressing infiltrates, worsening of gas exchange or an increase in the requirements of an intubated infant for ventilator support, and at least four of the following symptoms: fever or hypothermia, apnea/bradycardia, tachypnea, increased secretions, purulent secretions, increased CRP levels, and neutrophilia. Pyelonephritis was defined as the co-occurrence of the clinical signs of sepsis and CRP levels >10 mg/l within 12–60 h after the initial assessment of infection and by the presence in urine of $>10^6$ cells/l and $>10^5$ bacteria/ml.

Newborns were considered probably infected if they had clinical signs of infection, CRP $\geq$ 10 mg/l within 12–60 h after the initial assessment of infection, had no alternative diagnosis, and showed improvement in clinical status following treatment with antibiotics.

Newborns were considered probably not infected if an alternative diagnosis could explain their clinical signs or elevated CRP, if stool cultures or tracheal aspirates were positive for bacteria in the absence of clinical or biological signs of infection, if their blood culture was positive but CRP was <4 mg.L^{-1} or if they showed favorable outcomes following antibiotic treatment for <5 days.

Newborns were classified as certainly not infected if they showed clinical improvement and a normalization of CRP levels without antibiotics.

Statistical Analysis

Normally distributed quantitative values were expressed as means and standard deviations and compared using Fisher's t-tests, whereas non-normally distributed values were expressed as medians and ranges and compared using Mann-Whitney U-tests.

Diagnostic properties were analyzed using Bayes' theorem, with the results expressed as sensitivity, specificity, negative predictive value (NPV), positive predictive value (PPV), positive likelihood ratio (LR+), and negative likelihood ratio (LR-). Receiver operating characteristic (ROC) curve analyses of combinations of markers were performed using binary criteria: if one of the two levels exceeded its threshold value, the result was considered positive. Areas under the curve were compared using the DeLong test (15). In all statistical analyses, a P value <0.05 was considered statistically significant.

Ethics

The study protocol was approved by the institutional review board of each hospital and by the ethics committee East IV in June 2008 (approval number 08/30). Both parents of each newborn provided written informed consent.

RESULTS

A total of 130 infants were included in the study. There were 61 girls and 69 boys. The median gestational age was 28 weeks (24-41) and median birth weight was 1,037 grams (580–3,880). The characteristics of the study population are presented in **Table 2**. Of the 130 patients, 34 (26.2%) were classified as infected, including 18 certainly infected and 14 probably infected; and 96 (73.8%) were classified as not infected, including 65 certainly not infected and 31 probably not infected. The most frequently detected bacterium was methicillin resistant coagulase negative *Staphylococcus*. Seventeen children had septicemia, and one had pyelonephritis.The pathogens identified in the positive blood cultures are presented in **Table 3**. No child in this study died during the infectious episode.

The median time between the onset of clinical signs and blood sampling was 4.7 h (0–32 h).

Diagnostic Properties of Inflammatory Markers

Table 4 shows the diagnostic properties of the different markers and their combinations. The optimal threshold values were obtained using the ROC curve methods. Of all markers tested, both alone and combined, the combination of IL-6 and CRP_i has the highest sensitivity (78.12%; 95% confidence interval [CI] 60.03–90.72%), NPV (91.3%; 95% CI 82.38–96.32%) and LR- (0.29; 95% CI 0.12–0.49). Semi-quantitative measurement of IL-8 had the highest specificity (92.19%; 95% CI 82.70–97.41%), PPV (72.22%; 95% CI 46.52–90.30%), and LR+ (6.17; 95% CI 2.67–28.44) but had a low sensitivity (48.15%; 95% CI 28.67–68.05%).

In **Table 5**, we present the diagnostic properties of the different markers and their combination calculated only in certainly infected infants and after exclusion of probably infected ones.

TABLE 2 | Characteristics of the study population.

	Infected $n = 34$	Not infected $n = 96$	p
Male/Female	15/18	46/51	0.84
Gestational age (wk) Median (range)	27 (24–41)	28 (24–41)	0.06
Birthweight (g) Median (range)	888 (604–3,300)	1070 (580–3,880)	0.03
Duration of antibiotic treatment (d) Median (range)	9 (2–20)	0 (0–9)	0.0001
Postnatal age at onset of infection (d) Median (range)	11 (4–109)	12 (4–58)	0.83
CRIB score Mean ± *SD*	10.9 ± 3.8	8.8 ± 3.5	0.006

Comparison of the Areas Under the Curve

ROC curves for each of the markers or combination of markers are shown in **Figures 1, 2**. There were no significant differences between the AUCs of PCT and the combinations of CRP_i with quantitative and semi-quantitative measurement of IL-8. However, the AUC for the combination of IL-6 and CRP_i tended to be significantly superior to the AUC for PCT ($p = 0.055$; **Table 6**).

DISCUSSION

This study compared the performance of currently available inflammatory markers to diagnose NBI in all newborn infants suspected of NBI. The optimal assay should be rapid, available round the clock, and inexpensive. It should be reliable and reproducible with excellent diagnostic properties, including a clearly determined threshold value for the diagnosis of NBI. Moreover, because it is used for diagnosis in newborns, these assays should require as little blood as possible and identify all infected infants immediately after infection is suspected. Moreover, the real value of a diagnostic test should be determined by calculating likelihood ratios (16).

This study assessed two markers that can be measured separately and combination of markers. Semi-quantitative assays of IL8 have the potential advantages of rapidity and use at the bedside. This marker showed high specificity, with good LR+ and LR- close to the recommended optimal values of >10 and <0.1, respectively (16). However, the best threshold value determined in our study was higher than the one recommended by the developer of the technique (50 μg/l). Moreover, this test had relatively low sensitivity, <50%, limiting its usefulness. PCT had acceptable specificity, but low sensitivity, around 60%, and far from ideal LR + and LR-, findings similar to those observed in several studies (7, 12, 17). Although other studies have reported that PCT has better diagnostic properties for NBI (5, 10, 11), those studies included control groups consisting of healthy newborns with no suspicion of infection, a methodology found to artificially increase the diagnostic accuracy of the tested markers (6). Other studies, however, have reported that PCT is a better marker for NBI than CRP, with PCT found to have a greater sensitivity and a lower LR- than CRP during initial stages of infection (18–20). Another study reported also that this assay had a better global diagnostic performance (21). Thus, our finding of better diagnostic properties of CRP as

TABLE 3 | List of pathogens identified in positive blood cultures.

Bacteria	Methicillin-sensitive Coagulase Negative Staphylococci	Methicillin-resistant Coagulase Negative Staphylococci	*Bacillus cereus*	*Pseudomonas aeruginosa*	*Staphylococcus capitis*
Number of cases	3	9	1	1	3

TABLE 4 | Diagnostic properties of the different inflammatory markers.

Test	Threshold values	Se (%)	Sp (%)	PPV (%)	NPV (%)	LR+	LR-
CRP_i $n = 130$	4.05 mg/l	70.59 (52.52–84.90)	84.21 (75.30–90.88)	61.54 (44.62–76.64)	88.89 (80.51–94.54)	4.47 (2.79–8.38)	0.35 (0.17–0.54)
Quantitative IL-8 $n = 114$	107 ng/l	40,62 (23.70–59.36)	86.59 (77.26–93.11)	54.17 (32.82–74.44)	78.89 (69.01–86.79)	3.03 (1.54–6.66)	0.69 (0.48–0.89)
Semi-quantitative IL-8 $n = 91$	77.5 ng/l	48.15 (28.67–68.05)	92.19 (82.70–97.41)	72.22 (46.52–90.30)	80.82 (69.92–89.10)	6.17 (2.67–28.44)	0.56 (0.36–0.78)
PCT $n = 106$	0,69 μg/l	59.26 (38.80–77.61)	78.48 (67.80–86.94)	48.48 (30.80–66.46)	84.93 (74.6–92.23)	2.75 (1.61–4.95)	0.52 (0.29–0.78)
IL-6/CRP_i $n = 126$	21.7 ng/l–4.05 mg/l	78.12 (60.03–90.72)	76.34 (66.40–84.54)	53.19 (38.08–67.89)	91,03 (82.38–96.32)	3.30 (2.25–5.27)	0.29 (0.12–0.49)
Quantitative IL-8 / CRP_i $n = 114$	107 ng/l–4.05 mg/l	75.00 (56.60–88.54)	75.31 (64.47–84.22)	54.55 (38.85–69.61)	88,41 (78.43–94.86)	3.04 (2.01–5.06)	0.33 (0.13–0.55)
Semi–quantitative IL-8 / CRP_i $n = 91$	77.5 ng/l–4.05 mg/l	74.07 (53.72–88.89)	77.78 (65.54–87.28)	58,82 (40.70–75.35)	87,50 (75.93–94.82)	3.33 (2.09–6.13)	0.33 (0.13–0.57)

The values in brackets indicate the 95% confidence intervals.
Se, Sensitivity ; Sp, Specificity; PPV, Positive predictive values; NPV, Negative predictive values; LR+, Positive likelihood ratios; LR-, Negative likelihood ratios.

compared to PCT alone is intriguing. It could be explained by several factors. First, a delayed sampling in the course of infection, possibly suggested by the time elapsed between the onset of clinical signs determined retrospectively and the timing of sampling, could explain the better performances of CRP, which rises in the circulation 8–12 h after the onset of infection. Second, the inclusion of probably infected infants in the whole analysis, has certainly increased the diagnostic properties of CRP. This hypothesis is partly supported by the fact that the diagnostic properties of PCT are a bit better than the ones of CRP when calculated only in infants with proven NBI. Finally, we observed a threshold value between 0.5 and 1 μg/l, whereas a large multicenter study recommended the use of higher threshold values and that these values should vary according to the birthweight of the newborns (22). Anyway, the variability in LR and the large confidence intervals suggest the need for caution when using this single marker for the diagnosis of NBI.

Our results confirm that combinations of cytokine and CRP assays yielded a more accurate diagnosis than any individual marker. In our study, quantitative IL-8 plus CRP_i and IL-6 plus CRP_i had the best diagnostic properties. This finding appears logical based on the kinetics of inflammatory cascades. IL-6 is the main stimulator of hepatocyte synthesis of CRP, but has a short half-life, as does IL-8. The combination of these two cytokines with CRP can enable the continuous detection of inflammatory phenomena resulting from infection. The combination of IL-6 and CRP_i had the best sensitivity, specificity and LR-. Use of these assays in combination could reduce the number of antibiotics with an excellent NPV and good LR- while maintaining high sensitivity. This hypothesis is also supported by the strong LR- observed in other studies (3, 4, 9). The combination of IL-8 and CRP_i also showed excellent diagnostic performance, similar to that of IL-6 and CRP_i (8, 23).

Assays of other cytokines, including IL-10, TNF alpha, IL-1 beta, and IL-12 are currently available (24, 25). These techniques appear reliable, sensitive, reproducible and automatable, but are not yet used in clinical practice. The blood volumes required are very low (50–100 μL of serum), although assay times are somewhat longer (2–3 h). Lipopolysaccharide binding protein (LBP) has been reported to be a more accurate diagnostic marker than IL-6, IL-8 and PCT for the diagnosis of infections in neonates (26, 27). More recently, a new marker, presepsin, was identified; however, those studies included a small number of infants and used uninfected healthy newborn infants as a control group (28–30). Multiplex PCR assays using small volumes of blood are also being developed to detect the DNA of several bacterial species (31, 32). Although these assays were shown to be faster and more accurate than blood cultures, several hours were required to obtain their results (32).

TABLE 5 | Diagnostic properties of the different inflammatory markers in the certainly infected infants.

Test	Threshold values	Se (%)	Sp (%)	PPV (%)	NPV (%)	LR+	LR-
CRP_i $n = 83$	7.82 mg/l	66.67 (40.99; 86.66)	89.23 (79.06; 95.56)	63.16 (38.36; 83.71)	90.62 (80.70; 96.48)	6.19 (2.86; 13.40)	0.37 (0.19; 0.72)
Quantitative IL-8 $n = 69$	74.13 ng/l	43.75 (19.75; 70.12)	89.09 (77.75; 95.89)	53.85 (25.13; 80.78)	84.48 (72.58; 92.65)	4.01 (1.57; 10.24)	0.63 (0.41; 0.98)
Semi quantitative IL-8 $n = 52$	77.72 ng/l	53.85 (25.13; 80.78)	95.24 (83.84; 99.42)	77.78 (39.99; 97.19)	86.96 (73.74; 95.06)	11.31 (2.67; 47.88)	0.48 (0.27; 0.88)
PCT $n = 63$	1.5 μg/l	53.85 (25.13; 80.78)	98.04 (89.55; 99.95)	87.5 (47.35; 99.68)	89.29 (78.12; 95.97)	27.46 (3.70; 203.91)	0.47 (0.26; 0.85)
IL-6/CRP_i $n = 79$	21.4–7.82 mg/l	75 (47.62; 92.73)	84.13 (72.74; 92.12)	54.55 (32.21; 75.61)	92.98 (83.00; 98.05)	4.72 (2.50; 8.92)	0.3 (0.13; 0.70)
Semi quantitative IL-8/CRP_i $n = 52$	77.72 ng/l–7.82 mg/l	69.23 (38.57; 90.91)	88.1 (74.37; 96.02)	64.29 (35.14; 87.24)	90.24 (76.87; 97.28)	5.82 (2.37; 14.29)	0.35 (0.15; 0.80)

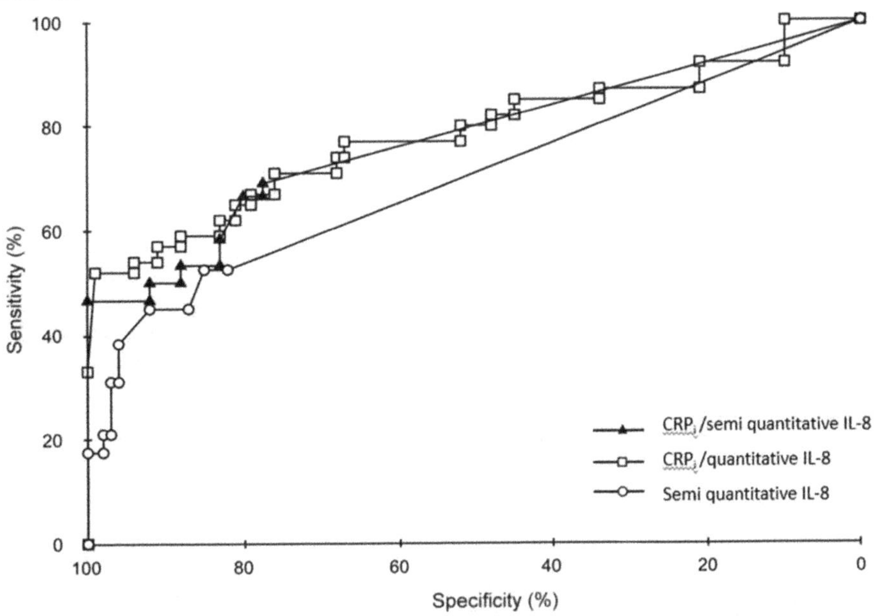

FIGURE 1 | Receiver operating characteristic (ROC) curves for CRPi plus semi quantitative determination of IL-8, CRPi plus quantitative determination of IL-8 and semi-quantitative determination of IL-8 alone.

The limitations of our study are first the relatively small number of certainly infected infants. Second, the classification into "infected" and "not infected" infants is very challenging and a possible limitation for observational studies. However, this challenge exists in all studies regarding neonatal infection. We think that it is essential to include also the group of probably infected infants in the determination of the diagnostic properties of inflammatory markers. We have to consider them as infected infants to encompass all the situations met in the daily clinical life. Finally, our study was not designed to assess the ability of markers to guide antibiotic treatment. The combination of IL-8 and CRP was found, however, to result in significant reductions in unnecessary antibiotics and cost of care, without risk to the study population (8). Similar results were found for early-onset neonatal infections, in a large multicenter randomized study involving 1291 infants admitted for suspected infections and clinically stable to wait the results of the assays (33). To our knowledge, however, no studies to date have confirmed the results of the latter study in neonates with NBI. The results of cytokine assays may be integrated into clinical and biological algorithms, similar to those proposed for early onset neonatal infection (34, 35). In these algorithms, PCT concentration in cord blood was found to be an efficient marker that could guide the treatment of newborns suspected of early onset neonatal sepsis (34–37). This approach could also include bacterial DNA load, as assessed by PCR multiplex assays (32).

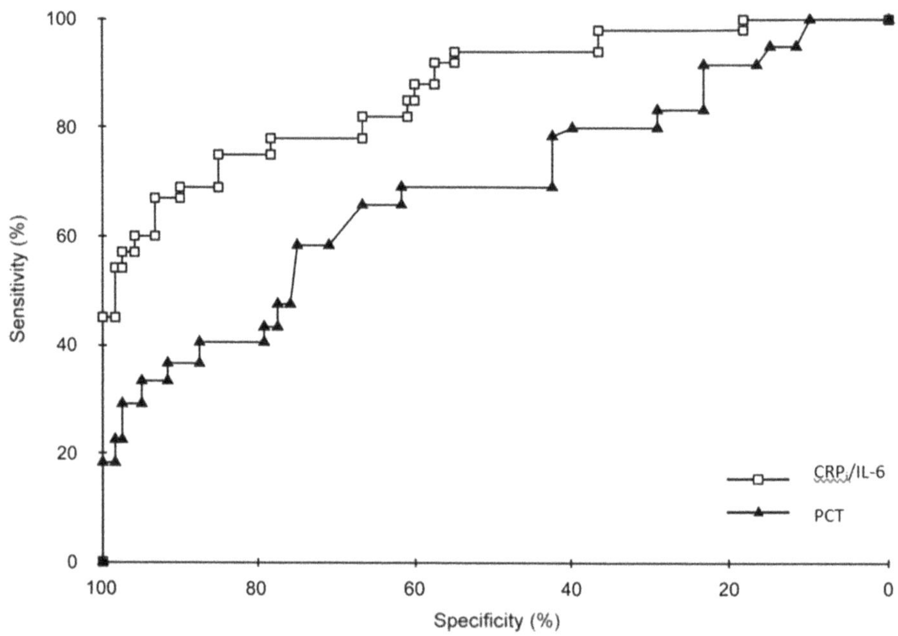

FIGURE 2 | Receiver operating characteristic (ROC) curves for CRP_i plus determination of IL-6, PCT alone.

TABLE 6 | Comparison of areas under the curves for the different marker.

Markers	AUC	CI 95%	*P**
PCT vs. IL-6/CRP_i	71.65–84.80	(57.74–85.56)–(75.03–96.58)	0.055
PCT vs. quantitative IL-8/CRP_i	71.65–80.51	(57.74–85.56)–(67.51–93.51)	0.330
PCT vs. Semi-quantitative IL-8/CRP_i	71.65–81.44	(57.74–85.56)–(69.88–93.00)	0.253
Semi-quantitative IL-8/CRP_i vs. IL-6/CRP_i	81.44–85.80	(69.88–93.00)–(75.03–96.58)	0.336
Quantitative IL-8/CRP_i vs. IL-6/CRP_i	80.51–85.80	(67.51–93.51)–(75.03–96.58)	0.288

**Delong test.*

CONCLUSION

The combinations of CRP_i with IL-6 and IL-8 were superior to individual assays in the early diagnosis of NBI. The combination of IL-6 plus CRP_i was especially useful, but was not sufficient for sole use, and PCT was inferior to the combination of IL-6 plus CRP_i. The semi-quantitative determination of IL-8 had good diagnostic properties but its sensitivity was too low for use in clinical practice. The benefit of this combination to rationalize antibiotic treatment should be evaluated with clinical and biological decision algorithms, while awaiting the identification of more efficient markers that are clinically usable.

AUTHOR CONTRIBUTIONS

LD contributed to the data recording and analysis, wrote the first draft of the manuscript and edited the tables and figures. CL reviewed, the data analysis, contributed to the patient enrollment, data recording, and analysis, contributed to the writing of the first draft of the manuscript. SI, ML, JG, and DA participated in the study protocol development, enrolled patients in their department, contributed to the data recording and approved the final draft of the manuscript. TL, and CR contributed to the study protocol development, performed the markers measurement and analysis, ensured the quality of the measurements and the anonnimity of the results. FS coordinated and performed the statistical analyses, contributed to the edition of the figures and approved the final draft of the manuscript. PK coordinated the study deveplomlent and wrote the initial protocol, participated in the study enrollment, contributed to the writing of the manuscript and reviewed and approved the final draft.

ACKNOWLEDGMENTS

We also thank the team of nurses for their assistance in acquiring data during the study period. We are especially grateful to the parents and their infants who participated in this research program. This work was supported by the Centre Hospitalier Universitaire de Strasbourg (Projet de Recherche Institutionnel n°4108).

REFERENCES

1. Boghossian NS, Page GP, Bell EF, Stoll BJ, Murray JC, Cotten CM, et al. Late-onset sepsis in very low birth weight infants from singleton and multiple-gestation births. *J Pediatr.*(2013) 162:1120–4. doi: 10.1016/j.jpeds.2012.11.089
2. Stoll BJ, Hansen NI, Adams-Chapman I, Fanaroff AA, Hintz SR, Vohr B, et al. Neurodevelopmental and growth impairment among extremely low-birth-weight infants with neonatal infection. *JAMA* (2004) 292:2357–65. doi: 10.1001/jama.292.19.2357
3. Ng PC, Cheng SH, Chui KM, Fok TF, Wong MY, Wong W, et al. Diagnosis of late onset neonatal sepsis with cytokines, adhesion molecule, and C-reactive protein in preterm very low birthweight infants. *Arch Dis Child Fetal Neonatal Ed.* (1997) 77:F221–7. doi: 10.1136/fn.77.3.F221
4. Laborada G, Rego M, Jain A, Guliano M, Stavola J, Ballabh P, et al. Diagnostic value of cytokines and C-reactive protein in the first 24 hours of neonatal sepsis. *Am J Perinatol.* (2003) 20:491–501. doi: 10.1055/s-2003-45382
5. Chiesa C, Pacifico L, Rossi N, Panero A, Matrunola M, Mancuso G. Procalcitonin as a marker of nosocomial infections in the neonatal intensive care unit. *Intensive Care Med.* (2000) 26:175–7. doi: 10.1007/s0013400 51139
6. Jaeschke R, Guyatt GH, Sackett DL: Users' guides to the medical literature. III. How to use an article about a diagnostic test. B. What are the results and will they help me in caring for my patients? The evidence-based medicine working group. *JAMA* (1994) 271:703–7. doi: 10.1001/jama.1994.035103300 81039
7. Franz AR, Kron M, Pohlandt F, Steinbach G. Comparison of procalcitonin with interleukin 8, C-reactive protein and differential white blood cell count for the early diagnosis of bacterial infections in newborn infants. *Pediatr Infect Dis J.* (1999) 18:666–71. doi: 10.1097/00006454-199908000-00003
8. Franz AR, Steinbach G, Kron M, Pohlandt F. Reduction of unnecessary antibiotic therapy in newborn infants using interleukin-8 and C-reactive protein as markers of bacterial infections. *Pediatrics* (1999) 104:447–53. doi: 10.1542/peds.104.3.447
9. Ceccon MEJR, Vaz FAC, Diniz EMA, Okay TS. Interleukins 6 and C-reactive protein for the diagnosis of late onset sepsis in the newborn infant. *Rev Assoc Med Bras.* (2006) 52:79–85. doi: 10.1590/S0104-423020060002 00016
10. Enguix A, Rey C, Concha A, Medina A, Coto D, Diéguez MA. Comparison of procalcitonin with C-reactive protein and serum amyloid for the early diagnosis of bacterial sepsis in critically ill neonates and children. *Intensive Care Med.* (2001) 27:211–15. doi: 10.1007/s0013400 00709
11. Pérez Solís D, López Sastre JB, Coto Cotallo GD, Diéguez Junquera MA, Deschamps Mosquera EM, Crespo Hernández M. Procalcitonin for the diagnosis of nosocomial neonatal sepsis. *An Pediatr.* (2006) 64:349–53. doi: 10.1157/13086523
12. López Sastre JB, Pérez Solís D, Roqués Serradilla V, Fernández Colomer B, Coto Cotallo GD, Krauel Vidal X, et al. Procalcitonin is not sufficiently reliable to be the sole marker of neonatal sepsis of nosocomial origin. *BMC Pediatr.* (2006) 6:16. doi: 10.1186/1471-2431-6-16
13. Garner JS, Jarvis WR, Emori TG, Horan TC, Hughes JM. CDC definitions for nosocomial infections 1988. *Z Arztl Fortbild.* (1991) 85:818–27.
14. Guerti K, Devos H, Ieven MM, Mahieu LM. Time to positivity of neonatal blood cultures: fast and furious? *J Med Microbiol.* (2011) 60:446–53. doi: 10.1099/jmm.0.020651-0
15. DeLong ER1, DeLong DM, Clarke-Pearson DL. Comparing the areas under two or more correlated receiver operating characteristic curves: a nonparametric approach. *Biometrics* (1988) 44:837–4516.
16. Halkin A, Reichman J, Schwaber M, Paltiel O, Brezis M. Likelihood ratios: getting diagnostic testing into perspective. *QJM* (1998) 91:247–58. doi: 10.1093/qjmed/91.4.247
17. Kuhn P, Escande B, Rivera S, Langlet C, Messer J. Procalcitonin and neonatal infection. *Arch Pediatr.* (2004) 11:585–6. doi: 10.1016/j.arcped.2004.03.092
18. Vazzalwar R, Pina-Rodrigues E, Puppala BL, Angst DB, Schweig L. Procalcitonin as a screening test for late-onset sepsis in preterm very low birth weight infants. *J Perinatol.* (2005) 25:397–402. doi: 10.1038/sj.jp.7211296
19. Jacquot A, Labaune JM, Baum TP, Putet G, Picaud JC. Rapid quantitative procalcitonin measurement to diagnose nosocomial infections in newborn infants. *Arch Dis Child Fetal Neonatal Ed.* (2009) 94:345–8. doi: 10.1136/adc.2008.155754
20. Fendler WM, Piotrowski AJ. Procalcitonin in the early diagnosis of nosocomial sepsis in preterm neonates. *J Paediatr Child Health* (2008) 44:114–8. doi: 10.1111/j.1440-1754.2007.01230.x
21. Isidor B, Caillaux G, Gilquin V, Loubersac V, Caillon J, Roze JC, et al. The use of procalcitonin in the diagnosis of late-onset infection in neonatal intensive care unit patients. *Scand J Infect Dis.* (2007) 39:1063–6. doi: 10.1080/00365540701466181
22. Auriti C, Fiscarelli E, Ronchetti MP, Argentieri M, Marrocco G, Quondamcarlo A, et al. Procalcitonin in detecting neonatal nosocomial sepsis. *Arch Dis Child Fetal Neonatal Ed.* (2012) 97:368–70. doi: 10.1136/fetalneonatal-2010-194100
23. Verboon-Maciolek MA, Thijsen SFT, Hemels MAC, Menses M, van Loon AM, Krediet TG, et al: Inflammatory mediators for the diagnosis and treatment of sepsis in early infancy. *Pediatr Res.* (2006) 59:457–61. doi: 10.1203/01.pdr.0000200808.35368.57
24. Berner R, Niemeyer CM, Leitits JU, Funke A, Schwab C, Rau U, et al. Plasma levels of granulocyte colony-stimulating factor, tumor necrosis factor alpha, interleukin-1ß, IL-6, IL-8, and soluble intercellular adhesion molecule-1 in neonatal early onset sepsis. *Pediatr Res.* (1998) 44:469–77. doi: 10.1203/00006450-199810000-00002
25. Santana-Reyes C, Garcia-Munoz F, Reyes D, González G, Dominguez C, Domenech E. Role of cytokines (interleukin-1b, 6, 8, tumor necrosis factor-1a and soluble-receptor of interleukin-2) and C-reactive protein in the diagnosis of neonatal sepsis. *Acta Paediatr.* (2003) 92, 221–27. doi: 10.1111/j.1651-2227.2003.tb00530.x
26. Pavcnik-Arnol M, Hojker S, Derganc M. Lipopolysaccharide-binding protein in critically ill neonates and children with suspected infection: comparison with procalcitonin, interleukin-6, and C-reactive protein. *Intensive Care Med.* (2004) 30:1454–60. doi: 10.1007/s00134-004-2307-4
27. Berner R, Fürll B, Stelter F, Dröse J, Müller H-P, Schütt C. Elevated levels of lipopolysaccharide-binding protein and soluble CD14 in plasma in neonatal early-onset sepsis. *Clin Diagn Lab Immunol.* (2002) 9:440–445. doi: 10.1128/CDLI.9.2.440-445.2002
28. Kumar N, Dayal R, Singh P, Pathak S, Pooniya V, Goyal A, et al. A comparative evaluation of presepsin with procalcitonin and CRP in diagnosing neonatal sepsis. *Indian J Pediatr.* (2018). doi: 10.1007/s12098-018-2744-7. [Epub ahead of print].
29. Miyosawa Y, Akazawa Y, Kamiya M, Nakamura C, Takeuchi Y, Kusakari M, et al. Presepsin as a predictor of positive blood culture in suspected neonatal sepsis. *Pediatr Int.* (2018) 60:157–61. doi: 10.1111/ped.13469
30. Seliem W, Sultan AM. Presepsin as a predictor of early onset neonatal sepsis in the umbilical cord blood of premature infants with premature rupture of membranes. *Pediatr Int.* (2018) 60: 428–32. doi: 10.1111/ped.13541
31. Van den Brand M, Peters RPH, Catsburg A, Rubenjan A, Broeke FJ, van den Dungen FAM, et al. Development of a multiplex real-time PCR assay for the rapid diagnosis of neonatal late onset sepsis. *J Microbiol Methods* (2014) 106:8–15. doi: 10.1016/j.mimet.2014.07.034
32. Van den Brand M, van den Dungen FAM, Bos MP, van Weissenbruch MM, van Furth AM, de Lange A, Rubenjan A, et al. Evaluation of a real-time PCR assay for detection and quantification of bacterial DNA directly in blood of preterm neonates with suspected late-onset sepsis. *Crit Care.* (2018) 22–105. doi: 10.1186/s13054-018-2010-4
33. Franz AR, Bauer K, Schalk A, Garland SM, Bowman ED, Rex K, et al. Measurement of interleukin 8 in combination with C-reactive protein reduced unnecessary antibiotic therapy in newborn infants: a multicenter, randomized, controlled trial. *Pediatrics* (2004) 114:1–8. doi: 10.1542/peds.114.1.1
34. Cabaret B, Laurans C, Launay E, Orsonneau JL, Roze JC, Gras-Le Guen C. Diagnostic value of a new procalcitonin cord sample-guided algorithm to manage newborns suspected of early-onset infection. *Arch Pediatr.* (2013) 20:954–62. doi: 10.1016/j.arcped.2013.06.020

35. Lencot S, Cabaret B, Sauvage G, Laurans C, Launay E, Orsonneau JL, et al. A new procalcitonin cord-based algorithm in early-onset neonatal infection: for a change of paradigm. *Eur J Clin Microbiol Infect Dis.* (2014) 33:1229–38. doi: 10.1007/s10096-014-2065-3
36. Gras-le Guen C, Launay E, Boscher C, Caillon J. What is new in neonatal infection? *Bull Acad Natl Med.* (2016) 200: 81–90.
37. Stocker M, van Herk W, El Helou S, Dutta S, Fontana MS, Schuerman FABA, et al. Procalcitonin-guided decision making for duration of antibiotic therapy in neonates with suspected early-onset sepsis: a multicentre, randomised controlled trial (NeoPIns). *Lancet* (2017) 390:871–81. doi: 10.1016/S0140-6736(17)31444-7

8

Time-to-Positivity of Blood Cultures in Children with Sepsis

*Alexa Dierig[1], Christoph Berger[2], Philipp K. A. Agyeman[3], Sara Bernhard-Stirnemann[4], Eric Giannoni[5,6], Martin Stocker[7], Klara M. Posfay-Barbe[8], Anita Niederer-Loher[9], Christian R. Kahlert[9], Alex Donas[7], Paul Hasters[10], Christa Relly[2], Thomas Riedel[11], Christoph Aebi[3], Luregn J. Schlapbach[3,12,13,14] and Ulrich Heininger[1]**

[1] Infectious Diseases and Vaccinology, University of Basel Children's Hospital, Basel, Switzerland, [2] Division of Infectious Diseases and Hospital Epidemiology, Children's Research Center, University Children's Hospital Zurich, Zurich, Switzerland, [3] Department of Pediatrics, Inselspital, Bern University Hospital, University of Bern, Bern, Switzerland, [4] Cantonal Hospital Aarau, Children's Hospital, Aarau, Switzerland, [5] Department Mother-Woman-Child, Service of Neonatology, Lausanne University Hospital, Lausanne, Switzerland, [6] Infectious Diseases Service, Lausanne University Hospital, Lausanne, Switzerland, [7] Department of Pediatrics, Children's Hospital Lucerne, Lucerne, Switzerland, [8] Pediatric Infectious Diseases Unit, Children's Hospital of Geneva, University Hospitals of Geneva, Geneva, Switzerland, [9] Children's Hospital of Eastern Switzerland St. Gallen, St. Gallen, Switzerland, [10] Department of Neonatology, University Hospital Zurich, Zurich, Switzerland, [11] Department of Pediatrics, Cantonal Hospital Graubuenden, Chur, Switzerland, [12] Faculty of Medicine, The University of Queensland, Brisbane, QLD, Australia, [13] Paediatric Critical Care Research Group, Mater Research Institute, University of Queensland, Brisbane, QLD, Australia, [14] Paediatric Intensive Care Unit, Lady Cilento Children's Hospital, Children's Health Queensland, Brisbane, QLD, Australia

***Correspondence:**
Ulrich Heininger
ulrich.heininger@ukbb.ch

Background: Blood cultures are essential for the diagnosis and further appropriate treatment in children with suspected sepsis. In most hospitals, children will be empirically treated or closely monitored for at least 48 h awaiting results of blood cultures. Several studies have challenged the optimal duration of empiric treatment in the era of continuously monitored blood culture systems. The aim of our study was to investigate time-to-positivity (TTP) of blood cultures in children with proven sepsis.

Methods: The Swiss Pediatric Sepsis Study prospectively enrolled children 0–16 years of age with blood culture positive sepsis between September 2011 and October 2015. TTP was prospectively assessed in six participating academic pediatric hospitals by fully automated blood culture systems.

Results: In 521 (93%) of 562 bacteremia episodes (493 children, median age 103 days, range 0 days–16.9 years) a valid TTP was available. Median TTP was 12 h (IQR 8–17 h, range 0–109 h). By 24, 36, and 48 h, 460 (88%), 498 (96%), and 510 (98%) blood cultures, respectively, were positive. TTP was independent of age, sex, presence of comorbidities, site of infection and severity of infection. Median TTP in all age groups combined was shortest for group B streptococcus (8.7 h) and longest for coagulase-negative staphylococci (16.2 h).

Conclusion: Growth of bacteria in blood cultures is detectable within 24 h in 9 of 10 children with blood culture-proven sepsis. Therefore, a strict rule to observe or treat all children with suspected sepsis for at least 48 h is not justified.

Keywords: sepsis, children, bacteremia, blood cultures, time-to-positivity

INTRODUCTION

Surviving Sepsis Campaign guidelines recommend obtaining blood cultures before initiation of antibiotic treatment in newborns, infants and children with suspected sepsis (1, 2). Due to globally increasing antibiotic resistance rates, the World Health Organization (WHO) has urged countries to develop action plans against antibiotic resistance (3). Blood cultures represent a cornerstone of antibiotic stewardship to streamline targeted treatment and to reduce unnecessary use of antibiotics. However, blood cultures in patients with suspected sepsis are often negative. For example, the number of neonates with suspected sepsis needed to treat for 1 culture proven neonatal sepsis varies between 44 and 100 (4–6).

In most hospitals, children with suspected sepsis will be empirically treated or closely monitored for at least 48 h awaiting results of the blood cultures. However, this measure is based on limited evidence. The American Academy of Pediatrics recommends stopping antibiotic therapy in neonates treated for suspected early-onset sepsis after 48 h if cultures remain negative (7). Several studies in infants <90 days of age have challenged whether this empiric treatment and observation period is still justified in the era of continuous monitoring blood culture systems (8–10): They demonstrated that ≥96% of all blood cultures were positive by 36 h (9, 10) and that ceasing antibiotic treatment after implementation of an evidence-based care process model including an empiric treatment period of 24–36 h did not show any adverse events (8).

Limitations of currently available data on optimal use of time-to-positivity (TTP) for decision making on empiric antibiotic treatment in suspected sepsis are (1) lack of data on pediatric age groups beyond early infancy, (2) lack of multicenter studies, and (3) lack of detailed characterization of host and pathogen features. The aim of this study was to analyse TTP in children with blood culture positive sepsis recruited through a large prospective multicenter population-based pediatric sepsis cohort study and to investigate host and pathogen factors associated with TTP.

METHODS

As part of the Swiss Pediatric Sepsis Study, we analyzed TTP values in children with blood culture positive sepsis between September 2011 and October 2015. Details of the Swiss Pediatric Sepsis Study have previously been reported (11, 12). The study was approved by the respective ethics committees of all participating centers (Cantonal Ethics Committee, Inselspital, University of Bern, no. KEK-029/11). Written informed consent from patients, and/or their legal guardians was obtained before study enrollment. In patients who fulfilled inclusion criteria but consent was not available (224 of 521), waiver from informed consent had been granted by the ethics commission for collection of anonymized clinical data.

Children 0–16 years of age with bacteremia in the presence of a systemic inflammatory response syndrome (SIRS) were enrolled in all 10 major pediatric hospitals in Switzerland during the study period. SIRS, severe sepsis and septic shock were defined according to the international consensus conference on pediatric sepsis (13). Briefly, for children beyond the neonatal period, SIRS was defined as the presence of at least 2 of the following four criteria, one of which had to be abnormal temperature or leukocyte count: body temperature <36°C or >38.5°C; abnormal heart rate for age; abnormal respiratory rate for age; leukocyte count elevated or depressed for age or >10% immature neutrophils. Age specific limits for heart rate, respiratory rate, and leukocyte count were applied as defined in the 2005 consensus definitions. For neonates (<28 days old, or <44 weeks postconceptional age in premature newborns) at least 2 of the following signs were required to be present: tachycardia >180/min, tachypnea >60/min or increased apnea frequency, temperature instability, leukocyte count 34 × 103 /mm^3 or immature:total neutrophil ratio >0.2, capillary refill >2 s, apathia or irritability.

Severe sepsis was defined as sepsis plus one of the following: cardiovascular organ dysfunction or acute respiratory distress syndrome or two or more other organ dysfunctions.

Septic shock was defined as sepsis and cardiovascular organ dysfunction.

Each bacteremia episode received a study number and was analyzed. The present sub-study is restricted to 6 of the 10 participating centers (designated A to F) where fully automated blood culture systems were used, which allowed prospective assessment of TTP. TTP was defined as the time interval between placement of the blood culture bottle into the automated system and detection of a positive signal. The following blood culture systems were used: Beckton Dickinson (BD), Allschwill, Switzerland, Bactec Aerob/Anaerob, Peds Plus/F und mycosis IC/F Mycosis und Pedi (center A), BD Bactec FX (center B), BD Bactec Lytic/10 Anaerobic/F, BD Bactec Aerobic Plus/F BD Bactec Peds Plus/F (center C), bioMerieux, Geneva, Switzerland, BacT/ALELRT PF Aerob/anaerob, BacT/ALERT FA Aerob, BacTALERT FN Anaerob (center D), BD Bactec peds plus/F, BD Bactec lytic/10 anaerobic/f, BD Bactec plus aerobic/F (center E), BD Bactec plus aerobic/F, BD Bactec plus anaerobic/F, BD Bactec peds plus (center F). Centers B to F used fully automated blood culture systems from the beginning of the study, center A introduced it mid-2013.

Early-onset neonatal sepsis was defined as sepsis occurring <72 h of age and late-onset neonatal sepsis as ≥72 h in term infants and 72 h of age to <44 weeks of gestational age in premature infants. Hospital-acquired infection (i.e., blood culture obtained >48 h after admission) and central line-associated bloodstream infection (CLABSI) were defined according to the criteria of the Centers for Disease Control and Prevention (CDC) (14). In patients with suspected sepsis, positive blood cultures were only included if contamination was ruled out by the treating physician. The definition of contamination was based on the following criteria: absence of a central line at the time the blood culture was taken; blood culture growing a mixed flora of different coagulase-negative staphylococci (CoNS); and blood cultures growing pathogens considered as contaminants by the treating physician.

Chronic inborn or acquired medical conditions, recent surgery, or burns where considered as comorbidities and were categorized according to the pediatric complex chronic conditions classification system, version 2 (15).

Pre-planned Subgroup Analyses and Statistics

For statistical data analysis all extracted data was stored in spreadsheets (Microsoft Excel 2010, version 14.0). For descriptive analyses, the total number of cases and all cases stratified by study center were analyzed. For comparative analyses of TTP, we analyzed cases from all study centers combined and all bacteria combined, stratified by sex. For further analyses, cases were stratified by study centers, the 5 most frequently isolated organisms, age (0–27 days, 28–365 days, 1–5 years, 6–10 years and >10 years), focus of infection, outcome/severity of infection, prematurity, comorbidity, and community-acquired vs. nosocomial infection.

Descriptive statistics are presented as median (IQR) for continuous variables and as frequencies (%) for categorical variables. We fitted a generalized linear model with a log-link function and Gamma distribution for potential determinants of TTP with age, gender, presence of comorbidity, sepsis severity, site of infection, and pathogens using a random effect to correct for correlation between multiple observations at the same hospital. We added 0.01 h to all TTP measurements to remove zero values. We separately fitted univariable models or all variables and a multivariable model containing all variables. We present the results of the multivariable model as estimates (multiplicative factor by which to multiply the TTP of the respective reference group) with 95% CIs and p-values of likelihood ratio testing. We additionally fitted a multilevel binomial regression model for potential determinants of death within the first 30 days after sepsis onset with the TTP (adjusting for patient age, sex, presence of comorbidity, severity of sepsis, site of infection, and pathogen) using a random effect to correct for correlation between multiple observations at the same hospital.

Statistical significance was defined at a two-sided p-value of <0.05. We did regression analyses with R version 3.4.3.

RESULTS

General Characteristics

During the study period, 493 patients with 562 bacteremia episodes were enrolled in study centers A-F. Of these, 521 (93%) had blood culture TTP recorded and they are the subject of these analyses; 311 (60%) of 521 episodes occurred in male patients with no difference between infants <90 days of age and patients >90 days of age (**Supplement Table 1**). Median age of patients was 103 days (range: 0 days–16.9 years; IQR 11 days–3.8 years); 196 (38%) were neonates (i.e., ≤28 days old), 257 (49%) were <90 days old and 125 (24%) were <365 days old.

In 291 (56%) episodes the sepsis was community-acquired and 86 (30%) of these patients had at least 1 comorbidity. In 230 (44%) episodes the sepsis was hospital-acquired and 205 (89%) of these patients had at least 1 comorbidity.

In 417 (80%) episodes a focus for sepsis could be identified and most commonly this was related to a central venous catheter

Case fatality rate was 7% ($N = 37$). Children <90 days of age had significantly more episodes with severe sepsis than children >90 days of age (**Supplement Table 1**).

Blood culture isolates by study center are summarized in **Table 1**. Overall 336 (64%) were Gram-positive and 185 (36%) were Gram-negative pathogens. The distribution of pathogens stratified by age, i.e., <90 days and >90 days, is shown in **Supplement Table 1**.

Time to Positivity and Associations With Pathogens and Host Characteristics

Median TTP was 11.7 h (IQR 8.3–17.1) with minimal variability between different study centers (**Supplement Table 2**).

Table 2 shows results of multivariable analysis of TTP by patient and disease characteristics. TTP was independent of age, sex, presence of a comorbidity (see **Table 3**), site of infection, and severity of sepsis. Compared to coagulase-negative staphylococci,

TABLE 1 | Bacterial pathogens isolated from blood cultures by study center (A-F).

	A n (%)	B n (%)	C n (%)	D n (%)	E n (%)	F n (%)	Total n (%)
Escherichia coli	21 (20)	6 (11)	18 (13)	21 (24)	23 (24)	8 (22)	97 (19)
Coagulase-negative-staphylococci	7 (7)	15 (28)	40 (29)	6 (7)	13 (13)	2 (5)	83 (16)
Staphylococcus aureus	13 (12)	9 (17)	18 (1)	11 (12)	13 (13)	8 (22)	77 (14)
Group B streptococcus	11 (10)	12 (22)	4 (3)	4 (4)	10 (10)	3 (8)	47 (9)
Streptococcus pneumoniae	13 (12)	1 (2)	9 (6)	8 (9)	8 (8)	8 (22)	47 (9)
Group A streptococcus	5 (5)	0 (0)	4 (3)	8 (9)	5 (5)	2 (5)	24 (5)
Enterococcus spp.	8 (8)	1 (2)	4 (3)	2 (2)	2 (2)	2 (5)	19 (4)
Klebsiella spp.	7 (7)	1 (2)	11 (8)	1 (1)	4 (4)	1 (3)	25 (5)
Neisseria meningitidis	2 (2)	0 (0)	4 (3)	3 (3)	4 (4)	2 (5)	13 (2)
Pseudomonas aeruginosa	4 (4)	0 (0)	3 (2)	1 (1)	2 (2)	0 (0)	11 (2)
Haemophilus influenzae	1 (1)	0 (0)	2 (1)	1 (1)	3 (3)	0 (0)	6 (1)
Other Gram-negative pathogens♦	11 (10)	2 (4)	10 (7)	2 (2)	4 (4)	0 (0)	29 (6)
Other Gram-positive pathogens•	2 (2)	7 (13)	15 (11)	6 (7)	6 (6)	1 (3)	38 (7)
Total	105	54	139	89	97	37	521

♦ *Stenotrophomonas maltophilia, Serratia marcescens, Serratia liquefaciens, Citrobacter Sedlakii, Citrobacter freundii, Elizabethkingia meningoseptica, Salmonella group B, Salmonella group C, Acinetobacter lwofii, Enterobacter cloacae, Capnocytophaga sp., Proteus mirabilis, Cardiobacterium hominis*

• *Bifidobacterium spp., Fusobacterium nucleatum, Fusobacterium necrophorum, Streptococcus bovis, Lactobacillus spp., Streptococcus mitis, Streptococcus equi, Streptococcus, salivarius, Streptococcus anginosus, Streptococcus sanguinis, Streptococcus viridans, Listeria monocytogenes, Micrococcus luteus, Bacillus cereus, Bacillus pumilus, Rothia mucilaginosa,*

TABLE 2 | Median (IQR) TTP by patient and infection characteristics and adjusted* estimates of TTP investigating potential predictive factors in a generalized linear model.

	n (%)	TTP, Median (IQR), h	Multivariable model	
			Estimated TTP (95% CI)[a]	Adjusted *p*-value[b]
Age groups				$p = 1.0$
<28 days	196 (38%)	11.3 (7.57–18.7)	Reference	
28–365 days	125 (24%)	11.0 (8.40–15.6)	0.95 (0.79–1.13)	
1–4 years	93 (18%)	12.0 (9.12–16.2)	1.01 (0.82–1.25)	
5–9 years	53 (10%)	11.9 (9.00–16.2)	0.97 (0.75–1.25)	
10–16 years	54 (10%)	12.0 (8.62–16.5)	0.94 (0.73–1.20)	
Sex				$p = 0.3$
Male sex	311 (60%)	11.3 (8.12–17.2)	Reference	
Female sex	210 (40%)	12.0 (8.50–16.8)	1.07 (0.94–1.22)	
Comorbidity				$p = 0.1$
No comorbidity	230 (44%)	12.0 (8.93–16.9)	Reference	
Comorbidity present	291 (56%)	11.0 (7.50–17.1)	0.85 (0.72–1.01)	
Severity of sepsis				$p = 0.9$
Sepsis	324 (62%)	11.7 (8.67–16.6)	Reference	
Severe sepsis	100 (19%)	12.4 (7.56–19.6)	0.96 (0.80–1.15)	
Septic shock	97 (19%)	11.3 (7.50–15.1)	1.00 (0.84–1.19)	
Site or type of infection				$p = 0.1$
Central-line associated bloostream	151 (29%)	11.9 (7.65–18.1)	Reference	
Primary bloodstream	104 (20%)	10.1 (7.17–14.4)	0.94 (0.76–1.17)	
Urinary tract	56 (11%)	11.0 (8.12–15.4)	1.27 (0.97–1.65)	
Pneumonia	45 (9%)	13.2 (10.3–16.2)	1.28 (0.95–1.74)	
Central nervous system	40 (8%)	10.0 (8.33–14.7)	0.94 (0.69–1.28)	
Gastrointestinal system	32 (6%)	11.8 (7.88–18.2)	1.32 (0.99–1.76)	
Bones and joints	30 (6%)	14.1 (11.3–20.1)	1.04 (0.72–1.49)	
Skin and soft tissue	30 (6%)	12.5 (9.35–16.7)	1.06 (0.79–1.42)	
Other specific infection type[b]	33 (6%)	12.0 (9.00–19.5)	1.20 (0.88–1.62)	
Pathogens				$p < 0.001$
Coagulase-negative staphylococci	84 (16%)	16.2 (10.4–23.1)	Reference	
Staphylococcus aureus	77 (15%)	14.0 (9.12–17.1)	0.74 (0.57–0.95)	
Group B streptococci	47 (9%)	8.70 (5.95–10.2)	0.44 (0.33–0.59)	
Streptococcus pneumoniae	46 (9%)	11.4 (9.05–13.9)	0.53 (0.37–0.74)	
Other Gram-positive bacteria[c]	82 (16%)	13.2 (10.0–19.8)	0.81 (0.63–1.03)	
Escherichia coli	97 (19%)	9.20 (6.68–12.0)	0.56 (0.43–0.71)	
Other Gram-negative bacteria[d]	88 (17%)	11.9 (8.54–18.7)	0.80 (0.62–1.04)	

*The adjusted model was adjusted for all variables listed

[a]Values and 95% CI are relative to the defined reference group

[b]P-value from likelihood ratio test. Endocarditis, toxic shock syndrome, ear, nose, and throat infection, and other non-specified focal infections.

[c]Enterococcus spp., group A streptococcus, viridans group streptococci, other Gram positive bacteria.

[d]Haemophilus influenzae, Klebsiella spp., Neisseria meningitidis, Pseudomonas aeruginosa, other Gram negative bacteria.

TTP was shorter in *Staphylococcus aureus* (−26%, 95% CI 5–43), group B streptococci (−56%, 95% CI 41–67), *Streptococcus pneumoniae* (−47%, 95% CI 26–63), and *Escherichia coli* (−44%, 95% CI 29–57). TTP of all organisms is demonstrated in **Figures 1A,B** and TTP of selected bacterial pathogens separated by different age groups in **Figure 2**.

Of the 521 sepsis episodes, 100 (19%) were severe and 97 (19%) presented with septic shock. There was no significant association between 30-day in hospital mortality and TTP: in children who died in the first 30 days after sepsis onset, median TTP was 12.0 (IQR 7.50–16.3) compared to 11.7 (IQR 8.4–17.1) in those who survived ($p = 0.8$).

TABLE 3 | Comorbidities detected in patients with 521 episodes of blood culture-proven sepsis.

	Number (%) of episodes[c]
Neurological or neuromuscular	17 (3)
Cardiovascular	35 (7)
Respiratory	30 (6)
Renal and urological	12 (2)
Gastrointestinal	37 (7)
Hematological or immunological	8 (2)
Metabolic	11 (2)
Other congenital or genetic defect	20 (4)
Malignant disease	46 (9)
Neonatal[a]	122 (23)
Surgery or burn	40 (8)
Technology dependence[b]	19 (4)
Solid organ transplantation	2 (<1)

[a]Gestational age <27 weeks, or birthweight <750 g, or history of mechanical ventilation, or history of necrotising colitis. [b]Central line or urinary catheter or ventriculoperitoneal shunt system present at sepsis onset, or total parental nutrition in a child that does not have any other comorbidity.
[c]More than one comorbidity might be present in a sepsis episode; therefore, numbers and percentages do not add up to 521 and 100, respectively.

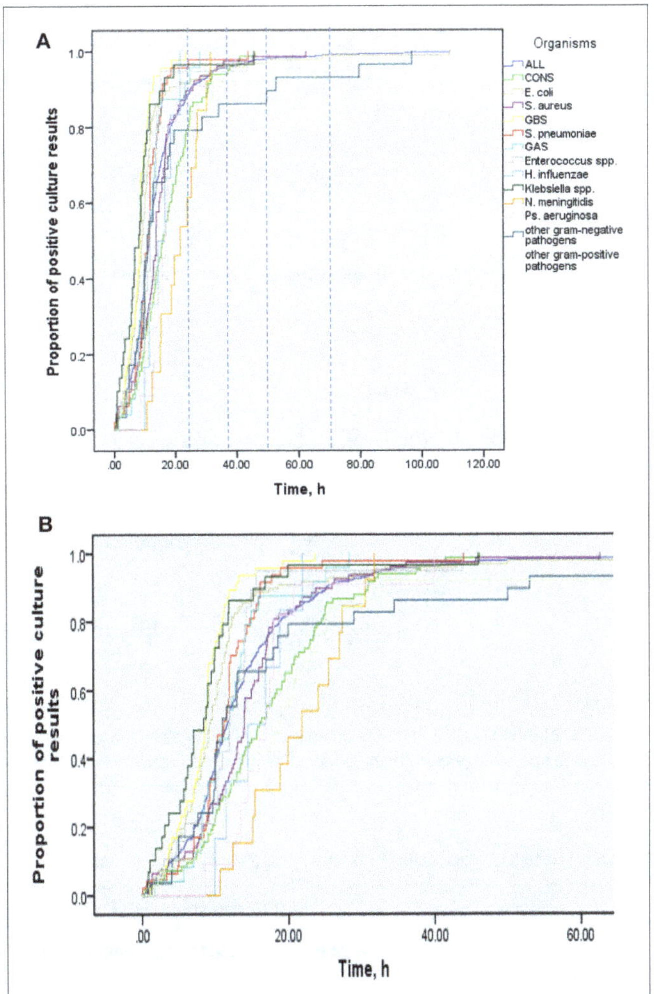

FIGURE 1 | (A) TTP of all organisms, Kaplan-Meier-Curve. **(B)** cutout of **(A)**.

Characteristics of Sepsis Episodes According to TTP Thresholds (TTP >24 to ≤36 h, >36 to ≤48 h and >48 h)

By 24 h, 460 (88%) of 521 blood cultures were positive as were 498 (96%) and 510 (98%) by 36 and 48 h, respectively (**Table 4**). When comparing infants <90 days of age with those >90 days of age, proportions of positive blood cultures within 24, 36, and 48 h were almost identical with 88% vs. 89%, 96% vs. 95%, and 98% vs. 97%, respectively. Of the 11 blood cultures which became positive after 48 h, 4 were obtained in infants <90 days of age including 3 preterm babies with a gestational age of 25+6 weeks, 26+2 weeks and 28+4 weeks, representing 1.6% of all positive blood cultures in this age group. Three each grew *E. coli, Bifidobacterium longum* and *Fusobacterium* species, one grew *Staphylococcus aureus* and one grew *Capnocytophaga* species. Two of the 3 children with *E. coli* septicemia and a TTP of >48 h had urinary tract infections and no organ dysfunction. The third child, without any comorbidities, suffered from peritonitis with septic shock. Of the other 8 episodes with TTP >48 h, 4 patients presented with signs of septic shock. One of them, an extremely premature baby (gestational age 25+6), died. Similar to the overall proportion of patients with comorbidities (69%), 6 (55%) of the 11 patients with TTP >48 h had a comorbidity and 2 of them developed severe sepsis with septic shock.

DISCUSSION

We report on prospectively assessed TTP in a large national prospective cohort of children with blood culture proven sepsis. In our multivariate analysis, TTP was only dependent on pathogens, whereas sex, age, site of infection, presence of a comorbidity and severity of sepsis were not relevant.

Nine of 10 blood cultures turned positive within 24 h and 19 of 20 turned positive within 36 h after incubation. These findings contrast with the wide practice to treat children with suspected sepsis with antibiotics for >48 h while waiting for blood culture results. This "48 h rule" has historically evolved in the era prior to automated TTP recording systems. Our results indicate the need to critically reevaluate this rule.

Blood cultures represent one of the most widely used test in pediatrics, despite a low positivity rate, issues related to false positive tests due to contaminations, and false negative tests due to antibiotic pre-treatment and small inocula (16–18)., These limitations are increased if the cultures are obtained incorrectly, especially if the volume is inadequate (19). However, if positive, they confirm the diagnosis of bacteremia or sepsis and appropriate antibiotic treatment can be initiated (20). Fully automated blood culture systems with recording of TTP have evolved and several studies have since then been conducted to challenge the minimum of 48 h to observe or even treat a child with suspected bacteremia used by many centers (9, 10).

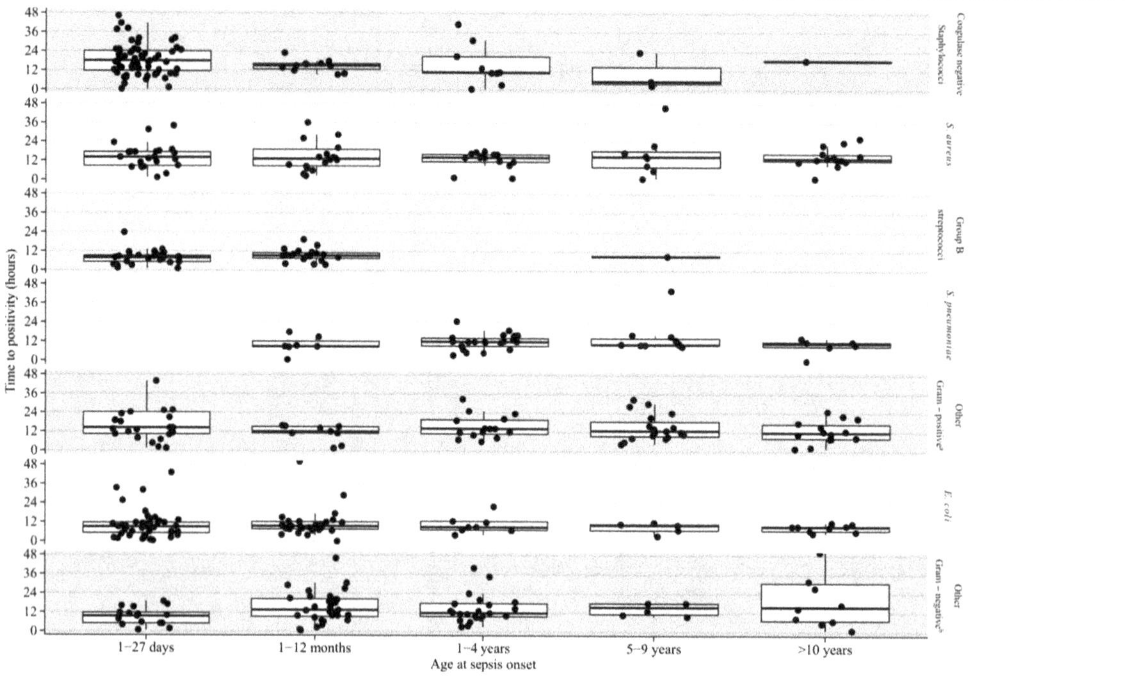

FIGURE 2 | Blood culture TTP in selected bacterial pathogens by age group. [a]Group A streptococcus, viridans group streptococci, other gram positive bacteria. [b]Klebsiella species, *Neisseria meningitides*, *Pseudomonas aeruginosa*, other gram negative bacteria.

TABLE 4 | Patient characteristics with sepsis episodes by TTP thresholds.

		TTP threshold n (%)			
		≤ 24 h	>24 - ≤36 h	>36 - ≤48 h	>48 h
Overall n		460	38	12	11
Age (d)	<90	226 (49%)	20 (53%)	7 (58%)	4 (36%)
Prematurity	≤28+0	66 (14%)	9 (16%)	4 (33%)	2 (18%)
	28+1 −31+6	32 (7%)	5 (13%)	1 (8%)	1 (9%)
	>32+0 – 36+6	35 (8%)	1 (3%)	1 (8%)	–
HAI		199 (43%)	18 (47%)	8 (67%)	5 (45%)
Severity	Severe sepsis	82 (18%)	13 (34%)	5 (42%)	–
	Septic shock	87 (19%)	5 (13%)	1 (8%)	4 (36%)
Fatal outcome		32 (7%)	2 (5%)	2 (17%)	1 (9%)
Comorbidity		257 (56%)	19 (50%)	9 (75%)	6 (55%)
Focus present		295 (64%)	27 (71%)	12 (100%)	10 (91%)

The recording of TTP in a large prospective population-based cohort of children with confirmed sepsis can inform clinicians in decision making about the appropriate length of empiric antibiotic treatment in the absence of a positive blood culture. Most clinicians stop antibiotic treatment if (a) the blood culture remains negative, (b) there is no focus of infection that would require continued antibiotic treatment, and (c) the clinical course of the disease is favorable. Yet, the chosen threshold of time after which blood cultures are highly unlikely to become positive will have a large influence on duration of antibiotic treatment. Longer periods of antibiotic treatment expose patients to risks such as medication errors, adverse events including selection of antibiotic resistance, nosocomial infections. Further, antibiotics increase the risk of necrotizing enterocolitis and death in preterm newborns (21). Moreover, prolonged hospital stays do increase health care costs and stress to patients, their relatives, and caregivers (22–24).

Our findings support previous studies performed in infants <90 days of age investigating TTP, which suggested that a shorter observation period and/or empiric antibiotic treatment, i.e., 24 or 36 h rather than the current practice of 48 h, might be appropriate (8–10). The decision by the treating physician to stop or continue antibiotics is not only based on blood culture result but also patient risk factors, clinical signs and severity of disease on presentation and during the course, response to treatment, inflammatory markers, and age. Procalcitonin-guided decision making has been shown to also guide the duration of antibiotic treatment in neonates with suspected early-onset sepsis (25, 26). It is well established that the likelihood to isolate an organism from blood culture increases with the amount of blood obtained for inoculation. Therefore, particularly in neonates blood cultures are often false negative (27). Unfortunately, there is limited data on the optimal volume in the pediatric age groups and different recommendations exist (28, 29).

In our study, the sensitivity of blood cultures increased only marginally (i.e., by 2%) when comparing a 48 h incubation threshold with a 36 h period. This demonstrates that the 48 h cut-off is arbitrary and based on tradition rather than strong evidence. However, the difficulty of decision making is exemplified by the fact that the longest TTP values in our study were 68 and 109 h for *E. coli* in the age groups 28–365 days and 1–5 years, respectively (**Figure 2**). Furthermore, our study was not designed to evaluate the prediction of which children, presenting with SIRS, will have a positive blood culture beyond 24 or 36 h. Hence, individual factors always need to be taken into account for decision making. Also, if the patient's clinical course is favorable and antibiotic treatment is stopped in the presence of a negative blood culture, parents still need to be advised to recognize signs and symptoms of concern and they need to be contactable for arrangement of a clinical reassessment as true pathogens might be detected after 36 or 48 h.

Not surprisingly, and also described in the literature, TTP varies by pathogen (30, 31). In our study, median TTP values were shortest for *E. coli* and GBS (approximately 9 h each) and longest for *S. aureus* and CoNS (14 and 16 h, respectively). While some studies found short TTP for organisms such as *Enterobacter,* E. coli or *S. aureus* correlated with poor outcomes in adults (30–32), median TTP value—irrespective of pathogen—did not predict poor outcome or admission and treatment on PICU in our study.

Also, a comparison of children <90 days of age and >90 days of age, as most studies in the literature investigated only children <90 days of age (9, 10), did not show any significant difference in their median TTP (11 h vs. 12 h). However, as infants <90 days of age and particularly neonates, represent a special pediatric cohort, especially in regards to their management, our data provides valuable information also on children >90 days of age. Children <90 days of age had significantly different sites of infection (e.g., primary blood stream infection) and sepsis episodes tend to be more severe. Also, as expected, pathogens differed significantly between these 2 groups, with *Escherichia coli* and CONS being the most common pathogens in infants <90 days of age and that is, in regards to *Escherichia coli* consistent with the literature (9, 10).

We did not see any significant differences in median TTP for children with or without comorbidity. A study in adults looking especially at patients with solid tumors or hematological disease found significantly lower TTPs in these patients compared with patients with benign tumors (33).

In our study, 42% of sepsis cases were hospital-acquired infections. Similar magnitudes have been reported before (34, 35). In a retrospective cohort study in South Africa investigating blood culture positive bacterial and fungal infections in children with a median age of 11.5 months, the proportion of hospital-acquired infections was 53.5% (34). Similarly, a study in South African neonates revealed a proportion of nosocomial infections of 62.2% of all positive blood cultures (35).

Whereas, as already mentioned above, most previous studies (retrospective or observational) investigated mainly neonates and infants <90 days of age or specific foci of infection (9, 10, 36), strengths of this study include the prospective, multicenter, population-based design and recruitment, use of a strict case definition, and inclusion of the entire pediatric age range with detailed capture of host and pathogen characteristics.

Our study had several limitations: Study centers that did not use automated laboratory systems had to be excluded. TTP "sensu strictu" (i.e., duration of incubation until blood culture becomes positive) must be distinguished from TTP "sensu latu" (i.e., time interval between collection of blood for culture and report of positive result to the treating physician). In our and most previously reported studies, TTP sensu strictu was analyzed. For patient management in the clinical context, TTP sensu latu reflects reality better than TTP sensu strictu and should be the subject of future studies. Also, the study protocol did not specify the maximum time allowed between obtaining blood cultures and processing them in the microbiology laboratory. Thus, bacteria may have started to replicate earlier in some episodes than formally measured, thereby leading to shorter TTP values. Furthermore, different blood culture systems were used in different study centers and the amount of inoculated blood, which is defined in each center according to the recommendations either given by the culture systems manufacturers or by local hospital guidelines, was not recorded. While these factors probably have increased heterogeneity of TTP findings in our study, they reflect a real world scenario in a pragmatic study design (37–39). Also, our study included children with comorbidities and it would have been interesting to carry out subgroup analyses on populations of special interest such as neutropenic patients. However, as numbers of specific comorbidities were low, such analyses would not have been meaningful. Finally, our study was based on children with positive blood cultures, and we cannot comment on blood culture negative bacterial infections. In addition, the study was not designed to analyse the performance of other clinical and laboratory criteria to guide antimicrobial therapy. As per international best practice, infectious diseases and/or antimicrobial stewardship team advice was routinely sought in the study centers once blood culture positivity was known.

In conclusion, blood cultures were positive within 36 h of incubation in 90% of children with sepsis. TTP was <24 h in the great majority of children with sepsis, but occasionally it was >36–48 h in individual sepsis episodes. Therefore, a strict and general rule to treat or observe all children for at least 48 h is not justified; rather, the decision to continue with empiric antibiotic treatment in the absence of a positive blood culture should be reconsidered after 24 and 36 h and antibiotic treatment should be stopped if the diagnosis of sepsis cannot be held up. Future studies are needed to test whether empiric antibiotic treatment in children with negative blood cultures can be safely reduced to <48 h and to identify factors that would allow to predict which children with SIRS will still have positive blood cultures beyond 36 h of incubation. Still, TTP is an important pillar on which the decisions for or against antibiotic treatment and its duration should be based. Therefore, standardized measurement of TTP in children with sepsis continues to be valuable, and ongoing analyses should be encouraged.

AUTHOR CONTRIBUTIONS

ADi, CB, EG, MS, LS and UH: conception or design of the work. ADi, CB, EG, MS, SB-S, and UH: data collection. ADi, CB, PA, LS, and UH: data analysis and interpretation. ADi: drafting the article. CB, SB-S, EG, MS, PA, LS, and UH: critical revision of the article. Final approval of the version to be published and agreement to be accountable for all aspects of the work in ensuring that questions related to the accuracy or integrity of any part of the work are appropriately investigated and resolved: all authors.

Society of Intensive Care, the Bangerter Foundation, the Vinetum and Borer Foundation, and the Foundation for the Health of Children and Adolescents.

REFERENCES

1. Dellinger RP, Levy MM, Rhodes A, Annane D, Gerlach H, Opal SM, et al. Surviving sepsis campaign: international guidelines for management of severe sepsis and septic shock, 2012. *Intensive Care Med.* (2013) 39:165–228. doi: 10.1007/s00134-012-2769-8
2. Davis AL, Carcillo JA, Aneja RK, Deymann AJ, Lin JC, Nguyen TC, et al. American College of Critical Care Medicine clinical practice parameters for hemodynamic support of pediatric and neonatal septic shock. *Crit Care Med.* (2017) 45:1061–93. doi: 10.1097/CCM.0000000000002425
3. World Health Organization. *Antimicrobial Resistance, Fact Sheet.* (2016). Available online at: http://www.who.int/mediacentre/factsheets/fs194/en/ (Accessed October 13, 2017).
4. Cohen-Wolkowiez M, Moran C, Benjamin DK, Cotten CM, Clark RH, Benjamin DK, et al. Early and late onset sepsis in late preterm infants. *Pediatr Infect Dis J.* (2009) 28:1052–6. doi: 10.1097/INF.0b013e3181acf6bd
5. Escobar GJ, Puopolo KM, Wi S, Wi S, Turk BJ, Kuzniewicz MW, et al. Stratification of risk of early-onset sepsis in newborns ≥34 weeks' gestation. *Pediatrics* (2014) 133:30–6. doi: 10.1542/peds.2013-1689
6. Fjalstad JW, Stensvold HJ, Bergseng H, Simonsen GS, Salvesen B, Rønnestad AE, et al. Early-onset sepsis and antibiotic exposure in term infants: a nationwide population-based study in Norway. *Pediatr Infect Dis J.* (2016) 35:1–6. doi: 10.1097/INF.0000000000000906
7. Polin RA, Committee on Fetus and Newborn. Management of neonates with suspected or proven early-onset bacterial sepsis. *Pediatrics* (2012) 129:1006–15. doi: 10.1542/peds.2012-0541
8. Byington CL, Reynolds CC, Korgenski K, Sheng X, Valentine KJ, Nelson RE, et al. Costs and infant outcomes after implementation of a care process model for febrile infants. *Pediatrics* (2012) 130:e16–24. doi: 10.1542/peds.2012-0127
9. Biondi EA, Mischler M, Jerardi KE, Statile AM, French J, Evans R, et al. Blood culture time to positivity in febrile infants with bacteremia. *JAMA Pediatr.* (2014) 168:844–9. doi: 10.1001/jamapediatrics.2014.895
10. Lefebvre CE, Renaud C, Chartrand C. Time to positivity of blood cultures in infants 0 to 90 days old presenting to the emergency department: is 36 hours enough? *J Pediatric Infect Dis Soc.* (2017) 6:28–32. doi: 10.1093/jpids/piv078
11. Giannoni E, Berger C, Stocker M, Agyeman P, Posfay-Barbe KM, Heininger U, et al. Incidence and outcome of group B streptococcal sepsis in infants in Switzerland. *Pediatr Infect Dis J.* (2015) 35:222–5. doi: 10.1097/INF.0000000000000974
12. Agyeman PAA, Schlapbach LJ, Giannoni E, Stocker M, Posfay-Barbe KM, Heininger U, et al. Epidemiology of blood culture-proven bacterial sepsis in children in Switzerland: a population-based cohort study. *Lancet Child Adolescent Health* (2017) 1:79–158. doi: 10.1016/S2352-4642(17)30010-X
13. Goldstein B, Giroir B, Randolp A. International Consensus Conference on Pediatric Sepsis. International pediatric sepsis consensus conference: definitions for sepsis and organ dysfunction in pediatrics. *Pediatr Crit Care Med.* (2005) 6:2–8. doi: 10.1097/01.PCC.0000149131.72248.E6
14. Centers for Disease Control and Prevention. *Central Line-Associated Bloodstream Infection (CLABSI) and Non-central Line-Associated Bloodstream Infection.* (2017). Available online at: https://www.cdc.gov/nhsn/PDFs/pscManual/2PSC_IdentifyingHAIs_NHSNcurrent.pdf (Accessed September 11, 2017).
15. Feudtner C, Feinstein JA, Zhong W, Hall M, Dai D. Pediatric complex chronic conditions classification system version 2: updated for ICD-10 and complex medical technology dependence and transplantation. *BMC Pediatr.* (2014) 14:199. doi: 10.1186/1471-2431-14-199
16. Iroh Tam PY, Bernstein E, Ma X, Ferrieri P. Blood culture in evaluation of pediatric community-acquired pneumonia: a systematic review and meta-analysis. *Hosp Pediatr.* (2015) 5:324–36. doi: 10.1542/hpeds.2014-0138
17. Jardine L, Davies MW, Faoagali J. Incubation time required for neonatal blood cultures to become positive. *J Paediatr Child Health* (2006) 42:797–802. doi: 10.1111/j.1440-1754.2006.00980.x
18. Buttery JP. Blood cultures in newborns and children: optimising an everyday test. *Arch Dis Child Fetal Neonatal Ed.* (2002) 87:F25–8. doi: 10.1136/fn.87.1.F25
19. Cantey JB, Baird SD. Ending the culture of culture-negative sepsis in the neonatal unit. *Pediatrics* (2017) 140:e20170044. doi: 10.1542/peds.2017-0044
20. Dien Bard J, McElvania TeKippe E. Diagnosis of bloodstream infections in children. *J Clin Microbiol.* (2016) 54:1418–24. doi: 10.1128/JCM.02919-15
21. Esaiassen E Fjalstad JW, Juvet LK, van den Anker N, Klingenberg C.Antibiotic exposure in neonates and early adverse outcomes: a systematic review and meta-analysis. *J Antimicrob Chermother.* (2017) 72:1858–70. doi: 10.1093/jac/dkx088
22. Condra CS, Parbhu B, Lorenz D, Herr SM. Charges and complications associated with the medical evaluation of febrile young infants. *Pediatr Emer Care* (2010) 26:186–91. doi: 10.1097/PEC.0b013e3181d1e180
23. Klevens RM, Edwards JR, Richards CL, Horan TC, Gaynes RP, Pollock DA. Estimating health care-associated infections and deaths in U.S. hospitals, 2002. *Public Health Rep.* (2007) 122:160–6. doi: 10.1177/0033354907122 00205
24. Nizzam M, Norzila MZ. Stress among parents with acutely ill children. *Med J Malaysia* (2001) 56:428–34.
25. Rossum van AMC, Wulkan RW, Oudesluys-Murphy AM. Procalcitonin as an early marker of infection in neonates and children. *Lancet Infect Dis.* (2004) 4:620–30. doi: 10.1016/S1473-3099(04)01146-6
26. Stocker M, Van Herk W, El Helou S, Dutta S, Fontana MS, Schuerman F. Procalcitonin-guided decision making for duration of antibiotic therapy in neonates with suspected early-onset sepsis: a multicenter, randomized controlled trial (NeoPlns). *Lancet* (2017) 390:871–81. doi: 10.1016/S0140-6736(17)31444-7
27. Connell TG, Rele M, Cowley D, Buttery JP, Curtis N. How reliable is a negative blood culture result? Volume of blood submitted for culture in routine practice in a children's hospital. *Pediatrics* (2007) 119:891–6. doi: 10.1542/peds.2006-0440
28. Baron EJ, Miller JM, Weinstein MP, Richter SS, Gilligan PH, Thomson RB, et al. A guide to utilization of the microbiology laboratory for diagnosis of infectious diseases: 2013 recommendations by the Infectious Diseases Society of America (IDSA) and the American Society for Microbiology (ASM). *Clin Infect Dis.* (2013) 57:e22–121. doi: 10.1093/cid/cit278
29. Sarkar S, Bhaga I, DeCristofaro JK, Wiswell TE, Spitzer AR. A study of the role of multiple site blood cultures in the evaluation of neonatal sepsis. *J Perinatol.* (2006) 26:28–22. doi: 10.1038/sj.jp.7211410
30. Ning Y, Hu R, Yao G, Bo S. Time to positivity of blood culture and its prognostic value in bloodstream infection. *Eur J Clin Microbiol Infect Dis.* (2016) 35:619–24. doi: 10.1007/s10096-016-2580-5
31. Peralta G, Roiz MP, Sanches MB, Garrido JC, Ceballos B, Rodriguez-Lera MJ, et al. Time-to-positivity in patients with *Escherichia coli* bacteraemia. *Clin Microbiol Infect.* (2007) 13:1077–82. doi: 10.1111/j.1469-0691.2007.01817.x

32. Sowden D, Anstey C, Faddy M. Blood culture time to positivity as a predictor of mortality in community acquired methicillin-susceptible Staphylococcus aureus bacteremia. *J Infect.* (2008) 56:295–6. doi: 10.1016/j.jinf.2008.01.005
33. Zhang Q, Li D, Bai C, Zhang W, Zheng S, Zhang P, et al. Clinical prognostic factors for time to positivity in cancer patients with bloodstream infections. *Infection* (2016) 44:583–8. doi: 10.1007/s15010-016-0890-2
34. Lochan H, Pillay V, Bamford C, Nuttall J, Eley B. Bloodstream infections at a tertiary level paediatric hospital in South Africa. *BMC Infect Dis.* (2017) 17:750. doi: 10.1186/s12879-017-2862-2
35. Dramowski A, Madide A, Bekker A. Neonatal nosocomial bloodstream infections at a referral hospital in a middle-income country: burden, pathogens, antimicrobial resistance and mortality. *Paediatr. Int Child Health* (2015) 35:265–72. doi: 10.1179/2046905515Y.0000000029
36. Chang MI, Carlson SJ, Nindivada P, O'Loughlin AA, Potemkin AK, Cowan E, et al. Challenging the 48-hour rule-out for central line-associated bloodstream infections in the pediatric intestinal failure population: a retrospective pilot study. *J Parenter Enteral Nutr.* (2016) 40:567–73. doi: 10.1177/0148607114567897
37. Zadroga R, Williams DN, Gotschall R, Hanson K, Nordberg V, Deike M, et al. Comparison of 2 blood culture media shows significant differences in bacterial recovery for patients on antimicrobial therapy. *Clin Infect Dis.* (2013) 56:790–7. doi: 10.1093/cid/cis1021
38. Isaacman DJ, Karasic RB, Reynolds EA, Kost SI. Effect of number of blood cultures and volume of blood on detection of bacteremia in children. *J Pediatr.* (1996) 128:190–5. doi: 10.1016/S0022-3476(96)70388-8
39. Yaacobi N, Bar-Meir M, Shchors I, Bromiker R. A prospective controlled trial of the optimal volume for neonatal blood cultures. *Pediatr Infect Dis J.* (2015) 34:351–4. doi: 10.1097/INF.0000000000000594

9

Invasive Meningococcal Disease in the Vaccine Era

Simon Nadel[1] and Nelly Ninis[2]*

[1] Paediatric Intensive Care Unit, St. Mary's Hospital and Imperial College London, London, United Kingdom, [2] Paediatrics, St Mary's Hospital, London, United Kingdom

***Correspondence:**
Simon Nadel
s.nadel@imperial.ac.uk

Infection with the meningococcus is one of the main causes of meningitis and septicaemia worldwide. Humans are the only natural reservoir for the meningococcus which is found primarily as a commensal inhabitant in the nasopharynx in ~10% of adults, and may be found in over 25% of individuals during adolescence. Prompt recognition of meningococcal infection and early aggressive treatment are essential in order to reduce mortality, which occurs in up to 10% of those with invasive meningococcal disease (IMD). This figure may be significantly higher in those with inadequate or delayed treatment. Early administration of effective parenteral antimicrobial therapy and prompt recognition and appropriate management of the complications of IMD, including circulatory shock and raised intracranial pressure (ICP), are critical to help improve patient outcome. This review summarizes clinical features of IMD and current treatment recommendations. We will discuss the evidence for immunization and effects of vaccine strategies, particularly following implementation of effective vaccines against Group B meningococcus.

Keywords: meningococcal, sepsis, meningitis, treatment, epidemiology, vaccine

EPIDEMIOLOGY OF MENINGOCOCCAL DISEASE

Neisseria meningitidis is an obligate human commensal which resides in the nasopharynx. The estimated carriage rate is estimated as between 0.6 and 34%. This figure may be higher in adolescents, young adults and in individuals living in overcrowded or confined spaces (1, 2).

There are several known serogroups of *N. meningitidis* which cause disease. The majority (more than 90%) of invasive disease is caused by just six serogroups A, B, C, W, X, and Y. The distribution of serogroups causing disease varies with age group and geographical location (1).

Approximately half a million cases of IMD occur worldwide each year, with a mortality rate of ~10% (3). Figures regarding incidence of IMD worldwide is difficult to ascertain because of inaccuracies in reporting and variations in bacteriological surveillance in different countries around the world, together with recognized under-reporting in many parts of the developing world. In the developed world, the known incidence of IMD has decreased to <1 case per 100,000 population per year.

In the meningitis belt of sub-Saharan Africa, pandemics of meningococcal disease occur regularly and attack rates may exceed 800 cases per 100,000 population per year. In some countries in this region attack rates may be as high as 1 person in every 100 (3).

The incidence of disease caused by the different serogroups is constantly changing, both around the world and in different countries, not only because of selection pressure following introduction of effective vaccines and differences in antimicrobial usage, but also due to stochastic variations in epidemiology due to unknown reasons, including changes in population behaviors and movements of large numbers of people due to air travel.

Serogroup A meningococcus (MenA) was very common in the developed world in the early part of the twentieth Century. However, for reasons that are unclear, since the 1970s it has virtually disappeared as a cause of invasive disease and nasopharyngeal colonization in Western Europe. MenA was the most common cause of IMD worldwide, due to it being the cause of major epidemics of IMD in sub-Saharan Africa, with an incidence approaching 1 case/100 population, and associated mortality rate reaching 75% in children, adolescents and young adults. However, following the introduction of a hugely successful vaccination campaign in the meningitis belt in sub-Saharan Africa, MenA has been virtually eliminated as a cause of epidemic meningitis (4).

Serogroup B meningococcus (MenB) is the cause of endemic disease in much of the developed world, including North America, Canada, Western Europe, Australasia and South America. Following the successful introduction of vaccines which are effective against serogroup C meningococcus (MenC) in many parts of the world, MenB is now causes ~60% of IMD in the developed world. Nearly half of this disease burden occurs in children <2 years of age (5). In the last 2 years MenB vaccine has been routinely introduced into the infant schedule in the UK and is available for university and other outbreaks in other parts of the world, including North America and Canada. Although initial reports of a reduction of disease incidence following infant immunization are encouraging, we await formal incidence data (6).

Serogroup C meningococcus (MenC) is common in the developed world and occasionally causes outbreaks and epidemics. The incidence of MenC disease has decreased in those countries which have introduced effective conjugate vaccines against MenC, including much of Western Europe and Canada (5).

In recent years there has been a dramatic increase in the number of cases of IMD caused by serogroup W (MenW). In 2016/2017, there were 225 cases of MenW disease in all ages in the UK (amounting to around a third of total reports). MenW may also contain the hypervirulent ST11 complex and has been associated with an atypical presentation of gastro-intestinal symptoms and shock without a rash. Misdiagnosis is therefore common and partly because of this, MenW is associated with a high case fatality rate (7).

Serogroup Y meningococcus (MenY) is becoming an increasingly important cause of meningococcal disease in the USA and is more recently being increasingly reported from the UK (7).

The changes in epidemiology of carriage and invasive disease of MenW and MenY has led to alterations in vaccine schedule, including introduction of MenACWY vaccine in adolescents in the UK.

Serogroup X meningococcus (MenX) is increasingly being reported in parts of sub-Saharan Africa as a cause of IMD (3).

The UK has the only national meningococcal disease vaccine programme in the World which covers serogroups A, B, C, W, and Y. However, IMD will continue to occur as the vaccine programme is not universal—i.e., not all ages are covered and no vaccine is 100% effective.

INVASIVE MENINGOCOCCAL DISEASE

Young children, adolescents, and young adults suffer the greatest burden of disease from the meningococcus. Children are particularly vulnerable to IMD because of their relative immune immaturity, in particular their relative under-responsiveness to pure polysaccharide antigens such as the meningococcal capsule. Over 75% of all cases of meningococcal meningitis and septicaemia occur in children <5 years of age. Adolescents and young adults are the group with the highest prevalence of nasopharyngeal carriage, and IMD is also relatively common in this age group (8).

The World Health Organization (WHO) estimates that ~170,000 deaths occur each year from meningococcal and other bacterial meningitis and meningococcal septicaemia worldwide; the case fatality rate from invasive disease can be up to 50%, even with appropriate treatment. In addition, the estimated median risk of at least one major or minor long-term sequelae is ~20% (with a range of 12.3–35.3%). In less developed low to middle income countries, IMD remains the fourth most common cause of disability (9).

The epidemiology of bacterial meningitis and septicaemia worldwide has changed dramatically in the last 20 years following introduction of highly effective conjugate protein/polysaccharide vaccines.

Before the introduction of the conjugated vaccine against Haemophilus influenzae type b (Hib), this was the most common cause of bacterial meningitis worldwide. More recently, introduction of highly effective multivalent conjugated vaccines against *Streptococcus pneumoniae* and against MenC have resulted in significant reduction in disease burden due to these organisms.

There remain considerable problems with diagnosis, particularly in the developing world with underdeveloped microbiological services and without up to date diagnostic methods such as polymerase chain reaction (PCR).

The advent of PCR diagnostics has dramatically improved detailed microbiological diagnosis, including serogroup and subtype, for microbiological confirmation and epidemiological tracing to aid public health and outbreak control (10).

Clinical Features of Meningococcal Disease

It is unclear why the meningococcus invades the bloodstream after nasopharyngeal colonization to cause invasive disease. It is likely that bacterial virulence factors, environmental conditions and innate host susceptibility all play important roles.

Clinical manifestations of IMD in any individual are determined by the extent of host inflammatory factors such as activation of the immune system and host inflammatory response. These are clearly influenced by host genetic differences in constituents of the host inflammatory response regulation including those factors in the complement system, cytokines, and chemokines and the coagulation cascade. Bacterial factors, such as capsular serogroup, the amount of endotoxin released from the cell wall during growth and proliferation and bacterial load are also likely to be extremely influential in determination of the host inflammatory response (11).

In some affected individuals there may be fulminant progression of disease, followed by multi-organ failure and death within just a few hours. Even when IMD is diagnosed early and appropriate treatment is rapidly initiated, mortality rate may be up to 10%.

Of those who survive IMD, approximately 30% suffer sequelae, particularly affecting physical, cognitive, and psychological functioning. This may lead to obvious neurological impairment, nerve deafness, amputation of limbs or digits, or skin scarring (9, 12). Prompt recognition of disease and early aggressive treatment with antibiotics and fluid resuscitation are most important. Rapid identification and treatment of disease complications such as shock, raised intracranial pressure (ICP) and seizures, are vitally important to improve outcome.

Presentation of Disease

In the early stages of disease, the clinical picture is non-specific and may be confused with common trivial viral illnesses. The finding of the classical haemorrhagic rash in a child with fever is highly suggestive of IMD, However, up to 20% of children with IMD will have no rash or a non-specific maculopapular rash, and in many cases appearance of the classical haemorrhagic rash may be delayed until the disease is well advanced (13).

Non-specific clinical features such as fever, tachycardia, cold hands and feet, leg pain, and mottled or blue skin color are often present in the first 12 h of disease. The onset of the characteristic haemorrhagic petechial/purpuric rash may be delayed beyond this point, sometimes appearing up to 24 h after the first symptoms.

The classical signs and symptoms of meningism are more common in older children with meningitis. The textbook symptoms and signs of meningitis such as fever, headache, photophobia, neck stiffness, and altered mental status may not be present completely or may not be present at all, particularly in infants and younger children. A high level of suspicion of meningitis is crucial to making an early diagnosis.

Disease Progression

Invasive meningococcal disease in infants, children and young adults usually presents as two main clinical syndromes—shock and meningitis—which may exist on their own or co-exist. It should be emphasized that these two specific syndromes may overlap to a certain extent and may occur simultaneously and determine the priorities for treatment.

Shock

Meningococcal septic shock is characterized by a fulminant host inflammatory response to bacterial invasion. The disease may rapidly progress to cardiovascular failure, disseminated intravascular coagulopathy (DIC), multi-organ failure, and death unless rapid and aggressive resuscitation, together with organ support is initiated. Shock is present in ~20% of patients with IMD and is associated with high mortality and morbidity.

Meningitis

Meningitis is the most common clinical manifestation of IMD. It may develop following a longer period of low-grade bacteraemia and has a less fulminant course than shock. Patients may exhibit signs of meningeal irritation (meningism) which may progress to a depression in the level of consciousness, coma, seizures, and features of raised intracranial pressure (ICP).

Rarely, patients with meningococcal meningitis may present very acutely after a short prodromal period, with acute signs of raised ICP which rapidly progresses to deep coma, brain-stem herniation, and death.

Shock and meningitis may co-exist and present a formidable management challenge.

Invasive meningococcal disease may progress and evolve rapidly, even after appropriate treatment has been initiated. Therefore, all children admitted with suspected meningococcal disease should be closely monitored for signs of disease progression and deterioration. An improved clinical outcome critically depends on the prompt recognition of life- or limb-threatening complications including shock and/or raised ICP.

We will focus on the management of shock, raised ICP, antibiotic treatment, and adjunctive treatment modalities (14).

Meningococcal Septic Shock (Figure 1)

Shock is defined as inadequate delivery of oxygen and nutrients to the tissues. In IMD it results from a combination of hypovolaemia secondary to development of capillary leak syndrome due to endothelial cell dysfunction, impaired myocardial function, abnormal vasomotor tone, and impaired cellular metabolism. In a proportion of patients, relative adrenal insufficiency is present.

The clinical features of compensated shock arise because perfusion of vital organs, including brain and heart is maintained at the expense of perfusion of more expendable organs such as the skin, kidneys, and gut. In the early phases of shock this redistribution of circulating blood volume compensates for the hypovolaemia and maintains circulating blood volume and cardiac output. As a result of these compensatory mechanisms, patients with meningococcal septicaemia often present with cold hands and feet, prolonged capillary refill time and reduced urine output. As the disease progresses, ischaemia of the skin or even whole limbs may occur. In addition, many patients with shock will develop acute kidney injury, oligo/anuria, and may require renal replacement therapy.

Despite the presence of shock, cerebral perfusion and therefore function will be preserved until decompensation occurs, so that the child's relatively alert state may make even experienced clinicians underestimate the degree of cardiovascular collapse.

Development of hypotension signifies the failure of the compensatory circulatory mechanisms. We must emphasize that to diagnose shock in children, one should not rely on the demonstration of systemic arterial hypotension. Children can compensate for the loss of a significant amount of their circulating blood volume without a reduction in their blood pressure and therefore they may have normal blood pressure until shock is well-advanced.

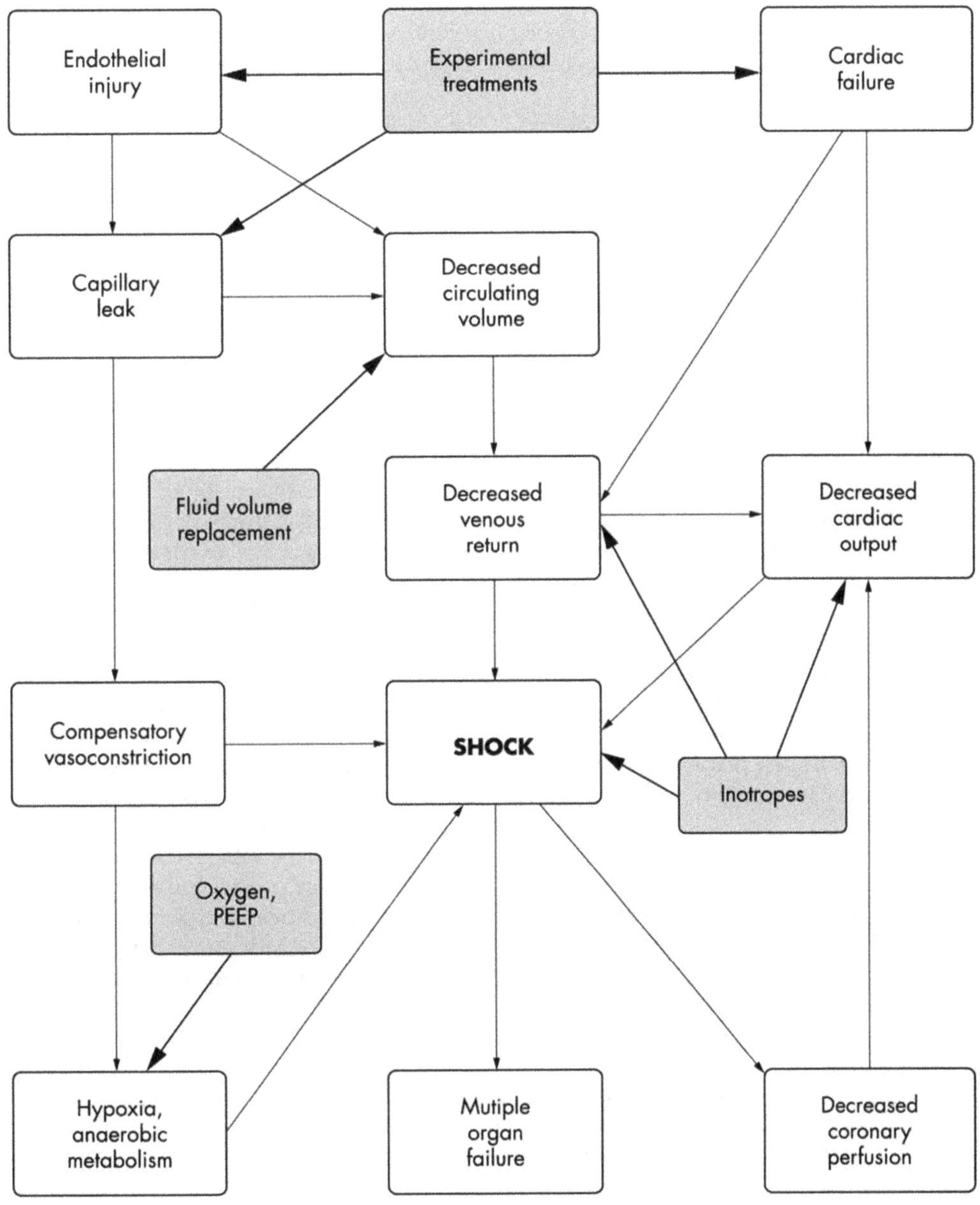

FIGURE 1 | Pathophysiology of septic shock. Filled boxes are the treatment options. Taken from Welch and Nadel (15).

Myocardial dysfunction is invariably present in children with meningococcal septicaemia and shock, and arises due to a number of different pathological processes.

Hypovolaemia (from capillary leak and abnormalities in vasomotor tone) leading to decreased cardiac filling; the presence of hypoxia (due to pulmonary dysfunction), acidosis and multiple electrolyte abnormalities including hypokalaemia, hypocalcaemia, hypophosphataemia, hypomagnesaemia, hypoglycaemia, and disturbed fatty acid metabolism all impair myocardial contractility; bacterial products and inflammatory mediators such as tumor necrosis factor and interleukin 1 directly suppress myocardial contractility. Interleukin 6 (IL-6) has been demonstrated to have specific myocardial depressant properties in IMD (16).

Cardiac output may improve with intravenous fluid volume resuscitation and correction of metabolic derangements. However, patients often require treatment with vasoactive agents and inotropes to improve myocardial function.

Initial Assessment and Management

Initial assessment of all patients with any potentially life-threatening illness follows the usual treatment algorithms which concentrate on management of "A, airway; B, breathing; C, circulation."

Clinical assessment should be aimed at detecting features of shock, raised ICP, DIC and the need for advanced organ support. Assessment should be repeated frequently to evaluate response to treatment and to identify clinical deterioration.

The "A"irway is usually patent in meningococcal disease, unless consciousness is impaired. "B"reathing may be compromised by development of pulmonary oedema due to capillary leakage of fluid in the lungs, leading to hypoxia, and respiratory distress. "C"irculation is affected as described above.

Management of Shock

There are many evidence-based treatment guidelines available for the appropriate management of children with septic shock, including that due to meningococcal disease.

Probably the most widely used are the Surviving Sepsis Guidelines, which incorporate guidelines for the management of shock in infants and children. The latest iteration of these were published in 2012 and have recently been updated (17, 18). These guidelines and more recent evidence pointing to improvement in outcome associated with complete bundle compliance suggests that implementation of treatment guidelines including a "recognition bundle" containing a trigger tool for rapid identification of patients with septic shock; a "resuscitation and stabilization bundle" to help adherence to best practice principles; and a "performance bundle" to identify and overcome perceived barriers to the pursuit of best practice principles, can lead to significant improvement in mortality and presumably morbidity (19).

The primary aim of circulatory support in shock is to maintain and replenish adequate tissue perfusion for the supply of oxygen and nutrients to the cells. To achieving this goal the clinician must adequately replenish the circulating volume with appropriate fluid resuscitation. Early and aggressive fluid resuscitation is associated with improved survival in pediatric septic shock (14). Inotropic support is often required in order to maintain adequate cardiac output and organ perfusion.

It is recommended that an initial bolus of 20 mL/kg of fluid should be given over 5–10 min to children with signs of shock. The expected response to this volume replacement is reduction in heart rate, improved peripheral perfusion, decreased capillary refill time, and improved urine output. In milder cases, shock is reversed by this initial fluid bolus, but regular repeated review is mandatory, as despite appropriate management, the disease may progress.

In patients with more advanced shock, aggressive fluid resuscitation may need to continue in order to reverse shock. In these patients, establishment of secure central venous access is a priority. This will aid and guide adequate fluid resuscitation, safe administration of vasoactive agents and measurement of central venous oxygen saturation ($ScvO_2$). Central venous oxygen saturation is a useful guide to the adequacy of oxygen delivery, with the goal of achieving $ScvO_2$ >70% and central venous pressure (CVP) of 8–12 mmHg (17).

If signs of shock persist after 40–60 mL/kg of fluid resuscitation given within an hour, there is a significant risk of pulmonary oedema developing with further fluid resuscitation. Elective tracheal intubation and initiation of mechanical ventilation is recommended at this stage, even without evidence of overt respiratory failure being present. If performed early, before respiratory failure is obvious, intubation and ventilation is associated with an improvement in outcome and is thought to be beneficial by allowing reduction of myocardial and respiratory muscle oxygen consumption and by facilitating delivery of positive end expiratory pressure (PEEP) to aid oxygenation (14). The sedation and muscle relaxation used in these circumstances also facilitates placement of arterial and central venous catheters.

Response to fluid resuscitation should be monitored continuously by repeated assessment of vital signs including heart rate, blood pressure, CVP, urine output, metabolic status, and peripheral perfusion. Fluid resuscitation with volumes in excess of 60 ml/kg are often needed for adequate enhancement of circulating volume. Development of pulmonary oedema and/or hepatomegaly suggest that further fluid resuscitation may not be beneficial, and may actually be harmful, as fluid overload may be present. Further support with vasoactive agents would be indicated if signs of fluid overload develop.

Controversy persists regarding the optimal fluid for resuscitation in children with septic shock. Our practice is to use 5% human albumin solution (HAS) as our preferred resuscitation fluid in septic shock of any cause. Use of 5% HAS has been associated with a reduction in morbidity and mortality in some adult studies (20). However, no equivalent studies have been performed in children with septic shock. Blood products may be required to correct anemia, thrombocytopenia, and coagulopathy, although there is controversy regarding correction of coagulation in the absence of overt bleeding.

To improve myocardial function which is invariably depressed in septic shock, treatment with adrenaline or noradrenaline should be initiated early, preferably via a central vein. It is usually impractical to gain central venous access in children before the child is sedated for tracheal intubation. Dilute dopamine or noradrenaline can be administered through a peripheral vein, or the intra-osseous route can be used to deliver concentrated solutions of adrenaline and noradrenaline until central venous access is obtained.

There is some evidence that shock refractory to inotropes may be more common in children with impaired adrenal responsiveness. Studies in adults with septic shock have documented adrenal hypo-responsiveness associated with inotrope unresponsiveness and suggested that low-dose steroid supplementation may improve survival. However, a more recent study failed to confirm these findings (21). A recently published study suggests that hydrocortisone together with fludrocortisone may confer a survival benefit in adults with septic shock (22). A meta-analysis of pediatric studies found no benefit for steroids in reducing mortality, duration of shock or length of hospital stay (23). The Surviving Sepsis campaign 2012 guidelines suggest use of low-dose replacement hydrocortisone therapy in children with fluid-refractory and catecholamine-resistant shock with suspected or proven adrenal insufficiency. It is suggested that a random cortisol level should be taken before steroids are given and a short ACTH test should be carried out at some stage to determine the need for ongoing steroid supplementation.

Most guidelines would suggest that advanced organ support for refractory shock should be implemented.

The use of renal replacement therapy or plasma exchange in sepsis has been recommended in some treatment guidelines. However, there is no evidence that these modalities improve outcomes in pediatric septic shock (24).

For children with shock refractory to increasing doses of inotropes who have severe cardio-respiratory failure, referral for Extra Corporeal Life Support (ECLS) may provide some survival benefit. However, reports of use of this modality are primarily anecdotal and ECLS is not widely available (25).

Respiratory Support

Facial oxygen should be delivered routinely from the outset in any child with sepsis. If no major airway or breathing problem is present, priority is given to assessment and management of the circulation. The indications for immediate endotracheal intubation and mechanical ventilation are hypoxia with respiratory distress, which may indicate progression of pulmonary oedema; persistent shock despite fluid resuscitation of >40 ml/kg and need for further fluid resuscitation; fluctuating or decreasing conscious level (Glasgow Coma Score < 8, or a decrease of 3 points within 1 h); or signs of raised ICP.

Induction of anesthesia for tracheal intubation in shocked children may exacerbate cardiovascular instability. The presence of an experienced pediatric anesthetist and/or intensivist should be available. When possible, the cardiovascular system should be stabilized before intubation by adequate fluid resuscitation and initiation of vasoactive agents but the potential for acute decompensation should be anticipated.

A cuffed endotracheal tube should be used for tracheal intubation, as pulmonary oedema is likely to develop, and high ventilator pressures may be needed to maintain oxygenation and ventilation.

Disseminated Intravascular Coagulopathy (DIC)

Disseminated intravascular coagulopathy (DIC) is common in severe sepsis, regardless of the etiology. Both pro-coagulant and anticoagulant pathways are dysregulated as a consequence of activation of the inflammatory and coagulation cascades, in addition to the presence of endothelial cell dysfunction (26).

The coagulopathy that is present in meningococcal septicaemia and shock arises from a combination of the loss of the anticoagulant proteins C and S from the plasma, and the failure of anticoagulant mechanisms on the endothelial surface due to loss of surface proteins and glycosamionoglycans. The endothelial receptors which regulate protein C activation (endothelial protein C receptor and thrombomodulin) have been found to be down-regulated in patients with meningococcal septicaemia (27). Levels of circulating activated protein C and antithrombin III are reduced; the normal fibrinolytic mechanisms are suppressed due to reduced production of endothelial tissue plasminogen activator, and increased production of plasminogen activator inhibitior-1 (PAI-1) and other fibrinolysis inhibitors such as thrombin-activatable fibrinolysis inhibitor (TAFI). Together, all of these abnormalities result in uncontrolled microvascular thrombosis, suppression of degradation of intravascular thrombi, resulting in the clinical syndrome of DIC and Purpura Fulminans.

This may result in spontaneous pulmonary, gastric or cerebral hemorrhage, particularly in the presence of any associated thrombocytopenia. Correction of severe coagulopathy with vitamin K, fresh frozen plasma, platelets and, cryoprecipitate may prevent life-threatening hemorrhage. To this end regular blood cell count and coagulation studies should be monitored.

Recombinant activated Protein C (aPC) was initially shown to reduce mortality in adults with severe sepsis and septic shock. However, a study of the use of aPC in children with severe sepsis, including purpura fulminans and meningococcal disease failed to show any benefit, and possibly showed harm in younger infants with thrombocytopaenia (28). Therefore, aPC is no longer available as a therapeutic option in sepsis.

Biochemical Derangements

Patients with septic shock often have severe derangements in blood biochemistry. These should be sought by repeated sampling and corrected when detected. Regular evaluation of blood electrolytes (including sodium which is particularly important in the context of raised ICP, potassium, phosphate, calcium, and magnesium) is important as derangements in homeostasis may impair cardiovascular status. Blood urea and creatinine should be monitored to assess renal function and need for renal replacement therapy.

Regular and repeated blood gas analysis should be carried out to identify evolving metabolic acidosis, monitor blood glucose, and electrolyte abnormalities and follow serial lactate levels. Correction of severe metabolic acidosis with Sodium Bicarbonate may result in improved cardiovascular status and improved response to inotropes.

Lactate clearance has been shown to be an important indicator of the adequacy of resuscitation. Failure to clear lactate has been shown to be a poor prognostic indicator in pediatric septic shock (29).

Skin and Limbs

Purpura fulminans is commonly associated with meningococcal septicaemia. The skin may be severely affected in meningococcal septicaemia because of inadequate skin perfusion and microvascular thrombosis. The capillary leak may exacerbate tissue oedema and cause a compartment syndrome.

The role of fasciotomy in preserving limb viability in purpura fulminans is a subject of debate, but is indicated in circumstances where there is ischaemia in the presence of documented increased compartment pressure. Multi-disciplinary input from intensivists, orthopedic, vascular, and plastic surgeons is vital before a decision regarding surgical intervention is taken. Amputation should not be performed until it is felt to be unavoidable and only following extensive multidisciplinary discussion (30).

Raised Intracranial Pressure

Raised ICP occurs due to inflammation of the meninges in meningitis and capillary leakage from cerebral blood vessels, leading to cerebral oedema. Clinically significant raised ICP is rare. Although most critically ill children with IMD have shock as their primary clinical presentation, a minority present with signs of raised ICP as their predominant clinical manifestation.

Raised ICP may restrict cerebral blood flow. To understand the physiologic impact of raised ICP on cerebral blood flow one must be familiar with the physiology of the intracranial vault.

Cerebral blood flow (CBF) supplies oxygen and nutrients to the brain. Three major factors regulate CBF: Cerebral perfusion pressure (CPP), partial pressure of arterial CO_2, and partial pressure of arterial O_2. Hypoxia causes cerebral vasodilation and increases CBF, and therefore ICP. Hypercapnia causes cerebral vasodilation and similarly affects CBF and ICP. Hypocapnia causes cerebral vasoconstriction, and thus reduces CBF and ICP.

CPP is the difference between mean arterial pressure (MAP) and ICP, and represents the pressure gradient across the cerebrovascular bed (CPP = MAP – ICP). In meningitis, normal cerebral vascular auto-regulation is lost, and therefore cerebral perfusion becomes critically dependent on CPP. MAP can be increased by vasopressors to increase CPP. A CPP of at least 50 mmHg has been associated with an improved outcome in traumatic brain injury, but no such correlation between CPP and outcome has been identified in non-traumatic brain injury (31).

Reduction of ICP—and thus increased CPP—may be accomplished by reducing intracranial fluid volume using agents such as the osmotic diuretic Mannitol or hypertonic saline to reduce cerebral oedema. In addition, maintaining the head elevated to 30° and in the midline facilitates cerebral venous drainage. Prevention of hypercarbia and hypoxia reduces intracerebral blood volume. All these measures may help to control ICP and therefore maintain CBF and reduce the risk of cerebral herniation and brain-stem death. However, there is no robust clinical trial data that suggests these measures improve outcome.

Signs of raised ICP include declining level of consciousness, focal neurological signs including unequal, dilated or poorly responsive pupils, systemic arterial hypertension, and associated bradycardia. Papilloedema is a late finding and is not uniformly present in acutely raised ICP.

Patients with shock without meningitis may present with impaired consciousness as a result of acidosis or cerebral hypoperfusion due to impaired cerebral perfusion due to shock. Conversely, patients without shock with meningitis may have reduced consciousness and peripheral vasoconstriction due to impaired cerebral perfusion due to raised ICP. These signs may cause confusion, with patients being misdiagnosed with shock. In this case, poor peripheral perfusion in the absence of metabolic acidosis and with normal blood lactate, together with relative bradycardia, normal, or high blood pressure and decreased level of consciousness or other neurological signs should be assumed to be due to raised ICP. If raised ICP is suspected, aggressive fluid resuscitation should be avoided, as excess fluid may exacerbate cerebral oedema.

If raised ICP is suspected, an intravenous infusion of Mannitol (0.25–0.5 g/kg over 5 min), or 3% saline (3 mL/kg over 5 min), together with urgent tracheal intubation and mechanical ventilation to control the airway and breathing and regulate blood oxygen and carbon dioxide, may prevent brain-stem herniation and may be life-saving.

Following tracheal intubation, adequate sedation must be employed in order to prevent acute waves of ICP caused by agitation or coughing. Muscle relaxants should be avoided if possible as seizures may be masked. If present, seizures should be rapidly and aggressively treated to avoid any further increase in ICP due to increased cerebral metabolism. Other neuroprotective measures include avoidance of hyperthermia, hypoxia, and by maintaining the $PaCO_2$ in the normal range.

In the child with raised ICP and coexistent shock, the priority is to correct the circulatory disturbance before instituting specific measures to control ICP, although attempts to limit fluid resuscitation and maintain mean arterial pressure and blood gases in the normal range should be made to protect brain perfusion.

Antibiotic Therapy

The optimal initial antimicrobial therapy in patients with a clinical diagnosis of IMD is intravenous Ceftriaxone (100 mg/kg) but Cefotaxime (80 mg/kg) is a reasonable alternative if Ceftriaxone is contraindicated. Until definitive microbiological confirmation is available, it remains possible that alternative bacterial diagnoses or penicillin resistance (although this is extremely rare for the meningococcus) may be present. Other bacterial causes of Purpura Fulminans include *Streptococcus pneumoniae*, invasive Group A Streptococcus, *Staphylococcus aureus* and some Gram-negative bacteria. Broader antimicrobial cover may be necessary depending on the local bacterial resistance patterns and history of foreign travel or other risk factors.

The recommended duration of parenteral antibiotic therapy for uncomplicated IMD is 7 days (10).

Adjunctive Therapies

High dose corticosteroids given prior to, or concurrently with the first dose of antibiotics, appear to reduce incidence of neurological sequelae following Haemophilus influenzae type b (Hib) and pneumococcal meningitis. In meningococcal meningitis there is a trend toward improved outcome (32). The current recommendation is to administer Dexamethasone 0.15 mg/kg 6 hourly for 4 days if started before or within 4 h of the initial dose of parenteral antibiotic in patients with proven or suspected bacterial meningitis (10).

Outcome

It is estimated that around 30% of survivors of IMD will have significant morbidity, including digital or limb amputation, skin loss or scarring, orthopedic abnormalities including abnormal bone growth, nerve deafness unilateral or bilateral, other neurological abnormalities including hemiplegia, neurodevelopmental delay, and epilepsy. Aside from these physical sequelae, a large number of affected children and their families may suffer significant neuropsychological sequelae, including post-traumatic stress disorder, depression, psychosis, reduced educational performance, and major anxiety (9, 12, 33).

Skin Scarring

Skin scarring is particularly associated with meningococcal septicaemia. Buysse et al. reported that nearly half of children with meningococcal septicaemia had skin scarring, mainly on their extremities, face, and the trunk. Of these, 33% underwent debridement and skin grafting because of skin necrosis resulting from purpura (34).

Amputations/Limb Length Discrepancies

Amputations are a consequence of meningococcal septicaemia and purpura fulminans. The prevalence of distal amputations among 515 survivors of IMD in The Netherlands was reported as 0.8% (35). Amputation appeared more common in a study from Canada, where 3.1% of 471 survivors of IMD due to serogroups B and C had amputations, which was noted to be more frequent due to serogroup C infections (36). Among Dutch childhood survivors of meningococcal septic shock, 8% had amputations of extremities, ranging from one toe to both legs and one arm (34).

Meningococcal septicaemia can also cause bone growth abnormalities, due to damage to growth plates. Of 122 Australian survivors of meningococcal septicaemia 16 patients had partial or complete physeal growth arrest (37). Limb-length discrepancies were identified in 6% of the 120 Dutch meningococcal septic shock survivors (34).

Other Sequelae

Many studies have described the incidence and severity of varying long-term sequelae associated with IMD. One report suggests median risk of at least one sequela (major or minor, present after hospital discharge) associated with IMD, of 9.5% (95% CI: 5.1–15.1%) based on a meta-analysis of 27 studies that included 18,183 survivors of bacterial meningitis (9). The most common long-term consequences following meningococcal meningitis specifically were hearing loss (4.6%), cognitive difficulties (2.9%), and visual disturbances (2.7%). The risk of major sequelae was higher in lower-income countries, indicating the importance of good medical care in reducing long-term consequences.

Neurological Deficits

The occurrence of long-term neurological sequelae is more common in children who have experienced more severe infections. Thirty-five percent of 120 children who survived meningococcal septic shock suffered neurological impairments on follow up 4–10 years after PICU discharge (34).

Typically, hearing loss is identified in 2–4% of IMD survivors (36, 38), including those who suffered meningococcal septic shock, not only those with meningitis. This same Dutch study identified severe mental retardation (total IQ <70) in 3 of 120 patients; these patients also had epilepsy and two had spastic quadriplegia after meningococcal septicaemia (34).

Cognitive impairment and behavioral disturbances.

Several studies have identified milder neurodevelopmental deficits following IMD. A case–control study in the UK evaluated 115 child survivors of IMD ~10 years after disease onset (39). Most of these children did not have gross neurological deficits and most attended mainstream school. However, using detailed psychometric testing, survivors of IMD showed significantly lower scores compared with controls in cognition and educational performance. Educational problems are reported in >30% of children in terms of school achievement or concentration (40).

Cognitive impairments may also become apparent in older survivors of IMD. For example, a cohort of 101 adolescent IMD survivors (aged 15–19 years at time of disease) in the UK followed-up over a period of 1.5–3 years showed poorer educational outcomes compared with controls (41).

Psychological problems.

Several studies have reported that IMD can lead to delayed psychological problems such as post-traumatic stress disorder (PTSD), anxiety and depression. A UK study in 56 children (aged 3–16 years) indicated that there were statistically significant increases in emotional distress, hyperactivity and attention deficit disorder and at 12 months after discharge 11% of the children were considered at risk for PTSD (33).

Experience of IMD has significant psychological consequences for the parents of the index child. In interviews carried out 3–12 months following admission, nearly half the mothers of children with IMD were considered to be at psychiatric risk with the possibility of developing PTSD (42) and nearly a third of the other mothers were seeking professional help for psychological difficulties.

PREVENTION OF MENINGOCOCCAL DISEASE

Invasive meningococcal disease is of great concern to physicians whenever assessing a child with a febrile illness. In its early stages, it often presents with non-specific symptoms and is therefore very difficult to diagnose early. If misdiagnosed, the disease can progress rapidly with the patient dying within 24–48 h. Because of these factors and the fact that most disease occurs in young children, effective immunization of vulnerable populations is desirable.

There are two main classes of vaccine used for protection against IMD: pure polysaccharide vaccines and protein/polysaccharide conjugate vaccines. Both of these types of vaccines are based on the capsular polysaccharide of the meningococcus, which is a major virulence factor and is primarily responsible for colonization and invasion by prevention of host-mediated bacterial killing.

The host immune response to pure polysaccharide vaccines is not efficient in young children under the age of 2 years, because of reduced immune responsiveness to T-cell-independent antigens such as polysaccharides. This is an important limitation of vaccines based on these structures given that the highest risk for acquisition of IMD is in children <5 years of age. In addition, pure polysaccharide vaccines do not induce mucosal immunity and thus fail to prevent nasopharyngeal carriage of meningococci, and therefore cannot influence herd immunity.

In summary, pure polysaccharide vaccines are poorly immunogenic in children under 2 years of age, and confer inadequate and only temporary immunity, lasting for ~3–5 years in older children and adults. They do not impact nasopharyngeal carriage of pathogenic meningococci and in recent years they have been superceded by the conjugate protein/polysaccharide vaccines (32).

In recent years, effective quadrivalent conjugate polysaccharide vaccines have become available against the meningococcal serogroups A, C, Y, and W.

As MenA was the primary cause of IMD in the meningitis belt of sub-Saharan Africa, and was responsible for thousands of epidemic cases and deaths each year, the WHO initiated the Meningitis Vaccine Project, which developed a low-cost conjugate vaccine against MenA (MenAfriVac). This vaccine was successfully launched in mass vaccination campaigns as a single dose in over 250 million people aged 1–29 years across 25 countries in the African meningitis belt (4). Following this, a major reduction in numbers of cases of MenA disease in sub-Saharan Africa was observed.

MenC conjugate vaccine has been successfully introduced into much of Europe, and is now part of the routine immunization schedule. This vaccine is strongly immunogenic, giving relatively long-lasting immunity and immunological memory, and it also has a significant impact on decreasing nasopharyngeal carriage in vaccines and therefore confers herd immunity or community protection.

Since the introduction of MenC conjugate vaccine into the UK infant schedule in 1999, the incidence of MenC disease has decreased by 94% in immunized populations and 67% in unimmunized populations due to herd immunity (43). There has been a demonstrated important decrease in nasopharyngeal carriage, with, importantly, no increase in the carriage of other disease causing serogroups (44). In the epidemiological year 2016–2017 in all ages in the UK, there were 37 cases of MenC disease in total (6). Because of these low numbers of reported cases of MenC (and the ongoing vaccination programme with MenACWY quadrivalent conjugate vaccine in teenagers), in 2018 all infant Men C vaccine doses have been removed from the UK schedule, leaving a priming dose at 1 year and a booster in adolescence (as part of the MenACWY vaccine).

Vaccines for Serogroup B Meningococcus

Following the successful introduction of MenC vaccine, MenB has remained the most common cause of IMD, accounting for more than 50% of cases in the USA and as many as 90% of cases in Europe (5).

MenB has a poorly immunogenic capsule due to its polysaccharide structure. The polysaccharide capsule of MenB is composed of polysialic acid (α2–8 N-acetylneuraminic acid) which has structural similarity to carbohydrates found in fetal brain tissue. Therefore, there is a degree of immune tolerance to this polysaccharide, and there are concerns regarding the effect of modifying the sugar structure in a vaccine to make it more immunogenic, in case of induction of auto-immunity. These factors have therefore hindered progress on developing an effective polysaccharide vaccine as this molecular similarity does not allow the development of an effective protein/polysaccharide conjugate vaccine for MenB (45).

Because of these factors, vaccine development for MenB has required a different approach. MenB vaccines have now been developed targeting non-capsular structures, such as outer membrane porins, vesicles, and lipopolysaccharide (LPS).

LPS is a universal component of the outer membrane of Gram-negative bacteria and contributes to pathogenicity of the meningococcus. *Neisseria meningitidis* also produces various surface proteins, one of which, factor H binding protein, fHbp, binds human complement factor H. Human Factor H is important in regulating the alternative complement pathway. Binding of human Factor H to the surface of meningococci by bacterial fHbp is thought to inhibit complement-mediated bacterial lysis. Variations in human Factor H and related proteins have been found to be important factors in determining susceptibility to meningococcal disease (46, 47).

Another meningococcal surface protein, Neisserial Surface Protein A (NspA), can also bind human complement Factor H (48). Other factors which mimic or bind host molecules also inhibit complement-mediated bacterial lysis and phagocytosis. For example, N meningitidis sheds blebs of outer membrane which contain these outer membrane proteins and LPS. These outer membrane vesicles (OMVs) have been shown to initiate complement activation and might redirect complement activation away from invading meningococci in the circulation, thereby hindering the bactericidal effects of human complement.

In order to try to develop a universal vaccine against MenB, researchers at Novartis Vaccines used the genomic sequence of a serogroup B strain (N meningitidis serogroup B strain MC58)—a process called "reverse vaccinology" (49). This eventually led to development of an immunogenic MenB vaccine with novel vaccine protein antigens (a 4 component vaccine).

This novel 4CmenB (Bexsero©) vaccine was introduced into the UK infant schedule in September 2015. Latest figures estimate a vaccine uptake of 92.6% for the 2 infant doses by 52 weeks of age. There has been a definite impact on incidence of MenB in infants, in 2015/16 there was an incidence of 17 per 100,000 which was reduced to 11/100,000, a fall of 11% overall, following vaccine introduction (6). It is unknown whether this vaccine will have any effect on nasopharyngeal carriage and therefore provide herd protection. Even if 4CMenB had a definite effect on carriage, herd immunity will not occur whilst only infants are vaccinated as this will have no impact on the main source of carriage, which are adolescents.

Another vaccine effective against MenB, manufactured by Pfizer, which contains antigenic components from subfamilies A and B of meningococcal fHbp has undergone extensive clinical evaluation in young adults and adolescents. This vaccine (Trumemba©) has been widely used in North America in outbreaks of MenB disease in universities and has been shown to be safe and effective (50).

Studies in vaccinees who have received either Bexsero© or Trumemba© are being carried out in the UK to establish whether either or both of these vaccines have any effect on nasopharyngeal carriage, a prerequisite for the establishment of herd immunity. However, the only way to truly assess the effects of these vaccines on disease incidence and indirect protection is to carry out enhanced surveillance following population-wide vaccine introduction. It is important to consider the possibility that any protein-based MenB vaccine would have negligible or no impact on nasopharyngeal carriage, in which case there would be no clear strategy to induce herd immunity. This may suggest that the only way to reduce MenB incidence would be widespread all age immunization which may be economically unviable. However, if an impact on nasopharngeal carriage is demonstrated, then strategies to provide herd immunity, such as immunization of adolescents or adults could be appropriate.

Another potential benefit of use if these sub-capsular outer-membrane protein vaccines is their potential to induce cross protection against other meningococcal strains because the components of these vaccines are highly conserved protein antigens present in a high proportion of meningococcal subtypes irrespective of their covering capsule. This raises the possibility of development of a universal meningococcal vaccine, potentially leading to eradication of meningococcal disease (51).

CONCLUSION

The impact of conjugated meningococcal vaccines on disease incidence has been enormous. Countless young lives have been saved or dramatically improved due to disease prevention.

The challenge now is to continue to be vigilant in those populations that remain unimmunized so that appropriate recognition and management of invasive meningococcal disease is prioritized. In the meantime, it is clear that following guidelines and implementation of treatment bundles can have a significant effect on outcome.

We await data regarding the effectiveness of the newer protein vaccines against serogroup B meningoocccus on carriage and their cross-reactivity against non-B serogroups of meningococcus.

We look forward to a world without meningitis and septicaemia.

DISCLOSURE

SN has received consulting fees from Novartis and Pfizer. NN has received consulting fees from GSK and Pfizer.

AUTHOR CONTRIBUTIONS

All authors listed have made a substantial, direct and intellectual contribution to the work, and approved it for publication.

REFERENCES

1. Stephens DS, Greenwood B, Brandtzaeg P. Epidemic meningitis, meningococcaemia, and Neisseria meningitidis. *Lancet* (2007) 369:2196–210. doi: 10.1016/S0140-6736(07)61016-2
2. Rosenstein NE, Perkins BA, Stephens DS, Popovic T, Hughes JM. Meningococcal disease. *N Engl J Med.* (2001) 344:1378–88. doi: 10.1056/NEJM200105033441807
3. Harrison LH, Trotter CL, Ramsay ME. Global epidemiology of meningococcal disease. *Vaccine* (2009) 27:B51–63. doi: 10.1016/j.vaccine.2009.04.063
4. World Health Organisation. *Meningitis A Nearly Eliminated in Africa Through Vaccination, Reaching More Than 235 Million People.* Available online at: http://www.afro.who.int/search/node?keys=meningitis (Accessed June 1, 2018).
5. European Centre for Disease Prevention and Control. *Invasive Meningococcal Disease.* Annual Epidemiological Report for 2015. Stockholm: ECDC (2017).
6. Parikh SR, Andrews NJ, Beebeejaun K, Campbell H, Ribeiro S, Ward C, et al. Effectiveness and impact of a reduced infant schedule of 4CMenB vaccine against group B meningococcal disease in England: a national observational cohort study. *Lancet* (2016) 388:2775–82. doi: 10.1016/S0140-6736(16)31921-3
7. Public Health England. *Invasive Meningococcal Disease in England: Annual Laboratory Confirmed Reports for Epidemiological Year 2016/2017.* Health Protection Report (2017).
8. World Health Organization. *Meningococcal Meningitis Fact Sheet.* Available online at: http://www.who.int/mediacentre/factsheets/fs141/en/# (Accessed June 1, 2018).
9. Edmond K, Clark A, Korczak VS, Sanderson C, Griffiths UK, Rudan I. Global and regional risk of disabling sequelae from bacterial meningitis: a systematic review and meta-analysis. *Lancet Infect Dis.* (2010) 10:317–28. doi: 10.1016/S1473-3099(10)70048-7
10. *Management of Bacterial Meningitis and Meningococcal Septicaemia in Children and Young People Younger Than 16 Years in Primary and Secondary Care.* National Institute for Health and Clinical Excellence. CG102 (2010).
11. Rouphael NG, Stephens DS. Neisseria meningitidis: biology, microbiology, and epidemiology. *Methods Mol Biol.* (2012) 799:1–20. doi: 10.1007/978-1-61779-346-2_1
12. Wright C, Wordsworth R, Glennie L. Counting the cost of meningococcal disease: scenarios of severe meningitis and septicemia. *Paediatr Drugs* (2013) 15:49–58. doi: 10.1007/s40272-012-0006-0
13. Thompson MJ, Ninis N, Perera R, Mayon-White R, Phillips C, Bailey L, et al. Clinical recognition of meningococcal disease in children and adolescents. *Lancet* (2006) 367:397–403. doi: 10.1016/S0140-6736(06)67932-4
14. Pollard AJ, Nadel S, Ninis N, Faust SN, Levin M. Emergency management of meningococcal disease: eight years on. *Arch Dis Child.* (2007) 92:283–6. doi: 10.1136/adc.2006.102384
15. Welch SB, Nadel S. Treatment of meningococcal infection. *Arch Dis Child.* (2003) 88:608–14. doi: 10.1136/adc.88.7.608
16. Pathan N, Hemingway CA, Alizadeh AA, Stephens AC, Boldrick JC, Oragui EE, et al. Role of interleukin 6 in myocardial dysfunction of meningococcal septic shock. *Lancet* (2004) 363:203–9. doi: 10.1016/S0140-6736(03)15326-3
17. Dellinger RP, Levy MM, Rhodes A, Annane D, Gerlach H, Opal SM, et al. Surviving sepsis campaign: international guidelines for management of severe sepsis and septic shock: 2012. *Crit Care Med.* (2013) 41:580–637. doi: 10.1097/CCM.0b013e31827e83af
18. Davis AL, Carcillo JA, Aneja RK, Deymann AJ, Lin JC, Nguyen TC, et al. American College of Critical Care Medicine Clinical Practice Parameters for hemodynamic support of pediatric and neonatal septic shock. *Crit Care Med.* (2017) 45:1061–93. doi: 10.1097/CCM.0000000000002425
19. Evans IVR, Phillips GS, Alpern ER, Angus DC, Friedrich ME, Kissoon N, et al. Association between the New York sepsis care mandate and in-hospital mortality for pediatric sepsis. *JAMA* (2018) 320:358–67. doi: 10.1001/jama.2018.9071
20. Patel A, Laffan MA, Waheed U, Brett SJ. Randomised trials of human albumin for adults with sepsis: systematic review and meta-analysis with trial sequential analysis of all-cause mortality. *BMJ* (2014) 349:g4561. doi: 10.1136/bmj.g4561
21. Sprung CL, Annane D, Keh D, Moreno R, Singer M, Freivogel K, et al. Hydrocortisone therapy for patients with septic shock. *N Engl J Med.* (2008) 358:111–24. doi: 10.1056/NEJMoa071366
22. Annane D, Renault A, Brun-Buisson C, Megarbane B, Quenot JP, Siami S, et al. Hydrocortisone plus fludrocortisone for adults with septic shock. *N Engl J Med.* (2018) 378:809–18. doi: 10.1056/NEJMoa1705716

23. Menon K, McNally D, Choong K, Sampson M. A systematic review and meta-analysis on the effect of steroids in pediatric shock. *Pediatr Crit Care Med.* (2013) 14:474–80. doi: 10.1097/PCC.0b013e31828a8125
24. Forni LG, Ricci Z, Ronco C. Extracorporeal renal replacement therapies in the treatment of sepsis: where are we? *Semin Nephrol.* (2015) 35:55–63. doi: 10.1016/j.semnephrol.2015.01.006
25. Solé A, Jordan I, Bobillo S, Moreno J, Balaguer M, Hernández-Platero L, et al. Venoarterial extracorporeal membrane oxygenation support for neonatal and pediatric refractory septic shock: more than 15 years of learning. *Eur J Pediatr.* (2018) 177:1191–1200. doi: 10.1007/s00431-018-3174-2
26. Sarfatti A, Nadel S. Management of meningococcal disease. *Paediatr Child Health* (2015) 25:203–9. doi: 10.1016/j.paed.2015.01.006
27. Faust SN, Levin M, Harrison OB, Goldin RD, Lockhart MS, Kondaveeti S, et al. Dysfunction of endothelial protein C activation in severe meningococcal sepsis. *N Engl J Med.* (2001) 345:408–16. doi: 10.1056/NEJM200108093450603
28. Nadel S, Goldstein B, Williams MD, Dalton H, Peters M, Macias WL, et al. Drotrecogin alfa (activated) in children with severe sepsis: a multicentre phase III randomised controlled trial. *Lancet* (2007) 369:836–43. doi: 10.1016/S0140-6736(07)60411-5
29. Scott HF, Brou L, Deakyne SJ, Fairclough DL, Kempe A, Bajaj L. Lactate clearance and normalization and prolonged organ dysfunction in pediatric sepsis. *J Pediatr.* (2016) 170:149–55.e1-4. doi: 10.1016/j.jpeds.2015.11.071
30. Davies MS, Nadel S, Habibi P, Levin M, Hunt DM. The orthopaedic management of peripheral ischaemia in meningococcal septicaemia in children. *J Bone Joint Surg Br.* (2000) 82:383–6. doi: 10.1302/0301-620x.82b3.9887
31. Forsyth RJ, Raper J, Todhunter E. Routine intracranial pressure monitoring in acute coma. *Cochrane Database Syst Rev.* (2015) CD002043. doi: 10.1002/14651858.CD002043.pub3
32. Sadarangani M, Pollard AJ. Can we control all-cause meningococcal disease in Europe? *Clin Microbiol Infect.* (2016) 22(Suppl. 5):S103–12. doi: 10.1016/j.cmi.2016.03.006
33. Garralda ME, Gledhill J, Nadel S, Neasham D, O'Connor M, Shears D. Longer-term psychiatric adjustment of children and parents after meningococcal disease. *Pediatr Crit Care Med.* (2009) 10:675–80. doi: 10.1097/PCC.0b013e3181ae785a
34. Buysse CM, Oranje AP, Zuidema E, Hazelzet JA, Hop WC, Diepstraten AF, et al. Long-term skin scarring and orthopaedic sequelae in survivors of meningococcal septic shock. *Arch Dis Child.* (2009) 94:381–6. doi: 10.1136/adc.2007.131862
35. Schildkamp RL, Lodder MC, Bijlmer HA, Dankert J, Scholten RJ. Clinical manifestations and course of meningococcal disease in 562 patients. *Scand J Infect Dis.* (1996) 28:47–51.
36. Erickson L, De Wals P. Complications and sequelae of meningococcal disease in Quebec, Canada, 1990–1994. *Clin Infect Dis.* (1998) 26:1159–64. doi: 10.1086/520303
37. Bache CE, Torode IP. Orthopaedic sequelae of meningococcal septicemia. *J Pediatr Orthop.* (2006) 26:135–9. doi: 10.1097/01.bpo.0000187991.71645.e7
38. Viner RM, Booy R, Johnson H, Edmunds WJ, Hudson L, Bedford H, et al. Outcomes of invasive meningococcal serogroup B disease in children and adolescents (MOSAIC): a case-control study. *Lancet Neurol.* (2012) 11:774–83. doi: 10.1016/S1474-4422(12)70180-1
39. Fellick JM, Thomson AP, Sills J, Hart CA. Neurological soft signs in mainstream pupils. *Arch Dis Child.* (2001) 85:371–4. doi: 10.1136/adc.85.5.371
40. Koomen I, Raat H, Jennekens-Schinkel A, Grobbee DE, Roord JJ, van Furth M. Academic and behavioral limitations and health-related quality of life in school-age survivors of bacterial meningitis. *Qual Life Res.* (2005) 14:1563–70. doi: 10.1007/s11136-004-7706-z
41. Borg J, Christie D, Coen PG, Booy R, Viner RM. Outcomes of meningococcal disease in adolescence: prospective, matched-cohort study. *Pediatrics* (2009) 123:e502–9. doi: 10.1542/peds.2008-0581
42. Judge D, Nadel S, Vergnaud S, Garrala ME. Psychiatric adjustment following meningococcal disease treated on a PICU. *Intens Care Med.* (2002) 28:648–65. doi: 10.1007/s00134-002-1237-2
43. Halperin SA, Bettinger JA, Greenwood B, Harrison LH, Jelfs J, Ladhani SN, et al. The changing and dynamic epidemiology of meningococcal disease. *Vaccine* (2012) 30(Suppl. 2):B26–36. doi: 10.1016/j.vaccine.2011.12.032
44. Borrow R, Alarcón P, Carlos J, Caugant DA, Christensen H, Debbag R, et al. The Global Meningococcal Initiative: global epidemiology, the impact of vaccines on meningococcal disease and the importance of herd protection. *Expert Rev Vaccines* (2017) 16:313–28. doi: 10.1080/14760584.2017.1258308
45. Nadel S. Prospects for eradication of meningococcal disease. *Arch Dis Child.* (2012) 97:993–8. doi: 10.1136/archdischild-2012-302036
46. Martinón-Torres F, Png E, Khor CC, Davila S, Wright VJ, Sim KS, et al. Natural resistance to Meningococcal Disease related to CFH loci: meta-analysis of genome-wide association studies. *Sci Rep.* (2016) 6:35842. doi: 10.1038/srep35842
47. Davila S, Wright VJ, Khor CC, Sim KS, Binder A, Breunis WB, et al. Genome-wide association study identifies variants in the CFH region associated with host susceptibility to meningococcal disease. *Nat Genet.* (2010) 42:772–6. doi: 10.1038/ng.640
48. Lewis LA, Ngampasutadol J, Wallace R, Reid JE, Vogel U, Ram S. The meningococcal vaccine candidate neisserial surface protein A (NspA) binds to factor H and enhances meningococcal resistance to complement. *PLoS Pathog.* (2010) 6:e1001027. doi: 10.1371/journal.ppat.1001027
49. Giuliani MM, Adu-Bobie J, Comanducci M, Aricò B, Savino S, Santini L, et al. A universal vaccine for serogroup B meningococcus. *Proc Natl Acad Sci USA.* (2006) 103:10834–9. doi: 10.1073/pnas.0603940103
50. Duffy J, Johnsen P, Ferris M, Miller M, Leighton K, McGilvray M, et al. Safety of a meningococcal group B vaccine used in response to two university outbreaks. *J Am Coll Health* (2017) 65:380–8. doi: 10.1080/07448481.2017.1312418
51. Bianchi A, Fantoni S, Prugnola A. Meningococcal B vaccine and the vision of a meningitis free world. *J Prev Med Hyg.* (2015) 56:E10-3. doi: 10.15167/2421-4248/jpmh2015.56.3.491

10

Sepsis-Induced Immunosuppression in Neonates

Julie E. Hibbert[1], *Andrew Currie*[1,2] *and Tobias Strunk*[1,3*]

[1] *Centre for Neonatal Research and Education, University of Western Australia, Perth, WA, Australia,* [2] *School of Veterinary and Life Sciences, Murdoch University, Perth, WA, Australia,* [3] *Neonatal Directorate, King Edward Memorial Hospital for Women, Subiaco, WA, Australia*

Correspondence:
Tobias Strunk
tobias.strunk@health.wa.gov.au

Neonates, especially those born preterm, are at increased risk of sepsis and adverse long-term effects associated with infection-related inflammation. Distinct neonatal immune responses and dysregulated inflammation are central to this unique susceptibility. The traditional separation of sepsis into an initial hyper-inflammatory response followed by hypo-inflammation is continually under review with new developments in this area of research. There is evidence to support the association of mortality in the early acute phase of sepsis with an overwhelming hyper-inflammatory immune response. Emerging evidence from adults suggests that hypo- and hyper-inflammation can occur during any phase of sepsis and that sepsis-immunosuppression is associated with increased mortality, morbidity, and risk to subsequent infection. In adults, sepsis-induced immunosuppression (SII) is characterised by alterations of innate and adaptive immune responses, including, but not limited to, a prominent bias toward anti-inflammatory cytokine secretion, diminished antigen presentation to T cells, and reduced activation and proliferation of T cells. It is unclear if sepsis-immunosuppression also plays a role in the adverse outcomes associated with neonatal sepsis. This review will focus on exploring if key characteristics associated with SII in adults are observed in neonates with sepsis.

Keywords: neonates, preterm infant, innate immunity, adaptive immunity, immune cell function, sepsis, infection, immunosuppression

INFLAMMATION AND SEPSIS—A NEW PARADIGM?

Sepsis, defined as life-threatening organ dysfunction caused by a dysregulated host response to infection, represents an enormous burden affecting more than 30 million people with potentially 6 million associated deaths per year (1). Until recently, adult sepsis complicated by organ dysfunction, was termed severe sepsis, but is now represented by an increase in the Sequential Organ Failure Assessment (SOFA) score, secondary to the infection cause (2). The SOFA score, based on respiratory, cardiovascular, hepatic, coagulation, renal, and neurological systems, determines the extent of organ function and an increase of two points or more is associated with in-hospital mortality of >10% (2). Septic shock is defined as sepsis with circulatory and cellular/metabolic abnormalities that substantially increase mortality (2). Recent evidence from critically ill adults with sepsis and septic shock suggests the extent of recovery from sepsis may depend on the host's ability to orchestrate both the pro-inflammatory and hypo-inflammatory responses to achieve immunological homoeostasis following infection (3, 4). Hotchkiss et al., described three potential inflammatory responses to sepsis, and acknowledged that the immune response to sepsis is determined by many factors, including pathogen virulence and comorbidities (4). Firstly, at the onset of sepsis the pro-inflammatory response can dominate, even though both the pro-inflammatory and anti-inflammatory responses are initiated, and lead to an overwhelming hyper-inflammatory state that may cause multiple organ dysfunction and death within 1–2 days. Secondly, in patients with impaired immune responses due to comorbidities, the hyper-inflammatory phase may be absent or reduced and a profound anti-inflammatory state may occur, which may lead to further impaired immunity with increased risk of nosocomial infections and higher risk of death 10–14 days following sepsis onset. Thirdly, the immune response cycles between hyper-inflammatory and hypo-inflammatory states and death can occur in either state. With this response, there is an increased probability of the patient developing overwhelming immunosuppression as the infection persists (4).

There is increasing evidence to support the role of immunosuppression in sepsis (4). Critically ill adults with sepsis and septic shock may develop *sepsis-induced immunosuppression (SII)*, a phenomenon of persistent systemic hypo-inflammation that compromises many immune functions, prevents bacterial elimination and immune homeostasis (3–7). Importantly, SII is associated with increased risk of multi-organ failure and mortality, and ongoing immunosuppression results in prolonged (10–14 days) susceptibility to secondary viral and bacterial infections (3–6, 8).

Immunologically, SII in adults is incompletely characterised, but is commonly associated with altered functions of the complex network of innate and adaptive immune responses to infection. Specifically, neutrophils, monocytes, macrophages, and dendritic cells (DCs) display a prominent shift of phenotype and function toward an impaired inflammatory response. This further includes decreased bactericidal defences in neutrophils (including oxidative burst and low intracellular expression of myeloperoxidase and lactoferrin), reduced neutrophil chemotaxis, biased anti-inflammatory cytokine secretion with an increased interleukin (IL)-10 to tumour necrosis factor alpha (TNFα) ratio. There is also reduced expression of the major histocompatibility complex (MHC) II cell surface receptor human leukocyte antigen-DR (HLA-DR) and consequently impaired antigen-presenting capacity of DCs and monocytes (3, 4, 6, 7). Changes to the adaptive immune response in adults with SII include: reduced activation of T cells through diminished cell surface expression of the co-stimulatory molecules CD80 and CD86 on antigen presenting cells (APCs); inhibition of T cell proliferation due to expansion of cell populations with immunosuppressive function, such as immature neutrophils, myeloid-derived suppressor cells (MDSCs), and regulatory T cells (Tregs); reduced effector functions of T cells, B cells, and natural killer cells; and T cell exhaustion, typified by decreased T cell activation, reduced ability to produce cytokines, and decreased cytotoxic functions (3, 4, 6, 7). Sepsis-induced apoptosis of DCs, CD4+ and CD8+ T cells and B cells occurs in primary immune organs such as blood, bone marrow, spleen, and thymus, resulting in an overwhelming depletion of immune cells (3, 4, 6, 7).

The suppressive effect of endotoxin tolerance, induced by repeat or long-term exposure to bacterial endotoxins, like lipopolysaccharide (LPS), mediates immune dysfunction through reprogramming of cell signalling and is associated with immunosuppression observed in the later-stage of adult sepsis (7, 9). Leukocytes from adult patients with sepsis behave similarly to *in vitro* endotoxin-tolerised cells, with a reduced responsiveness to produce cytokines, especially TNFα, upon re-challenge with LPS (10). The molecular mechanism is unclear, but Pena and colleagues have recently identified an endotoxin tolerance gene signature that may predict sepsis and organ dysfunction in adults with sepsis (9). Murine macrophages challenged with Gram-positive bacteria can also induce endotoxin tolerance, termed as cross-tolerance, to a lesser extent than LPS (11), but no associated gene signature has yet been reported.

SEPSIS-INDUCED IMMUNOSUPPRESSION AND THE NEONATE

Neonatal immune development is complex, incompletely understood and orchestrated by many factors, including intra- and extra-uterine exposure to antigens and commensal organisms (12–16). Immune development in infants born preterm (<37 weeks' gestation) may be further altered by perinatal exposures to corticosteroids and antibiotics and the unique environmental influences associated with prolonged hospital stay (e.g., mechanical ventilation, use of indwelling plastic devices, parenteral nutrition, invasive procedures, and exposure to nosocomial microbes) (14, 15, 17–19).

Despite advances in neonatal care, sepsis remains a significant cause of morbidity among neonates and is one of the most common causes of neonatal death, accounting for over four-hundred and twenty thousand deaths per year (20). Sepsis is a common complication that affects up to 40% of neonates born <28 weeks' gestation (21, 22). Chronic long-term morbidities, such as lung disease and neurodevelopmental impairment, are further increased among infants who acquire nosocomial sepsis (23, 24). Inflammation-related brain injury and the associated long-term effects are clearly evident in preterm infants with sepsis (23), and have also been observed in adults with sepsis (25).

The increased risk of sepsis-associated morbidity and mortality in neonates is largely attributed to immature innate immune functions resulting in dysregulated pro-inflammatory responses to systemic infection—often referred to as a "cytokine storm" (26–30). The mortality rate in infants with sepsis is 10–16%, with 50–57% of neonates die within the first 3 days of sepsis onset, 12–20% within 4–7 days and 23–39% after 7 days (31, 32). Similar to adults (4), there is strong evidence to support the association of mortality in the acute phase, i.e., within first days of sepsis, with a dysregulated pro-inflammatory immune response (28–30, 33, 34). However, emerging evidence suggests that the immature immune response to infection in neonates is characteristically similar to the endotoxin tolerance phenotype observed in critically ill adults with sepsis (7, 35). This is evident despite Gram-positive bacteria being the major causative organisms in neonatal sepsis (36), unlike in adult sepsis

(37). In the neonatal setting, the risk of sepsis may be mediated by a relative inability to initiate appropriate hyper-inflammatory responses which, along with a predominant hypo-inflammatory response, actively causes immunosuppression (35). In keeping with findings in adult SII, Gervassi and colleagues proposed that the distinct neonatal responses to invasive microbes, as well as to vaccines, may be at least partly explained by active immune suppression, such as inhibition of T cell proliferation and function by Tregs and MDSCs, and the potential for B cells to skew the immune response toward an anti-inflammatory T helper 2 response (38).

Sepsis-induced immunosuppression has not yet been defined in neonates. In adults, SII signifies sepsis severity, septic shock, and mortality (3, 4, 6, 7). Identifying immunosuppression in neonates may not be as straight forward for several reasons, namely: the lack of a globally accepted definition for neonatal sepsis, including grading of severity; the distinct patterns of immune development; and the sparse data available on immune function and response to infection at the time of neonatal sepsis.

Firstly, neonatal sepsis, especially in those born preterm, is not clearly defined. The recently updated Third International Consensus Definitions for sepsis and septic shock in adults are not applicable to children, infants and neonates (2, 39, 40), and there is no equivalent SOFA score for determining sepsis severity in neonatal sepsis. Further to this, the international paediatric consensus definition for sepsis specifically excludes preterm neonates (39) and performs poorly in term neonates (40). This has widespread implications not only for reporting incidence and prevalence of neonatal sepsis, but for clinical management (accurate diagnosis and appropriate treatment) and the short- and long-term impact on clinical outcomes (41, 42). Further to this, the lack of a clear neonatal sepsis definition creates a substantial barrier to identifying predictive markers for sepsis, and improving diagnostic accuracy and speed (41, 43). To date, there is no consensus definition of neonatal sepsis and the current "gold standard" of positive blood culture plus clinical symptoms for the definition of "confirmed sepsis" has significant limitations (41, 44, 45). To further complicate diagnosis, sepsis can also be classified as "clinical sepsis," with a negative culture in a symptomatic newborn (41).

Secondly, development of immunoregulation is distinct in neonates compared with adults. This includes differences in: (a) absolute numbers of immune cells (e.g., lower neutrophil counts and higher natural killer cell counts in neonates) (12, 46, 47); (b) the proportions of immune cell subtypes (e.g., higher immature/total neutrophil ratio in neonates) (48, 49), and (c) levels of various immune plasma proteins (e.g., lower complement, immunoglobulin, antimicrobial peptide levels in neonates) (12, 13).

Lastly, there is limited data on neonatal innate immune responses during sepsis, and studies relating immune function to sepsis severity are lacking. Neonatal immune studies commonly utilise cord blood, which is not representative of the immune system at 1–3 weeks of age, when the most common form of neonatal invasive infection, late-onset sepsis (LOS), typically occurs (50). Data available from the time of sepsis can be limited by low number of neonates and confounded by multiple factors, such timing of sample collection, volume of blood sample collection, pathogenesis of the causative organism, time of sepsis onset [e.g., early-onset sepsis (EOS) <72 h after birth and LOS >72 h after birth], and sepsis definition (e.g., confirmed vs. clinical). Further to this, time from sepsis onset to death is poorly reported and therefore causative attribution not consistently possible.

Confirming and describing SII in neonates may be instrumental in better defining the immune pathophysiology of neonatal sepsis. This could also aid in the identification of unique biomarkers that could be of clinical utility for immunomonitoring, prediction of outcomes, or even targeted therapeutics. The remainder of this review focusses on characterising immunosuppression in neonatal sepsis and their associated clinical implications. The principal immune functions characterised include cytokine secretion, antigen presentation, expansion of immunosuppressive cells, effector cell function, and sepsis-induced immune cell apoptosis. Information on gestational age (GA), postnatal age at onset of sepsis, classification (i.e., confirmed and clinical sepsis) and age at sepsis-related death in many studies were incomplete and may confound the interpretation. Available data were included in this review and in **Tables 1–5** and **Supplementary Tables 1, 2**. For clarity, when neonatal GA was not described in the publication, we considered any infant born ≥37 weeks' gestation as term and any infant born <37 weeks' gestation as preterm.

INFLAMMATORY CYTOKINE SECRETION IN RESPONSE TO INFECTION IN ADULTS AND NEONATES

Circulating Inflammatory Cytokines in Adult Sepsis

Together, pro- and anti-inflammatory cytokines influence the innate immune responses to infection (88). Plasma levels of pro-inflammatory cytokines, including TNFα, IL-6, IL-8, IL-1β, interferon gamma (IFNγ), and the anti-inflammatory cytokines IL-10 and IL-4 are elevated in adults with sepsis and septic shock (52, 56–58, 72, 89)—study details described in **Table 1**. Interestingly, those with septic shock had both higher pro- and anti-inflammatory levels than patients without shock (57), with the levels of IL-6 and IL-8 positively associated with IL-10 levels (56), indicating a correlation with sepsis severity. Further support for the positive association between sepsis severity and immunosuppression are provided by reports of increased mortality in septic patients with elevated IL-10 levels or a high IL-10/TNFα ratio (52, 57–59). Additionally, patients who regained organ function by day 4 following sepsis onset had a significantly higher TNFα production capacity compared to those with ongoing organ failure by day 6 (51). While there is concomitant secretion of pro- and anti-inflammatory cytokines during sepsis, the increased ratio of IL-10 to TNFα is associated with sepsis mortality and immunosuppression (52,

TABLE 1 | Sepsis-induced immunosuppression—association of secreted cytokine concentration with sepsis severity in neonates and adults with sepsis.

Adult or neonatal GA	Cohort sepsis characteristics (*n*) and mortality (if applicable)	Time of blood sampling and age at sepsis	Observation in septic cohort	References
TNFα				
Adult	Organ dysfunction during sepsis: 24 - Organ failure recovery by day 4: 11 - Organ failure ongoing: 13	Blood samples were taken within 24 h of initial suspicion of sepsis and on hospital days 4 and 6 Mean (median) age at sepsis 55 (55) years	Increased TNFα production capacity is associated with organ failure recovery	(51)
Adult	Septic shock: 38 - Survivors: 22 - Non-survivors: 16 Mortality within 28 days after diagnosis. Time from sepsis onset not described	Blood samples were taken on days 1–2, 3–4, 5–7, and 8–15 days following initial suspicion of sepsis Mean age at sepsis 64 years (95% CI 59–69)	TNFα levels were increased in non-survivors compared to survivors, but not significantly	(52)
Term (GA range 37–42 weeks)	Clinical ($n = 10$) and confirmed ($n = 3$) LOS: 13 - Sepsis: 4 - Severe sepsis: 6 - Septic shock: 3	Blood sample was taken at initial suspicion of sepsis Median age at sepsis: 10 days (IQR 7–22 days)	TNFα levels were not associated with sepsis severity	(53)
Mix of preterm and Term (mean GA not described)	Sepsis: 50 (EOS: 41 and LOS: 9) - Survivors: 33 - Non-survivors:17 Non-sepsis inflammation: 50 Controls: 50 Time from sepsis onset to death not described	Blood samples were taken at sepsis evaluation (time 0) and on days 1 and 2 Age at sepsis not described	TNFα was significantly elevated in non-survivors, compared to survivors, at time 0, but not on days 1 or 2	(54)
Mix of preterm and Term (mean GA 35.8 ± 4.1)	Confirmed sepsis: 26 (EOS $n = 3$ and LOS $n = 13$) - Survivors: 17 - Non-survivors: 9 Controls: 29 Mortality: EOS deaths <2 days: 5 LOS deaths >7 days: 4 Time from sepsis onset to death not described	Blood samples were taken at sepsis evaluation before antimicrobial therapy (time 0) and on days 3 and 7 Mean (±SD) age at sepsis: EOS 1.9 (±1.1) days LOS 20.6 (±8.4) days	TNFα significantly increased progressively during sepsis in the non-survivors TNFα significantly decreased progressively during sepsis in the survivors	(55)
IL-6				
Adult	Septic shock: 20 SIRS: 11 Healthy controls: 10	Blood sample was taken within 24 h initial suspicion of sepsis Age at septic shock: 68 years	IL-6 levels higher in septic shock than controls. Increased levels of IL-6 were positively associated with IL-10 levels in septic shock, indicating correlation with sepsis severity	(56)
Adult	Sepsis:32 - Sepsis: 19 - Septic shock: 13 Healthy controls: 15	Blood sample was taken at initial suspicion of sepsis Mean age (±SD) at sepsis: 70.8 (±12.7) years	Significantly elevated IL-6 levels in septic patients compared to controls Significantly elevated levels in septic shock compared to sepsis without shock	(57)
Term (GA range 37–42 weeks)	Clinical ($n = 10$) and confirmed ($n = 3$) LOS: 13 - Sepsis: 4 - Severe sepsis: 6 - Septic shock: 3	Blood sample was taken within 24 h initial suspicion of sepsis Median (IQR) age at sepsis: 10 (7–22) days	Increased IL-6 levels are associated with septic shock	(53)
Mix of preterm and Term (mean GA 35.8 ± 4.1)	Confirmed sepsis: 26 (EOS $n = 13$ and LOS $n = 13$) - Survivors: 17 - Non-survivors: 9 Controls: 29 Mortality: EOS deaths <2 days: 5 LOS deaths >7 days: 4 Time from sepsis onset to death not described	Blood samples were taken at sepsis evaluation before antimicrobial therapy (time 0) and on days 3 and 7 following Mean (±SD) age at sepsis: EOS 1.9 (±1.1) days LOS 20.6 (±8.4) days	IL-6 significantly increased progressively during sepsis episode in the non-survivors IL-6 significantly decreased progressively during sepsis episode in the survivors	(55)

(Continued)

TABLE 1 | Continued

Adult or neonatal GA	Cohort sepsis characteristics (*n*) and mortality (if applicable)	Time of blood sampling and age at sepsis	Observation in septic cohort	References
Mix of preterm and Term (mean GA not described)	Confirmed sepsis: 50 (EOS $n = 41$ and LOS $n = 9$) - Survivors: 33 - Non-survivors: 17 Non-sepsis inflammation: 50 Controls: 50 Time from sepsis onset to death not described	Blood samples were taken at sepsis evaluation (time 0) and on days 1 and 2 following Age at sepsis not described	IL-6 was significantly elevated in non-survivors compared to survivors, at time all three timepoints	(54)
IL-8				
Adult	Septic shock: 20 SIRS: 11 Healthy controls: 10	Blood sample was taken within 24 h initial suspicion of sepsis Age at septic shock: 68 years	IL-8 levels elevated compared to SIRS and control. Increased levels of IL-8 are positively associated with IL-10 levels in septic shock, indicating correlation with sepsis severity	(56)
Term (GA range 37–42 weeks)	Clinical ($n = 10$) and confirmed ($n = 3$) LOS: 13 - Sepsis: 4 - Severe sepsis: 6 - Septic shock: 3	Blood sample was taken at initial suspicion of sepsis Median age at sepsis: 10 (IQR 7–22) days	Increased IL-8 levels gradually increased with sepsis severity, but not significantly	(53)
Mix of preterm and Term (mean GA 35.8 ± 4.1)	Confirmed sepsis: 26 (EOS $n = 13$ and LOS $n = 13$) - Survivors: 17 - Non-survivors: 9 Controls: 29 - Mortality: EOS deaths <2 days: 5 LOS deaths >7 days: 4 Time from sepsis onset to death not described	Blood samples were taken at sepsis evaluation before antimicrobial therapy (time 0) and on days 3 and 7 Mean (±SD) age at: EOS 1.9 (±1.1) days LOS 20.6 (±8.4) days	IL-8 increased progressively during sepsis episode in the non-survivors (only significantly between time 0 and day 3) IL-8 significantly decreased progressively during sepsis episode in the survivors	(55)
Mix of preterm and Term (mean GA not described)	Sepsis: 50 (EOS $n = 41$ and LOS $n = 9$) - Survivors: 33 - Non-survivors:17 Non-sepsis inflammation: 50 Controls: 50 Time from sepsis onset to death not described	Blood samples were taken at sepsis evaluation (time 0) and on days 1 and 2 Age at sepsis not described	IL-8 was significantly elevated in non-survivors compared to survivors, at time all three timepoints	(54)
IL-10				
Adult	Septic shock: 38 - Survivors: 22 - Non-survivors: 16 Mortality within 28 days after diagnosis. Time from sepsis onset to death not described	Blood samples were taken on days 1–2, 3–4, 5–7, and 8–15 days following initial suspicion of sepsis Mean age at sepsis: 64 years (95% CI 59–69)	IL-10 levels were significantly elevated throughout the septic episode in non-survivors compared to survivors	(52)
Adult	Infection (includes more than only sepsis): 399 - Survivors: 366 - Non-survivors: 33 Time from sepsis onset to death unclear	Blood sample was taken when empirical antibiotics commenced Median (IQR) age at sepsis: 61 (45–77) years	IL-10 levels were significantly higher in the non-survivors. Increased IL-10 levels were associated with increased risk of mortality	(58)
Adult	Septic shock: 20 SIRS: 11 Healthy controls: 10	Blood sample was taken within 24 h initial suspicion of sepsis Age at septic shock: 68 years	IL-10 levels more elevated than controls. Increased levels of IL-6 and IL-8 are positively associated with IL-10 levels in septic shock, indicating correlation with sepsis severity	(56)
Adult	Sepsis:32 - Sepsis: 19 - Septic shock: 13 Healthy controls: 15	Blood sample was taken at time of initial suspicion of sepsis Mean (±SD) age at sepsis: 70.8 (±12.7) years	Significantly elevated IL-10 levels in septic patients compared to controls. Significantly elevated levels in septic shock compared to sepsis without shock	(57)

(Continued)

TABLE 1 | Continued

Adult or neonatal GA	Cohort sepsis characteristics (*n*) and mortality (if applicable)	Time of blood sampling and age at sepsis	Observation in septic cohort	References
Adult	Sepsis: 61 - Survivors: 41 - Non-survivors: 20 Time from sepsis onset to death not described	Blood sample was taken on day of admission and the next day Median (IQR) age at sepsis in years: Survivors 52.5 (36–61.5) Non-survivors 54.5 (42.5–62.5)	Significantly elevated IL-10 levels in non-survivors compared to survivors	(59)
Adult	Post-operative sepsis: 35 - Survivors: 24 - Non-survivors: 11 Post-operative non-sepsis controls: 85 Mean time to mortality 22.3 (±6.6) days. Time from sepsis onset to death not described	Blood sample was taken at time of initial suspicion of sepsis Mean (±SEM) age at sepsis: 61 (±2) years	Sepsis is associated with deficient IL-10 production. Sepsis survival correlated with recovery of pro-inflammatory secretion, but not IL-10	(60)
Term (GA range 37–42 weeks)	Clinical (*n* = 10) and confirmed (*n* = 3) LOS: 13 - Sepsis: 4 - Severe sepsis: 6 - Septic shock: 3	Blood sample was taken at time of initial suspicion of sepsis Median (IQR) age at sepsis: 10 (7–22) days	Increased IL-10 levels gradually increased are with sepsis severity, but not significantly	(53)
IL-10/TNFα RATIO				
Adult	Septic shock: 38 - Survivors: 22 - Non-survivors: 16 Mortality within 28 days after diagnosis. Time from sepsis onset to death not described	Blood samples were taken on days 1–2, 3–4, 5–7, and 8–15 days following initial suspicion of sepsis Mean age at sepsis: 64 years (95% CI 59–69)	IL-10/TNFα ratio was significantly increased during the first days of sepsis in non-survivors compared to survivors	(52)
Adult	Infection (includes more than only sepsis): 399 - Survivors: 366 - Non-survivors: 33 Time from sepsis onset to death unclear	Blood sample was taken when empirical antibiotics commenced Median (IQR) age at sepsis: 61 (45–77) years	IL-10/TNFα ratio was significantly higher in non-survivors compared to survivors	(58)
Neonate of any GA	Not assessed	–	–	–

GA, gestational age; LOS, late-onset sepsis; EOS, early-onset sepsis; VLBW, very low birth weight; SIRS, systemic inflammatory response syndrome; IL, interleukin; TNFα, tumour necrosis factor alpha; IFNγ, type II interferon; IQR, interquartile range; SD, standard deviation; CI, confidence interval.

58), however, the mechanism for this association has yet to be elucidated.

Functional Assessment of Cytokine Secretion in Adult Sepsis

Pro-inflammatory (TNFα, IL-1β, IL-6, IL-12) and anti-inflammatory (IL-10) responses occur concomitantly in stimulated whole blood and isolated monocytes from septic adults, albeit at a reduced capacity compared to healthy adults (60, 84, 89–91). Interestingly survival in these patients was associated with the recovery of pro-inflammatory cytokine production, but not IL-10 production—the IL-10/TNFα ratio was not reported (60). A similar pattern of decreased TNFα, IL-6, IFNγ, and IL-10 was also observed in a post-mortem study of stimulated splenocytes from patients who died of sepsis (84). These results suggest patients with sepsis have a sub-optimal capacity to produce pro- and anti-inflammatory cytokines, which is inversely associated with sepsis severity, especially when IL-10 levels remain relatively higher, eventually leading to organ failure, septic shock, and/or death.

Circulating Inflammatory Cytokines in Neonatal Sepsis

In both preterm and term neonates with EOS or LOS, the circulating levels of pro-inflammatory cytokines, IL-6 (28, 53–55, 92–96), IL-8 (53–55), and IFNγ (92, 94, 95) are consistently elevated compared to non-septic neonates. Whereas, TNFα and IL-1β levels are more variable (28, 53, 95, 96) or increased (28, 53–55, 92, 94, 96). The inconsistent reports of TNFα and IL-1β concentrations in neonatal sepsis may be a confounded by the kinetics and short half-life of circulating TNFα and IL-1β and the timing of sample collection relative to the onset of sepsis (97, 98). Circulating anti-inflammatory IL-10 concentrations (28, 53, 92, 94, 95) are elevated in preterm and term neonates with EOS or LOS compared to non-septic neonates, whereas the concentration of IL-4 is more variable (28, 92, 94, 95). These studies did not report the ratio of IL-10 to TNFα. Neonatal and sepsis characteristics, and relevant outcomes of these studies not in relation to sepsis severity are described in the **Supplementary Table 1**.

TABLE 2 | Sepsis-induced immunosuppression—association of monocyte surface HLA-DR expression with sepsis severity in neonates and adults with sepsis.

Adult or neonatal GA	Cohort sepsis characteristics (*n*) and mortality (if applicable)	Time of blood sampling and age at sepsis	Observation in septic cohort	References
Adult	Septic shock: 38 - Survivors: 22 - Non-survivors: 16 Mortality within 28 days after diagnosis. Time from sepsis onset to death not described	Blood samples were taken on days 1–2, 3–4, 5–7, and 8–15 days following initial suspicion of sepsis Mean age at sepsis: 64 years (95% CI 59–69)	Decreased % HLA-DR expression in septic shock Significantly lower % HLA-DR expression in non-survivors compared to survivors	(52)
Adult	Sepsis: 61 - Survivors: 41 - Non-survivors: 20 Time from sepsis onset to death not described	Blood sample was taken on day of admission and the next day Median (IQR) age at sepsis in years: Survivors 52.5 (36–61.5) Non-survivors 54.5 (42.5–62.5)	Decreased HLA-DR expression in sepsis. Significantly lower in non-survivors compared to survivors	(59)
Adult	Organ dysfunction during sepsis: 37 SIRS: 13 Healthy control: 20	Blood sample was taken within 24 h of sepsis development Median (IQR) age at sepsis: 69.4 (±2.7) years	Progressive significant decrease in CD14/HLA-DR expression in the organ dysfunction during sepsis group	(61)
Adult	Sepsis/septic shock: 20 Post-surgical inflammation: 20 Non-sepsis controls: 10	Blood sample was taken within 24 h of study inclusion Median (IQR) age at sepsis: 60 (53–67) years	Decreased HLA-DR surface protein and mRNA expression in sepsis/septic shock TNFα:HLA-DR ratio correlates negatively with SOFA score	(62)
Adult	Sepsis: 17 - Survivor: 6 - Non-survivors: 11 Non-sepsis controls: 10 Healthy control: 12 Time to mortality: During 1st septic episode $n = 9$ During 2nd septic episode $n = 2$ Time from sepsis onset to death not described	Blood sample was taken upon admission to the study Mean (±SEM) age at sepsis: 71 (±5) years	HLA-DR expression significantly decreased in sepsis group. HLA-DR expression was significantly lower in non-survivors, compared to survivors 6 of 17 with sepsis later developed nosocomial infections	(63)
Mix of preterm and Term (mean GA 37.5 ± 3.8)	Clinical ($n = 22$) and confirmed ($n = 18$) LOS: 40 - Survivor: 32 - Non-survivor: 8 Non-sepsis disorder: 24 Controls: 25 Time to mortality: during hospital stay. Time from sepsis onset to death not described	Sample collection time not described Mean (±SD) age at sepsis: 16.3 (±5.8) days	Significantly lower HLA-DR expression in sepsis group HLA-DR expression was significantly lower in non-survivors compared to survivors No significant difference HLA-DR expression between term and preterm No significant difference HLA-DR expression between clinical and confirmed LOS	(64)
Mix of moderate preterm and term (median GA 36; IQR 32–39 wks)	Clinical ($n = 42$) and confirmed ($n = 21$) EOS and LOS: 63 -Survivor: 50 -Non-survivor: 13 Non-sepsis: 37 Controls: 29 Mortality < 30 days $n = 13$ Time from sepsis onset to death not described	Blood sample taken upon initial suspicion of sepsis Median (IQR) age at sepsis: 4 (2–11) days	HLA-DR expression was significantly decreased in the sepsis group. Lower, but not significantly, in non-survivors compared to survivors	(65)
Preterm (mean GA 31 ± 2 weeks)	EOS: 22 - Mild sepsis: not described -Severe sepsis: not described Controls: Not described	Blood samples taken at admission to NICU during first 48 h of life, during infection, and recovery Mean age at sepsis: Not described	Percent of HLA-DR positive monocytes significantly recovered in those with mild sepsis. Percent expression of HLA-DR on monocytes significantly dropped followed by a significant recovery in those with severe sepsis	(66)*

*HLA-DR, Human Leukocyte Antigen-DR isotype; GA, gestational age; LOS, late-onset sepsis; EOS, early-onset sepsis; VLBW, very low birth weight; SIRS, systemic inflammatory response syndrome; SD, standard deviation; IQR, inter-quartile range. *Conference abstract only, limited data available.*

TABLE 3 | Sepsis-induced immunosuppression—association of immunosuppressive cell expansion with sepsis severity in neonates and adults with sepsis.

Adult or neonatal GA	Cohort sepsis characteristics (*n*) and mortality (if applicable)	Time of blood sampling and age at sepsis	Observation in septic cohort	References
IMMATURE NEUTROPHILS				
Adult	Sepsis: 177 - Sepsis: 82 - Organ dysfunction during sepsis: 66 - Septic shock: 29 Outpatient control: 50 Community-acquired infection without SIRS: 15	Blood sampling was done as part of routine haematological analysis. Sample collection time not described Mean (±SD) age at sepsis: Sepsis: 57 (±22) years Organ dysfunction during sepsis: 62 (±17) years Septic shock: 63 (±14) years	Sepsis group had increased immature granulocytes compared to the two control groups	(67)
Adult	Sepsis: 83 - Confirmed sepsis: 51 - Clinical sepsis: 32 Non-infection SIRS: 39 Non-SIRS: 14 Healthy control: 20	Blood sample was taken within 48 h of admission to the intensive care unit Mean (±SD) age at sepsis: Confirmed sepsis: 62 (±16) years Clinical sepsis: 66 (±13) years	Immature neutrophils were elevated in the sepsis group. Immature neutrophils frequency was significantly higher in confirmed sepsis compared to clinical sepsis and non-infection inflammation	(68)
Adult	Septic shock: 43 - Survivor: 35 - Non-survivors: 8 Healthy controls: 23 Time to mortality: within 28 days of sepsis onset. Time from sepsis onset to death not described	Blood samples were taken at days 3–4 and 6–8 after onset of septic shock Median (IQR) age at septic shock in years: 70 (65–80)	Increased circulating immature granulocytes associated with increased risk of death	(69)
Mix of: Preterm ≤28 weeks GA (*n* = 21) Preterm >28–36 weeks GA (*n* = 123) Term >36 weeks GA (*n* = 141)	Clinical and confirmed EOS (*n* = 76) and LOS (*n* = 134): 210 - Survivor: 222 - Non-survivor: 63 No sepsis: 75 Time from sepsis onset to death not described	Blood sample was taken upon initial suspicion of sepsis Mean (±SD) age at sepsis: 6.7 (±7.4) days	Severity of neutrophil left shift correlates with increased sepsis mortality risk in both preterm and term neonates	(70)
VLBW <1500g (approximate mean GA 27 weeks)	EOS: 5 - Survivor: 0 - Non-survivors: 5 LOS: 15 - Survivor: 0 - Non-survivors: 15 Controls: NA Mean (±SD) age of death: EOS:1.6 (±0.5) days LOS:17.8 (±12.1) days Time from sepsis onset to death not described	Post-mortem examination completed within 2 h of death Mean (±SD) age at sepsis: EOS: 0 (±0) days LOS: 14.1 (±9.9) days	EOS: Slightly elevated, but not significantly, circulating immature neutrophils during early phase of sepsis LOS: Elevated circulating immature neutrophils. Significantly elevated during terminal stages	(71)
T REGULATORY CELLS				
Adult	Sepsis: 80 - Sepsis: 31 - Organ dysfunction during sepsis: 33 - Septic shock: 16 Healthy controls: 18	Blood sample was taken within 24 h after sepsis diagnosis Median (IQR) age at sepsis: Sepsis: 45 (28–72) years Organ dysfunction during sepsis: 54 (18–87) years Septic shock: 64 (18–84) years	Increased Treg mRNA in sepsis patients	(72)
Adult	Sepsis: 32 - Sepsis:19 - Septic shock: 13 Healthy controls: 10	Blood sample was taken at time of sepsis diagnosis Mean (±SD) age at sepsis: 70.8 (±12.7) years	Significantly increased Tregs in $CD4^+$ T cells in sepsis group. Significantly higher in septic shock than sepsis without shock	(57)
Adult	Septic shock: 16 - Survivor: 7 - Non-survivor: 9 Healthy controls: 36	Blood sampling was taken on days 1, 3, 5 and 7–10 following sepsis onset Mean age at sepsis: 54 years	Elevated circulating $CD4^+$ Treg cells in the sepsis group. $CD4^+$ Treg more elevated in non-survivors compared to survivors	(73)
Adult	Sepsis: 118 - Sepsis: 78 - Septic shock: 40 Healthy control: 21	Blood sample was taken the day of study inclusion Median (IQR) age at: Sepsis: 73.5 (62–81) years Septic shock: 78.5 (60–84) years	Increased Tregs in $CD4^+$ T cells in the sepsis group	(74)

(Continued)

TABLE 3 | Continued

Adult or neonatal GA	Cohort sepsis characteristics (*n*) and mortality (if applicable)	Time of blood sampling and age at sepsis	Observation in septic cohort	References
Adult	Sepsis: 42 - Survivor: 23 - Non-survivor: 19 Healthy control: 14 Time to mortality: <28 days. Time from sepsis onset to death not described	Blood samples were taken days 0 and day 5 Mean (±SD) age at sepsis: 49.1 (±10.2) years	Increased CD39+ Tregs in the sepsis group. Higher Treg expression in those with organ failure and non-survivors	(75)
Neonate of any GA	Not assessed	–	–	–
MYELOID DERIVED SUPPRESSOR CELLS				
Adult	Sepsis: 94 - Organ dysfunction during sepsis: 22 - Septic shock: 72 Non-septic ICU: 11 Healthy controls: 67	Blood sample taken within 3 days of sepsis diagnosis Median (IQR) age, in years, at: Organ dysfunction during sepsis: 57 (41–75) Septic shock: 63 (53–73)	In the sepsis group MDSC genes are up-regulated, G-MDSCs expanded and plasma MDSC mediator levels are increased	(76)
Adult	Septic shock: 74 Healthy controls: 18	Blood samples were taken within 12 h of sepsis diagnosis, and on days 1, 4, 7, 14, 21 and 28 Mean age at sepsis: 60 years	MDSCs persistently increased in the septic shock group. MDSCs were functionally immunosuppressive	(77)
Adult	Sepsis: 24 - Sepsis: 12 - Septic shock: 12 Non-sepsis: 12	Blood samples were taken at enrolment, and on days 2–4 and 7-discharge Median (IQR) age at: Sepsis: 45 (39–55) years Septic shock: 52 (45–57) years	G-MDSCs were increased in the sepsis group. G-MDSCs were significantly higher in septic shock compared to sepsis without shock. G-MDSCs were functionally immunosuppressive	(78)
Neonate of any GA	Not assessed	–	–	–

GA, gestational age; LOS, late-onset sepsis; EOS, early-onset sepsis; VLBW, very low birth weight; ICU, intensive care unit; Treg, T regulatory cells; MDSC, myeloid derived suppressor cells; G-MDSC, granulocytic-myeloid derived suppressor cells; SIRS, systemic inflammatory response syndrome; SD, standard deviation; IQR, inter-quartile range.

Gestational age may significantly influence the neonatal cytokine response to infection. In 14 very preterm (mean GA 28.7 ± 1.3 weeks) and 12 moderately preterm (mean GA 34.6 ± 1.8 weeks) neonates with confirmed or clinical sepsis (including LOS and EOS), the cytokine profiles differed (92). During sepsis, the levels of IFNγ, IL-6, IL-10, and IL-4 were significantly elevated in the moderate preterm group only. In contrast, the levels of TNFα did not significantly change from pre-sepsis to during sepsis in either group. These results suggest that increasing GA may be associated with a more robust pro- and anti-inflammatory response. While the lack of inflammatory response in very preterm infants may explain the increased incidence and severity of sepsis (99). The results from this small study do not allow firm conclusions on neonatal clinical outcomes.

Increased IL-6, IL-1β, and IL-8 cytokine production might be associated with sepsis severity and/or mortality in neonates with sepsis (53–55)—study details described in **Table 1**. Silveira-Lessa and colleagues investigated cytokine production in 13 term (GA range 37–42 weeks) neonates with confirmed ($n = 3$) and clinical ($n = 10$) LOS, including 6 with severe sepsis [classified as per the international paediatric consensus definition for sepsis (39)] and 3 with septic shock (53). Higher IL-6 and IL-1β levels were significantly associated with septic shock ($n = 3$) and mortality ($n = 2$), respectively (53). Increased levels of IL-8 and IL-10 were associated with sepsis, whereas TNFα was not changed. The sample size in this study was small, thus limiting the interpretation of significant changes in cytokine levels associated with sepsis severity. Similarly, increased levels of IL-6 and IL-8 persisted for longer in preterm and term neonates with fatal LOS and EOS (combined $n = 26$), whereas the duration of elevated TNFα levels was variable (54, 55). Similar to adults (100, 101), it has been suggested that IL-6 concentrations are a strong indicator of sepsis prognosis in neonates (53, 54). The results from these studies, summarised in **Table 1**, suggest increased and persistent levels of pro-inflammatory mediators correlate with greater neonatal sepsis severity. However, evidence as to the association between persistent anti-inflammatory mediator levels and clinical sepsis severity in neonates remains inconclusive.

The focus of the above neonatal studies was to characterise patterns of cytokine production in septic neonates as potential predictive or diagnostic tools or markers of development, and not necessarily to associate cytokine responses to clinical outcomes. From these results, we can acknowledge that neonates are capable of eliciting a cytokine response similar to that of adults in response to infection (52, 56–58, 72, 89). We cannot, however, infer that the pattern of cytokine production associated with SII and sepsis severity in adults, is also present in these neonates.

Functional Assessment of Cytokine Secretion in Neonatal Sepsis

One study has assessed monocyte cytokine production in 32 extremely (median gestation 25.5 weeks, range <28 weeks) and 44 very (median gestation 29 weeks, range 28–32 weeks) preterm

TABLE 4 | Sepsis-induced immunosuppression—association of effector cell function and programmed cell death-1 receptor expression with sepsis severity in neonates and adults with sepsis.

Adult or neonatal GA	Cohort sepsis characteristics (*n*) and mortality (if applicable)	Time of blood sampling and age at sepsis	Observation in septic cohort	References
Adult	Sepsis: 118 - Sepsis: 78 - Septic shock: 40 Healthy control: 21	Blood sample was taken on day of study inclusion Median (IQR) age at: Sepsis: 73.5 (62–81) years Septic shock: 78.5 (60–84) years	Increased PD-1 expression on Tregs in sepsis group	(74)
Adult	Septic shock: 64 Trauma control: 13 Healthy control: 49	Blood samples were taken on days 1–2, 3–5, and 6–10 after diagnosis Median (IQR) age at septic shock: 64 (54–73) years	Increased PD-1, PD-L1 expression on monocytes, and $CD4^+$ T cells in septic shock group	(79)
Adult	Sepsis: 135 - Sepsis: 59 - Septic shock: 76 Healthy control: 29	Blood samples were taken 3–4 days after onset of symptoms Median (IQR) age at: Sepsis: 71 (66–78) years Septic shock: 71 (61–78) years	Increased PD-L1 expression on monocytes in the sepsis group	(80)
VLBW <1,500 g and ≤32 weeks GA (mean GA 26.8 weeks)	LOS: 39 - Sepsis: 28 - Septic shock: 5 Non-survivors: 6 Control: NA Time to mortality during hospitalisation Time from sepsis onset to death not described	Blood sample was taken within 24 h of symptom onset Age at sepsis not described	Increased PD-L1 expression on monocytes in sepsis group. Significant increases in those with septic shock and/or death compared to survivors of sepsis without shock	(81)

GA, gestational age; LOS, late-onset sepsis; VLBW, very low birth weight; PD-1, programmed cell death protein-1; PD-L1, programmed cell death ligand-1; Tregs, T regulatory cells; SD, standard deviation; IQR, inter-quartile range.

neonates with confirmed ($n = 38$) and clinical ($n = 38$) LOS (102). The authors of this report found that following monocyte stimulation with Pam3Cys, both groups produced equivalent IL-1β, but extremely preterm neonates produced higher IL-18 (102). These results highlight the influence GA has on neonatal immune regulation, but outcomes are limited. There is a need to further investigate if immune cell dysfunction at the time of sepsis underpins immunosuppression in neonatal sepsis.

REDUCED MHC CLASS II EXPRESSION IN ADULT AND NEONATAL SEPSIS

HLA-DR Expression in Adult Sepsis

The upregulation of HLA-DR cell surface expression on APCs is a hallmark of APC activation and essential for increased presentation of antigens to naïve T cells, a critical step for initiating the adaptive immune response (103). Low HLA-DR expression associated with SII is often referred to as immunoparalysis (6, 104, 105) and the established cut-off for identifying immunoparalysis in adult patients with sepsis is <30% HLA-DR positive monocytes (6, 106, 107). In adults, sepsis and septic shock have been shown to negatively affect HLA-DR cell surface expression and cause immunosuppression (52, 61–63, 73, 76, 108)—study details summarised in **Table 2.** Low HLA-DR expression on monocytes and immunoparalysis are related to sepsis severity as shown by a significant increase in SOFA scores in adults with sepsis (61, 62). Monocyte HLA-DR expression is also significantly lower in sepsis non-survivors compared to survivors (52, 59, 61, 63).

Low HLA-DR expression on adult monocytes during sepsis is associated with altered immune responses, including imbalanced secretion of pro- and anti-inflammatory mediators and reduced antigen presentation capacity, and importantly sepsis severity and mortality (52, 59, 61–63). Decreased monocyte HLA-DR expression in critically ill adults with sepsis or septic shock has also been associated with a prominent shift toward significantly increased circulating levels of IL-10 (52, 59, 63). Interestingly, IL-10 mediates HLA-DR expression on monocytes (109–111), suggesting that HLA-DR expression could be a marker of SII-related cytokine changes.

In a study of 17 critically ill adults with sepsis, decreased expression of HLA-DR and CD86 on monocytes and CD28 on lymphocytes was significantly associated with reduced antigen presentation (63). Although the authors did not find any association between the levels of HLA-DR expression or antigen presentation and development of secondary infections, 6 of the 8 patients who survived sepsis went on to develop a secondary infection, 2 of whom later died (63).

Low HLA-DR Expression in Neonatal Sepsis

Several studies reported a decrease in monocyte HLA-DR expression in preterm and term neonates with confirmed or clinical sepsis (including EOS and LOS) (64–66, 93, 112). Neonatal and sepsis characteristics, and relevant outcomes of these studies not in relation to sepsis severity are described in the **Supplementary Table 2.** Decreased HLA-DR expression

TABLE 5 | Sepsis-induced immunosuppression—association of sepsis-induced immune cell apoptosis and depletion with sepsis severity in neonates and adults with sepsis.

Adult or neonatal GA	Cohort sepsis characteristics (*n*) and mortality (if applicable)	Time of blood sampling and age at sepsis	Observation in septic cohort	References
Adult	Prospective study: Sepsis: 71 Non-sepsis:55 Healthy control: 6	Blood samples were collected at various times during sepsis Mean age range at sepsis: 57–59	Increased T cell, B cell, and dendritic cell apoptosis in the sepsis group	(82)
Adult	Prospective study: Septic shock: 19 Healthy control: 22	Blood sample was collected at time of study inclusion Mean (±SD) age at sepsis: 58 (±4) years	Marked increase in apoptosis of $CD4^+$ and $CD8^+$ T cells and B cells in the septic shock group	(83)
Adult	Post-mortem study: Organ dysfunction during sepsis: 40 Trauma control: 29 Median (range) days of sepsis: 4 (1–40). Time from sepsis onset to death not described	Post-mortem sample collection occurred 30–180 min following death Mean (±SD) age at organ dysfunction during sepsis: 71.7 (±15.9) years	Extensive depletion of splenic $CD4^+$ and $CD8^+$ T cells and HLA-DR cells in the organ dysfunction during sepsis group	(84)
Adult	Prospective and post-mortem study Sepsis: 27 - Survivor: 2 - Non-survivors: 25 Non-septic critically ill: 16 Trauma control: 25 Mean age of death and time from sepsis onset to death not described	Sample collection was either intraoperatively (survivors) or post-mortem (15 min to 6 h following death) Mean age as sepsis not described	Depletion of splenic $CD4^+$ T helper cells and B cells in the sepsis group	(85)
VLBW <1,500 g (approximate mean GA 27 weeks)	EOS: 5 - Survivor: 0 - Non-survivors: 5 LOS: 15 - Survivor: 0 - Non-survivors: 15 Controls: NA Mean (±SD) age of death: EOS:1.6 (±0.5) days LOS:17.8 (±12.1) days Time from sepsis onset to death not described	Post-mortem examination completed within 2 h of death Mean (±SD) age at sepsis: EOS: 0 (±0) days LOS: 14.1 (±9.9) days	EOS: No cell depletion LOS: Depletion of thymus lymphocytes	(71)
Moderate preterm (GA range 35–37 weeks)	Sepsis: 6 - Survivor: 0 - Non-survivor:6 Control mortality: 6 Mean age of death and time from sepsis onset to death not described	Post-mortem examination time not described Age at sepsis not described	Depletion of neutrophils in the sepsis group	(86)
Mix of preterm and term (GA mean 29.2 (range 24–38) weeks)	EOS: 10 - Survivor: 0 - Non-survivor: 10 Control mortality: 20 Time to mortality within 48 h after birth. Time from sepsis onset to death not described	Post-mortem examination occurred between 4 and 12 h following death Age at sepsis <48 h after birth	Depletion of T cells and B cells	(87)

GA, gestational age; LOS, late-onset sepsis; EOS, early-onset sepsis; VLBW, very low birth weight; HLA-DR, Human Leukocyte Antigen-DR isotype.

observed in mixed cohorts of preterm and term with neonatal sepsis appears unrelated to the GA (64, 93, 112). Serial assessment of HLA-DR expression during neonatal sepsis demonstrated that 3 days after sepsis onset, HLA-DR expression in both preterm and term neonates were similar to those without sepsis (93). However, low HLA-DR expression is a possible marker of sepsis-related mortality, as monocyte HLA-DR expression is down-regulated in term and preterm non-survivors of sepsis compared to survivors (64, 65)—study details summarised in **Table 2**. In this small study, Genel et al reported a significant decrease in monocyte HLA-DR expression between non-survivor ($n = 8$) and survivor ($n = 32$) preterm and term (median GA 36 weeks) neonates with confirmed ($n = 18$) and clinical ($n = 22$) LOS (mean postnatal age 16.3 days) (64). The preterm and term neonates with ≤30% HLA-DR positive monocytes had a 30-fold higher risk of mortality (Odds ratio 30); with 53.8% mortality among those with ≤30% HLA-DR positive monocytes compared to only 3.7% in neonates with >30% HLA-DR positive monocytes (64), similar to adults with confirmed immunoparalysis (61). Unlike for HLA-DR surface expression levels, the proportion of cells expressing any HLA-DR in neonates is correlated with GA and acts as a predisposing factor for sepsis as reported in 31 very low birth weight infants (VLBW; GA range 23–31 weeks) with clinical (n = 14) and confirmed (n = 17) sepsis (EOS n = 2 and LOS n = 29) (113). Pradhan et al. suggested that monocyte HLA-DR expression, combined with CD64 expression on neutrophils, may be a useful prognostic marker for neonatal sepsis (65).

There is a decrease in HLA-DR positive monocytes among preterm and term neonates with sepsis, compared to non-septic neonates (64, 66, 93, 112, 114, 115). Decreased HLA-DR positive monocytes in neonates with sepsis appears unrelated to the GA (64, 93, 112). Fotopoulos et al. monitored the proportion of HLA-DR positive monocytes over the course of a septic episode in preterm neonates (mean GA 31 weeks), with and without EOS (66). They reported that the percentage of HLA-DR positive monocytes significantly recovered over the course of sepsis in those neonates with mild sepsis, while those with severe sepsis showed a significant drop followed by a rise only upon recovery (66). While the authors did not provide the criteria for defining sepsis severity, this data may suggest that a decreased percentage of HLA-DR positive monocytes is associated with sepsis severity in neonates, however additional research in this area is essential.

EXPANSION OF IMMUNOSUPPRESSIVE CELLS IN ADULT AND NEONATAL SEPSIS

Immature Neutrophils in Adult Sepsis

The ability of immature neutrophils to suppress T cell proliferation was first observed by Pillay et al. (116), although the mechanism for suppression remains unclear. An increased frequency of immature neutrophils has been observed in adults with sepsis and is associated with sepsis severity, poor clinical outcomes, and increased risk of septic shock and mortality (67–69)—study details summarised in **Table 3**. As sepsis becomes more severe in adults, the increased frequency in immature neutrophil has been shown to be associated with a decrease in T cell proliferation (67).

Immature Neutrophils in Neonatal Sepsis

While neonates with sepsis have increased numbers of circulating immature neutrophils compared to neonates without sepsis, this is not a reliable diagnostic marker (117–121). There is a paucity of data on whether the T cell suppressive function of immature neutrophils contributes to sepsis severity, adverse outcomes, and increased mortality in neonatal sepsis. Saied and colleagues evaluated neutrophil left shift for its predictive value in sepsis outcomes in extremely preterm (n = 21; GA range ≤28 weeks), very/moderate preterm (n = 123; GA range >28–36 weeks), and term (n = 141; GA range >36 weeks) neonates with confirmed or clinical sepsis (EOS n = 76; LOS n = 134) (70). Although T cell function was not assessed in this study, they found that an increase in left shift (and hence proportions of immature neutrophils) correlates with increased sepsis mortality risk in preterm and term neonates (70). Further to this, Itoh et al. found a high number of circulating immature neutrophils, in addition to depleted lymphocytes in the thymus and hypertrophic spleen, in 15 VLBW infants (<1,500 g) that died from confirmed LOS (mean time from sepsis onset to death 3.7 ± 3.3 days) (71). Yet, the number of circulating immature neutrophils was only slightly elevated during the initial stage of sepsis the neonates that died from confirmed EOS (n = 5; mean time from sepsis onset to death 1.6 ± 0.5 days) (71). However, the number of neonates with sepsis were low and a non-septic control group was lacking for comparison. The frequency of immature neutrophils and its relation to sepsis severity observed in both neonates and adults are summarised in **Table 3.** These two studies suggest that immature neutrophils may be associated with worse outcomes with neonatal sepsis, however, further studies with larger sample size and non-septic controls are essential. Whether increased numbers of immature neutrophils are a consequence of sepsis or whether they cause more severe infection due to their immunosuppressive function on T cells remains to be determined in neonatal sepsis.

Regulatory T Cells (Tregs) in Adult Sepsis

Tregs play an important role in the maintenance of immune homeostasis, however their role in immunosuppression during sepsis is not entirely clear (7, 122, 123). Several studies have reported an elevated proportion of Tregs following the onset of sepsis or septic shock in adults, and associated this with an increased risk of immunosuppression, mortality, and morbidity (57, 72–75)—study details summarised in **Table 3**. The increased risk of mortality associated with sepsis and sepsis shock may be attributed to the immunosuppressive functions of Tregs by: (a) directly inhibiting effector CD4+ T cell proliferation and cytokine secretion (124–126); (b) indirectly supressing APC/T-cell receptor mediated CD4+ and CD8+ T cell activation (125–127); (c) suppressing T cell activation through increased expression of programmed cell death-1 (PD-1) receptor (128); or (d) suppressing other immune effector cells such as natural killer cells, B cells, and monocytes (129–131).

Regulatory T Cells (Tregs) in Neonatal Sepsis

Identifying the role of Tregs in neonatal sepsis is an emerging area of research. The proportion of Tregs is elevated in term neonates with confirmed sepsis (n = 30) (132). Likewise, the proportion of Tregs is higher in 22 preterm neonates (mean GA 28.1 ± 3.7 weeks) with clinical EOS (133). Sepsis severity and mortality were not discussed in these studies, nor was the age of sepsis onset. Surprisingly, unlike cord blood (134–137), the elevated proportion of Tregs reported in septic neonates may not be affected by GA (133), suggesting sepsis alone, and not gestation, influences Treg frequency, postnatally. There are no data on the potential impact of Tregs on sepsis severity, immunosuppression, or mortality during neonatal sepsis. Treg frequencies and further functional analysis is required to determine whether Tregs suppress T cell proliferation and function during neonatal sepsis, as observed in adults with SII (74, 122, 123, 125).

Myeloid-Derived Suppressor Cells (MDSCs) in Adult Sepsis

In healthy adults, the immature cells of the myeloid lineage, namely monocytic- and granulocytic-MDSCs, rapidly differentiate into DCs, macrophages, and granulocytes and act to preserve innate immunity (138). The expansion of MDSCs to suppress both the innate and adaptive immune responses is a phenomenon under investigation in adults with SII (77, 138). MDSC expansion has been observed in adults with sepsis and septic shock (76–78, 138), as summarised in **Table 3**. The immune suppressive characteristics of MDSC expansion, namely inhibition of T cell proliferation (76–78, 138) and increased secretion of immunosuppressive mediator IL-10 (78, 138), have been observed in adults with sepsis. MDSC expansion is associated with sepsis severity (77, 78) and adverse outcomes, such as chronic immune suppression following prolonged MDSC expansion in critically ill adults with sepsis (77). Expansion of MDSCs has also been shown to be associated with higher risk for subsequent nosocomial infections (76, 77), a characteristic found among patients with SII. However, the frequency of MDSCs among sepsis survivors and non-survivors was found to be similar, suggesting MDSC expansion alone does not influence mortality (76).

Myeloid-Derived Suppressor Cells (MDSCs) in Neonatal Sepsis

Only one group has investigated the frequency of MDSCs during neonatal sepsis, and found a significant increase in the frequency of MDSCs in 10 preterm neonates (mean GA 25 ± 3 weeks) with early- and late-onset clinical (80%) and confirmed (20%) sepsis compared to preterm neonates (GA range 23 to <37 weeks) without sepsis (139). No associations with severity or sepsis outcomes were made in this study. With the limited data and small sample size in this publication the characterisation of MDSCs during neonatal sepsis requires further evaluation.

PROLONGED IMMUNOSUPPRESSION AND ALARMINS

Alarmins (also referred to as damage-associated molecular patterns), such as S100A8 and S100A9, are pro-inflammatory mediators present in low levels in circulating myeloid cells, namely monocytes and granulocytes, even in healthy subjects. S100A8 and S1009A are up-regulated in response to bacterial products, as well as pro- (e.g., TNFα and IL-1β) and anti-inflammatory cytokines (e.g., IL-10 and transforming growth factor β) (140). Up-regulation of S100A8 and S100A9 positively regulates MDSC frequency and function (141, 142), stimulates Treg expansion (140), and induces endotoxin tolerance by rendering phagocytes unresponsive to secondary Toll-Like Receptor-4 stimulation (143). Whether S100A8 and S100A9 function to enhance inflammation or to support immunosuppression is still unclear.

Alarmins in Adult Sepsis

Plasma levels of S100A8 and S100A9 were elevated, as was up-regulation of S100A12, S100A9, and arginase-1 gene expression, in adults with sepsis, compared to non-septic patients in intensive care (76). The increased levels of S100A12, S100A9, and arginase-1 were associated with MDSC expansion, and high initial levels of granulocytic-MDSCs, arginase-1 and S100A12 were associated with subsequent infections (76). Alarmins, such as the S100 proteins, may therefore, play multiple roles in adult SII.

Alarmins in Neonatal Sepsis

S100A8/A9 levels were elevated in eight neonates with confirmed sepsis (144). Gestational age, postnatal age at sepsis onset and relation of alarmin levels to the severity of the sepsis were not discussed. Whether alarmins, such as S100A8/S100A9, play a role in MDSC expansion and immunosuppression in neonatal sepsis requires further investigation.

COMPROMISED T CELL EFFECTOR CELL FUNCTION IN ADULT AND NEONATAL SEPSIS

Immune Checkpoint Molecule Expression in Adult Sepsis

The increased expression of the negative co-stimulatory molecule PD-1, and its associated ligand (PD-L1), on circulating monocytes, neutrophils and effector T cells may contribute to SII (79). Increased expression of PD-1/PD-L1 on monocytes and lymphocytes is associated with decreased monocyte HLA-DR expression, increased proportions of Tregs, and T cell exhaustion (3, 4, 79, 145–147). Several groups have reported an over-expression of PD-1 on T cells, including CD4+ and Tregs, and PD-L1 on monocytes in adults with sepsis and septic shock compared to healthy adults (74, 79, 80, 83, 84). Increased expression of PD-1 and PD-L1 on lymphocytes and monocytes is associated with more organ dysfunction during sepsis and increased risk of secondary infections and mortality (74, 79, 80), as summarised in **Table 4**. In addition, increased PD-L1 expression on monocytes has been shown to be an independent predictor of mortality in septic shock patients (80).

PD-1/PD-1L are inhibitory immune checkpoint molecules and blockade of their function to interact with other immune cells is being explored as a therapeutic agent for reversing the effects of immunosuppression (148). Pre-clinical models of sepsis, have shown that blockade of the PD-1/PD-L1 pathway with an antagonistic anti-PD-L1 antibody improves survival by inhibiting lymphocyte apoptosis and T cell exhaustion (145, 149, 150). Further to this, *in vitro* blockade of the PD-1/PD-L1 pathway in the blood from septic adults, decreases lymphocyte apoptosis, increases pro-inflammatory cytokine production and decreases IL-10 production (83, 146). Antibody blockade of PD-1 or PD-L1 as an immunomodulatory therapy for reversing immunosuppression is being trialled to improve survival in human patients with cancer (151). This promising therapy may spark exploration for PD-1 blockade immunotherapy in sepsis.

Immune Checkpoint Molecule Expression in Neonatal Sepsis

Despite the interest in exploring PD-1 blockade for reversing immunosuppression in septic adults, there is a paucity of data pertaining to PD-1 and PD-L1 expression or T cell exhaustion in neonates, and importantly neonates with sepsis. PD-1 expression was increased in 34 VLBW (<1,500 g and GA range ≤32 weeks) with confirmed LOS, and expression was significantly increased in 5 preterm infants with septic shock (identified using the international paediatric consensus criteria) and/or mortality ($n = 6$) compared to surviving preterm infants without shock (81). The role of GA on PD-1 expression during neonatal sepsis has not been explored. The results from this study, summarised in **Table 4**, suggest increased PD-1 expression may have an immunosuppressive function in neonatal sepsis, however with the limited available data this interpretation remains inconclusive.

Interestingly, Young and colleagues recently investigated the role of PD-1 in murine neonates and found improved survival in septic PD-1 knockout mice, further supporting the functional importance of PD-1 in neonatal sepsis and related mortality (152). The therapeutic potential for targeted blockade of PD-1 means that this is an area that deserves urgent exploration.

Up-regulation of carcinoembryonic antigen-related cell-adhesion molecule 1 (CEACAM1), another inhibitory immune checkpoint molecule (153), on T cells leads to reduced proliferation and cytokine secretion causing T cell suppression and subsequent prolonged immunosuppression (154, 155). Although not reported in adults with SII, the percentage of CEACAM1-positive CD4+ T cells in 12 preterm neonates with LOS is increased compared to 16 non-septic controls (155). With the small sample size and limited available data it is inconclusive as to whether increased expression of CEACAM1 on CD4+ T cells contributes to immunosuppression in septic neonates and thus requires further investigation.

SEPSIS-INDUCED IMMUNE CELL APOPTOSIS IN ADULTS AND NEONATES

Immune Cell Apoptosis in Adult Sepsis

Cell death is an important step for resolving infection and maintaining immune homeostasis. However, sepsis-induced immune cell apoptosis, resulting in an overwhelming depletion of immune cells, including T cells (CD4+ and CD8+), B cells, and DCs, is evident in prospective studies of adults with sepsis (82, 83). Similar findings have been reported in post-mortem studies of adults who died from sepsis, septic shock, and sepsis-related multiple organ dysfunction (84, 85, 156, 157)—study details summarised in **Table 5**. The degree of immune cell apoptosis has been shown to be correlated with sepsis severity, supporting a role for apoptosis in SII (82). In support of this concept, in mice *in vivo* prevention of cell death improves sepsis survival (158–162).

Immune Cell Apoptosis in Neonatal Sepsis

Three post-mortem studies have reported lymphocyte depletion in the spleen, thymus, and bone marrow in both preterm and term neonates that died from EOS and LOS compared to neonates that died of causes other than sepsis (71, 86, 87). The sample size in all three studies was small, with 5–15 neonates in the sepsis groups. There were conflicting results between the two studies that reported on lymphocyte depletion following EOS (71, 87). Only two of the three studies described the time from sepsis onset to death; death occurred within 48 h after sepsis onset for EOS (71, 87) and, on average, 3.7 (± 3.3) days following sepsis onset for LOS (71). These results, summarised in **Table 5**, suggest both term and preterm neonates with severe sepsis may develop sepsis-induced immune cell apoptosis, however there are no prospective studies to support this conclusion. Sepsis-induced immune cell apoptosis in relation to disease severity has not been assessed in neonates. A mouse model of neonatal sepsis found that blocking necroptosis, programmed cell death triggered by the caspase-independent pathway through death receptors, by inhibition of receptor-interacting protein kinase 1 with necrostatin-1, reduced lung injury associated with sepsis and improved survival (162).

IS SEPSIS-INDUCED IMMUNOSUPPRESSION A FEATURE OF NEONATAL SEPSIS?

In adults, SII is associated with increased risk of multi-organ failure and mortality as well as susceptibility to secondary viral and bacterial infections (3, 4, 6, 8). Similar clinical characteristics, including increased risk of multi-organ failure and mortality, are observed in neonatal sepsis (31, 163–165). It is unclear if these adverse outcomes observed in neonates are due to an overwhelming hyper-inflammatory immune response and/or SII. From the limited data available, it appears that fatal neonatal sepsis may be associated with alterations in immune function that are in agreement with SII findings in adults (3, 4, 6). The dysregulated immune responses observed in various neonatal studies include imbalanced secretion of pro- and anti-inflammatory mediators (53–55), diminished HLA-DR monocyte surface expression (64), expansion of immature neutrophils (70, 71), increased expression of PD-1/PD-L1 (81), and depletion of leukocytes (71, 86, 87). Published neonatal studies are limited by: (i) small sample size of neonates, (ii) incomplete reporting of time from sepsis onset to death, and (iii) the lack of consistent neonatal sepsis definition and objective measures for the degree of severity.

Despite distinct patterns of causative pathogens in adult and neonatal sepsis, similar immune function alterations are observed and endotoxin tolerance appears to be a feature in both adult and neonatal sepsis (9, 35). Therefore, SII may occur independently as a feature of the subsequent host response to inflammation.

In adults, SII is associated with increased susceptibility to secondary bacterial infections and associated late mortality (166, 167). Whether this is a result of organ damage or persistent SII is unclear. Interestingly, one study reported that the immune alterations associated with SII in adult septic shock survivors continued until discharge from the intensive care unit, but resolved by 6 months (168). It is unclear if survivors of neonatal sepsis remain at increased risk of developing subsequent infections (31, 163, 169–171). Preterm infants may have more than one episode of sepsis (~20%) during their NICU admission, and it is uncertain whether having a previous episode of sepsis contributes to the overall risk compared to the major risk factor that is degree of immaturity (31, 163, 169). Preterm neonates, remain at increased risk of infection-related admissions to hospital well into childhood (inversely related to both GA and birth weight) (172), however if neonatal sepsis contributes to infection-related hospital readmissions in childhood has not been studied. Increased risk of subsequent, more severe infections is a hallmark of SII in adults, but it is unclear if this clinical outcome is observed in neonates with sepsis.

CONCLUSIONS

Sepsis mortality in neonates may be associated with alterations in immune function that are in agreement with SII findings in adults. Whether immune cell dysfunction or impairment underpins immunosuppression in neonatal sepsis requires further investigation and stronger evidence. Large, collaborative longitudinal studies, from birth through to childhood, are essential to evaluate immune changes in neonates with sepsis, including the role for SII. Yet, first a definitive consensus on the definition of neonatal sepsis and severity needs to be established. Until then, sepsis severity could be measured by mortality. Advances in further understanding the immunological mechanisms behind immunosuppression may lead to effective targeted treatment therapies for reversing or modulating SII and improve outcomes. Immunosuppression reversal with PD-1/PD-L1 antibody blockade is currently being trialled in adult cancer patients who share similar immune defects as those with SII (151). Furthermore, pentoxifylline, an immune modulatory drug, is currently being trialled to improve long-term outcomes, primarily neurodevelopment impairment, associated with neonatal sepsis (ANZCTR ACTRN12616000405415). Assessing the impact of such interventions on SII-associated markers may provide a mechanistic insight into the success or failure of these interventions in preventing short and long-term negative sepsis outcomes.

AUTHOR CONTRIBUTIONS

JH conceived and wrote the first and subsequent drafts. TS and AC conceived and revised the manuscript.

ACKNOWLEDGMENTS

TS is supported by a Raine Medical Research Foundation Clinician Research Fellowship.

REFERENCES

1. Fleischmann C, Scherag A, Adhikari NK, Hartog CS, Tsaganos T, Schlattmann P, et al. Assessment of global incidence and mortality of hospital-treated sepsis. Current estimates and limitations. *Am J Respir Crit Care Med.* (2016) 193:259–72. doi: 10.1164/rccm.201504-0781OC
2. Singer M, Deutschman CS, Seymour CW, Shankar-Hari M, Annane D, Bauer M, et al. The Third International Consensus Definitions for Sepsis and Septic Shock (Sepsis-3). *JAMA.* (2016) 315:801–10. doi: 10.1001/jama.2016.0287
3. Hotchkiss RS, Monneret G, Payen D. Sepsis-induced immunosuppression: from cellular dysfunctions to immunotherapy. *Nat Rev Immunol.* (2013) 13:862–74. doi: 10.1038/nri3552
4. Hotchkiss RS, Monneret G, Payen D. Immunosuppression in sepsis: a novel understanding of the disorder and a new therapeutic approach. *Lancet Infect Dis.* (2013) 13:260–8. doi: 10.1016/S1473-3099(13)70001-X
5. Lyle NH, Pena OM, Boyd JH, Hancock RE. Barriers to the effective treatment of sepsis: antimicrobial agents, sepsis definitions, and host-directed therapies. *Ann N Y Acad Sci.* (2014) 1323:101–14. doi: 10.1111/nyas.12444
6. Pfortmueller CA, Meisel C, Fux M, Schefold JC. Assessment of immune organ dysfunction in critical illness: utility of innate immune response markers. *Intensive Care Med Exp.* (2017) 5:49. doi: 10.1186/s40635-017-0163-0
7. Venet F, Monneret G. Advances in the understanding and treatment of sepsis-induced immunosuppression. *Nat Rev Nephrol.* (2018) 14:121–37. doi: 10.1038/nrneph.2017.165
8. Arens C, Bajwa SA, Koch C, Siegler BH, Schneck E, Hecker A, et al. Sepsis-induced long-term immune paralysis–results of a descriptive, explorative study. *Crit Care* (2016) 20:93. doi: 10.1186/s13054-016-1233-5
9. Pena OM, Hancock DG, Lyle NH, Linder A, Russell JA, Xia J, et al. An endotoxin tolerance signature predicts sepsis and organ dysfunction at initial clinical presentation. *EBioMedicine* (2014) 1:64–71. doi: 10.1016/j.ebiom.2014.10.003
10. Cavaillon JM, Adib-Conquy M. Bench-to-bedside review: endotoxin tolerance as a model of leukocyte reprogramming in sepsis. *Crit Care* (2006) 10:233. doi: 10.1186/cc5055
11. Dobrovolskaia MA, Medvedev AE, Thomas KE, Cuesta N, Toshchakov V, Ren T, et al. Induction of *in vitro* reprogramming by Toll-like receptor (TLR)2 and TLR4 agonists in murine macrophages: effects of TLR "homotolerance" versus "heterotolerance" on NF-kappa B signaling pathway components. *J Immunol.* (2003) 170:508–19. doi: 10.4049/jimmunol.170.1.508
12. Levy O. Innate immunity of the newborn: basic mechanisms and clinical correlates. *Nat Rev Immunol.* (2007) 7:379–90. doi: 10.1038/nri2075
13. Basha S, Surendran N, Pichichero M. Immune responses in neonates. *Expert Rev Clin Immunol.* (2014) 10:1171–84. doi: 10.1586/1744666X.2014.942288
14. MacGillivray DM, Kollmann TR. The role of environmental factors in modulating immune responses in early life. *Front Immunol.* (2014) 5:434. doi: 10.3389/fimmu.2014.00434
15. Shah BA, Padbury JF. Neonatal sepsis: an old problem with new insights. *Virulence* (2014) 5:170–8. doi: 10.4161/viru.26906

16. van Well GTJ, Daalderop LA, Wolfs T, Kramer BW. Human perinatal immunity in physiological conditions and during infection. *Mol Cell Pediatr.* (2017) 4:4. doi: 10.1186/s40348-017-0070-1
17. Melville JM, Moss TJ. The immune consequences of preterm birth. *Front Neurosci.* (2013) 7:79. doi: 10.3389/fnins.2013.00079
18. Sharma AA, Jen R, Butler A, Lavoie PM. The developing human preterm neonatal immune system: a case for more research in this area. *Clin Immunol.* (2012) 145:61–8. doi: 10.1016/j.clim.2012.08.006
19. Raymond SL, Rincon JC, Wynn JL, Moldawer LL, Larson SD. Impact of early-life exposures to infections, antibiotics, and vaccines on perinatal and long-term health and disease. *Front Immunol.* (2017) 8:729. doi: 10.3389/fimmu.2017.00729
20. Liu L, Oza S, Hogan D, Perin J, Rudan I, Lawn JE, et al. Global, regional, and national causes of child mortality in 2000–13, with projections to inform post-2015 priorities: an updated systematic analysis. *Lancet* (2015) 385:430–40. doi: 10.1016/S0140-6736(14)61698-6
21. Greenberg RG, Kandefer S, Do BT, Smith PB, Stoll BJ, Bell EF, et al. Late-onset sepsis in extremely premature infants: 2000–2011. *Pediatr Infect Dis J.* (2017) 36:774–9. doi: 10.1097/INF.0000000000001570
22. Barton L, Hodgman JE, Pavlova Z. Causes of death in the extremely low birth weight infant. *Pediatrics* (1999) 103:446–51. doi: 10.1542/peds.103.2.446
23. Strunk T, Inder T, Wang X, Burgner D, Mallard C, Levy O. Infection-induced inflammation and cerebral injury in preterm infants. *Lancet Infect Dis.* (2014) 14:751–62. doi: 10.1016/S1473-3099(14)70710-8
24. Stoll BJ, Hansen NI, Adams-Chapman I, Fanaroff AA, Hintz SR, Vohr B, et al. Neurodevelopmental and growth impairment among extremely low-birth-weight infants with neonatal infection. *JAMA* (2004) 292:2357–65. doi: 10.1001/jama.292.19.2357
25. Sonneville R, Verdonk F, Rauturier C, Klein IF, Wolff M, Annane D, et al. Understanding brain dysfunction in sepsis. *Ann Intensive Care* (2013) 3:15. doi: 10.1186/2110-5820-3-15
26. Strunk T, Currie A, Richmond P, Simmer K, Burgner D. Innate immunity in human newborn infants: prematurity means more than immaturity. *J Matern Fetal Neonatal Med.* (2011) 24:25–31. doi: 10.3109/14767058.2010.482605
27. Wynn JL, Wong HR. Pathophysiology and treatment of septic shock in neonates. *Clin Perinatol.* (2010) 37:439–79. doi: 10.1016/j.clp.2010.04.002
28. Khaertynov KS, Boichuk SV, Khaiboullina SF, Anokhin VA, Andreeva AA, Lombardi VC, et al. Comparative assessment of cytokine pattern in early and late onset of neonatal sepsis. *J Immunol Res.* (2017) 2017:8601063. doi: 10.1155/2017/8601063
29. Schultz C, Rott C, Temming P, Schlenke P, Moller JC, Bucsky P. Enhanced interleukin-6 and interleukin-8 synthesis in term and preterm infants. *Pediatr Res.* (2002) 51:317–22. doi: 10.1203/00006450-200203000-00009
30. Rittirsch D, Flierl MA, Ward PA. Harmful molecular mechanisms in sepsis. *Nat Rev Immunol.* (2008) 8:776–87. doi: 10.1038/nri2402
31. Stoll BJ, Hansen N, Fanaroff AA, Wright LL, Carlo WA, Ehrenkranz RA, et al. Late-onset sepsis in very low birth weight neonates: the experience of the NICHD Neonatal Research Network. *Pediatrics* (2002) 110(2 Pt 1):285–91. doi: 10.1542/peds.110.2.285
32. Stoll BJ, Hansen NI, Sanchez PJ, Faix RG, Poindexter BB, Van Meurs KP, et al. Early onset neonatal sepsis: the burden of group B Streptococcal and *E. coli* disease continues. *Pediatrics* (2011) 127:817–26. doi: 10.1542/peds.2010-2217
33. Wynn JL, Wilson CS, Hawiger J, Scumpia PO, Marshall AF, Liu JH, et al. Targeting IL-17A attenuates neonatal sepsis mortality induced by IL-18. *Proc Natl Acad Sci USA.* (2016) 113:E2627–35. doi: 10.1073/pnas.1515793113
34. Roger T, Schneider A, Weier M, Sweep FC, Le Roy D, Bernhagen J, et al. High expression levels of macrophage migration inhibitory factor sustain the innate immune responses of neonates. *Proc Natl Acad Sci USA.* (2016) 113:E997–1005. doi: 10.1073/pnas.1514018113
35. Maddux AB, Douglas IS. Is the developmentally immature immune response in paediatric sepsis a recapitulation of immune tolerance? *Immunology* (2015) 145:1–10. doi: 10.1111/imm.12454
36. Cortese F, Scicchitano P, Gesualdo M, Filaninno A, De Giorgi E, Schettini F, et al. Early and late infections in newborns: where do we stand? A review. *Pediatr Neonatol.* (2016) 57:265–73. doi: 10.1016/j.pedneo.2015.09.007
37. Vincent JL, Rello J, Marshall J, Silva E, Anzueto A, Martin CD, et al. International study of the prevalence and outcomes of infection in intensive care units. *JAMA.* (2009) 302:2323–9. doi: 10.1001/jama.2009.1754
38. Gervassi AL, Horton H. Is infant immunity actively suppressed or immature? *Virology* (2014) 2014:1–9. doi: 10.4137/VRT.S12248
39. Goldstein B, Giroir B, Randolph A. International pediatric sepsis consensus conference: definitions for sepsis and organ dysfunction in pediatrics. *Pediatr Crit Care Med.* (2005) 6:2–8. doi: 10.1097/00130478-200501000-00049
40. Hofer N, Zacharias E, Muller W, Resch B. Performance of the definitions of the systemic inflammatory response syndrome and sepsis in neonates. *J Perinat Med.* (2012) 40:587–90. doi: 10.1515/jpm-2011-0308
41. Wynn JL. Defining neonatal sepsis. *Curr Opin Pediatr.* (2016) 28:135–40. doi: 10.1097/MOP.0000000000000315
42. Wynn JL, Wong HR, Shanley TP, Bizzarro MJ, Saiman L, Polin RA. Time for a neonatal-specific consensus definition for sepsis. *Pediatr Crit Care Med.* (2014) 15:523–8. doi: 10.1097/PCC.0000000000000157
43. Ng S, Strunk T, Jiang P, Muk T, Sangild PT, Currie A. Precision medicine for neonatal sepsis. *Front Mol Biosci.* (2018) 5:70. doi: 10.3389/fmolb.2018.00070
44. Meem M, Modak JK, Mortuza R, Morshed M, Islam MS, Saha SK. Biomarkers for diagnosis of neonatal infections: a systematic analysis of their potential as a point-of-care diagnostics. *J Glob Health* (2011) 1:201–9.
45. Dong Y, Speer CP. Late-onset neonatal sepsis: recent developments. *Arch Dis Child Fetal Neonatal Ed.* (2015) 100:F257–63. doi: 10.1136/archdischild-2014-306213
46. Melvan JN, Bagby GJ, Welsh DA, Nelson S, Zhang P. Neonatal sepsis and neutrophil insufficiencies. *Int Rev Immunol.* (2010) 29:315–48. doi: 10.3109/08830181003792803
47. Guilmot A, Hermann E, Braud VM, Carlier Y, Truyens C. Natural killer cell responses to infections in early life. *J Innate Immun.* (2011) 3:280–8. doi: 10.1159/000323934
48. Lawrence SM, Eckert J, Makoni M, Pereira HA. Is the use of complete blood counts with manual differentials an antiquated method of determining neutrophil composition in newborns? *Ann Clin Lab Sci.* (2015) 45:403–13.
49. Simon AK, Hollander GA, McMichael A. Evolution of the immune system in humans from infancy to old age. *Proc Biol Sci.* (2015) 282:20143085. doi: 10.1098/rspb.2014.3085
50. Camacho-Gonzalez A, Spearman PW, Stoll BJ. Neonatal infectious diseases: evaluation of neonatal sepsis. *Pediatr Clin North Am.* (2013) 60:367–89. doi: 10.1016/j.pcl.2012.12.003
51. Maddux AB, Hiller TD, Overdier KH, Pyle LL, Douglas IS. Innate immune function and organ failure recovery in adults with sepsis. *J Intensive Care Med.* 2017:885066617701903. doi: 10.1177/0885066617701903
52. Monneret G, Finck ME, Venet F, Debard AL, Bohe J, Bienvenu J, et al. The anti-inflammatory response dominates after septic shock: association of low monocyte HLA-DR expression and high interleukin-10 concentration. *Immunol Lett.* (2004) 95:193–8. doi: 10.1016/j.imlet.2004.07.009
53. Silveira-Lessa AL, Quinello C, Lima L, Redondo ACC, Ceccon M, Carneiro-Sampaio M, et al. TLR expression, phagocytosis and oxidative burst in healthy and septic newborns in response to Gram-negative and Gram-positive rods. *Hum. Immunol.* (2016) 77:972–80. doi: 10.1016/j.humimm.2016.07.230
54. Prashant A, Vishwanath P, Kulkarni P, Sathya Narayana P, Gowdara V, Nataraj SM, et al. Comparative assessment of cytokines and other inflammatory markers for the early diagnosis of neonatal sepsis-a case control study. *PLoS ONE* (2013) 8:e68426. doi: 10.1371/journal.pone.0068426
55. Kocabas E, Sarikcioglu A, Aksaray N, Seydaoglu G, Seyhun Y, Yaman A. Role of procalcitonin, C-reactive protein, interleukin-6, interleukin-8 and tumor necrosis factor-alpha in the diagnosis of neonatal sepsis. *Turk J Pediatr.* (2007) 49:7–20.
56. Tamayo E, Fernandez A, Almansa R, Carrasco E, Heredia M, Lajo C, et al. Pro- and anti-inflammatory responses are regulated simultaneously from the first moments of septic shock. *Eur Cytokine Netw.* (2011) 22:82–7. doi: 10.1684/ecn.2011.0281

57. Ono S, Kimura A, Hiraki S, Takahata R, Tsujimoto H, Kinoshita M, et al. Removal of increased circulating CD4+CD25+Foxp3+ regulatory T cells in patients with septic shock using hemoperfusion with polymyxin B-immobilized fibers. *Surgery* (2013) 153:262–71. doi: 10.1016/j.surg.2012.06.023
58. van Dissel JT, van Langevelde P, Westendorp RG, Kwappenberg K, Frolich M. Anti-inflammatory cytokine profile and mortality in febrile patients. *Lancet* (1998) 351:950–3. doi: 10.1016/S0140-6736(05)60606-X
59. Hynninen M, Pettila V, Takkunen O, Orko R, Jansson SE, Kuusela P, et al. Predictive value of monocyte histocompatibility leukocyte antigen-DR expression and plasma interleukin-4 and−10 levels in critically ill patients with sepsis. *Shock* (2003) 20:1–4. doi: 10.1097/01.shk.0000068322.08268.b4
60. Weighardt H, Heidecke CD, Emmanuilidis K, Maier S, Bartels H, Siewert JR, et al. Sepsis after major visceral surgery is associated with sustained and interferon-gamma-resistant defects of monocyte cytokine production. *Surgery* (2000) 127:309–15. doi: 10.1067/msy.2000.104118
61. Papadopoulos P, Pistiki A, Theodorakopoulou M, Christodoulopoulou T, Damoraki G, Goukos D, et al. Immunoparalysis: clinical and immunological associations in SIRS and severe sepsis patients. *Cytokine* (2017) 92:83–92. doi: 10.1016/j.cyto.2017.01.012
62. Winkler MS, Rissiek A, Priefler M, Schwedhelm E, Robbe L, Bauer A, et al. Human leucocyte antigen (HLA-DR) gene expression is reduced in sepsis and correlates with impaired TNFα response: a diagnostic tool for immunosuppression? *PLoS ONE* (2017) 12:e0182427. doi: 10.1371/journal.pone.0182427
63. Manjuck J, Saha DC, Astiz M, Eales LJ, Rackow EC. Decreased response to recall antigens is associated with depressed costimulatory receptor expression in septic critically ill patients. *J Lab Clin Med.* (2000) 135:153–60. doi: 10.1067/mlc.2000.104306
64. Genel F, Atlihan F, Ozsu E, Ozbek E. Monocyte HLA-DR expression as predictor of poor outcome in neonates with late onset neonatal sepsis. *J Infect.* (2010) 60:224–8. doi: 10.1016/j.jinf.2009.12.004
65. Pradhan R, Jain P, Paria A, Saha A, Sahoo J, Sen A, et al. Ratio of neutrophilic CD64 and monocytic HLA-DR: a novel parameter in diagnosis and prognostication of neonatal sepsis. *Cytometry B Clin Cytom.* (2016) 90:295–302. doi: 10.1002/cyto.b.21244
66. Fotopoulos S, Debonera F, Stamokosta E, Paterakis G, Stavropoulos-Giokas C, Germenis A, et al., (eds.). The monocyte HLA-DR expression of healthy and infected premature neonates. *Pediatr Res* (1999) 45:763.
67. Guerin E, Orabona M, Raquil MA, Giraudeau B, Bellier R, Gibot S, et al. Circulating immature granulocytes with T-cell killing functions predict sepsis deterioration*. *Crit Care Med.* (2014) 42:2007–18. doi: 10.1097/CCM.0000000000000344
68. Mare TA, Treacher DF, Shankar-Hari M, Beale R, Lewis SM, Chambers DJ, et al. The diagnostic and prognostic significance of monitoring blood levels of immature neutrophils in patients with systemic inflammation. *Crit Care* (2015) 19:57. doi: 10.1186/s13054-015-0778-z
69. Demaret J, Venet F, Friggeri A, Cazalis MA, Plassais J, Jallades L, et al. Marked alterations of neutrophil functions during sepsis-induced immunosuppression. *J Leukoc Biol.* (2015) 98:1081–90. doi: 10.1189/jlb.4A0415-168RR
70. Saied DA. Can we rely on the neutrophil left shift for the diagnosis of neonatal sepsis? Need for re-evaluation. *Egypt Pediatr Assoc Gaz.* (2018) 66. doi: 10.1016/j.epag.2017.12.002
71. Itoh K, Aihara H, Takada S, Nishino M, Lee Y, Negishi H, et al. Clinicopathological differences between early-onset and late-onset sepsis and pneumonia in very low birth weight infants. *Pediatr Pathol.* (1990) 10:757–68. doi: 10.3109/15513819009064710
72. Li J, Li M, Su L, Wang H, Xiao K, Deng J, et al. Alterations of T helper lymphocyte subpopulations in sepsis, severe sepsis, and septic shock: a prospective observational study. *Inflammation* (2015) 38:995–1002. doi: 10.1007/s10753-014-0063-3
73. Monneret G, Debard AL, Venet F, Bohe J, Hequet O, Bienvenu J, et al. Marked elevation of human circulating CD4+CD25+ regulatory T cells in sepsis-induced immunoparalysis. *Crit Care Med.* (2003) 31:2068–71. doi: 10.1097/01.CCM.0000069345.78884.0F
74. Liu Q, An L, Qi Z, Zhao Y, Li C. Increased expression of programmed cell death-1 in regulatory T cells of patients with severe sepsis and septic shock: an observational clinical study. *Scand J Immunol.* (2017) 86:408–17. doi: 10.1111/sji.12612
75. Huang H, Xu R, Lin F, Bao C, Wang S, Ji C, et al. High circulating CD39(+) regulatory T cells predict poor survival for sepsis patients. *Int J Infect Dis.* (2015) 30:57–63. doi: 10.1016/j.ijid.2014.11.006
76. Uhel F, Azzaoui I, Gregoire M, Pangault C, Dulong J, Tadie JM, et al. Early expansion of circulating granulocytic myeloid-derived suppressor cells predicts development of nosocomial infections in patients with sepsis. *Am J Respir Crit Care Med.* (2017) 196:315–27. doi: 10.1164/rccm.201606-1143OC
77. Mathias B, Delmas AL, Ozrazgat-Baslanti T, Vanzant EL, Szpila BE, Mohr AM, et al. Human myeloid-derived suppressor cells are associated with chronic immune suppression after severe sepsis/septic shock. *Ann Surg.* (2017) 265:827–34. doi: 10.1097/SLA.0000000000001783
78. Darcy CJ, Minigo G, Piera KA, Davis JS, McNeil YR, Chen Y, et al. Neutrophils with myeloid derived suppressor function deplete arginine and constrain T cell function in septic shock patients. *Crit. Care* (2014) 18:R163. doi: 10.1186/cc14003
79. Guignant C, Lepape A, Huang X, Kherouf H, Denis L, Poitevin F, et al. Programmed death-1 levels correlate with increased mortality, nosocomial infection and immune dysfunctions in septic shock patients. *Crit Care* (2011) 15:R99. doi: 10.1186/cc10112
80. Shao R, Fang Y, Yu H, Zhao L, Jiang Z, Li CS. Monocyte programmed death ligand-1 expression after 3–4 days of sepsis is associated with risk stratification and mortality in septic patients: a prospective cohort study. *Crit Care* (2016) 20:124. doi: 10.1186/s13054-016-1301-x
81. Zasada M, Lenart M, Rutkowska-Zapala M, Stec M, Durlak W, Grudzien A, et al. Analysis of PD-1 expression in the monocyte subsets from non-septic and septic preterm neonates. *PLoS ONE.* (2017) 12:e0186819. doi: 10.1371/journal.pone.0186819
82. Hotchkiss RS, Osmon SB, Chang KC, Wagner TH, Coopersmith CM, Karl IE. Accelerated lymphocyte death in sepsis occurs by both the death receptor and mitochondrial pathways. *J Immunol.* (2005) 174:5110–8. doi: 10.4049/jimmunol.174.8.5110
83. Zhang Y, Li J, Lou J, Zhou Y, Bo L, Zhu J, et al. Upregulation of programmed death-1 on T cells and programmed death ligand-1 on monocytes in septic shock patients. *Crit Care* (2011) 15:R70. doi: 10.1186/cc10059
84. Boomer JS, To K, Chang KC, Takasu O, Osborne DF, Walton AH, et al. Immunosuppression in patients who die of sepsis and multiple organ failure. *JAMA.* (2011) 306:2594–605. doi: 10.1001/jama.2011.1829
85. Hotchkiss RS, Tinsley KW, Swanson PE, Schmieg RE, Jr., Hui JJ, Chang KC, et al. Sepsis-induced apoptosis causes progressive profound depletion of B and CD4+ T lymphocytes in humans. *J Immunol.* (2001) 166:6952–63. doi: 10.4049/jimmunol.166.11.6952
86. Christensen RD, Rothstein G. Exhaustion of mature marrow neutrophils in neonates with sepsis. *J Pediatr.* (1980) 96:316–8. doi: 10.1016/S0022-3476(80)80837-7
87. Toti P, De Felice C, Occhini R, Schuerfeld K, Stumpo M, Epistolato MC, et al. Spleen depletion in neonatal sepsis and chorioamnionitis. *Am J Clin Pathol.* (2004) 122:765–71. doi: 10.1309/RV6E9BMC9954A2WU
88. Striz I, Brabcova E, Kolesar L, Sekerkova A. Cytokine networking of innate immunity cells: a potential target of therapy. *Clin Sci.* (2014) 126:593–612. doi: 10.1042/CS20130497
89. Munoz C, Carlet J, Fitting C, Misset B, Bleriot JP, Cavaillon JM. Dysregulation of *in vitro* cytokine production by monocytes during sepsis. *J Clin Invest.* (1991) 88:1747–54. doi: 10.1172/JCI115493
90. Rigato O, Salomao R. Impaired production of interferon-gamma and tumor necrosis factor-alpha but not of interleukin 10 in whole blood of patients with sepsis. *Shock* (2003) 19:113–6. doi: 10.1097/00024382-200302000-00004
91. Sinistro A, Almerighi C, Ciaprini C, Natoli S, Sussarello E, Di Fino S, et al. Downregulation of CD40 ligand response in monocytes from sepsis patients. *Clin Vacc Immunol.* (2008) 15:1851–8. doi: 10.1128/CVI.00184-08
92. Segura-Cervantes E, Mancilla-Ramirez J, Gonzalez-Canudas J, Alba E, Santillan-Ballesteros R, Morales-Barquet D, et al. Inflammatory response in

preterm and very preterm newborns with sepsis. *Mediat inflamm.* (2016) 2016:6740827. doi: 10.1155/2016/6740827
93. Drossou-Agakidou V, Kanakoudi-Tsakalidou F, Sarafidis K, Tzimouli V, Taparkou A, Kremenopoulos G, et al. *In vivo* effect of rhGM-CSF And rhG-CSF on monocyte HLA-DR expression of septic neonates. *Cytokine* (2002) 18:260–5. doi: 10.1006/cyto.2002.1037
94. Ng PC, Li K, Wong RP, Chui K, Wong E, Li G, et al. Proinflammatory and anti-inflammatory cytokine responses in preterm infants with systemic infections. *Arch Dis Child Fetal Neonatal Ed.* (2003) 88:F209–13. doi: 10.1136/fn.88.3.F209
95. Ye Q, Du LZ, Shao WX, Shang SQ. Utility of cytokines to predict neonatal sepsis. *Pediatr Res.* (2017) 81:616–21. doi: 10.1038/pr.2016.267
96. Silveira RC, Procianoy RS. Evaluation of interleukin-6, tumour necrosis factor-alpha and interleukin-1beta for early diagnosis of neonatal sepsis. *Acta Paediatr.* (1999) 88:647–50. doi: 10.1080/08035259950169314
97. Engelberts I, Stephens S, Francot GJ, van der Linden CJ, Buurman WA. Evidence for different effects of soluble TNF-receptors on various TNF measurements in human biological fluids. *Lancet* (1991) 338:515–6. doi: 10.1016/0140-6736(91)90591-C
98. van Deuren M. Kinetics of tumour necrosis factor-alpha, soluble tumour necrosis factor receptors, interleukin 1-beta and its receptor antagonist during serious infections. *Eur J Clin Microbiol Infect Dis.* (1994) 13(Suppl. 1):S12–6. doi: 10.1007/BF02390680
99. Afonso EDP, Blot S. Effect of gestational age on the epidemiology of late-onset sepsis in neonatal intensive care units - a review. *Expert Rev Anti Infect. Ther.* (2017) 15:917–24. doi: 10.1080/14787210.2017.1379394
100. Jekarl DW, Lee SY, Lee J, Park YJ, Kim Y, Park JH, et al. Procalcitonin as a diagnostic marker and IL-6 as a prognostic marker for sepsis. *Diagn Microbiol Infect Dis.* (2013) 75:342–7. doi: 10.1016/j.diagmicrobio.2012.12.011
101. Barre M, Behnes M, Hamed S, Pauly D, Lepiorz D, Lang S, et al. Revisiting the prognostic value of monocyte chemotactic protein 1 and interleukin-6 in the sepsis-3 era. *J Crit Care* (2018) 43:21–8. doi: 10.1016/j.jcrc.2017.08.024
102. Zasada M, Lenart M, Rutkowska-Zapala M, Stec M, Mol N, Czyz O, et al. Analysis of selected aspects of inflammasome function in the monocytes from neonates born extremely and very prematurely. *Immunobiology* (2018) 223:18–24. doi: 10.1016/j.imbio.2017.10.019
103. Parihar A, Eubank TD, Doseff AI. Monocytes and macrophages regulate immunity through dynamic networks of survival and cell death. *J Innate Immun.* (2010) 2:204–15. doi: 10.1159/000296507
104. Hamers L, Kox M, Pickkers P. Sepsis-induced immunoparalysis: mechanisms, markers, and treatment options. *Mine Anestesiol.* (2015) 814)426–39.
105. Sundar KM, Sires M. Sepsis induced immunosuppression: implications for secondary infections and complications. *Ind J Crit Care Med.* (2013) 17:162–9. doi: 10.4103/0972-5229.117054
106. Docke WD, Hoflich C, Davis KA, Rottgers K, Meisel C, Kiefer P, et al. Monitoring temporary immunodepression by flow cytometric measurement of monocytic HLA-DR expression: a multicenter standardized study. *Clin Chem.* (2005) 51:2341–7. doi: 10.1373/clinchem.2005.052639
107. Frazier WJ, Hall MW. Immunoparalysis and adverse outcomes from critical illness. *Pediatr Clin North Am.* (2008) 55:647–68, xi. doi: 10.1016/j.pcl.2008.02.009
108. Lukaszewicz AC, Grienay M, Resche-Rigon M, Pirracchio R, Faivre V, Boval B, et al. Monocytic HLA-DR expression in intensive care patients: interest for prognosis and secondary infection prediction. *Crit Care Med.* (2009) 37:2746–52. doi: 10.1097/CCM.0b013e3181ab858a
109. de Waal Malefyt R, Haanen J, Spits H, Roncarolo MG, te Velde A, Figdor C, et al. Interleukin 10 (IL-10) and viral IL-10 strongly reduce antigen-specific human T cell proliferation by diminishing the antigen-presenting capacity of monocytes via downregulation of class II major histocompatibility complex expression. *J Exp Med.* (1991) 174:915–24. doi: 10.1084/jem.174.4.915
110. Koppelman B, Neefjes JJ, de Vries JE, de Waal Malefyt R. Interleukin-10 down-regulates MHC class II alphabeta peptide complexes at the plasma membrane of monocytes by affecting arrival and recycling. *Immunity* (1997) 7:861–71. doi: 10.1016/S1074-7613(00)80404-5
111. Fumeaux T, Pugin J. Role of interleukin-10 in the intracellular sequestration of human leukocyte antigen-DR in monocytes during septic shock. *Am J Respir Crit Care Med.* (2002) 166:1475–82. doi: 10.1164/rccm.200203-217OC
112. Kanakoudi-Tsakalidou F, Debonera F, Drossou-Agakidou V, Sarafidis K, Tzimouli V, Taparkou A, et al. Flow cytometric measurement of HLA-DR expression on circulating monocytes in healthy and sick neonates using monocyte negative selection. *Clin Exp Immunol.* (2001) 123:402–7. doi: 10.1046/j.1365-2249.2001.01471.x
113. Palojarvi A, Petaja J, Siitonen S, Janer C, Andersson S. Low monocyte HLA-DR expression as an indicator of immunodepression in very low birth weight infants. *Pediatr Res.* (2013) 73(4 Pt 1):469–75. doi: 10.1038/pr.2012.199
114. Juskewitch JE, Abraham RS, League SC, Jenkins SM, Smith CY, Enders FT, et al. Monocyte HLA-DR expression and neutrophil CD64 expression as biomarkers of infection in critically ill neonates and infants. *Pediatr Res.* (2015) 78:683–90. doi: 10.1038/pr.2015.164
115. Skrzeczynska J, Kobylarz K, Hartwich Z, Zembala M, Pryjma J. CD14+CD16+ monocytes in the course of sepsis in neonates and small children: monitoring and functional studies. *Scand J Immunol.* (2002) 556):629–38. doi: 10.1046/j.1365-3083.2002.01092.x
116. Pillay J, Kamp VM, van Hoffen E, Visser T, Tak T, Lammers JW, et al. A subset of neutrophils in human systemic inflammation inhibits T cell responses through Mac-1. *J Clin Invest.* (2012) 122:327–36. doi: 10.1172/JCI57990
117. Newman TB, Draper D, Puopolo KM, Wi S, Escobar GJ. Combining immature and total neutrophil counts to predict early onset sepsis in term and late preterm newborns: use of the I/T2. *Pediatr Infect Dis J.* (2014) 33:798–802. doi: 10.1097/INF.0000000000000297
118. Mikhael M, Brown LS, Rosenfeld CR. Serial neutrophil values facilitate predicting the absence of neonatal early-onset sepsis. *J Pediatr.* (2014) 164:522 -528.e3. doi: 10.1016/j.jpeds.2013.10.080
119. Murphy K, Weiner J. Use of leukocyte counts in evaluation of early-onset neonatal sepsis. *Pediatr Infect Dis J.* (2012) 31:16–9. doi: 10.1097/INF.0b013e31822ffc17
120. Cimenti C, Erwa W, Herkner KR, Kasper DC, Muller W, Resch B. The predictive value of immature granulocyte count and immature myeloid information in the diagnosis of neonatal sepsis. *Clin Chem Lab Med.* (2012) 50:1429–32. doi: 10.1515/cclm-2011-0656
121. Hornik CP, Benjamin DK, Becker KC, Benjamin DK, Jr., Li J, Clark RH, et al. Use of the complete blood cell count in late-onset neonatal sepsis. *Pediatr Infect Dis J.* (2012) 31:803–7. doi: 10.1097/INF.0b013e31825691e4
122. Cao C, Ma T, Chai YF, Shou ST. The role of regulatory T cells in immune dysfunction during sepsis. *World J Emerg Med.* (2015) 6:5–9. doi: 10.5847/wjem.j.1920-8642.2015.01.001
123. Wan YY. Regulatory T cells: immune suppression and beyond. *Cell Mol Immunol.* (2010) 7:204–10. doi: 10.1038/cmi.2010.20
124. Dieckmann D, Plottner H, Berchtold S, Berger T, Schuler G. *Ex vivo* isolation and characterization of CD4(+)CD25(+) T cells with regulatory properties from human blood. *J Exp Med.* (2001) 193:1303–10. doi: 10.1084/jem.193.11.1303
125. Schmidt A, Oberle N, Krammer PH. Molecular mechanisms of treg-mediated T cell suppression. *Front Immunol.* (2012) 3:51. doi: 10.3389/fimmu.2012.00051
126. Sakaguchi S, Wing K, Onishi Y, Prieto-Martin P, Yamaguchi T. Regulatory T cells: how do they suppress immune responses? *Int Immunol.* (2009) 21:1105–11. doi: 10.1093/intimm/dxp095
127. Levings MK, Sangregorio R, Roncarolo MG. Human cd25(+)cd4(+) t regulatory cells suppress naive and memory T cell proliferation and can be expanded *in vitro* without loss of function. *J Exp Med.* (2001) 193:1295–302. doi: 10.1084/jem.193.11.1295
128. Parry RV, Chemnitz JM, Frauwirth KA, Lanfranco AR, Braunstein I, Kobayashi SV, et al. CTLA-4 and PD-1 receptors inhibit T-cell activation by distinct mechanisms. *Mol Cell Biol.* (2005) 25:9543–53. doi: 10.1128/MCB.25.21.9543-9553.2005
129. Ghiringhelli F, Menard C, Terme M, Flament C, Taieb J, Chaput N, et al. CD4+CD25+ regulatory T cells inhibit natural killer cell functions in a transforming growth factor-beta-dependent

manner. *J Exp Med.* (2005) 202:1075–85. doi: 10.1084/jem.20051511
130. Taams LS, van Amelsfort JM, Tiemessen MM, Jacobs KM, de Jong EC, Akbar AN, et al. Modulation of monocyte/macrophage function by human CD4+CD25+ regulatory T cells. *Hum Immunol.* (2005) 66:222–30. doi: 10.1016/j.humimm.2004.12.006
131. Lim HW, Hillsamer P, Banham AH, Kim CH. Cutting edge: direct suppression of B cells by CD4+ CD25+ regulatory T cells. *J Immunol.* (2005) 175:4180–3. doi: 10.4049/jimmunol.175.7.4180
132. Behrendt J, Karpe J, Mazur B, Stojewska M, Sadownik B, Wasek A, et al. [Quantitative changes of CD3+, CD4+, CD8+, HLA-DR+, T lymphocytes and CD25+ cells in eutrophic full-term neonates with staphylococcal septicemia]. *Przegl lek.* (2002) 59(Suppl. 1):50–3.
133. Pagel J, Hartz A, Figge J, Gille C, Eschweiler S, Petersen K, et al. Regulatory T cell frequencies are increased in preterm infants with clinical early-onset sepsis. *Clin Exp Immunol.* (2016) 185:219–27. doi: 10.1111/cei.12810
134. Takahata Y, Nomura A, Takada H, Ohga S, Furuno K, Hikino S, et al. CD25+CD4+ T cells in human cord blood: an immunoregulatory subset with naive phenotype and specific expression of forkhead box p3 (Foxp3) gene. *Exp Hematol.* (2004) 32:622–9. doi: 10.1016/j.exphem.2004.03.012
135. Dirix V, Vermeulen F, Mascart F. Maturation of CD4+ regulatory T lymphocytes and of cytokine secretions in infants born prematurely. *J Clin. Immunol.* (2013) 33:1126–33. doi: 10.1007/s10875-013-9911-4
136. Luciano AA, Arbona-Ramirez IM, Ruiz R, Llorens-Bonilla BJ, Martinez-Lopez DG, Funderburg N, et al. Alterations in regulatory T cell subpopulations seen in preterm infants. *PLoS ONE* (2014) 9:e95867. doi: 10.1371/journal.pone.0095867
137. Rueda CM, Moreno-Fernandez ME, Jackson CM, Kallapur SG, Jobe AH, Chougnet CA. Neonatal regulatory T cells have reduced capacity to suppress dendritic cell function. *Eur J Immunol.* (2015) 45:2582–92. doi: 10.1002/eji.201445371
138. Janols H, Bergenfelz C, Allaoui R, Larsson AM, Ryden L, Bjornsson S, et al. A high frequency of MDSCs in sepsis patients, with the granulocytic subtype dominating in gram-positive cases. *J Leukoc Biol.* (2014) 96:685–93. doi: 10.1189/jlb.5HI0214-074R
139. Schwarz J, Scheckenbach V, Kugel H, Spring B, Pagel J, Hartel C, et al. Granulocytic myeloid-derived suppressor cells (GR-MDSC) accumulate in cord blood of preterm infants and remain elevated during the neonatal period. *Clin Exp Immunol.* (2018) 191:328–37. doi: 10.1111/cei.13059
140. El Gazzar M. Immunobiology of S100A8 and S100A9 proteins and their role in acute inflammation and sepsis. *Int J Immunol Immunother.* (2015) 2:2. doi: 10.23937/2378-3672/1410013
141. Cheng P, Corzo CA, Luetteke N, Yu B, Nagaraj S, Bui MM, et al. Inhibition of dendritic cell differentiation and accumulation of myeloid-derived suppressor cells in cancer is regulated by S100A9 protein. *J Exp Med.* (2008) 205:2235–49. doi: 10.1084/jem.20080132
142. Sinha P, Okoro C, Foell D, Freeze HH, Ostrand-Rosenberg S, Srikrishna G. Proinflammatory S100 proteins regulate the accumulation of myeloid-derived suppressor cells. *J Immunol.* (2008) 181:4666–75. doi: 10.4049/jimmunol.181.7.4666
143. Austermann J, Friesenhagen J, Fassl SK, Petersen B, Ortkras T, Burgmann J, et al. Alarmins MRP8 and MRP14 induce stress tolerance in phagocytes under sterile inflammatory conditions. *Cell Rep.* (2014) 9:2112–23. doi: 10.1016/j.celrep.2014.11.020
144. Decembrino L, De Amici M, Pozzi M, De Silvestri A, Stronati M. Serum calprotectin: a potential biomarker for neonatal sepsis. *J Immunol Res.* (2015) 2015:147973. doi: 10.1155/2015/147973
145. Brahmamdam P, Inoue S, Unsinger J, Chang KC, McDunn JE, Hotchkiss RS. Delayed administration of anti-PD-1 antibody reverses immune dysfunction and improves survival during sepsis. *J Leukoc Biol.* (2010) 88:233–40. doi: 10.1189/jlb.0110037
146. Chang K, Svabek C, Vazquez-Guillamet C, Sato B, Rasche D, Wilson S, et al. Targeting the programmed cell death 1: programmed cell death ligand 1 pathway reverses T cell exhaustion in patients with sepsis. *Crit Care* (2014) 18:R3. doi: 10.1186/cc13176
147. de Kleijn S, Langereis JD, Leentjens J, Kox M, Netea MG, Koenderman L, et al. IFN-gamma-stimulated neutrophils suppress lymphocyte proliferation through expression of PD-L1. *PLoS ONE* (2013) 8:e72249. doi: 10.1371/journal.pone.0072249
148. Patil NK, Guo Y, Luan L, Sherwood ER. Targeting immune cell checkpoints during sepsis. *Int J Mol Sci.* (2017) 18:2413. doi: 10.3390/ijms18112413
149. Zhang Y, Zhou Y, Lou J, Li J, Bo L, Zhu K, et al. PD-L1 blockade improves survival in experimental sepsis by inhibiting lymphocyte apoptosis and reversing monocyte dysfunction. *Crit Care* (2010) 14:R220. doi: 10.1186/cc9354
150. Huang X, Venet F, Wang YL, Lepape A, Yuan Z, Chen Y, et al. PD-1 expression by macrophages plays a pathologic role in altering microbial clearance and the innate inflammatory response to sepsis. *Proc Natl Acad Sci USA.* (2009) 106:6303–8. doi: 10.1073/pnas.0809422106
151. Topalian SL, Hodi FS, Brahmer JR, Gettinger SN, Smith DC, McDermott DF, et al. Safety, activity, and immune correlates of anti-PD-1 antibody in cancer. *New Engl J Med.* (2012) 366:2443–54. doi: 10.1056/NEJMoa1200690
152. Young WA, Fallon EA, Heffernan DS, Efron PA, Cioffi WG, Ayala A. Improved survival after induction of sepsis by cecal slurry in PD-1 knockout murine neonates. *Surgery* (2017) 161:1387–93. doi: 10.1016/j.surg.2016.11.008
153. Markel GS, Y.; Mandel, I.; Hakim, M.; Shaked, R.;. Inhibition of the novel immune checkpoint CEACAM1 to enhance anti-tumor immunological activity. *J Clin Oncol.* (2016) 34(15 Suppl.):3044. doi: 10.1200/JCO.2016.34.15_suppl.3044
154. Chen CJ, Shively JE. The cell-cell adhesion molecule carcinoembryonic antigen-related cellular adhesion molecule 1 inhibits IL-2 production and proliferation in human T cells by association with Src homology protein-1 and down-regulates IL-2 receptor. *J Immunol.* (2004) 172:3544–52. doi: 10.4049/jimmunol.172.6.3544
155. van der Flier M, Sharma DB, Estevao S, Emonts M, Rook D, Hazelzet JA, et al. Increased CD4(+) T cell co-inhibitory immune receptor CEACAM1 in neonatal sepsis and soluble-CEACAM1 in meningococcal sepsis: a role in sepsis-associated immune suppression? *PLoS ONE* (2013) 8:e68294. doi: 10.1371/journal.pone.0068294
156. Hotchkiss RS, Swanson PE, Freeman BD, Tinsley KW, Cobb JP, Matuschak GM, et al. Apoptotic cell death in patients with sepsis, shock, and multiple organ dysfunction. *Crit Care Med.* (1999) 27:1230–51. doi: 10.1097/00003246-199907000-00002
157. Hotchkiss RS, Tinsley KW, Swanson PE, Grayson MH, Osborne DF, Wagner TH, et al. Depletion of dendritic cells, but not macrophages, in patients with sepsis. *J Immunol.* (2002) 168:2493–500. doi: 10.4049/jimmunol.168.5.2493
158. Hotchkiss RS, Swanson PE, Knudson CM, Chang KC, Cobb JP, Osborne DF, et al. Overexpression of Bcl-2 in transgenic mice decreases apoptosis and improves survival in sepsis. *J Immunol.* (1999) 162:4148–56.
159. Hotchkiss RS, Chang KC, Grayson MH, Tinsley KW, Dunne BS, Davis CG, et al. Adoptive transfer of apoptotic splenocytes worsens survival, whereas adoptive transfer of necrotic splenocytes improves survival in sepsis. *Proc Natl Acad Sci USA.* (2003) 100:6724–9. doi: 10.1073/pnas.1031788100
160. Inoue S, Unsinger J, Davis CG, Muenzer JT, Ferguson TA, Chang K, et al. IL-15 prevents apoptosis, reverses innate and adaptive immune dysfunction, and improves survival in sepsis. *J Immunol.* (2010) 184:1401–9. doi: 10.4049/jimmunol.0902307
161. Meng Y, Zhao Z, Zhu W, Yang T, Deng X, Bao R. CD155 blockade improves survival in experimental sepsis by reversing dendritic cell dysfunction. *Biochem Biophys Res Commun.* (2017) 490:283–9. doi: 10.1016/j.bbrc.2017.06.037
162. Bolognese AC, Yang WL, Hansen LW, Denning NL, Nicastro JM, Coppa GF, et al. Inhibition of necroptosis attenuates lung injury and improves survival in neonatal sepsis. *Surgery.* (2018) 2018:S0039-6060(18)30096-5. doi: 10.1016/j.surg.2018.02.017
163. Tsai MH, Hsu JF, Chu SM, Lien R, Huang HR, Chiang MC, et al. Incidence, clinical characteristics and risk factors for adverse outcome in

neonates with late-onset sepsis. *Pediatr Infect Dis J.* (2014) 33:e7–e13. doi: 10.1097/INF.0b013e3182a72ee0

164. Qazi SA, Stoll BJ. Neonatal sepsis: a major global public health challenge. *Pediatr Infect Dis J.* (2009) 28(1 Suppl.):S1–2. doi: 10.1097/INF.0b013e31819587a9
165. Liu L, Johnson HL, Cousens S, Perin J, Scott S, Lawn JE, et al. Global, regional, and national causes of child mortality: an updated systematic analysis for 2010 with time trends since 2000. *Lancet* (2012) 379:2151–61. doi: 10.1016/S0140-6736(12)60560-1
166. Prescott HC, Osterholzer JJ, Langa KM, Angus DC, Iwashyna TJ. Late mortality after sepsis: propensity matched cohort study. *BMJ* (2016) 353:i2375. doi: 10.1136/bmj.i2375
167. Ou SM, Chu H, Chao PW, Lee YJ, Kuo SC, Chen TJ, et al. Long-term mortality and major adverse cardiovascular events in sepsis survivors. A nationwide population-based study. *Am J Res Crit Care Med.* (2016) 194:209–17. doi: 10.1164/rccm.201510-2023OC
168. Zorio V, Venet F, Delwarde B, Floccard B, Marcotte G, Textoris J, et al. Assessment of sepsis-induced immunosuppression at ICU discharge and 6 months after ICU discharge. *Ann Intens Care* (2017) 7:80. doi: 10.1186/s13613-017-0304-3
169. Makhoul IR, Sujov P, Smolkin T, Lusky A, Reichman B. Epidemiological, clinical, and microbiological characteristics of late-onset sepsis among very low birth weight infants in Israel: a national survey. *Pediatrics* (2002) 109:34–9. doi: 10.1542/peds.109.1.34
170. Lin CB, Hornik CP, Clark R, Cotten CM, Benjamin DK, Jr., Cohen-Wolkoweiz M, et al. Very low birth weight neonates who survive early-onset sepsis do not have an increased risk of developing late-onset sepsis. *Early Hum Dev.* (2012) 88:905–9. doi: 10.1016/j.earlhumdev.2012.07.009
171. Wynn JL, Hansen NI, Das A, Cotten CM, Goldberg RN, Sanchez PJ, et al. Early sepsis does not increase the risk of late sepsis in very low birth weight neonates. *J Pediatr.* (2013) 162:942 -948.e3 doi: 10.1016/j.jpeds.2012.11.027
172. Miller JE, Hammond GC, Strunk T, Moore HC, Leonard H, Carter KW, et al. Association of gestational age and growth measures at birth with infection-related admissions to hospital throughout childhood: a population-based, data-linkage study from Western Australia. *Lancet Infect. Dis.* (2016) 16:952–61. doi: 10.1016/S1473-3099(16)00150-X

11

Predictors of Mortality in Neonates and Infants Hospitalized with Sepsis or Serious Infections in Developing Countries

Li(Danny) Liang[1]*, Naima Kotadia*[2]*, Lacey English*[3]*, Niranjan Kissoon*[4,5]*, J. Mark Ansermino*[5,6,7]*, Jerome Kabakyenga*[8,9]*, Pascal M. Lavoie*[10] *and Matthew O. Wiens*[5,6,9*]

[1] Faculty of Medicine, University of Toronto, Toronto, ON, Canada, [2] Faculty of Medicine, University of British Columbia, Vancouver, BC, Canada, [3] School of Medicine, University of North Carolina, Chapel Hill, NC, United States, [4] Department of Pediatrics, University of British Columbia, Vancouver, BC, Canada, [5] Center for International Child Health, British Columbia Children's Hospital, Vancouver, BC, Canada, [6] Department of Anesthesiology, Pharmacology and Therapeutics, Faculty of Medicine, University of British Columbia, Vancouver, BC, Canada, [7] Department of Anesthesia, British Columbia Children's Hospital and University of British Columbia, Vancouver, BC, Canada, [8] Maternal Newborn and Child Health Institute, Mbarara University of Science and Technology, Mbarara, Uganda, [9] Faculty of Medicine, Mbarara University of Science and Technology, Mbarara, Uganda, [10] Division of Neonatology, Department of Pediatrics, University of British Columbia, Vancouver, BC, Canada

***Correspondence:**
Matthew O. Wiens
matthew.wiens@cw.bc.ca

Background: Neonates and infants comprise the majority of the 6 million annual deaths under 5 years of age around the world. Most of these deaths occur in low/middle income countries (LMICs) and are preventable. However, the clinical identification of neonates and infants at imminent risk of death is challenging in developing countries.

Objective: To systematically review the literature on clinical risk factors for mortality in infants under 12 months of age hospitalized for sepsis or serious infections in LMICs.

Methods: MEDLINE and EMBASE were systematically searched using MeSH terms through April 2017. Abstracts were independently screened by two reviewers. Subsequently, full-text articles were selected by two independent reviewers based on PICOS criteria for inclusion in the final analysis. Study data were qualitatively synthesized without quantitative pooling of data due to heterogeneity in study populations and methodology.

Results: A total of 1,139 abstracts were screened, and 169 full-text articles were selected for text review. Of these, 45 articles were included in the analysis, with 21 articles featuring neonatal populations (under 28 days of age) exclusively. Most studies were from Sub-Saharan Africa and South Asia. Risk factors for mortality varied significantly according to study populations. For neonatal deaths, prematurity, low birth-weight and young age at presentation were most frequently associated with mortality. For infant deaths, malnutrition, lack of breastfeeding and low oxygen saturation were associated with mortality in the highest number of studies.

Conclusions: Risk factors for mortality differ between the neonatal and young infant age groups and were also dependant on the study population. These data can serve as a starting point for the development of individualized predictive models for in-hospital and post-discharge mortality and for the development of interventions to improve outcomes among these high-risk groups.

Keywords: risk prediction, neonatal mortality, infant mortality, systematic review, developing countries, infectious disease, sepsis, hospital mortality

INTRODUCTION

Significant progresses have been made over the past two decades in reducing global under-5 mortality from 91 deaths per 1,000 live births in 1990 to 43 deaths per 1,000 live births in 2015 (1). However, mortality in neonates (under 28 days of age) and infants (under 1 year of age) remains disproportionately high, representing over two-thirds of under-5 deaths in children below 5 years of age (2). Of these deaths, 90% occur in developing countries (3), with the highest neonatal mortality rates occurring in Sub-Saharan Africa. Thus, interventions among neonates and infants are urgently needed in these countries if the recent UN Sustainable Development Goals are to be achieved, targeting to decrease under-5 mortality to <25 per 1,000 live births and neonatal mortality to <12 per 1,000 live births by 2030 (4, 5).

Reducing mortality in neonates and young infants has lagged significantly behind that of older pediatric populations (6). Although no consensus has been made, some studies suggest preterm birth, intrapartum complications, and sepsis are leading causes of death among neonates (7). The relative risk of death from these events ranges from 10 to 36 times greater in LMICs, as compared to high income countries (3).

A population-based health survey in 56 countries from 1990 to 2002 identified main factors contributing to infant mortality around the world, including first births, shorter birth interval, male sex, gestational multiplicity, and rural setting (8, 9). Infants of mothers with less education or who lived further away from health care resources were also at greater risk of death (8, 9).

However, in spite of this knowledge, our ability to develop effective interventions for this age group remains limited, as causes of death are multi-factorial and often involve a greater social context. Published systematic reviews have attempted to discern more age-specific factors, but these studies have largely focused on high resource settings (10). Given that the greatest burden of neonatal and infant deaths occur in LMICs, this is an important limitation (11). Finally, underserved populations tend to have limited research, making the benefits of systematic reviews in the identification of gaps in these cases all the more impactful (12, 13).

The objective of this systematic review was to develop an evidence base of studies assessing risk factors for mortality among newborns and infants who are hospitalized in LMICs. The focus of this literature review was serious infections and sepsis, as they are the most commonly identified, and potentially highly preventable (14), causes of neonatal and infant deaths in LMICs.

METHODS

Study Eligibility Criteria and Systematic Search

This systematic review focused on children <1 year old evaluated for sepsis or other serious infections in LMICs. Study eligibility was defined according to the conventional Populations, Interventions, Comparators, Outcomes, and Study Design (PICOS) criteria, determined *a priori* (**Table 1**).

A study was included if (i) it presented original data from either a prospective or retrospective cohort study or from a randomized controlled trial, (ii) the majority of the subjects were under 1 year of age or a multivariate analysis adjusting for age was conducted, or a subgroup analysis for specific mortality risk factors was collected for patients <1 year old,

TABLE 1 | PICOS criteria outlining study eligibility.

Criteria	Inclusion
Population	Newborns and young infants hospitalized with sepsis or other serious infection in a resource poor/developing country (majority of patients must be <1 year of age, or a multivariate analysis adjusting for age must be conducted) • Studies conducted in developed countries will be excluded • Studies involving non-admitted patients (ex. Ambulatory or community) or surgical patients will be excluded
Interventions	Usual care, or care during an intervention of any kind*
Comparisons	N/A
Outcomes	Studies must evaluate and report risk factors, along with a risk estimate (OR, RR, etc) or valid statistical analysis for at least one of the following outcomes: • In-hospital mortality prior to discharge • Post-discharge mortality occurring either in community or upon readmission
Study designs	Studies must be one of the following: • Single arm or multi-arm trials • Prospective cohort study • Retrospective cohort studies • One case-control study
Language	English language only

**Please note that in all studies included except one, the intervention was usual care. If any additional interventions were employed and the results showed statistical significance, the relative risks for the control arm as well as the intervention arm will be described separately in the results section.*

(iii) the study was conducted in a developing country (defined as countries classified by the United Nations Development Program (UNDP) in its 2016 report as having a low or medium Human Development Index (15)), and (iv) published in English.

Studies were excluded if (i) some or all of the patients were not admitted (ex. ambulatory or community health facilities), (ii) it represented a surgical population since mortality risk factors for surgeries would likely differ from those of acute illness, or (iii) the study population included nosocomial infections (**Table 1**).

MEDLINE and EMBASE databases were searched with the assistance of a medical librarian (**Appendix 1** and **Appendix 2**), using the Ovid platform. The search dates were from database inception to April 2017.

Study Selection and Data Extraction

Two investigators (LL and NK) independently conducted two rounds of review to determine study eligibility among identified articles. Articles were first screened based on the abstract using the PICOS criteria defined in **Table 1**, where articles clearly meeting exclusion criteria were immediately discarded. A second round of review involved screening the remaining manuscripts in full text, to determine final eligibility. At both stages, discrepancies were resolved by consensus or by arbitration by a third investigator (MW).

For all included articles in the analysis, the following study characteristics were extracted, including: country/region, study period, study design, study population, number of subjects, number of deaths, proportion of participants under 12 months and under 1 month of age, type of analyses conducted for risk factors (i.e., multivariate vs. univariate) and length of post-discharge follow-up. All variables included in the mortality risk factor analyses were recorded. If both univariate and multivariate analyses were performed, only the results from the multivariate analysis were recorded. Data extraction was completed by one investigator and checked by a second investigator for accuracy and consistency.

Outcomes and Data Analysis

The primary aim of this systematic review was to determine the risk factors for mortality among neonates and infants hospitalized with an infectious process in developing countries. All risk estimates pertain to in-patient mortality, except those specifically noted as risk factors for outpatient (i.e., post-discharge) mortality.

As all studies were interpreted from a cohort design perspective, their quality was assessed using the Newcastle-Ottawa Scale (16). Each study was reviewed by one investigator (LE) for criteria related to selection, comparability, and outcome assessment.

Due to expected heterogeneity in study population, risk factors and analysis, it was determined *a priori* that formal meta-analysis would not be conducted. The primary form of analysis was therefore descriptive and conducted using Microsoft Excel (Redmond, WA). Studies were grouped according to both participant age group (neonatal vs. infant) and underlying population (i.e., disease etiology).

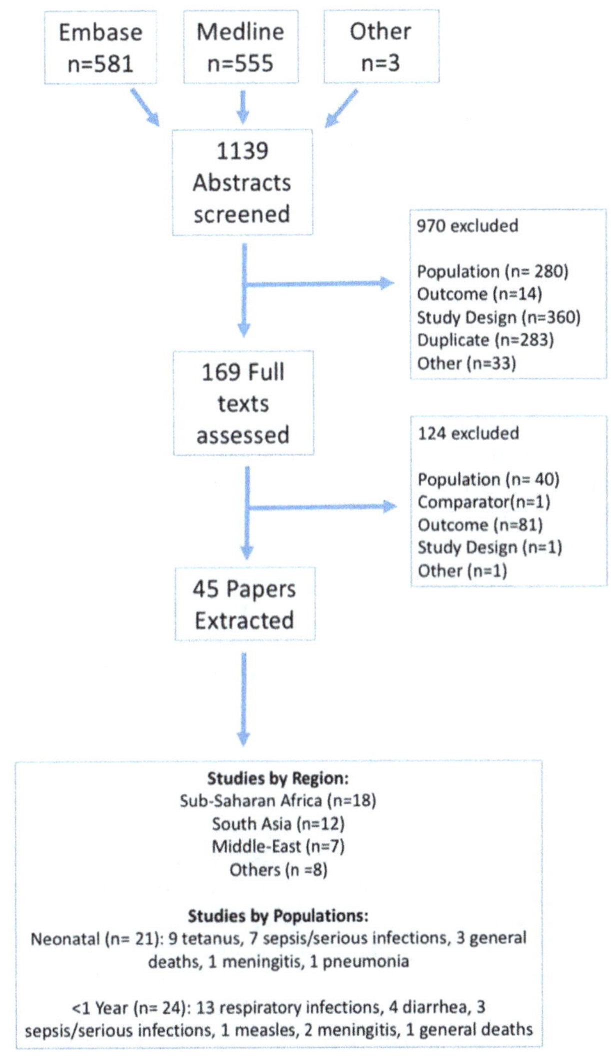

FIGURE 1 | Systematic review flowchart.

RESULTS

Summary of Included Articles

Through the systematic literature search, 1,139 abstracts were identified. Of these, 970 were excluded during the abstract screening stage. The full-text of the remaining 169 articles were reviewed, after which an additional 124 articles were excluded. Thus, a total of 45 articles were included (**Figure 1**) (17–62).

Among these 45 studies, the majority of studies were prospective or retrospective cohort studies (**Tables 3, 4**). Upon assessment using the Newcastle-Ottawa scale, the average score for included studies was 6.3 out of 9 stars, based on selection criteria, comparability of cohorts, and assessment of outcomes encompassing attrition. Included studies were found to have low comparability, with only 40% controlling for confounders in the study design or statistical analysis. Approximately 70% of studies chose representative samples and reported reliable inclusion criteria.

Among the 45 included studies, multiple geographic regions were represented: 18 from Sub-Saharan Africa, 12 from South Asia, 7 from the Middle-East and 8 from other regions (**Table 2**). Twenty-one (46.6%) focused exclusively on the neonatal populations, whereas the other 24 studies (53.3%) focused on children under 1 year of age (**Table 2**). Nearly all of the studies ($n = 42$, 93.3%) focused exclusively on in-hospital deaths, while two (4.4%) studies focused exclusively on post-discharge death and one study (2.2%) on both in-hospital and post-discharge death. Seventeen (37.8%) of the included studies were published before 2000. The median number of study participants was 201 children (IQR 102-697).

Among 21 neonatal studies, nine focused on tetanus, seven on sepsis, one on meningitis, one on respiratory infections, and three on general admissions (**Table 2**). Among the 24 infant studies, 13 focused on children with respiratory infections. The remaining focused on diarrhea ($n = 4$), sepsis or serious infections ($n = 3$), meningitis ($n = 2$), measles ($n = 1$) and general admissions ($n = 1$; **Table 2**). Key results, along with definitions for all parameters, are highlighted in **Tables 3**, **4**. For each illness, the most common risk factors, prioritized by frequency, are presented in these tables to ensure conciseness. Risk factors discussed only in a single study were not included in these tables, but are reported in the **Supplementary Table 1**.

Neonatal Mortality

Tetanus

A total of nine studies evaluated predictors of mortality for neonatal tetanus. Mortality rates ranged from 10.3 to 67.9% in these studies. The most consistent predictors of mortality were young age of presentation and onset, presence of fever and risus sardonicus. For young age at presentation, the adjusted odds ratios ranged from 1.64 (95% CI: 1.22–2.18) to 5.29 (95% CI: 1.73–16.17). The presence of fever was associated with increased odds of mortality, ranging from 4.6 (95% CI: 2.8–7.6) to 17.92 (95% CI: 2.29–135.53). Three of the five studies reported fever as a statistically significant variable, but did not provide odds ratios. The odds of mortality among patients with risus sardonicus study were 4.5 (95% CI: 2.4–8.6) in one study. Two studies also found risus sardonicus and young age of onset to be significantly associated with mortality, although specific values were not provided.

Variables frequently assessed as potential risk factors, but which consistently showed no association with mortality in this population included sex, tetanic spasms/spasticity, umbilical inflammation, sepsis, trismus, maternal tetanus immunization status, lack of sucking, omphalitis, irritability, high heart rate and high respiratory rate.

Sepsis/Serious Infections

Seven studies evaluated mortality among populations of neonates with sepsis or severe infection. Mortality rates were very high, ranging from 14.6 to 36.0% of admitted patients. Prematurity and low birth weight were significantly associated with mortality in two studies for each of these factors. The odds ratio for prematurity was 2.22 (95% CI: 1.07–4.63) for one study and not given for another study. Similarly, the odds ratio for low birth weight was 6.1 (95% CI: 0.8–44.4) in one study and not given for another study. Platelet count, weight at presentation, sex and white blood cell counts did not show statistically significant correlations with mortality in these studies.

General Hospital Admissions

Three studies assessed mortality among general neonatal hospital admissions. These studies have included neonatal populations with diarrhea, malaria, pneumonia, jaundice, convulsions, soft-tissue infections, asphyxia, tetanus, omphaitis, congenital malformations, intrapartum abnormalities and hypothermia. Low admission weight and hypothermia were found to be statistically significant predictors of mortality in both studies in which they were assessed. The odds of mortality for children with low admission weight was 1.61 (95% CI: 1.15–2.26) and 5.88 (95% CI: 3.03–11.1), and for children with hypothermia was 2.48 (95% CI: 1.76–3.49) and 7.14 (95% CI: 2.22–40). Maternal age, sex and time of day at presentation were not significant correlates of mortality in these studies.

Other Studies

In the single study assessing mortality among neonates with meningitis, a bulging anterior fontanelle was the only significant predictor of mortality, with an odds ratio of 7.7 (95% CI: 1.7–35.4). Hypothermia, feeding difficulties, jaundice, cyanosis, vomiting, convulsions and respiratory distress showed no significant correlation with mortality among meningitis patients. It is worth mentioning that the above study only contained a total of 17 deaths, so was likely underpowered. In the single study focused on respiratory infections among neonates, an alveolar-arterial carbon dioxide gradient (AaCO2 gradient) >250 mmHg was the only statistically significant predictor of mortality, with an odds ratio of 71.1 (95% CI: 1.1–4,395). Weight, gestational age, lethargy, age at presentation, pH <7.2, absent neonatal reflexes, shock, fraction of inspired oxygen (FiO2), blood base excess, blood culture, C-reactive protein level, arterial alveolar oxygen ratio, and ventilatory support showed little or no correlation with mortality among patients with respiratory infections. Many of these variables were significant correlates of mortality in univariate analysis but lost significance in multivariate analysis. However, it is possible that the study is underpowered since only a total of 22 deaths were reported in the study.

Infant (<1 Year) Mortality

Respiratory Infections

In the 13 studies evaluating respiratory tract infections, mortality rates ranged from 1.2 to 15.3% among admitted infants. Malnutrition, low oxygen saturation, younger age and positive Human Immunodeficiency Virus (HIV) status were top predictors of mortality in these patients. The odds of mortality among malnourished patients varied from 3.8 (95% CI: 2.7–5.4) to 6.32 (95% CI: 2.72–14.57). Among four studies, the odds of mortality among patients with lower oxygen saturation were 2.7 (95% CI: 2.1–3.5), 2.46 (95% CI: 1.3–4.65), and significant, but not provided, in the two remaining studies. The odds ratios of mortality among younger infants with respiratory infections, defined as <4 months in one study and <6 months in another,

TABLE 2 | Study characteristics.

Author and year	Study countries	Study period[a]	Study type	Study population	Mortality type (IP/PD)[b]	Total No. of patients	No. of patients who died	No. of patients <1 month	No. of patients <1 year
NEONATAL STUDIES (<1 MONTH)									
Basu et al. (18)	India	1997–2003	Retrospective	Neonatal tetanus	IP + PD	101	67	101	101
Ballot et al. (17)	South Africa	2007–2011	Retrospective	Neonatal fungal sepsis	IP	63	27	63	63
Chiabi et al. (20)	Cameroon	2008–2009	Prospective	Neonatal sepsis	IP	218	46	218	218
Daoud et al. (22)	Jordan	1992–1994	Prospective	Neonatal meningitis	IP	53	17	53	53
Davies-Adetugbo et al. (23)	Nigeria	1991–1995	Retrospective	Neonatal tetanus	IP	174	96	174	174
Dikici et al. (25)	Turkey	1991–2006	Retrospective	Neonatal tetanus	IP	67	27	67	67
Ertem et al. (28)	Turkey	1994–2001	Retrospective	Neonatal tetanus	IP	56	38	56	56
Ghiorghis et al. (29)	Ethiopia	1992–1993	Retrospective	Neonatal sepsis	IP	542	195	542	542
Gurkan et al. (31)	Turkey	1991–1997	Retrospective	Neonatal tetanus	IP	55	22	55	55
Gurses et al. (32)	Turkey	1978–1988	Retrospective	Neonatal tetanus	IP	133	54	133	133
Ibinda et al. (33)	Kenya	1999–2013	Retrospective	Neonatal tetanus	IP	191	118	191	191
Mathur et al. (37)	India	NA	Prospective	Neonatal respiratory distress	IP	150	48	150	150
Mugalu et al. (40)	Uganda	2002	Prospective	Neonatal septicemia	IP	110	20	110	110
Okomo et al. (44)	Gambia	2009–2013	Retrospective	All neonatal deaths	IP	5,285	1,734	5,285	5,285
Okoromah et al. (45)	Nigeria	NA	Retrospective	Neonatal tetanus	IP	39	4	39	39
Ozkan et al. (46)	Turkey	2003–2010	Retrospective	Neonatal sepsis (preterm)	IP	151	22	151	NA
Sarna et al. (52)	India	1988	Retrospective	All neonatal deaths	IP	7,309	328	328	328
Saleem et al. (50)	Pakistan	2006–2011	Retrospective	Neonatal sepsis	IP	104	17	104	104
Sheikh et al. (55)	Pakistan	2012	Prospective	Neonatal sepsis	IP	125	20	125	125
Simiyu et al. (56)	Kenya	2000	Retrospective	All neonatal deaths	IP	308	97	308	308
Yaramis et al. (60)	Turkey	1990–1999	NA	Neonatal tetanus	IP	73	38	73	73
INFANT STUDIES (<12 MONTHS)									
Bhatnagar et al. (19)	India	2005–2008	RCT	Serious bacterial infection	IP	848	7	182	848
Coakley et al. (21)	Papua New Guinea	1989	Prospective	Measles	IP	282	48	NA	NA
Demers et al. (24)	Central African Republic	1996–1997	Prospective	Acute respiratory infections	IP	395	49	14	222
Djelantik et al. (26)	Indonesia	1999–2001	Retrospective	Pneumonia	IP	4,351	505	NA	NA
Duke et al. (27)	Papua New Guinea	1998–1999	Prospective	Pneumonia	IP	703	46	NA	NA
Goel et al. (30)	South Africa	1989–1995	Retrospective	Staphylococcal pneumonia	IP	100	7	NA	78
Islam et al. (62)	Bangladesh	1991–1992	Prospective	Diarrhea	PD	427	30	NA	329
Khan et al. (34)	Pakistan	2007–2008	Retrospective	Sepsis	IP	133	32	NA	NA
Kuti et al. (35)	Nigeria	2011–2013	Retrospective	Bacterial meningitis	IP	81	22	NA	NA
Lehmann et al. (36)	Papua New Guinea	1989–1992	Prospective	Bacterial meningitis	IP	696	96	NA	535
Moisi et al. (39)	Kenya	2004–2008	Prospective	General mortality	PD	14,971	535	NA	NA
Mulholland et al. (41)	Gambia	1990–1991	Prospective	Serious infections	IP	697	64	NA	697
Nantanda et al. (42)	Uganda	2005–2006	Prospective	Pneumonia	IP	157	24	87	NA
Nathoo et al. (43)	Zimbabwe	1989–1990	Prospective	Lower respiratory infection	IP	704	104	0	502
Ramakishna et al. (47)	Malawi	2005–2006	Prospective	Pneumonia	IP	233	25	0	117
Rodriguez et al. (48)	Columbia	2009–2011	Retrospective	Respiratory syncytial virus infection	IP	2,147	25	NA	1,549
Sachdev et al. (49)	India	1988	Prospective	Diarrhea	IP	382	37	NA	NA

(Continued)

TABLE 2 | Continued

Author and year	Study countries	Study period[a]	Study type	Study population	Mortality type (IP/PD)[b]	Total # of patients	# of patients who died	# of patients <1 month	# of patients <1 year
Sehgal et al. (53)	India	1993–1994	Prospective	Lower respiratory infection	IP	201	21	NA	105
Santhanakrishnan et al. (51)	India	NA	NA	Diarrhea, acute	IP	575	64	NA	441
Shann et al. (54)	Papua New Guinea	NA	Prospective	Pneumonia	IP	47	7	NA	NA
Smyth et al. (57)	Zambia	1994–1995	Prospective	Pneumonia	IP	167	23	NA	104
Tupasi et al. (59)	Philippines	1981–1983	Prospective	ALRI	IP	726	34	NA	361
Teka et al. (58)	Bangladesh	1990–1994	Case-control	Diarrhea	IP	928	46	NA	NA
Zhang et al. (61)	China	2007–2010	Prospective	Pneumonia	IP	707	41	NA	535

[a]*All studies cohort unless otherwise specified.*
[b]*IP, inpatient; PD, post-discharge.*

varied from 2.4 (95% CI: 1.6–3.5) to 3.6 (95% CI: 2.8–4.6). One study showed an association between high respiratory rate and mortality, while another showed high respiratory rates to be significantly associated with mortality. Cyanosis (four studies), wheezing (four studies), duration of breastfeeding (two studies) and congenital cardiac abnormalities (two studies) were not found to be correlates of mortality in these studies.

Diarrhea

In the four studies focused on infants admitted with diarrhea, the mortality rate was between 5 and 11.1%. Malnutrition and the absence of breastfeeding were the top predictors of mortality among both in-hospital and post-discharge populations, showing statistically significant correlations with mortality. The odds of mortality varied widely from 1.9 (95% CI: 1.6–2.3) to 84.16 (95% CI: 9.1–775.9) among malnourished patients, and from 2.35 (95% CI: 1.44–3.84) to 4.2 (95% CI: 1.3–13.2) among non-breastfed patients. Dehydration status, blood in stools, xerophthalmia, and concurrent pneumonia did not appear as statistically significant correlates of mortality.

Sepsis/Serious Infections

In the three studies focused on sepsis or serious infection, organ dysfunction, the need for more than 2 inotropes and bacterial isolates in blood showed significant correlations with mortality. The odds of mortality was 18 (95% CI 2.2–144) for organ dysfunction, 3.5 (95% CI 1.3–9.2) for those needing for more than 2 inotropes and significant, although not specifically provided, for those with bacteremia. Zinc intake and a Pediatric Risk of Mortality (PRISM) score >10 were not statistically significantly correlated in these studies.

Other Studies

Two studies assessed predictors of mortality among patients with meningitis. Low hemoglobin (OR 2.9, 95% CI: 1.5–5.3), refusal or inability to feed (OR 3.3, 95% CI: 2.1–5.6), vomiting (OR 1.7, 95% CI: 1.2–2.7), and drowsiness (OR 2.9, 95% CI: 1.7–5) were significant predictors of mortality. In addition, high WBC count and low CSF glucose were significantly associated with increased odds of mortality, although odds ratios were not specifically stated. Multiple seizures, coma at presentation, neck stiffness, hyponatremia, hyperglycemia, hypoglycorrhachia, and turbid CSF showed no significant correlation with mortality. This is likely underpowered as only 22 deaths were reported in the study describing the above risk factors.

One study focused on mortality among a post-discharge population. This study found malnutrition defined as weight-for-age Z score < −3 (OR 3.42, 95% CI 2.5–4.68), hypoxia (OR 2.3, 95% CI: 1.64–3.23), bacteremia (OR 1.77, 95% CI: 1.15–2.74), jaundice (OR 1.77, 95% CI: 1.08–2.91), hepatomegaly (OR 2.34, 95% CI: 1.6–3.42), and hospitalization length <13 days (OR 1.83, 95% CI: 1.33–2.52) showed significant correlations with post-discharge mortality. Age and parasitemia showed no correlation with mortality outcomes.

Lastly, in one study on infants with measles, low birth weight and nosocomial infections showed significant correlations with mortality, although the odds ratios were not provided. Infant age and vitamin A supplementation did not correlate with mortality.

DISCUSSION

This systematic review focused on risk factors of mortality among hospitalized neonates and infants under 1 year of age due to infectious causes in LMICs. To the best of our knowledge, this is the first systematic literature review that focuses of clinical predictors of mortality from severe infection among hospitalized neonates and infants in developing countries. Most previous work on these populations consist of single population-based studies (11, 63). Previous systematic reviews of clinical predictors of mortality from severe infections have included infants in developed countries, which may not applicable to areas of the world where the majority of the disease burden occurs (10). Furthermore, other systematic reviews have examined predictors of severe illness and/hospitalization rather than mortality (64, 65), the latter which is a more objective, directly actionable outcome for use in intervention trials. Moreover,

TABLE 3 | Summary of risk factors for neonatal mortality by underlying disease.

Risk factor	**Included study**	**Risk estimate^{+}(95%CI)**	**Risk factor definitions**
TETANUS (*n* = 9 STUDIES)			
Cyanosis	Dikici et al. (25)	1.1 (0.2–7)	NR
	Gurkan et al. (31)	**NSS, estimate NR**	NR
	Gurses et al. (32)	**NSS, estimate NR**	NR
	Okoromah et al. (45)	**SS > 1, estimate NR**	NR
Fever	Basu et al. (18)*	**4.6 (2.8–7.6)**	Not reported
	Ertem et al. (28)	**17.92 (2.29–135.53)**	NR
	Gurses et al. (32)	**SS > 1, estimate NR**	NR
	Okoromah et al. (45)	**SS > 1, estimate NR**	>40°C
	Yaramis et al. (60)	**SS > 1, estimate NR**	NR
	Dikici et al. (23)	0.4 (0.4–5)	CV
	Gurkan et al. (31)	NSS, estimate NR	NR
Risus sardonicus	Basu et al. (18)*	**4.5 (2.4–8.6)**	NR
	Gurkan et al. (31)*	**SS > 1, estimate NR**	NR
	Gurses et al. (32)	**SS > 1, estimate NR**	NR
	Dikici et al. (23)	1.8 (0.1–20)	NR
Sex	Davies-Adetugbo et al. (23)	NSS, estimate NR	Male
	Dikici et al. (23)	1.2 (0.3–4)	Male
	Ibinda et al. (33)	0.67 (0.72–1.25)	Male
	Gurses et al. (32)	NSS, estimate NR	Male
	Okoromah et al. (45)	NSS, estimate NR	Male
Tetanic spasms, spasticity	Basu et al. (18)*	0.9 (0.5–1.9)	NR
	Dikici et al. (23)	1.1 (0.2–7)	NR
	Gurkan et al. (31)	NSS, estimate NR	NR
	Ibinda et al. (33)	**1.15 (1.04–1.26)**	NR
Young age	Davies-Adetugbo et al. (23)	**3.11 (1.04–5.8)**	<6 days
	Dikici et al. (23)	**5.28 (1.73–16.165)**	NR
	Gurkan et al. (31)	**SS > 1, estimate NR**	NR
	Gurses et al. (32)	**SS > 1, estimate NR**	NR
	Ibinda et al. (33)	**1.64 (1.22–2.18)**	NR
	Okoromah et al. (45)	NSS, estimate NR	NR
Young age at onset of symptoms	Gurses et al. (32)	**SS > 1, estimate NR**	NR
	Yaramis et al. (60)	**SS > 1, estimate NR**	NR
	Dikici et al. (23)	0.6 (0.3–1)	CV
	Ertem et al. (28)	0.6 (0.55–1)	CV
	Okoromah et al. (45)	NSS, estimate NR	NR
NEONATAL SEPSIS/SEPTICEMIA (*n* = 6 STUDIES)			
Gender	Sheikh et al. (55)	**SS > 1, estimate NR**	Male
	Saleem et al. (50)	3 (0.9–9.5)	Male
Late onset of sepsis	Ozkan et al. (46)	**1.2 (1–2.7)**	Late onset: 3–30 days
	Sheikh et al. (55)	**SS < 1, estimate NR**	Late onset: 3–30 days
Low birthweight	Chiabi et al. (20)	**SS > 1, estimate NR**	<2,500 g
	Ghiorghis et al. (29)	NSS, estimate NR	NR
	Saleem et al. (50)	6.1 (0.8–44.4)	<1,000 g
Positive blood culture	Chiabi et al. (20)	NSS, estimate NR	NR
	Sheikh et al. (55)	**SS > 1, estimate NR**	NR
Prematurity/low gestation age	Chiabi et al. (20)	NSS, estimate NR	<37 weeks
	Ghiorghis et al. (29)	**2.22 (1.07–4.63)**	<38 weeks
	Sarna et al. (52)	NSS, estimate NR	CV

(Continued)

TABLE 3 | Continued

Risk factor	Included study	Risk estimate+(95%CI)	Risk factor definitions
GENERAL DEATHS (*n* = 3 STUDIES)			
Hypothermia	Okomo et al. (44)	**2.48 (1.76–3.49)**	<36.5°C
	Simiyu et al. (56)	**7.14 (2.22–40)**	<36.5°C
Lack of maternal antenatal care	Okomo et al. (44)	**1.68 (1.17–2.41)**	NA
Low admission weight	Okomo et al. (44)	**1.61 (1.15–2.26)**	<1,500 g
	Simiyu et al. (56)	**5.88 (3.03–11.1)**	<2,500 g
Low birthweight	Sarna et al. (52)	**SS > 1, estimate NR**	<2,000 g
Prematurity, low gestation age	Sarna et al. (52)	**SS > 1, estimate NR**	<37 weeks

All risk estimates are odds ratios, unless relative risk ratio denoted by RR.
Bolded risk factors are statistically significant.
+Denotes all risk estimates are odds ratios, unless relative risk ratio denoted by RR.
**Denotes that post-discharge populations were assessed.*
SS>1, statistically significant association with risk estimate>1.
NR denotes "Not Reported."
NA denotes "Not Applicable."
NSS denotes not statistically significant.

other previous work have focused on on all-cause mortality from sepsis as universally preventable disease, rather than more specific illness populations (7). This evidence base is complementary to publications from the WHO, CDC, and other international organizations, which approach neonatal and infant mortality from a population perspective. This systematic review consolidates mortality outcomes on the individual and community level, by focusing on clinical, laboratory and socio-demographic risk factors. It can be used to guide interventions to address the epidemic of early mortality among over 4 million infants and neonates in developing countries.

Comprehensive understanding of the clinical risk factors for mortality in these populations is important for several reasons. First, compilation of risk factors will help to drive the development risk prediction models aimed at the identification of high-risk infants, in order to triage resources to improve health outcomes and health care efficiency. This precision public-health approach has previously been utilized to derive risk-prediction models. For example, the miniPIERS, a prediction model to identify women at risk of hypertensive-related death, was developed to intervene among high-risk pregnant women in LMICs (66). Similar models have been created to identify high-risk patients with Chagas disease and to predict pediatric post-discharge mortality (67–69). Second, expanding our understanding of clinical risk factors for mortality in this age group could highlight key diagnostic approaches and research gaps in these areas. Lastly, specific populations or diseases may have limited research, and the benefits of systematic reviews in the identification of such gaps is well-described (12, 13).

The predictors of mortality were assessed for two distinct age groups: neonates (<28 days old) and infants (28 days to 12 months old). Overall, the most frequent predictors of mortality in neonates were young age, fever or hypothermia, low birth weight and prematurity, while the most frequent predictors of mortality in infants were malnutrition, breast-feeding status and low oxygen saturation. It appears that perinatal variables play a larger role in predicting mortality during the neonatal period, whereas nutritional factors play a larger role among infants. Although both age groups encompassed a variety of disease populations, these risk factors found commonality in predicting mortality despite the heterogeneity in underlying conditions. Some of these predictors, such as temperature instability, young age, low birth weight, and prematurity, may not be surprising from a diagnostic perspective, as they are directly related to inherent causes of neonatal mortality. However, other predictors, such as a low oxygen saturation and breastfeeding, are more interesting from an interventional point of view. For instance, our results suggest that substantial efforts should be directed toward reducing malnutrition, promoting breastfeeding (parallel to HIV prevention) and developing affordable technologies for identifying oxygenation status among neonates and infants.

On the whole, included studies in this systematic review upheld strong research designs and maintained internal validity, based on the Newcastle-Ottawa scale. The primary limitation was comparability, as many studies did not adequately control for confounders, possibly due to small sample sizes. Retrospective studies utilizing medical record review were often faced with incomplete records, and the included studies may or may not have addressed this issue adequately. Other limitations of cohort studies often include recall and reporting bias, which were not assessed by this scale.

It is relevant to note that many of the studies identified for full text review assessed risk factors for serious illness, rather than mortality, and these studies were ultimately excluded (11, 70, 71). This systematic review focused primarily on predictors of mortality, since this downstream outcome is critical to the development of prediction tools or interventions to improve child health and survival. Furthermore, the definition of mortality is more consistent as compared to serious illness, which can have broad and heterogeneous definitions.

Although the definition of mortality is more objective, a major source of heterogeneity between studies was the variable definitions of risk factors. For example, malnutrition definitions varied from weight-for-age Z score <3 standard deviations to

TABLE 4 | Summary of risk factors for infant mortality by underlying disease.

Risk factor	Included study	Risk estimate+ (95%CI)	Risk factor definitions
DIARRHEA (n = 4 STUDIES)			
Dehydration	Sachdev et al. (49)	1.96 (0.5–8.2)	Severe dehydration
	Islam et al. (62)*	NSS, estimate NR	Severe dehydration
Maternal education	Islam et al. (62)*	**2.12 (1.37–3.28)**	<1 year of schooling
	Teka et al. (58)	1.96 (0.5–0.82)	No education
Non-breastfed	Santhanakrishnan et al. (51)	**2.29, estimate NR**	Not exclusively breastfed
	Teka et al. (58)	**4.19 (1.3–13.2)**	Non-breastfed
	Islam et al. (62)*	**2.35 (1.44–3.84)**	Non-breastfed
Poor nutritional status	Sachdev et al. (49)	**3.3 (2.7–4)**	Weight for age <50%
	Sachdev et al. (49)	**1.9 (1.6–23)**	Height for age <85%
	Santhanakrishnan et al. (51)	**4.94, estimate NR**	Degree of malnutrition of 2 or 3 on Gomez scale
	Teka et al. (58)	**84.16 (9.1–775.9)**	Weight for height <70%
	Islam et al. (62)*	**2.97 (1.43–6.16)**	Height for age <85%
Young age	Islam et al. (62)*	**4.57 (2.9–7.18)**	Age <6 months
	Santhanakrishnan et al. (51)	NSS, estimate NR	Age <6 months
	Sachdev et al. (49)	NSS, estimate NR	Age <6 months
ACUTE RESPIRATORY INFECTION OR PNEUMONIA (n = 13 STUDIES)			
Alteration of status	Demers et al. (24)	**3.23 (1.17–8.94)**	Moderate/severe mental alteration
	Sehgal et al. (53)	NSS, estimate NR	NR
	Sehgal et al. (53)	NSS, estimate NR	NR
	Zhang et al. (61)	NSS, estimate NR	NR
Cyanosis	Zhang et al. (61)	NSS, estimate NR	Central cyanosis
	Duke et al. (27)	1.46 (0.79–3.45)	NR
	Sehgal et al. (53)	NSS, estimate NR	NR
	Nantada et al. (42)	NSS, estimate NR	NR
Low oxygen saturation	Djelantik et al. (26)	**2.7 (2.1–3.5)**	SpO_2 <85%
	Duke et al. (27)	**2.46 (1.3–4.65)**	SpO_2 <70%
	Nantanda et al. (42)	**SS > 1, estimate NR**	NR
	Smyth et al. (57)	**SS > 1, estimate NR**	NR
	Ramakishna et al. (47)	**2.96 (0.94–0.29)**	SpO_2 <90%
	Zhang et al. (61)	NSS, estimate NR	SpO_2 <90%
Low respiratory rate	Djelantik et al. (26)	**4.6 (2.5–8.5)**	<40 breaths per minute
	Shann et al. (54)	NSS, estimate NR	<40 breaths per minute
Malnutrition	Djelantik et al. (26)	1.1(0.93–1.3)	Weight for age <5th percentile
	Demers et al. (24)	**2.74 (0.96–7.76)**	Weight for height >2SD less than median for age
	Nantanda et al. (42)	**SS > 1, estimate NR**	NR
	Nathoo et al. (43)	**3.8 (2.7–5.4)**	Weight for age <60%
	Sehgal et al. (53)*	**3.9 (1.01–9.07)**	WAZ < −3
	Tupasi et al. (59)	**4.4 (2–9.52)**	First degree malnutrition on Gomez Scale
	Duke et al. (27)	**6.32 (2.74–14.57)**	Weight for age <60%
	Smyth et al. (57)	**SS > 1, estimate NR**	Low WAZ[&]
	Shann et al. (54)	NSS, estimate NR	Weight for age <80%
Young age	Djelantik et al. (26)	**3.6 (2.8–4.6)**	Age <4 months
	Nathoo et al. (43)	**2.4 (1.6–3.5)**	Age <6 months
	Rodriguez et al. (48)	1.11(0.51–2.41)	Age <6 months
	Smyth et al. (57)	NSS, estimate NR	Age <6 months

(Continued)

TABLE 4 | Continued

Risk factor	Included study	Risk estimate+ (95%CI)	Risk factor definitions
SERIOUS INFECTION OR SEPSIS (*n* = 3 STUDIES)			
Bacteremia	Mulholland et al. (41)	**SS > 1, estimate NR**	NR
Need for >2 inotropes	Khan et al. (34)	**3.5 (1.3–9.2)**	>2 inotropes
Organ dysfunction	Khan et al. (34)	**18 (2.2–144)**	>2 dysfunctional organs
PRISM score >10	Bhatnagar et al. (19)[Intervention]	0.57 (0.27–1.23)	10 mg zinc intake daily
Zinc intake	Khan et al. (34)	1.5 (0.6–4)	>10

**Denotes that post-discharge populations were assessed.*
Bolded risk factors are statistically significant.
+Denotes all risk estimates are odds ratios, unless relative risk ratio denoted by RR.
&Denotes low weight-for-age Z score.
NR denotes "Not Reported."
NA denotes "Not Applicable."
SS>1, statistically significant association with risk estimate >1.
SS<1, statistically significant association with risk estimate <1.
[Intervention] In this study, the intervention was zinc intake and the comparator was normal care. The exposure (suspected bacterial infection) was the same for both groups. In all other studies included in this systematic review, the intervention is usual care with exposure to the risk factor, and the comparator is intervention without exposure to risk factor.

weight-for-age Z score <60% to first degree malnutrition on the Gomez scale (corresponding to <90% expected weight-for-age). Likewise, definitions for low oxygen saturation varied substantially between studies. Low oxygen saturation ranged from SpO_2 <70 to <92%. This heterogeneity was pervasive among sub-populations and limited the ability to perform meta-analyses. A further source of heterogeneity is the differences in inclusion criteria for populations with the same illness. For example, one study on if late-onset sepsis (defined as 3–30 days of life) is a risk factor for mortality looked at pre-term neonates whereas another study looked at at-term ones. This difference may be partially responsible for one studying showing a statistically significant positive correlation with mortality whereas the other showed a statistically significant negative correlation.

Although uncommon, a small proportion of included studies did not provide definition for the evaluated risk factors, such as fever and young age. The provision of clear definitions for risk factors is crucial for generalizability and study replication. Moreover, increased standardization of these definitions would allow future data to be more amenable to meta-analyses. This would greatly enhance the translation potential of these studies, especially since many of the existing individual studies are underpowered for statistical analysis.

This systematic review has several limitations. First, some studies identified in this review only conducted univariate analyses while others conducted multivariate analyses. Thus, risk factors identified as statistically significant in the univariate analyses may cease to be statistically significant if multivariate analyses were performed. Second, most studies focus on single disease populations, resulting in risk factors that may not be generalizable across multiple illness populations. Since sepsis is associated with most disease-related deaths (72), it may provide an overarching framework within which to assess mortality predictors that are applicable across different acute illness processes. Third, few studies focused on post-discharge mortality, resulting in a critical knowledge gap in child mortality research. Post-discharge mortality rates have been shown to be equal or greater than in-hospital mortality rates in pediatric populations (67). More post-discharge studies on neonates and infants would be useful in determining if there are additional risk factors relevant to this population. Fourth, many risk factors which we evaluated did not demonstrate statistical significance. Frequently, small sample sizes may have limited the ability to evaluate the association of important variables on mortality. These results underscore the need for adequately powered studies, but also clearly demonstrate the importance of those variables which did achieve statistical significance. Furthermore, some clinically important risk factors, such as maternal HIV status, maternal malnutrition and implementation of TB or HIV preventative therapy during pregnancy, may have not been captured as statistically significant risk factors as a result of many included studies being underpowered as well as the focus on hospitalized patients as an inclusion criteria. Lastly, many parameters found to be important predictors of mortality among infants, such as hemoglobin level, oxygen saturation and nutritional status, were not assessed in studies focused on serious infections among neonatal patients. The inclusion of these parameters in future studies has the potential to elucidate strong predictors of infant mortality.

CONCLUSIONS

This systematic review summarizes risk factors for mortality among neonates and infants in LMICs. Our data highlight major risk factors that could be incorporated into risk-prediction models to identify children at risk for in-hospital or post-discharge mortality. This data also points toward specific interventions that could be further incorporated into healthcare systems or policies. Targeted, evidence-based interventions have the potential to vastly reduce the burden of preventable mortality among neonates and infants around the world. Future studies in this area should incorporate precise definitions and risk estimates for mortality, including larger sample sizes, detailed statistical analysis, and overlapping risk factors between these high-risk age groups.

AUTHOR CONTRIBUTIONS

LL prepared first draft of manuscript, conducted systematic search and data extraction, assisted in analysis of data, approved final version of manuscript. NaK and LE conducted systematic search and data extraction, assisted in analysis of data, approved final version of manuscript. NiK, PL, JA, and JK reviewed and edited manuscript and provided critical interpretation of data, assisted in analysis of data, approved final version of manuscript. MW conceived study idea, assisted in systematic search and data extraction, assisted in analysis of data, reviewed and edited manuscript and provided critical interpretation of data, approved final version of manuscript.

REFERENCES

1. You D, Hug L, Ejdemyr S. Global, regional, and national levels and trends in under-5 mortality between 1990 and 2015, with scenario-based projections to 2030: a systematic analysis by the UN Inter-agency Group for child mortality estimation. *Lancet* (2015) 386:2275–86. doi: 10.1016/S0140-6736(15)00120-8
2. Rajaratnam JK, Marcus JR, Flaxman AD, Wang H, Levin-Rector A, Dwyer L, et al. Neonatal, postneonatal, childhood, and under-5 mortality for 187 countries, 1970–2010: a systematic analysis of progress towards millennium development goal 4. *Lancet* (2010) 375:1988–2008. doi: 10.1016/S0140-6736(10)60703-9
3. Ehret DY, Patterson JK, Bose CL. Improving neonatal care: a global perspective. *Clin Perinatol.* (2017) 44:567–82. doi: 10.1016/j.clp.2017.05.002
4. Zupan J. Perinatal mortality in developing countries. *N Engl J Med.* (2005) 352:2047–8. doi: 10.1056/NEJMp058032
5. *Children: Reducing Mortality.* World Health Organization (2016). Available online at: http://www.who.int/news-room/fact-sheets/detail/children-reducing-mortality (Accessed September 22, 2018).
6. Lawn JE, Cousens S, Zupan J. 4 million neonatal deaths: when? Where? Why? *Lancet* (2005) 365:891–900. doi: 10.1016/S0140-6736(05)71048-5
7. World Health Organization. Global *Health Observatory (GHO) Data: Causes of Child Mortality* (2016). Available online at: http://www.who.int/gho/child_health/mortality/causes/en/ (Accessed September 22, 2018).
8. Mahy M. *DHS Comparative Reports: Childhood Mortality in the Developing World.* Calverton, MD: ORC Macro (2003). Available Online at: https://dhsprogram.com/pubs/pdf/CR4/CR4.pdf
9. Rutstein SO. Factors associated with trends in infant and child mortality in developing countries during the 1990s. *Bull World Health Organ.* (2000) 78:1256–70.
10. Van den Bruel A, et al., Diagnostic value of clinical features at presentation to identify serious infection in children in developed countries: a systematic review. *Lancet* (2010) 375:834–45. doi: 10.1016/S0140-6736(09)62000-6
11. Young Infants Clinical Signs Study Group. Clinical signs that predict severe illness in children under age 2 months: a multicentre study. *Lancet* (2008) 371:135–42. doi: 10.1016/S0140-6736(08)60106-3
12. Saha S, Chant D, and McGrath J. A systematic review of mortality in schizophrenia: is the differential mortality gap worsening over time? *Arch Gen Psychiatr.* (2007) 64:1123–31. doi: 10.1001/archpsyc.64.10.1123
13. Jayne Wilson JG, Moroz V, Gaze M, Wheatley K. Using systematic reviews to identify research gaps–a case study: mIBG for the treatment of neuroblastoma in children. *Trials* (2013) 14(Suppl. 1):126. doi: 10.1186/1745-6215-14-S1-P126
14. Kissoon N, Reinhart K, Daniels R, Machado MFR, Schachter RD, Finfer S. Sepsis in children: global implications of the world health assembly resolution on sepsis. *Pediatr Crit Care Med.* (2017) 18:e625–7. doi: 10.1097/PCC.0000000000001340
15. Jahan S, *Human Development Report 2016: Human Development for Everyone.* New York, NY: UNDP (2016).
16. *The Newcastle-Ottawa Scale (NOS) for Assessing the Quality of Nonrandomised Studies in Meta-Analyses* (2018). Available online at: http://www.ohri.ca/programs/clinical_epidemiology/oxford.asp
17. Ballot DE, Bosman N, Nana T, Ramdin T, Cooper PA. Background changing patterns of neonatal fungal sepsis in a developing country. *J Trop Pediatr.* (2013) 59:460–4. doi: 10.1093/tropej/fmt053
18. Basu S, Paul DK, Ganguly S, Chandra PK. Risk factors for mortality from neonatal tetanus: 7 years experience in North Bengal, India. *Ann Trop Paediatr.* (2006) 26:233–239. doi: 10.1179/146532806X120336
19. Bhatnagar S, Wadhwa N, Aneja S, Lodha R, Kabra SK, Natchu UC, et al. Zinc as adjunct treatment in infants aged between 7 and 120 days with probable serious bacterial infection: a randomised, double-blind, placebo-controlled trial. *Lancet* (2012) 379:2072–8. doi: 10.1016/S0140-6736(12)60477-2
20. Chiabi A, Djoupomb M, Mah E, Nguefack S, Mbuagbaw L, Zafack J, et al. The clinical and bacteriogical spectrum of neonatal sepsis in a tertiary hospital in Yaounde, Cameroon. *Iran J Pediatr.* (2011) 21:441–8.
21. Coakley KJ, Coakley CA, Spooner V, Smith TA, Javati A, Kajoi M. A review of measles admissions and deaths in the paediatric ward of Goroka Base Hospital during 1989. *PNG Med J.* (1991) 34:6–12.
22. Daoud AS, Al-Sheyyab M, Abu-Ekteish F, Obeidat A, Ali AA, El-Shanti H. Neonatal meningitis in northern Jordan. *J Trop Pediatr.* (1996) 42:267–70.
23. Davies-Adetugbo AA, Torimiro SE, Ako-Nai KA, Prognostic factors in neonatal tetanus. *Trop Med Int Health* (1998) 3:9–13. doi: 10.1046/j.1365-3156.1998.00162.x
24. Demers AM, Morency P, Mberyo-Yaah F, Jaffar S, Blais C, Somsé P, et al. Risk factors for mortality among children hospitalized because of acute respiratory infections in Bangui, Central African Republic. *Pediatr Infect Dis J.* (2000) 19:424–32.
25. Dikici B, Uzun H, Yilmaz-Keskin E, Tas T, Gunes A, Kocamaz H, et al. Neonatal tetanus in Turkey; what has changed in the last decade? *BMC Infect Dis.* (2008) 8:112. doi: 10.1186/1471-2334-8-112
26. Djelantik IG, Gessner BD, Sutanto A, Steinhoff M, Linehan M, Moulton LH, et al. Case fatality proportions and predictive factors for mortality among children hospitalized with severe pneumonia in a rural developing country setting. *J Trop Pediatr.* (2003) 49:327–32. doi: 10.1093/tropej/49.6.327
27. Duke T, Mgone J, Frank D. Hypoxaemia in children with severe pneumonia in Papua New Guinea. *Int J Tuberculosis Lung Dis.* (2001) 5:511–9.
28. Ertem M, Cakmak A, Saka G, Ceylan A. Neonatal tetanus in the South-Eastern region of Turkey: changes in prognostic aspects by better health care. *J Trop Pediatr.* (2004) 50:297–300. doi: 10.1093/tropej/50.5.297
29. Ghiorghis B, Neonatal sepsis in Addis Ababa, Ethiopia: a review of 151 bacteremic neonates. *Ethiop Med J.* (1997) 35:169–76.
30. Goel A, Bamford L, Hanslo D, Hussey G. Primary staphylococcal pneumonia in young children: a review of 100 cases. *J Trop Pediatr.* (1999) 45:233–6.
31. Gürkan F, Boşnak M, Dikici B, Boşnak V, Taş MA, Haspolat K, et al. Neonatal tetanus: a continuing challenge in the southeast of Turkey: risk factors, clinical features and prognostic factors. *Eur J Epidemiol.* (1999) 15:171–4.
32. Gürses N, Aydin M. Factors affecting prognosis of neonatal tetanus. *Scand J Infect Dis.* (1993) 25:353–5.
33. Ibinda F, Bauni E, Kariuki SM, Fegan G, Lewa J, Mwikamba M, et al. Incidence and risk factors for neonatal tetanus in admissions to Kilifi County Hospital, Kenya. *PLoS ONE* (2015) 10:e0122606. doi: 10.1371/journal.pone.0122606

34. Khan MR, Maheshwari PK, Masood K, Qamar FN, Haque AU. Epidemiology and outcome of sepsis in a tertiary care PICU of Pakistan. *Indian J Pediatr.* (2012) 79:1454–8. doi: 10.1007/s12098-012-0706-z
35. Kuti BP, Bello EO, Jegede TO, Olubosede O. Epidemiological, clinical and prognostic profile of childhood acute bacterial meningitis in a resource poor setting. *J Neurosci Rural Pract.* (2015) 6:549–57. doi: 10.4103/0976-3147.165424
36. Lehmann D, Yeka W, Rongap T, Javati A, Saleu G, Clegg A, et al. Aetiology and clinical signs of bacterial meningitis in children admitted to Goroka Base Hospital, Papua New Guinea, 1989–1992. *Ann Trop Paediatr.* (1999) 19:21–32.
37. Mathur NB, Garg K, Kumar S. Respiratory distress in neonates with special reference to pneumonia. *Indian Pediatr.* (2002) 39:529–37.
38. Islam MA, Rahman MM, Mahalanabis D, Rahman AK. Death in a diarrhoeal cohort of infants and young children soon after discharge from hospital-risk factors and causes by verbal autopsy. *J Trop Pediatr.* (1996) 42:342–7.
39. Moïsi JC, Gatakaa H, Berkley JA, Maitland K, Mturi N, Newton CR. Excess child mortality after discharge from hospital in Kilifi, Kenya: a retrospective cohort analysis. *Bull World Health Organ.* (2011) 89:725–32, 732A. doi: 10.2471/BLT.11.089235
40. Mugalu J, Nakakeeto M, Kiguli S, Mulindwa DH. Aetiology, risk factors and immediate outcome of bacteriologically confirmed neonatal septicaemia in Mulago hospital, Uganda. *Afr Health Sci.* (2006) 6:120–6.
41. Mulholland EK, Ogunlesi OO, Adegbola RA, Weber M, Sam BE, Palmer A, et al. Etiology of serious infections in young Gambian infants. *Pediatr Infect Dis J.* (1999) 18(10 Suppl.):S35–41.
42. Nantanda R, Hildenwall H, Peterson S, Kaddu-Mulindwa D, Kalyesubula I, Tumwine JK. Bacterial aetiology and outcome in children with severe pneumonia in Uganda. *Ann Trop Paediatr.* (2008) 28:253–60. doi: 10.1179/146532808X375404
43. Nathoo KJ, Nkrumah FK, Ndlovu D, Nhembe M, Pirie DJ, Kowo H. Acute lower respiratory tract infection in hospitalized children in Zimbabwe. *Ann Trop Paediatr.* (1993) 13:253–61.
44. Okomo UA, Dibbasey T, Kassama K, Lawn JE, Zaman SM, Kampmann B, et al. Neonatal admissions, quality of care and outcome: 4 years of inpatient audit data from the Gambia's teaching hospital. *Paediatr Int Child Health* (2015) 35:252–64. doi: 10.1179/2046905515Y.0000000036
45. Okoromah CN, Lesi FE, Egri-Okwaji MT, Iroha E. Clinical and management factors related to outcome in neonatal tetanus. *Niger Postgrad Med J.* (2003) 10:92–5.
46. Ozkan H, Cetinkaya M, Koksal N, Celebi S, Hacimustafaoglu M. Culture-proven neonatal sepsis in preterm infants in a neonatal intensive care unit over a 7 year period: Coagulase-negative Staphylococcus as the predominant pathogen. *Pediatr Int.* (2014) 56:60–6. doi: 10.1111/ped.12218
47. Ramakrishna B, Graham SM, Phiri A, Mankhambo L, Duke T. Lactate as a predictor of mortality in Malawian children with WHO-defined pneumonia. *Arch Dis Child.* (2012) 97:336–42. doi: 10.1136/archdischild-2011-300920
48. Rodríguez DA, Rodríguez-Martínez CE, Cárdenas AC, Quilaguy IE, Mayorga LY, Falla LM, et al. Predictors of severity and mortality in children hospitalized with respiratory syncytial virus infection in a tropical region. *Pediatr Pulmonol.* (2014) 49:269–76. doi: 10.1002/ppul.22781
49. Sachdev HP, Kumar S, Singh KK, Satyanarayana L, Puri RK. Risk factors for fatal diarrhea in hospitalized children in India. *J Pediatr Gastroenterol Nutr.* (1991) 12:76–81.
50. Saleem AF, Qamar FN, Shahzad H, Qadir M, Zaidi AK. Trends in antibiotic susceptibility and incidence of late-onset Klebsiella pneumoniae neonatal sepsis over a six-year period in a neonatal intensive care unit in Karachi, Pakistan. *Int J Infect Dis.* (2013) 17:961–5. doi: 10.1016/j.ijid.2013.04.007
51. Santhanakrishnan BR, Ramalingam R. Risk factors for mortality in children with diarrhoeal disease in Madras, India. *J Diarrhoeal Dis Res.* (1987) 5:36–9.
52. Sarna MS, Saili A, Dutta AK, Kumari S. Neonatal mortality patterns in an urban hospital. *Indian Pediatr.* (1991) 28:719–24.
53. Sehgal V, Sethi GR, Sachdev HP, Satyanarayana L. Predictors of mortality in subjects hospitalized with acute lower respiratory tract infections. *Indian Pediatr.* (1997) 34:213–9.
54. Shann F, MacGregor D, Richens J, Coakley J. Cardiac failure in children with pneumonia in Papua New Guinea. *Pediatr Infect Dis J.* (1998) 17:1141–3.
55. Sheikh AN, Sajjad A, Hanif S. Neonatal sepsis: an evaluation of bacteriological spectrum, antibiotic susceptibilities and prognostic predictors at Civil Hospital, Karachi. *Pak Paediatr J.* (2014) 38:143–55.
56. Simiyu DE. Morbidity and mortality of neonates admitted in general paediatric wards at Kenyatta National Hospital. *East Afr Med J.* (2003) 80:611–6.
57. Smyth A, Carty H, Hart CA. Clinical predictors of hypoxaemia in children with pneumonia. *Ann Trop Paediatr.* (1998) 18:31–40. doi: 10.1080/02724936.1998.11747923
58. Teka T, Faruque AS, Fuchs GJ. Risk factors for deaths in under-age-five children attending a diarrhoea treatment centre. *Acta Paediatr.* (1996) 85:1070–5. doi: 10.1111/j.1651-2227.1996.tb14219.x
59. Tupasi TE, Velmonte MA, Sanvictores ME, Abraham L, De Leon LE, Tan SA, et al. Determinants of morbidity and mortality due to acute respiratory infections: Implications for intervention. *J Infect Dis.* (1988) 157:615–23.
60. Yaramis A, Tas MA. Neonatal tetanus in the southeast of Turkey: risk factors, and clinical and prognostic aspects. review of 73 cases, 1990–1999. *Turk J Pediatr.* (2000) 42:272–4.
61. Zhang Q, Guo Z, Bai Z, MacDonald NE. A 4 year prospective study to determine risk factors for severe community acquired pneumonia in children in southern China. *Pediatr Pulmonol.* (2013) 48:390–7. doi: 10.1002/ppul.22608
62. Islam MA, Rahman MM, Mahalanabis D, Rahman AK. Death in a diarrhoeal cohort of infants and young children soon after discharge from hospital: risk factors and causes by verbal autopsy. *J Trop Pediatr.* (1996) 42:342–7.
63. Weber MW, Carlin JB, Gatchalian S, Lehmann D, Muhe L, Mulholland EK, et al. Predictors of neonatal sepsis in developing countries. *Pediatr Infect Dis J.* (2003) 22:711–7. doi: 10.1097/01.inf.0000078163.80807.88
64. Coghill JE, Simkiss DE. Which clinical signs predict severe illness in children less than 2 months of age in resource poor countries? *J Trop Pediatr.* (2011) 57:3–8. doi: 10.1093/tropej/fmr001
65. Opiyo N, English M. What clinical signs best identify severe illness in young infants aged 0–59 days in developing countries? a systematic review. *Arch Dis Child.* (2011) 96:1052–9. doi: 10.1136/adc.2010.186049
66. Payne BA, Hutcheon JA, Ansermino JM, Hall DR, Bhutta ZA, Bhutta SZ, et al. A risk prediction model for the assessment and triage ofwomen with hypertensive disorders of pregnancy in low-resourced settings: the miniPIERS (Pre-eclampsia Integrated Estimate of RiSk) multi-country prospective cohort study. *PLoS Med.* (2014) 11:e1001589. doi: 10.1371/journal.pmed.1001589
67. Rassi A Jr., Rassi A, Little WC, Xavier SS, Rassi SG, Rassi AG, et al. Development and validation of a risk score for predicting death in Chagas' heart disease. *N Engl J Med.* (2006) 355:799–808. doi: 10.1056/NEJMoa053241
68. Wiens MO, Kumbakumba E, Larson CP, Ansermino JM, Singer J, Kissoon N, et al. Postdischarge mortality in children with acute infectious diseases: derivation of postdischarge mortality prediction models. *BMJ Open* (2015) 5:e009449. doi: 10.1136/bmjopen-2015-009449
69. Wiens MO, Kissoon N, Kabakyenga J. Smart hospital discharges to address a neglected epidemic in sepsis in low- and middle-income countries. *JAMA Pediatr.* (2018) 172:213–4. doi: 10.1001/jamapediatrics.2017.4519
70. Shitaye D, Asrat D, Woldeamanuel Y, Worku B. Risk factors and etiology of neonatal sepsis in Tikur Anbessa University Hospital, Ethiopia. *Ethiop Med J.* (2010) 48:11–21.
71. Pengsaa K, Lumbiganon P, Taksaphan S, Pairojkul S, Sookpranee T, Kosuwon P, et al. Risk factors for neonatal Klebsiella septicemia in Srinagarind Hospital. *Southeast Asian J Trop Med Public Health* (1996) 27:102–6.
72. Kissoon N, Uyeki T. Sepsis and the global burden of disease in children. *JAMA Pediatr.* (2016) 170:107–8. doi: 10.1001/jamapediatrics.2015.3241

12

Viral Sepsis in Children

Neha Gupta[1], *Robert Richter*[1], *Stephen Robert*[2] *and Michele Kong*[1*]

[1] Division of Pediatric Critical Care Medicine, Department of Pediatrics, University of Alabama at Birmingham, Birmingham, AL, United States, *[2] Division of Pediatric Critical Care Medicine, Cedars-Sinai Medical Center, Los Angeles, CA, United States*

***Correspondence:**
Michele Kong
mkong@peds.uab.edu

Sepsis in children is typically presumed to be bacterial in origin until proven otherwise, but frequently bacterial cultures ultimately return negative. Although viruses may be important causative agents of culture-negative sepsis worldwide, the incidence, disease burden and mortality of viral-induced sepsis is poorly elucidated. Consideration of viral sepsis is critical as its recognition carries implications on appropriate use of antibacterial agents, infection control measures, and, in some cases, specific, time-sensitive antiviral therapies. This review outlines our current understanding of viral sepsis in children and addresses its epidemiology and pathophysiology, including pathogen-host interaction during active infection. Clinical manifestation, diagnostic testing, and management options unique to viral infections will be outlined.

Keywords: viral sepsis, sepsis, viral infections, viral coinfections, secondary bacterial infections, pediatric, children

INTRODUCTION

Sepsis is a leading cause of pediatric mortality (1). Defined as systemic inflammatory response syndrome in the presence of a suspected or confirmed infection, it is a clinical syndrome principally characterized by dysregulation of the host innate immune response and may result in an immune phenotype of coexistent systemic inflammation and immunosuppression (2). Pathological cross-talk between inflammatory and coagulation cascades, complement activation, and neuroendocrine signals wreak havoc on homeostatic controls. This hyperinflammatory response has untoward effects on the cardiopulmonary system, vascular endothelium, and gut, precipitating progressive organ dysfunction until the host succumbs (3). The morbidity, mortality, and costs associated with pediatric sepsis impose a significant burden on the healthcare community and global economy (4, 5). Watson et al reported a mean hospital length of stay of 31 days, with approximately $2 billion spent annually in healthcare cost associated with severe pediatric sepsis (1). International guidelines for management of sepsis and septic shock stress the importance of rapid resuscitation, prompt antimicrobial administration, and supportive care of organ dysfunction as the mainstays of pediatric sepsis treatment (6).

Viral sepsis can be defined as a severe inflammatory response to a suspected or confirmed viral infection. However, making the definitive diagnosis of viral sepsis in a child is particularly challenging for clinicians. The astute clinician must incorporate the patient's history of present illness, physical exam, laboratory and radiographic data to determine the likelihood of a viral etiology for sepsis. Even with a positive viral test, limitations of the testing result should be considered. Despite these challenges, timely diagnosis of viral sepsis has significant implications on clinical management, including guiding the use of appropriate antiviral therapy and informing isolation and containment strategies. Moreover, timely diagnosis of viral sepsis may prevent unnecessarily prolonged antibacterial treatment exposure and thus could help prevent consequent antibacterial resistance and deleterious effects on the host microbiome. This review outlines our current understanding of viral sepsis in children, including its epidemiology and the pathophysiology of the viral-host response during active infection. The clinical manifestations, appropriate diagnostic testing, and management unique to viral infections are outlined.

Epidemiology

The true incidence of viral sepsis, particularly in the pediatric population, remains unknown. Since bacterial sepsis is amenable to treatment and is presumably more common, viral testing is frequently foregone in the acute presentation of sepsis. However, a recent study of adult patients with sepsis showed that viral respiratory pathogens, namely influenza A virus, human metapneumovirus, coronavirus, and respiratory syncytial virus (RSV), were overlooked in 70% of patients (7). In a multinational epidemiological study of children with severe sepsis, an infectious etiology was only proven in 65% of patients and out of these, approximately one-third had a viral infection (8). The most frequent sites of infection were the respiratory tract (40%) and bloodstream (20%), with rhinovirus, RSV, and adenovirus most commonly isolated. In contrast, the Australia and New Zealand sepsis study group identified a pathogen in approximately 50% of patients with sepsis and septic shock (9). Of these patients, only one-fifth had a viral etiology, with RSV, cytomegalovirus (CMV), Epstein-Barr virus (EBV), herpes simplex virus (HSV), varicella zoster virus (VZV) and influenza being the most common viruses identified in this study. Recently, Ames et al. reported that 16% of pediatric patients who presented with septic shock had a primary viral disease (10). In another study of neonates with sepsis, bacterial etiology was found in only approximately 15% of cases, making viral infection more likely as a plausible cause of sepsis in these patients (11).

In the pediatric intensive care unit (PICU), influenza virus is a leading cause of viral sepsis and caries an especially high mortality rate (12). RSV has also been found to cause severe bronchiolitis and may present with sepsis, especially in children with history of premature birth, chronic lung disease, congenital heart disease or primary immunodeficiency (13, 14). Sepsis has also been observed in neonates with HSV, human parechovirus (HPeV) and enteroviral infection (15–18). Patients with immunodeficiency due to human immunodeficiency virus (HIV) infection are highly susceptible to viral sepsis depending on the stage of disease and access and response to the treatment (19). In these patients, common viral infections observed to cause sepsis include RSV, influenza, parainfluenza, adenovirus, CMV, EBV, and VZV (19). Diarrheal diseases secondary to viral infections can also lead to sepsis, especially in developing countries (20). Although rare, rotavirus has been associated with sepsis due to bacterial coinfection (21). Despite several large studies on viral sepsis in general (ref as above), as well as on specific viruses, in the absence of routine viral testing during the diagnostic evaluation of sepsis, the true incidence of viral infection as the cause of sepsis remains unclear.

Pathophysiology and Host Response to Viral Sepsis

The host response to infection consists of a multitude of simultaneous processes designed to neutralize the infectious threat and initiate repair of injured tissue. Sepsis is characterized by systemic and dysregulated inflammation, which can lead to a vicious cycle of vascular endotheliopathy, microcirculatory hypoperfusion, intestinal barrier dysfunction, circulatory shock, mitochondrial failure, and death (22–24). Moreover, the concomitant compensatory anti-inflammatory response syndrome that is characterized by lymphocyte apoptosis and immune paralysis predisposes the host to secondary nosocomial infection and latent viral activation (25, 26). The type of mechanisms employed vary by virus but generally result in some combination of (1) cytokine release, (2) endotheliopathy, and (3) host cytotoxicity (27). While an in-depth review of the pathogenesis of all human disease-causing viruses is beyond the scope of this manuscript, we have outlined the general pathophysiology below, highlighting major illustrative viral examples where possible.

Cytokine Release (Figure 1)

Pathogen-recognition receptors (PRRs) are cellular sensors that recognize specific molecular structure of a pathogen (28). Toll-like receptors (TLRs) and retinoic acid-inducible gene-I (RIG-I)-like receptors (RLRs) are two types of PRRs that are involved in viral sensing (28). TLRs, which are found on the cell surface or within endosomes of monocytes, macrophages, dendritic, epithelial and endothelial cells, encounter pathogen-associated molecular patterns (PAMPs) (29, 30). Intracellular TLR-7 and TLR-8 recognize single-stranded Ribonucleic Acid (RNA) of viruses like HPeV, the enteroviruses, human metapneumovirus, and influenza; intracellular TLR-9 recognizes double-stranded (ds) DNA of viruses like the herpes viruses (e.g., HSV-1 and -2, EBV), adenovirus, and CMV; and TLR-3 recognizes dsRNA produced during intracellular viral replication (31). TLR activation culminates in myeloid differentiation primary response 88 (MyD88, through TLR-7,-8, and -9) or Toll/Interleukin (IL)-1 receptor domain-containing adapter protein inducing IFN-β (TRIF, through TLR-3) activation (32). These proteins, in turn, activate nuclear factor kappa-light-chain-enhancer of activated B cells (NF-κB) and IFN-regulatory factor (IFR)-mediated cytokine transcription (33–35). RLRs are cytosolic innate immunity sensors for viral RNA. Three members of RLRs have been identified: RIG-I, melanoma differentiation associated factor 5 (MDA5], and laboratory of genetics and physiology 2 (LGP2) (36). RIG-I and MDA5 recognize dsRNAs in response to different RNA viruses and signal the production of pro-inflammatory cytokines and type-1 IFNs (37). Cytokine proliferation instigates a pro-inflammatory cascade that results in complement activation, neutrophil chemotaxis, cytotoxic cluster of differentiation (CD) 8+ T-cell recruitment, and protease release from leukocytes and endothelial cells, particularly trypsin (38) and heparanase (39). Trypsin is upregulated and released by the vascular endothelium (38) and has been shown to cleave circulating pro-matrix metalloproteinase (pro-MMP) released from macrophages to form activated MMPs (40). MMPs, in conjunction with heparanase, degrade the endothelial glycocalyx (41, 42). Moreover, viral particles induce reactive oxygen species generation by circulating neutrophils, eosinophils, and macrophages (43, 44) that further injure the endothelial glycocalyx (45) and activate NF-κB cell-signaling

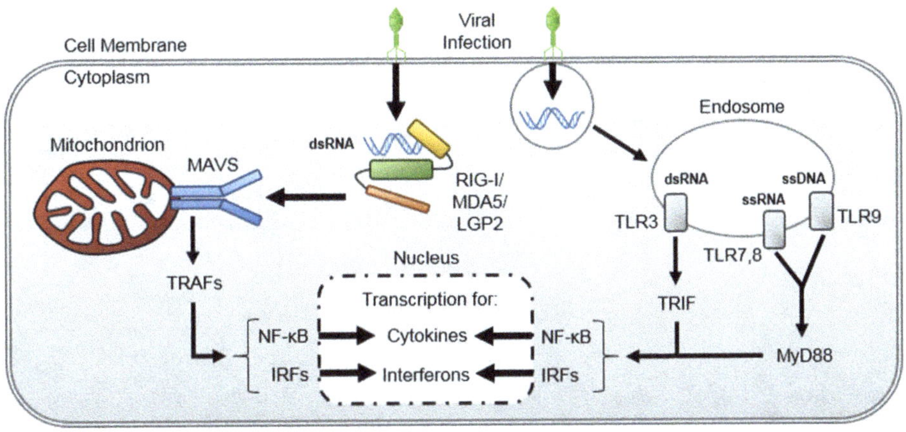

FIGURE 1 | Viral-induced cytokine upregulation and release. Double stranded viral ribonucleic acids are (dsRNA) recognized within the host cellular cytosol by retinoic acid-inducible gene-I (RIG-I)-like receptors (RLRs)- RIG-I, MDA5, and LGP2. The RLRs bound to viral dsRNA undergo conformational change and complex with mitochondrial antiviral signaling (MAVS) protein on the mitochondrion surface. The RLR-MAVS interaction instigates an assembly of host proteins to activate TNF-receptor-associated factors (TRAFs), thereby inducing nuclear factor kappa-light-chain-enhancer of activated B cells (NF-κB) and interferon regulator factor (IRF)-mediated cytokine transcription in the host cell nucleus. Viral nucleic acids are also recognized within Toll-like receptors (TLRs) within host cell endosomes, triggering myeloid differentiation primary response 88 (MyD88) and Toll/interleukin-1 receptor-domain-containing adaptor-inducing interferon-β (TRIF) pathways that also activate NF-κB and IRF-mediated cytokine transcription in the host cell nucleus.

(46), propagating a positive-feedback loop that results in endotheliopathy and end-organ damage.

Endotheliopathy (Figure 2)

Systemic viral dissemination appears to be the etiology of viral sepsis. The exact mechanisms by which viruses that are normally isolated to the respiratory or integumentary epithelium reach the bloodstream are not known. However, it is plausible that viremia occurs through direct invasion of epithelial cells (or neurons as in case of HSV or varicella disease) to reach the surrounding vasculature (47). Once in the blood, the virus may induce endothelial glycocalyx degradation by activating leukocytes, platelets, and endothelial cells to secrete MMPs and heparanase that target glycocalyx components (39, 48). Endothelial glycocalyx disruption exposes selectins and intracellular adhesion molecules, making them available for leukocyte adhesion and activation (49). Glycocalyx degradation also releases heparan sulfate that may bind and activate antithrombin III and exposes membrane-bound glycoprotein Ib/IX/V complexes (50) that can bind circulating von Willebrand factor (51) and P-selectins on platelets (52, 53), precipitating coagulopathy. Moreover, loss of integrity of the protein-rich glycocalyx alters the microvascular fluid equilibrium between the vascular lumen and subglycocalyx, increasing fluid and macromolecule filtration through the endothelium to the surrounding interstitium (54). The end result of endothelial glycocalyx damage is pro-inflammatory propagation and vascular leak that can compromise organ function.

Circulating viral particles may also induce endothelial cell structural changes that lead to barrier disruption and further vascular leak. Endothelial cells are anchored to each other through adherens junctions comprised predominantly of vascular endothelial (VE)-cadherin, which is attached to the endothelial cytoskeleton through beta-catenin and p120-catenin (55, 56). In human endothelial cells, pathogenic strains of hantavirus appear to bind to cellular surface β3-integrins, thereby promoting VE-cadherin internalization and adherens junction destabilization (57). VE-cadherin destabilization may also be mediated through the cellular membrane Tie2 receptor. Tie2 receptor is activated by angiopoietin-1 (Agpt-1) that is derived by periendothelial cells (58, 59). When activated, the Tie2 receptor activates PI3K/Akt cell-survival signaling and Rac1-mediated cytoskeletal stabilization (60). Inflammatory mediators, such as thrombin (61), reactive oxygen species (62), and VEGF (63), stimulate endothelial cell Weibel-Palade body exocytosis, releasing the Tie2 antagonist Agpt-2 (64). Agpt-2 acts in an autocrine fashion to inhibit Tie2 signaling, thereby promoting RhoA kinase activity and VE-cadherin destabilization (60). Mice infected with a pathogenic strain of H3N2 influenza virus develop acute lung injury that is rescued by the Tie2 agonist vasculotide (65), suggesting that the Tie2 receptor is integral in the development of endotheliopathy during viral sepsis. The exact mechanisms each virus employs to induce endothelial cell dysfunction are not clear; however, the typical presentation of capillary leak with viral sepsis suggests a common pathway by which endothelial integrity is compromised.

Host Cytotoxicity (Figure 3)

Viral-induced host cytotoxicity is mediated by cytopathic effects, cellular reprogramming, and/or initiation of host immune cytotoxic responses. Viruses take over and utilize host intracellular machinery to replicate, depleting host cells of energy stores and transcription potential. Furthermore, viral-infected cells may be activated for caspase-dependent apoptosis (66). Viruses may also indirectly promote apoptosis through macrophage reprogramming. Macrophages infected with H5N1

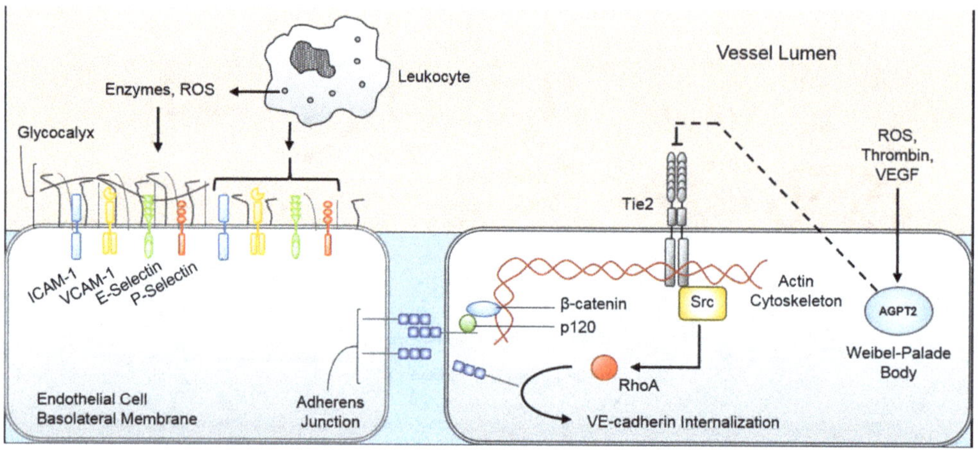

FIGURE 2 | Pathophysiologic mechanisms of viral-induced endotheliopathy. Innate immune system activation during viral sepsis precipitates leukocyte degranulation and release of enzymes and reactive oxygen species (ROS) that degrade the endothelial glycocalyx. Denuded endothelial glycocalyx exposes cellular adhesion molecules (e.g., ICAM-1, VCAM-1, E-selectin, P-selectin) that increase the margination and activation of leukocytes, further promoting the inflammatory response. Additionally, inflammatory mediators, namely thrombin, ROS, and vascular endothelial growth factor (VEGF), promote Weibel-Palade body exocytosis, releasing angiopoietin-2 (Agpt-2) into the circulation. Agpt-2 antagonizes the endothelial cell Tie2 receptor, allowing the Src-mediated RhoA enzyme to reconfigure the endothelial cell cytoskeleton and promote VE-cadherin internalization from the adherens junction. Loss of glycocalyx and adherens junction integrity permits increased trans-cellular protein and fluid movement from the vascular lumen to the interstitium. ICAM-1, intercellular adhesion molecule 1; VCAM-1, vascular cell adhesion molecule 1.

avian influenza have been shown to upregulate production and release of tumor necrosis factor (TNF)-related apoptosis-inducing ligand (TRAIL) that promote T-cell apoptosis (67). Though the effect of TRAIL on other cell lineages was not determined, it is plausible that the effect seen in T-cells may be more diffuse. Systemic viral dissemination from sites of primary infection (e.g., human metapneumovirus in the respiratory tract or HPeV in the gastrointestinal tract) may occur through these apoptotic mechanisms, whereby new virions are released, infect local endothelial cells, and cause further cellular apoptosis and systemic viral spread. The invasiveness and pervasiveness of the viral infection is likely dictated by cell tropism and genetically determined virulence as viruses with greater cytopathogenicity, such as H5N1 avian influenza (66) and HPeV-3 (68), are more likely to cause sepsis in immunocompetent hosts than viruses with typically minimal associated cytopathology (e.g., RSV or parainfluenza) (69). Lastly, effectors of the host immune system, such as natural killer (NK), cytotoxic CD8+ T cells and complement, attack, and destroy virally infected host cells.

Viral pathogenesis in children also varies according to the degree of host immunocompetence. Generally, young infants have significantly reduced TLR expression, antigen-presenting cell activity, NK cell responsiveness, T-cell functionality, B-cell maturity, and complement concentration (70). This immaturity of the developing immune system places young infants at significantly higher risk for severe disease from viruses that would typically cause minimal harm to older children and adults (e.g., HSV, HPeV, enteroviruses, CMV). Similarly, children with congenital or acquired immunodeficiencies are more susceptible to viral pathogens. Specific immunodeficiencies that place children at higher risk for viral sepsis include NK cell deficiency, interferon (IFN)-γ receptor deficiency, TLR-3 deficiency, nuclear factor-kappa B essential modulator deficiency, severe combined immunodeficiency, severe T-cell lymphopenia in DiGeorge syndrome, agammaglobulinemia, and hyperIgM syndrome (71). Severe RNA viral infections have also been observed in patients with loss-of-function mutation of the IFN induced with helicase C domain 1 (IFIH1) gene that encodes the RLR MDA5 (36, 37, 72). Moreover, children receiving immunomodulatory or immunosuppressive therapies due to malignancy, transplantation, or autoimmune disease are more susceptible to viral infection or reactivation.

Clinical Features and Risk Factors for Viral Sepsis

The constitutional symptoms and clinical features of viral sepsis are frequently indistinguishable from bacterial or fungal sepsis. Presenting symptoms and signs include fever, chills, rash, respiratory distress, nausea, vomiting, diarrhea, dysuria, confusion, and altered mental status. None of these symptoms is pathognomonic of sepsis, let alone viral induced sepsis. Moreover, classic features of systemic inflammation might not be seen in every individual, especially in immunocompromised children. Fever is one of the most common symptoms seen in septic children, attributable to the pyrogenic activity of IL-1, IL-6, IFNs, and TNF-α. It has been observed that these substances increase prostaglandin E2 synthesis in the hypothalamus (73, 74), resulting in the elevation in the host central nervous system core temperature set-point regulated by the pre-optic and dorsomedial hypothalamic nuclei (75). Hypothermia, on the other hand, is a less frequent but more specific indicator of sepsis that may be predictive of illness severity and death, especially in younger children and chronically debilitated patients (74). Injury to the vascular endothelium may result in broad array of failing

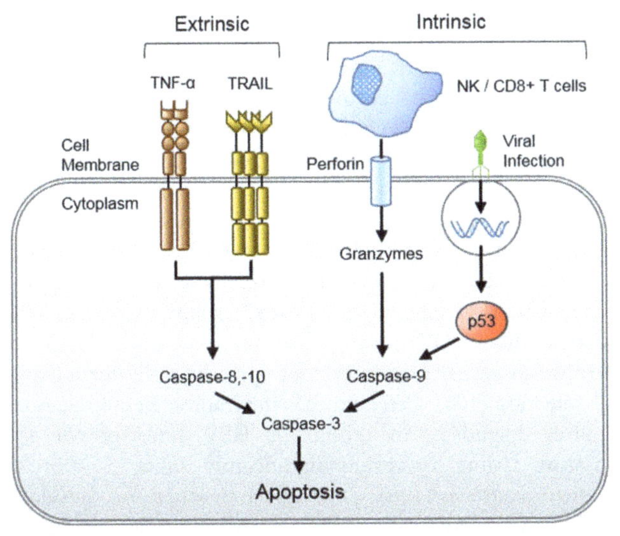

FIGURE 3 | Viral-induced host cytotoxicity through the extrinsic and intrinsic apoptotic pathways. Tumor necrosis factor-alpha (TNF-α) is released after viral recognition by the innate immune system, and TNF-related apoptosis-inducing ligand (TRAIL) is released from viral-reprogrammed macrophages, both of which bind their respective host cell surface death receptors to activate the extrinsic apoptotic pathway. Natural killer (NK) and cluster of differentiation 8 (CD8+) T cells inject perforin into the membranes of infected host cells, through which they secrete granzymes that elicit the intrinsic apoptotic pathway. The intrinsic pathway may be activated after viral protein recognition by the host cell or suicide gene insertion by cytotoxic viruses.

organs that manifests as confusion, nausea, vomiting, diarrhea, oliguria, and coagulopathy. A myriad of cardiopulmonary manifestations ranging from mild tachypnea and tachycardia to acute respiratory distress syndrome and shock can be seen (76). The presenting symptoms usually depend on the type of virus. Clinical presentation in patients with respiratory viral infections can range from completely asymptomatic to severe respiratory distress due to pneumonia. Diarrheal illness has been observed in patients infected with rotavirus, norovirus, enterovirus, and adenovirus. VZV and HSV infection may present with vesicular rash. Children with HSV or arbovirus infection may have confusion, altered mental status or seizures from encephalitis. Elevated transaminases are common with HSV and enteroviral infections which may be complicated by hepatitis, coagulopathy and encephalitis. Neonatal HPeV infection can mimic other enteroviral infections in the initial presentation. Often these patients present with fever, rash, irritability, feeding intolerance, and seizures (17). They can develop sepsis like illness and encephalitis. Patients with acute HIV infection often have flu-like symptoms such as fever, headache and rash, which usually resolve spontaneously. These patients soon enter a phase of clinical latency until they develop acquired immunodeficiency syndrome, usually heralded by acquisition of an opportunistic infection.

As with other types of sepsis, virus-induced sepsis requires a high index of suspicion, especially in very young children and those with chronic medical conditions. Neonates and young infants are at higher risk of sepsis from HSV, HPeVs, and enterovirus. HSV is usually acquired perinatally from mothers with genital herpes. Mothers with primary herpes are more likely to transmit the infection when compared to those with recurrent and non-primary herpes (77). Nielsen et al reported that second born children are at higher risk of HPeV-3 infection than the firstborn (78). Seizures, drowsiness and lethargy, and absence of oral lesions are associated with severe enteroviral infection in children (79). In RSV infection, comorbid conditions reported to increase the risk for severe infection include the history of prematurity, congenital heart disease, chronic lung disease, and immunodeficiency (13). In a recent study, Eggleston et al found that patients with metapneumovirus infection were more likely to be older and have congenital heart disease compared to RSV infected patients (80). In contrast, asthmatics and premature infants were at higher risk for rhinovirus infection (81). Finally, predisposing conditions for severe pediatric influenza infection include age less than 2 years; asthma; cardiac, renal, hepatic, hematologic, neurologic or neuromuscular conditions; long-term aspirin therapy; immunosuppressive therapy and residence in a chronic care facility (82). Risk of mother-to-child perinatal HIV transmission is higher in mothers with CD4 count < 200 cells/μL and lower in infants receiving antiretroviral prophylaxis (83, 84). If patients with any of these conditions present with sepsis, diagnostic viral testing and appropriate empiric antiviral treatment should be strongly considered according to the individual's risk factors.

Association With Secondary Bacterial Infections and Viral Coinfections

Secondary bacterial infections are commonly associated with respiratory viral infections (85). In the winter of 1995–96, an outbreak of *Streptococcus pneumoniae* pneumonia developed in otherwise healthy children who had a preceding influenza A viral illness (86). During the 2009–10 influenza A pandemic, one third of critically ill children afflicted with influenza were diagnosed with concurrent bacterial infections (87). In this study, the leading three bacterial coinfections were *Staphylococcus aureus*, *Pseudomonas spp.*, and *Haemophilus influenza* (87). In children hospitalized for RSV, *Haemophilus influenzae* and *Streptococcus pneumoniae* were the most common organisms isolated in those who developed bacteremia (88). These secondary bacterial infections may exacerbate innate immune dysfunction (89) and convey substantially increased risk of worse outcomes (90, 91). However, to date, the mechanisms underlying bacterial synergism and increased susceptibility to secondary bacterial infection in the setting of a preceding respiratory viral infection remain unclear. In general, this phenomenon appears to involve impairment of respiratory epithelial and innate immune system defenses. Viral destruction of the airway epithelium affects mucociliary clearance, allowing bacterial attachment to mucins and eventual colonization of the respiratory tract (92, 93). Additionally, viral-induced upregulation of IFN-γ and TNF-α may lead to a dysregulated host T-cell response, decreased neutrophil chemotaxis, and impaired macrophage phagocytosis that increases the host susceptibility to secondary bacterial pathogens (94). Upregulation of the surface platelet-activating factor receptor on epithelial cells and leukocytes by pro-inflammatory cytokines may also increase adhesion and invasion of certain virulent pneumococcal strains (95).

Rotavirus infection has also been associated with secondary bacterial infections (21). Although, the exact mechanisms leading to sepsis and organ dysfunction are unknown, a leading hypothesis entails translocation of bacteria and endotoxin through damaged intestinal epithelium into the splanchnic circulation, systemically increasing production of nitric oxide and circulating pro-inflammatory cytokines like TNF and IL-1β, and high mobility group box 1 protein, resulting in sequential organ failure (96). HIV infection can lead to apoptosis of CD4 T-lymphocytes, defective T and B lymphocyte function, decreased production of IFN-γ, IL-2 and immunoglobulins, and decreased NK cell activity (97–99). This leads to not only increased risk of secondary bacterial infections but also increased susceptibility to other viruses and intracellular organisms such as mycobacteria and *Pneumocystis jiroveci*.

Similar to bacterial coinfections, critically ill children can be simultaneously infected by multiple viruses. The course of illness in patients with viral coinfections depend on virus-virus interaction. Various mechanisms for disease virulence in viral coinfections have been proposed, including viral gene interactions, immunologic interactions and alteration in host environment (100). Even though the clinical significance such interactions is unknown, a study by Rhedin et al. reported increased risk of severe respiratory disease in patients with viral coinfections compared to those with single viral infections (101). Approximately 20% of the patients had viral coinfection and RSV, bocavirus and adenovirus were the most common viruses associated with coinfections (101).In another study performed in Canada on patients with respiratory viral infections, approximately 17% of the patients had viral coinfections (102). There was no difference in the risk of hospitalization or the severity of illness in patients with single viral infections and those with viral coinfections (102). Another study done in Greece revealed a much higher viral coinfection rate (42%) with most common coinfections with RSV, influenza, rhinovirus and parainfluenza viruses (103). Increased risk of hospitalization has been observed in patients with viral coinfections (103). However, systematic reviews and meta-analyses of children with viral coinfections have not shown any association with increased clinical severity (104, 105). Patients infected with HIV are at high risk of secondary viral infections such as CMV, HSV and respiratory viruses like RSV, influenza and metapneumovirus.

Diagnostic Testing

The diagnosis of viral sepsis is typically one of exclusion. Bacterial sepsis, whether primary or secondary, is usually of higher initial concern because failure to recognize this diagnosis and promptly administer systemic antibiotics has lethal consequences. Unfortunately, in our current state of limited antiviral therapies, even the prompt recognition and treatment of viral sepsis may not quickly improve a patient's clinical course. Nonetheless, early, definitive diagnosis of a primary viral septic process may inform treatment decision-making and help limit unnecessary systemic antibiotic administration. In symptomatic critically ill children, identification of a viral etiology can play an important role in the management and impact the outcome of these patients.

There are currently no standard approaches to viral diagnostic testing. Point-of-care (POC) antigen-based testing is relatively inexpensive and provides rapid detection of common respiratory viruses from a nasopharyngeal swab, such as RSV or common strains of human influenza. However, POC testing may lack the sensitivity needed to determine the etiology of life-threatening sepsis (106). Direct fluorescent antibody (DFA) testing may provide better specificity and a broader range of viral strain detection than POC testing, but the test depends on the collection of sufficient numbers of epithelial cells for adequate viral detection (107). Cell culture is the traditional gold-standard for viral diagnoses, including for HSV, however the long turn-around time for results significantly limits its utility for expedient diagnosis (108). Commercial or laboratory-developed nucleic acid amplification tests (NAATs) (e.g., polymerase chain reaction, PCR, or reverse transcription-loop-mediated isothermal amplification) may provide greater sensitivity and specificity than POC or DFA testing but requires sophisticated equipment and specially trained laboratory staff to complete (109, 110). NAATs have the added benefit of being highly multiplexed with new commercially available technology like Biofire® FilmArray® multiplex PCR (111). Unfortunately, the use of NAATs is limited by the high cost, delay in results and the inability to distinguish between viral nucleic acids from live viruses (112). Ultimately, the methods available for timely viral detection are limited by technique of sample collection and institutional resource availability.

Several limitations to the current diagnostic testing for causative viruses are worth noting, and results of viral testing always need to be interpreted with caution. For instance, although a type of enterovirus, HPeV cannot be detected on routine enterovirus PCR assay. HPeV-specific PCR is required to detect this virus in respiratory, CSF and stool samples of infected children and should be considered as a part of workup for neonates and young children presenting with sepsis (113). The clinical utility of viral respiratory PCR panels is also limited by their high rates of positive detections without clinical correlates. Detection of a virus in a patient with sepsis does not necessarily indicate causation. Some studies have shown that a respiratory virus can be detected in about one third of asymptomatic children (114, 115). Viral PCR testing is particularly difficult to interpret due to its high sensitivity for viral nucleic acids, making it challenging for the clinician to distinguish between active viral disease and viral nucleic acid or live viral carriage (112, 116, 117). A positive test could be a result of asymptomatic colonization, prolonged viral shedding or viral coinfection. In a study by Rhedin et al. comparing PCR results between symptomatic and asymptomatic patients, RSV, metapneumovirus and parainfluenza viruses had a significantly higher detection rate in children with acute respiratory infection, suggesting causation; however, other viruses (enterovirus, coronavirus, bocavirus, rhinovirus, and adenovirus) had an equally high detection rates in asymptomatic children (101). Because of these positive viral detections in asymptomatic children, it is important that clinicians consider the big picture, and factor in other pertinent information that may indicate an active ongoing bacterial infection before discontinuing antibacterial agents based on a viral assay. The use of serum biomarkers (see section below) and whole blood gene expression analysis (118) may serve a crucial role in this setting to discern viral from bacterial sepsis. When faced with a septic child who has an unusual sepsis presentation, does not respond to usual therapies, or has persistently negative diagnostic evaluations, a viral etiology must be considered and consultation with an infectious disease expert is recommended.

Biomarkers for Viral Sepsis

Several serum biomarkers, including lactate, C-reactive protein (CRP), and procalcitonin (PCT), are used to guide management in sepsis and are an important part of early goal directed therapy (119). PCT is more commonly used in the ICU setting for early determination of the likelihood of a bacterial etiology for sepsis and to guide antimicrobial duration (120, 121). Serum PCT has been shown to be elevated in bacterial infections and is superior to CRP in assessing the severity and course of the disease (122). However, the mean sensitivity of PCT as a biomarker of sepsis remains low at 77%, with a specificity of 79% (123, 124). Unfortunately, in general, these biomarkers are non-specific in distinguishing bacterial vs. viral infection (125).

In recent years, several viral-specific biomarkers have been identified. Many transcriptional signatures have been designed to distinguish viral infections from bacterial infections as well as non-infectious conditions (126, 127). Zaas et al. identified a 30-gene signature to discriminate symptomatic influenza A-infected subjects from both healthy and bacterially-infected subjects (128). In a recent study by Herberg et al., a 2-transcript RNA signature [*FAM89A* and *IFI44L*) showed promising results in its ability to distinguish between bacterial and viral infections, demonstrating that the expression of *IFI44L* was increased in patients with viral infection, whereas expression of *FAM89A* was increased in patients with bacterial infection (118). Another recent study identified a four-gene expression signature in whole blood to distinguish viral infections from other etiologies (129). Human myxovirus resistance protein 1 (MxA) is an important intermediate product in the IFN-mediated antiviral response against a variety of viruses. Serum MxA levels are significantly higher in patients with viral infections compared to bacterial infections in pediatric population and thus may be an additionally useful biomarker to discriminate viral from bacterial illness (130).

Preventive Strategies and Management

There is a paucity of data regarding treatment and management of viral infection. Supportive care is the current mainstay of therapy for most viral infections, particularly for respiratory viruses. Though broad-spectrum antibiotic therapy may be prudent until a bacterial source for sepsis has been definitively ruled-out, sustained antibiotic treatment has no role in the management of viral sepsis except in the case of bacterial coinfections. Many viral infections can be prevented with the use of hand hygiene, environmental decontamination, use of personal protective equipment, elimination of second-hand smoke, and isolation of infected children (131). Additional protection can be conferred by administering vaccines for common communicable viruses. These preventive strategies are of particular importance in high-risk patients. As the scope of available vaccines and anti-viral therapies remains rather limited, development of novel vaccines and treatment is critical (131).

For RSV infection, management is currently limited to passive immunization for at-risk infants. Palivizumab, an RSV-specific monoclonal antibody, is Food and Drug Administration (FDA) approved for the prevention of infection in high-risk infants during RSV season. The American Academy of Pediatrics has issued more clear recommendations for palivizumab use, stating that it should be administered as a monthly injection during RSV season in children born less than 29 weeks, 0 days gestation and are less than 12 months of age or in children with congenital heart disease, chronic lung disease (132). Studies have shown variable efficacy of palivizumab, with reduction in RSV hospitalization rate by approximately 60% (133). Currently, aerosolized ribavirin is the only FDA-approved treatment available for the management of RSV infection, though its use remains controversial (134). To date, RSV vaccines and antiviral therapies remain an active area of investigation (135). A randomized, controlled trial performed in adult patients with RSV infection compared the RSV entry inhibitor GS-5806 to placebo and demonstrated a decrease in both viral load and the clinical severity of infection in patients treated with GS-5806 (136). Similar fusion inhibitors such as ALX-0171 (137), JNJ-2408068 (138), MDT-637 (139), and VP14637 (138) demonstrate efficacy *in vitro*, and ALX-0171 is undergoing a phase II clinical trial in infants hospitalized for RSV (clinicaltrials.gov registration no. NCT02979431). The use of ALS-008176, an RSV polymerase inhibitor, has similarly been shown to reduce viral load, rapidly clear RSV, and improve the severity of disease in adults with RSV infection (140). ALN-RSV01 is a lipid-based nanoparticulate system, containing small-interfering RNA (siRNA] that demonstrates promising antiviral effects against RSV in lung transplant patients (141) by targeting the mRNA of the RSV nucleocapsid protein, thereby limiting viral replication (142). However, until these novel treatments have undergone appropriate clinical trials, the pediatric medical community must continue to wait for effective RSV antiviral therapy.

Unlike RSV, seasonal vaccines and several antiviral therapies are available to treat influenza viral infections. The seasonal influenza vaccine has demonstrated reasonable efficacy at attenuating influenza A and B viral disease (143). Currently, two forms of the influenza vaccine are available for use in children: a live attenuated vaccine in the form of a nasal spray and an inactivated vaccine in an injectable form. Antiviral agents used in the treatment and post-exposure prophylaxis of influenza infections include neuraminidase inhibitors (oseltamivir and zanamivir) and the adamantanes (amantadine and rimantadine). Oseltamivir is the most commonly used medication due to high prevalence of adamantane resistance. Oseltamivir has shown to be beneficial and tolerable in children with influenza if received within first 48 h of illness (144, 145). However, in cases of severe infection, initiation of oseltamivir beyond 48 h of symptom onset may still provide benefit (146). Nanotechnology-based vaccines are also being developed for influenza virus. InflexalR V and InfluvacR are two virosomal vaccines that have been shown to be efficacious against influenza infection (147, 148). STP702, another nanotherapeutic agent, is an siRNA under development designed to inhibit conserved regions in H1N1 and H5N1 strains of the influenza virus and prevent viral replication (116). Nanotraps such as sialylneolacto-N-tetraose c (LSTc)-bearing liposomal decoys bind to hemagglutinins on the influenza virus and prevent viral spread *in* vitro, demonstrating the potential have shown to be effective against influenza virus (117). The influenza polymerase inhibitor T-705 (favipiravir) has been demonstrated significant attenuation of influenza virus activity (149). Interestingly, at higher concentration, it has also shown to be effective against poliovirus, rhinovirus and RSV (149). Other agents under investigation include CS-8958, a long-acting neuraminidase inhibitor, and DAS181, an attachment inhibitor (150). Animal studies have also shown promising results with combination therapy (150). Various immunomodulatory agents have also been posited to temper the dysregulated host inflammatory response in severe influenza (151), including cyclooxygenase-2 inhibitors (152), doxycycline (153), glucocorticoids (154), macrolides (155, 156), peroxisome proliferator-activated receptor agonists such as gemfibrozil (157), sphingosine-1-phosphate (158), and the Tie2 receptor activator vasculotide (65). Further studies are needed to determine the efficacy of these treatments in human influenza infection.

Pleconaril, an orally administered viral capsid inhibitor, has shown to be effective against picornaviruses, especially enteroviruses and rhinoviruses (159). Abzug et al. reported greater survival in patients with neonatal enteroviral sepsis who received pleconaril (159). Similarly, patient with rhinovirus infection treated with pleconaril have shorter duration of symptoms, depending on susceptibility of the virus to the medication (160). No antiviral activity has been observed from pleconaril against HPeV (18). Intravenous immunoglobulin has shown potential benefit in management of enteroviral infections (161).

Prevention of neonatal HSV infection is more elusive as neonatal HSV disease often occurs after transmission from asymptomatic women with primary HSV infection (162). In cases of active maternal genital herpes, cesarean sections can decrease the incidence of neonatal HSV infection, especially when performed within 4 h of rupture of membranes (163). A subunit HSV vaccine has shown promising results in prevention of genital herpes and is currently under Phase III trial (164). Although not routinely recommended, antiviral prophylaxis with acyclovir in late pregnancy has been demonstrated to decrease viral shedding, leading to reduction in cesarean rates and recurrent herpes (165, 166). Patients with severe neonatal HSV infection (those with disseminated disease and CNS infection) should be treated with intravenous acyclovir for 21 days (167).

Viral sepsis may occur in HIV-infected children due to opportunistic or other secondary viral infections (19). Increasing use of highly active antiretroviral therapy (HAART) has significantly improved survival of HIV infected children by decreasing the progression to acquired immunodeficiency syndrome (AIDS), thereby maintaining host immunocompetence that protects against the development of viral sepsis (168–171). However, HAART is associated with potentially deleterious sequelae, making timing of the therapy very controversial in patients with active sepsis (19).

Outcomes

Extensive studies have not been done to characterize the effect of viral sepsis on outcomes. In a recent study, Hon et al. found no difference in mortality between patients with and without viral infections who were admitted to PICU (172). Shi et al performed a systematic review of RSV infections in 2015 and estimated case fatality rates in children with RSV infection to be around 2.2% (<6 months of age) and 2.4% (6–11 months of age) in developing countries. Case fatality rates in higher income countries were significantly lower (0.2 for <6 months and 0.9 for 6–11 months) (173). In another study, the highest mortality from RSV infection was seen at mean age of 6.2–7.5 months with three quarters of these cases associated with comorbid conditions (174).

Seasonal influenza epidemics and various pandemics have historically led to significant morbidity and mortality in the past, either due to exacerbation of an underlying condition or due to secondary bacterial infections. Mortality with influenza varies not only with season, but with predominant influenza strain and effectiveness of influenza vaccine each season. During the first year of the pandemic 2009 H1N1, global mortality in children aged 0–17 years was estimated to be as high as $\sim$ 45,000 cases, with majority of deaths occurring in Southeast Asia and Africa (175). Both pediatric and adult patients during this pandemic had a very rapid progression to respiratory failure and required prolonged mechanical ventilation and vasopressor support (176, 177). Various extrapulmonary complications secondary to influenza sepsis have been reported in the literature. These include, but are not limited to renal failure, rhabdomyolysis, encephalopathy, myocarditis, and multiorgan failure. These complications also lead to poorer outcomes (178).

Sepsis from HPeV can lead to significant morbidity in neonates and young children. Although, most infections are self-limited, long-term neurological deficits such as learning disability, developmental delay, paralysis and epilepsy have been observed in these patients (179, 180). HPeV infections have also been associated with encephalitis, hepatitis and coagulopathy (18). In addition, rare complications have also been observed in these patients including necrotizing enterocolitis, myocarditis, myositis, hemolytic uremic syndrome, and Reye's syndrome (18). Other enteroviral infections can lead to similar complications and long-term neurological deficits. Hepatic and cardiac dysfunction can also be observed in these patients (181–183). In HSV infection, neurological complications such as developmental delay and seizures have been observed in infected neonates (15). Mortality from systemic HSV infection is usually due to severe coagulopathy, hepatitis and pneumonitis (15). In a multicenter study, Spaeder et al. observed a mortality rate of 9% in patients with severe metapneumovirus infection (184). Increased mortality from metapneumovirus infection has been observed in children with chronic medical conditions, female gender and patients who acquired the infection in the hospital

(184). Similarly, RSV, parainfluenza and influenza infections, when acquired in hospital, have been associated with increased mortality (185). Rotavirus infection can lead to extraintestinal complications like seizures and meningoencephalitis (186, 187). In HIV patients, likelihood of progression to AIDS and of mortality are impacted by time of acquisition of HIV, viral load, CD4 count and timing of HAART initiation. Approximately 80% mortality has been observed in developing countries with limited access to HAART (188). Complications that lead to increased morbidity and mortality in these patients include severe CMV infection, encephalopathy, recurrent life-threatening bacterial infections, tuberculosis, and pneumocystis infection (189).

End-organ failure is a major contributor to mortality in sepsis and septic shock, including virus-induced sepsis. Complications such as acute respiratory distress syndrome, disseminated intravascular coagulation, and acute renal injury often leads to a worse prognosis. Developing countries often have disproportionately higher mortality in patients with viral infections (190), likely due to delayed diagnosis and treatment. Risk of severe sepsis is also related to the site of infection, with endocarditis and CNS infections being associated with mortality as high as 20% (1). Besides the site of infection, the type of virus also determines the risk of mortality. For example, meningitis from HPeVs is a common cause of sepsis in neonates and young children but consequent mortality is low in these patients (179). HPeV3 is associated with more severe disease than HPeV1 (113). Moreover, the extent of systemic involvement can predict the development of multiple organ failure and thus mortality (191). Sepsis related mortality has been reported in other viral infections including dengue fever (192). However, further studies are necessary in order to estimate the burden of viral sepsis on outcomes including morbidity, mortality, and health care related costs.

SUMMARY

Although the incidence of viral-induced sepsis is not precisely known, it is suspected to be common and may represent an important subset of children with "culture-negative sepsis." It is therefore critical for clinicians to suspect and test for viral infection in children with culture-negative sepsis if appropriate infection containment measures are to be instituted in a timely fashion and in the interest of early identification of children with viral infections amenable to treatment. These considerations are especially urgent for high-risk children, such as those born prematurely or those having congenital heart disease, chronic lung disease, or immunodeficiency. Appropriate diagnosis of viral sepsis may provide the clinician added confidence to limit the duration of empiric antibacterial exposure in children with sepsis, and therefore may be helpful in the fight against antibiotic-resistant bacteria. Further studies are needed to identify novel viral-specific biomarkers and therapeutics.

AUTHOR CONTRIBUTIONS

NG, RR, SR, and MK contributed to the conception, writing, and final edits of this manuscript.

REFERENCES

1. Watson RS, Carcillo JA, Linde-Zwirble WT, Clermont G, Lidicker J, Angus DC. The epidemiology of severe sepsis in children in the United States. *Am J Respir Crit Care Med.* (2003) 167:695–701. doi: 10.1164/rccm.200207-682OC
2. Singer M, Deutschman CS, Seymour CW, Shankar-Hari M, Annane D, Bauer M, et al. The third international consensus definitions for sepsis and septic shock (Sepsis-3). *JAMA* (2016) 315:801–10. doi: 10.1001/jama.2016.0287
3. Bone RC. The sepsis syndrome. Definition and general approach to management. *Clin Chest Med.* (1996) 17:175–81.
4. Marshall JC. Understanding the global burden of pediatric sepsis. *Am J Respir Crit Care Med.* (2015) 191:1096–8. doi: 10.1164/rccm.201503-0594ED
5. Fleischmann-Struzek C, Goldfarb DM, Schlattmann P, Schlapbach LJ, Reinhart K, Kissoon N. The global burden of paediatric and neonatal sepsis: a systematic review. *Lancet Respir Med.* (2018) 6:223–30. doi: 10.1016/S2213-2600(18)30063-8
6. Rhodes A, Evans LE, Alhazzani W, Levy MM, Antonelli M, Ferrer R, et al. Surviving sepsis campaign: international guidelines for management of sepsis and septic shock: 2016. *Intensive Care Med.* (2017) 43:304–77. doi: 10.1007/s00134-017-4683-6
7. Ljungstrom LR, Jacobsson G, Claesson BEB, Andersson R, Enroth H. Respiratory viral infections are underdiagnosed in patients with suspected sepsis. *Eur J Clin Microbiol Infect Dis.* (2017) 36:1767–76. doi: 10.1007/s10096-017-2990-z
8. Weiss SL, Fitzgerald JC, Pappachan J, Wheeler D, Jaramillo-Bustamante JC, Salloo A, et al. Global epidemiology of pediatric severe sepsis: the sepsis prevalence, outcomes, and therapies study. *Am J Respir Crit Care Med.* (2015) 191:1147–57. doi: 10.1164/rccm.201412-2323OC
9. Schlapbach LJ, Straney L, Alexander J, MacLaren G, Festa M, Schibler A, et al. Mortality related to invasive infections, sepsis, and septic shock in critically ill children in Australia and New Zealand, 2002–13: a multicentre retrospective cohort study. *Lancet Infect Dis.* (2015) 15:46–54. doi: 10.1016/S1473-3099(14)71003-5
10. Ames SG, Workman JK, Olson JA, Korgenski EK, Masotti S, Knackstedt ED, et al. Infectious etiologies and patient outcomes in pediatric septic shock.*J Pediatric Infect Dis Soc.* (2017) 6:80–6. doi: 10.1093/jpids/piv108
11. Byington CL, Enriquez FR, Hoff C, Tuohy R, Taggart EW, Hillyard DR, et al. Serious bacterial infections in febrile infants 1 to 90 days old with and without viral infections. *Pediatrics* (2004) 113:1662–6.
12. Bhat N, Wright JG, Broder KR, Murray EL, Greenberg ME, Glover MJ, et al. Influenza-associated deaths among children in the United States, 2003-2004. *N Engl J Med.* (2005) 353:2559–67. doi: 10.1056/NEJMoa051721
13. Caballero MT, Polack FP. Respiratory syncytial virus is an "opportunistic" killer. *Pediatr Pulmonol.* (2018) 53:664–7. doi: 10.1002/ppul.23963
14. Law BJ, Carbonell-Estrany X, Simoes EA. An update on respiratory syncytial virus epidemiology: a developed country perspective. *Respir Med.* (2002) 96 (Suppl. B):S1–7. doi: 10.1016/S0954-6111(02)90064-8
15. Kimberlin DW. Herpes simplex virus infections in neonates and early childhood. *Semin Pediatr Infect Dis.* (2005) 16:271–81. doi: 10.1053/j.spid.2005.06.007

16. Sharp J, Harrison CJ, Puckett K, Selvaraju SB, Penaranda S, Nix WA, et al. Characteristics of young infants in whom human parechovirus, enterovirus or neither were detected in cerebrospinal fluid during sepsis evaluations. *Pediatr Infect Dis J.* (2013) 32:213–6. doi: 10.1097/INF.0b013e318276b328
17. Verboon-Maciolek MA, Krediet TG, Gerards LJ, de Vries LS, Groenendaal F, van Loon AM. Severe neonatal parechovirus infection and similarity with enterovirus infection. *Pediatr Infect Dis J.* (2008) 27:241–5. doi: 10.1097/INF.0b013e31815c1b07
18. Harvala H, Wolthers KC, Simmonds P. *Parechoviruses* in children: understanding a new infection. *Curr Opin Infect Dis.* (2010) 23:224–30. doi: 10.1097/QCO.0b013e32833890ca
19. Hatherill M. Sepsis predisposition in children with human immunodeficiency virus. *Pediatr Crit Care Med.* (2005) 6(Suppl. 3):S92–8. doi: 10.1097/01.PCC.0000161579.39050.6B
20. Randolph AG, McCulloh RJ. Pediatric sepsis: important considerations for diagnosing and managing severe infections in infants, children, and adolescents. *Virulence* (2014) 5:179–89. doi: 10.4161/viru.27045
21. Scheier E, Aviner S. Septicemia following rotavirus gastroenteritis. *Isr Med Assoc J.* (2013) 15:166–9.
22. Klingensmith NJ, Coopersmith CM. The gut as the motor of multiple organ dysfunction in critical illness. *Crit Care Clin.* (2016) 32:203–12. doi: 10.1016/j.ccc.2015.11.004
23. Singer M. The role of mitochondrial dysfunction in sepsis-induced multi-organ failure. *Virulence* (2014) 5:66–72. doi: 10.4161/viru.26907
24. Lewis AJ, Billiar TR, Rosengart MR. Biology and metabolism of sepsis: innate immunity, bioenergetics, and autophagy. *Surg Infect.* (2016) 17:286–93. doi: 10.1089/sur.2015.262
25. Florescu DF, Kalil AC. Cytomegalovirus infections in non-immunocompromised and immunocompromised patients in the intensive care unit. *Infect Disord Drug Targets* (2011) 11:354–64.
26. Carcillo JA, Podd B, Aneja R, Weiss SL, Hall MW, Cornell TT, et al. Pathophysiology of pediatric multiple organ dysfunction syndrome. *Pediatr Crit Care Med.* (2017) 18(Suppl. 1):S32–45. doi: 10.1097/PCC.0000000000001052
27. Steinberg BE, Goldenberg NM, Lee WL. Do viral infections mimic bacterial sepsis? The role of microvascular permeability: a review of mechanisms and methods. *Antiviral Res.* (2012) 93:2–15. doi: 10.1016/j.antiviral.2011.10.019
28. Ng CS, Kato H, Fujita T. Recognition of viruses in the cytoplasm by RLRs and other helicases–how conformational changes, mitochondrial dynamics and ubiquitination control innate immune responses. *Int Immunol.* (2012) 24:739–49. doi: 10.1093/intimm/dxs099
29. Jensen S, Thomsen AR. Sensing of RNA viruses: a review of innate immune receptors involved in recognizing RNA virus invasion. *J Virol.* (2012) 86:2900–10. doi: 10.1128/JVI.05738-11
30. Iwasaki A, Pillai PS. Innate immunity to influenza virus infection. *Nat Rev Immunol.* (2014) 14:315–28. doi: 10.1038/nri3665
31. Chaturvedi A, Pierce SK. How location governs toll-like receptor signaling. *Traffic* (2009) 10:621–8. doi: 10.1111/j.1600-0854.2009.00899.x
32. Kaisho T, Akira S. Toll-like receptor function and signaling. *J Allergy Clin Immunol.* (2006) 117:979–87; quiz 88. doi: 10.1016/j.jaci.2006.02.023
33. Wang JQ, Jeelall YS, Ferguson LL, Horikawa K. Toll-like receptors and cancer: myd88 mutation and inflammation. *Front Immunol.* (2014) 5:367. doi: 10.3389/fimmu.2014.00367
34. Nimmerjahn F, Dudziak D, Dirmeier U, Hobom G, Riedel A, Schlee M, et al. Active NF-kappaB signalling is a prerequisite for influenza virus infection. *J Gen Virol.* (2004) 85:2347–56. doi: 10.1099/vir.0.79958-0
35. Sprague AH, Khalil RA. Inflammatory cytokines in vascular dysfunction and vascular disease. *Biochem Pharmacol.* (2009) 78:539–52. doi: 10.1016/j.bcp.2009.04.029
36. Loo YM, Gale M, Jr. Immune signaling by RIG-I-like receptors. *Immunity* (2011) 34:680–92. doi: 10.1016/j.immuni.2011.05.003
37. Kato H, Takeuchi O, Sato S, Yoneyama M, Yamamoto M, Matsui K, et al. Differential roles of MDA5 and RIG-I helicases in the recognition of RNA viruses. *Nature* (2006) 441:101–5. doi: 10.1038/nature04734
38. Wang S, Le TQ, Kurihara N, Chida J, Cisse Y, Yano M, et al. Influenza virus-cytokine-protease cycle in the pathogenesis of vascular hyperpermeability in severe influenza. *J Infect Dis.* (2010) 202:991–1001. doi: 10.1086/656044
39. Puerta-Guardo H, Glasner DR, Harris E. Dengue virus NS1 disrupts the endothelial glycocalyx, leading to hyperpermeability. *PLoS Pathog.* (2016) 12:e1005738. doi: 10.1371/journal.ppat.1005738
40. Duncan ME, Richardson JP, Murray GI, Melvin WT, Fothergill JE. Human matrix metalloproteinase-9: activation by limited trypsin treatment and generation of monoclonal antibodies specific for the activated form. *Eur J Biochem.* (1998) 258:37–43. doi: 10.1046/j.1432-1327.1998.2580037.x
41. Ramnath R, Foster RR, Qiu Y, Cope G, Butler MJ, Salmon AH, et al. Matrix metalloproteinase 9-mediated shedding of syndecan 4 in response to tumor necrosis factor alpha: a contributor to endothelial cell glycocalyx dysfunction. *FASEB J.* (2014) 28:4686–99. doi: 10.1096/fj.14-252221
42. Chappell D, Jacob M, Rehm M, Stoeckelhuber M, Welsch U, Conzen P, et al. Heparinase selectively sheds heparan sulphate from the endothelial glycocalyx. *Biol Chem.* (2008) 389:79–82. doi: 10.1515/BC.2008.005
43. Schwarz KB. Oxidative stress during viral infection: a review. *Free Radic Biol Med.* (1996) 21:641–9.
44. Perrone LA, Belser JA, Wadford DA, Katz JM, Tumpey TM. Inducible nitric oxide contributes to viral pathogenesis following highly pathogenic influenza virus infection in mice. *J Infect Dis.* (2013) 207:1576–84. doi: 10.1093/infdis/jit062
45. Rubio-Gayosso I, Platts SH, Duling BR. Reactive oxygen species mediate modification of glycocalyx during ischemia-reperfusion injury. *Am J Physiol Heart Circ Physiol.* (2006) 290:H2247–56. doi: 10.1152/ajpheart.00796.2005
46. Garofalo RP, Kolli D, Casola A. Respiratory syncytial virus infection: mechanisms of redox control and novel therapeutic opportunities. *Antioxid Redox Signal.* (2013) 18:186–217. doi: 10.1089/ars.2011.4307
47. Armstrong SM, Mubareka S, Lee WL. The lung microvascular endothelium as a therapeutic target in severe influenza. *Antiviral Res.* (2013) 99:113–8. doi: 10.1016/j.antiviral.2013.05.003
48. Chen HR, Chao CH, Liu CC, Ho TS, Tsai HP, Perng GC, et al. Macrophage migration inhibitory factor is critical for dengue NS1-induced endothelial glycocalyx degradation and hyperpermeability. *PLoS Pathog.* (2018) 14:e1007033. doi: 10.1371/journal.ppat.1007033
49. Constantinescu AA, Vink H, Spaan JA. Endothelial cell glycocalyx modulates immobilization of leukocytes at the endothelial surface. *Arterioscler Thromb Vasc Biol.* (2003) 23:1541–7. doi: 10.1161/01.ATV.0000085630.24353.3D
50. Wu G, Essex DW, Meloni FJ, Takafuta T, Fujimura K, Konkle BA, et al. Human endothelial cells in culture and *in vivo* express on their surface all four components of the glycoprotein Ib/IX/V complex. *Blood* (1997) 90:2660–9.
51. Ruggeri ZM. Von Willebrand factor, platelets and endothelial cell interactions. *J Thromb Haemost.* (2003) 1:1335–42.
52. Koedam JA, Cramer EM, Briend E, Furie B, Furie BC, Wagner DD. P-selectin, a granule membrane protein of platelets and endothelial cells, follows the regulated secretory pathway in AtT-20 cells. *J Cell Biol.* (1992) 116:617–25.
53. Berndt MC, Shen Y, Dopheide SM, Gardiner EE, Andrews RK. The vascular biology of the glycoprotein Ib-IX-V complex. *Thromb Haemost.* (2001) 86:178–88.
54. Levick JR, Michel CC. Microvascular fluid exchange and the revised Starling principle. *Cardiovasc Res.* (2010) 87:198–210. doi: 10.1093/cvr/cvq062
55. Xiao K, Allison DF, Kottke MD, Summers S, Sorescu GP, Faundez V, et al. Mechanisms of VE-cadherin processing and degradation in microvascular endothelial cells. *J Biol Chem.* (2003) 278:19199–208. doi: 10.1074/jbc.M211746200
56. Potter MD, Barbero S, Cheresh DA. Tyrosine phosphorylation of VE-cadherin prevents binding of p120- and beta-catenin and maintains the cellular mesenchymal state. *J Biol Chem.* (2005) 280:31906–12. doi: 10.1074/jbc.M505568200
57. Gorbunova E, Gavrilovskaya IN, Mackow ER. Pathogenic hantaviruses Andes virus and Hantaan virus induce adherens junction disassembly by directing vascular endothelial cadherin internalization in human endothelial cells. *J Virol.* (2010) 84:7405–11. doi: 10.1128/JVI.00576-10

58. Davis S, Aldrich TH, Jones PF, Acheson A, Compton DL, Jain V, et al. Isolation of angiopoietin-1, a ligand for the TIE2 receptor, by secretion-trap expression cloning. *Cell* (1996) 87:1161–9.
59. Brindle NP, Saharinen P, Alitalo K. Signaling and functions of angiopoietin-1 in vascular protection. *Circ Res.* (2006) 98:1014–23. doi: 10.1161/01.RES.0000218275.54089.12
60. Milam KE, Parikh SM. The angiopoietin-Tie2 signaling axis in the vascular leakage of systemic inflammation. *Tissue Barriers* (2015) 3:e957508. doi: 10.4161/21688362.2014.957508
61. Levine JD, Harlan JM, Harker LA, Joseph ML, Counts RB. Thrombin-mediated release of factor VIII antigen from human umbilical vein endothelial cells in culture. *Blood* (1982) 60:531–4.
62. Vischer UM, Jornot L, Wollheim CB, Theler JM. Reactive oxygen intermediates induce regulated secretion of von Willebrand factor from cultured human vascular endothelial cells. Blood (1995) 85:3164–72.
63. Matsushita K, Yamakuchi M, Morrell CN, Ozaki M, O'Rourke B, Irani K, et al. Vascular endothelial growth factor regulation of Weibel-Palade-body exocytosis. *Blood* (2005) 105:207–14. doi: 10.1182/blood-2004-0break4-1519
64. Fiedler U, Scharpfenecker M, Koidl S, Hegen A, Grunow V, Schmidt JM, et al. The Tie-2 ligand angiopoietin-2 is stored in and rapidly released upon stimulation from endothelial cell Weibel-Palade bodies. *Blood* (2004) 103:4150–6. doi: 10.1182/blood-2003-10-3685
65. Sugiyama MG, Armstrong SM, Wang C, Hwang D, Leong-Poi H, Advani A, et al. The Tie2-agonist vasculotide rescues mice from influenza virus infection. *Sci Rep.* (2015) 5:11030. doi: 10.1038/srep11030
66. Daidoji T, Koma T, Du A, Yang CS, Ueda M, Ikuta K, et al. H5N1 avian influenza virus induces apoptotic cell death in mammalian airway epithelial cells. *J Virol.* (2008) 82:11294–307. doi: 10.1128/JVI.01192-08
67. Zhou J, Law HK, Cheung CY, Ng IH, Peiris JS, Lau YL. Functional tumor necrosis factor-related apoptosis-inducing ligand production by avian influenza virus-infected macrophages. *J Infect Dis.* (2006) 193:945–53. doi: 10.1086/500954
68. Olijve L, Jennings L, Walls T. Human parechovirus: an increasingly recognized cause of sepsis-like illness in young infants. *Clin Microbiol Rev.* (2018) 31:e00047-17. doi: 10.1128/CMR.00047-17
69. Zhang L, Peeples ME, Boucher RC, Collins PL, Pickles RJ. Respiratory syncytial virus infection of human airway epithelial cells is polarized, specific to ciliated cells, and without obvious cytopathology. *J Virol.* (2002) 76:5654–66. doi: 10.1128/JVI.76.11.5654-5666.2002
70. Simon AK, Hollander GA, McMichael A. Evolution of the immune system in humans from infancy to old age. *Proc Biol Sci.* (2015) 282:20143085. doi: 10.1098/rspb.2014.3085
71. Orange JS. Congenital immunodeficiencies and sepsis. *Pediatr Crit Care Med.* (2005) 6(Suppl—3):S99–107. doi: 10.1097/01.PCC.0000164488.19810.DB
72. Asgari S, Schlapbach LJ, Anchisi S, Hammer C, Bartha I, Junier T, et al. Severe viral respiratory infections in children with IFIH1 loss-of-function mutations. *Proc Natl Acad Sci USA.* (2017) 114:8342–7. doi: 10.1073/pnas.1704259114
73. Dinarello CA, Kent EF, Jr. Chemical characterization of an interleukin-1-inducing substance derived from human mixed leukocyte reactions: IL-1-inducing substance is not gamma interferon. *Yale J Biol Med.* (1985) 58:101–13.
74. Harris RL, Musher DM, Bloom K, Gathe J, Rice L, Sugarman B, et al. Manifestations of sepsis. *Arch Intern Med.* (1987) 147:1895–906.
75. Zhao ZD, Yang WZ, Gao C, Fu X, Zhang W, Zhou Q, et al. A hypothalamic circuit that controls body temperature. *Proc Natl Acad Sci USA.* (2017) 114:2042–7. doi: 10.1073/pnas.1616255114
76. Krausz MM, Perel A, Eimerl D, Cotev S. Cardiopulmonary effects of volume loading in patients in septic shock. *Ann Surg.* (1977) 185:429–34.
77. Brown ZA, Wald A, Morrow RA, Selke S, Zeh J, Corey L. Effect of serologic status and cesarean delivery on transmission rates of herpes simplex virus from mother to infant. *JAMA* (2003) 289:203–9.
78. Nielsen NM, Midgley SE, Nielsen AC, Christiansen CB, Fischer TK. Severe human parechovirus infections in infants and the role of older siblings.*Am J Epidemiol.* (2016) 183:664–70. doi: 10.1093/aje/kwv206
79. Owatanapanich S, Wutthanarungsan R, Jaksupa W, Thisyakorn U. Risk factors for severe enteroviral infections in children. *J Med Assoc Thai.* (2016) 99:322–30.
80. Eggleston HA, Gunville CF, Miller JI, Sontag MK, Mourani PM. A comparison of characteristics and outcomes in severe human metapneumovirus and respiratory syncytial virus infections in children treated in an intensive care unit. *Pediatr Infect Dis J.* (2013) 32:1330–4. doi: 10.1097/INF.0b013e3182a2261b
81. Drysdale SB, Mejias A, Ramilo O. Rhinovirus - not just the common cold. *J Infect.* (2017) 74(Suppl 1):S41–6. doi: 10.1016/S0163-4453(17)30190-1
82. Committee on Infectious Diseases. Recommendations for prevention and control of influenza in children, 2017 - 2018. *Pediatrics* (2017) 140:e20172550. doi: 10.1542/peds.2017-2550
83. Ngwende S, Gombe NT, Midzi S, Tshimanga M, Shambira G, Chadambuka A. Factors associated with HIV infection among children born to mothers on the prevention of mother to child transmission programme at Chitungwiza Hospital, Zimbabwe, 2008. *BMC Public Health* (2013) 13:1181. doi: 10.1186/1471-2458-13-1181
84. de Lemos LM, Lippi J, Rutherford GW, Duarte GS, Martins NG, Santos VS, et al. Maternal risk factors for HIV infection in infants in northeastern Brazil. *Int J Infect Dis.* (2013) 17:e913–8. doi: 10.1016/j.ijid.2013.04.015
85. Hendaus MA, Jomha FA, Alhammadi AH. Virus-induced secondary bacterial infection: a concise review. *Ther Clin Risk Manag.* (2015) 11:1265–71. doi: 10.2147/TCRM.S87789
86. O'Brien KL, Walters MI, Sellman J, Quinlisk P, Regnery H, Schwartz B, et al. Severe pneumococcal pneumonia in previously healthy children: the role of preceding influenza infection. *Clin Infect Dis.* (2000) 30:784–9. doi: 10.1086/313772
87. Randolph AG, Vaughn F, Sullivan R, Rubinson L, Thompson BT, Yoon G, et al. Critically ill children during the 2009-2010 influenza pandemic in the United States. *Pediatrics* (2011) 128:e1450–8. doi: 10.1542/peds.2011-0774
88. Cebey-Lopez M, Pardo-Seco J, Gomez-Carballa A, Martinon-Torres N, Martinon-Sanchez JM, Justicia-Grande A, et al. Bacteremia in children hospitalized with respiratory syncytial virus infection. *PLoS ONE* (2016) 11:e0146599. doi: 10.1371/journal.pone.0146599
89. Hall MW, Geyer SM, Guo CY, Panoskaltsis-Mortari A, Jouvet P, Ferdinands J, et al. Innate immune function and mortality in critically ill children with influenza: a multicenter study. *Crit Care Med.* (2013) 41:224–36. doi: 10.1097/CCM.0b013e318267633c
90. Morens DM, Taubenberger JK, Fauci AS. Predominant role of bacterial pneumonia as a cause of death in pandemic influenza: implications for pandemic influenza preparedness. *J Infect Dis.* (2008) 198:962–70. doi: 10.1086/591708
91. Finelli L, Fiore A, Dhara R, Brammer L, Shay DK, Kamimoto L, et al. Influenza-associated pediatric mortality in the United States: increase of *Staphylococcus aureus* coinfection. *Pediatrics* (2008) 122:805–11. doi: 10.1542/peds.2008-1336
92. Wilson R, Dowling RB, Jackson AD. The biology of bacterial colonization and invasion of the respiratory mucosa. *Eur Respir J.* (1996) 9:1523–30.
93. Avadhanula V, Rodriguez CA, Devincenzo JP, Wang Y, Webby RJ, Ulett GC, et al. Respiratory viruses augment the adhesion of bacterial pathogens to respiratory epithelium in a viral species- and cell type-dependent manner. *J Virol.* (2006) 80:1629–36. doi: 10.1128/JVI.80.4.1629-1636.2006
94. Rynda-Apple A, Robinson KM, Alcorn JF. Influenza and bacterial superinfection: illuminating the immunologic mechanisms of disease. *Infect Immun.* (2015) 83:3764–70. doi: 10.1128/IAI.00298-15
95. Cundell DR, Gerard NP, Gerard C, Idanpaan-Heikkila I, Tuomanen EI. *Streptococcus pneumoniae* anchor to activated human cells by the receptor for platelet-activating factor. *Nature* (1995) 377:435–8. doi: 10.1038/377435a0
96. Lowenthal A, Livni G, Amir J, Samra Z, Ashkenazi S. Secondary bacteremia after rotavirus gastroenteritis in infancy. *Pediatrics* (2006) 117:224–6. doi: 10.1542/peds.2005-0177
97. Goulder PJ, Jeena P, Tudor-Williams G, Burchett S. Paediatric HIV infection: correlates of protective immunity and global perspectives in prevention and management. *Br Med Bull.* (2001) 58:89–108.

98. Tudor-Williams G, Pizzo PA. Pediatric human immunodeficiency virus infection. In: Stiehm ER, editor. *Immunologic Disorders in Infants and Children. 4th edn.* Philadelphia, PA: WB Saunders Company (1996). p. 510–52.
99. Hogan CM, Hammer SM. Host determinants in HIV infection and disease. Part 1: cellular and humoral immune responses. *Ann Intern Med.* (2001) 134:761–76.
100. DaPalma T, Doonan BP, Trager NM, Kasman LM. A systematic approach to virus-virus interactions. *Virus Res.* (2010) 149:1–9. doi: 10.1016/j.virusres.2010.01.002
101. Rhedin S, Lindstrand A, Rotzen-Ostlund M, Tolfvenstam T, Ohrmalm L, Rinder MR, et al. Clinical utility of PCR for common viruses in acute respiratory illness. *Pediatrics* (2014) 133:e538–45. doi: 10.1542/peds.2013-3042
102. Asner SA, Rose W, Petrich A, Richardson S, Tran DJ. Is virus coinfection a predictor of severity in children with viral respiratory infections? *Clin Microbiol Infect.* (2015) 21:264.e1–6. doi: 10.1016/j.cmi.2014.08.024
103. Kouni S, Karakitsos P, Chranioti A, Theodoridou M, Chrousos G, Michos A. Evaluation of viral co-infections in hospitalized and non-hospitalized children with respiratory infections using microarrays. *Clin Microbiol Infect.* (2013) 19:772–7. doi: 10.1111/1469-0691.12015
104. Lim FJ, de Klerk N, Blyth CC, Fathima P, Moore HC. Systematic review and meta-analysis of respiratory viral coinfections in children. *Respirology* (2016) 21:648–55. doi: 10.1111/resp.12741
105. Scotta MC, Chakr VC, de Moura A, Becker RG, de Souza AP, Jones MH, et al. Respiratory viral coinfection and disease severity in children: a systematic review and meta-analysis. *J Clin Virol.* (2016) 80:45–56. doi: 10.1016/j.jcv.2016.04.019
106. Aslanzadeh J, Zheng X, Li H, Tetreault J, Ratkiewicz I, Meng S, et al. Prospective evaluation of rapid antigen tests for diagnosis of respiratory syncytial virus and human metapneumovirus infections. *J Clin Microbiol.* (2008) 46:1682–5. doi: 10.1128/JCM.00008-08
107. Griffiths C, Drews SJ, Marchant DJ. Respiratory syncytial virus: infection, detection, and new options for prevention and treatment. *Clin Microbiol Rev.* (2017) 30:277–319. doi: 10.1128/CMR.00010-16
108. Leland DS, Ginocchio CC. Role of cell culture for virus detection in the age of technology. *Clin Microbiol Rev.* (2007) 20:49–78. doi: 10.1128/CMR.00002-06
109. Shirato K, Nishimura H, Saijo M, Okamoto M, Noda M, Tashiro M, et al. Diagnosis of human respiratory syncytial virus infection using reverse transcription loop-mediated isothermal amplification. *J Virol Methods* (2007) 139:78–84. doi: 10.1016/j.jviromet.2006.09.014
110. de-Paris F, Beck C, Machado AB, Paiva RM, da Silva Menezes D, de Souza Nunes L, et al. Optimization of one-step duplex real-time RT-PCR for detection of influenza and respiratory syncytial virus in nasopharyngeal aspirates. *J Virol Methods* (2012) 186:189–92. doi: 10.1016/j.jviromet.2012.07.008
111. Couturier MR, Barney T, Alger G, Hymas WC, Stevenson JB, Hillyard D, et al. Evaluation of the filmarray(R) respiratory panel for clinical use in a large children's hospital. *J Clin Lab Anal.* (2013) 27:148–54. doi: 10.1002/jcla.21576
112. Gill PJ, Richardson SE, Ostrow O, Friedman JN. Testing for respiratory viruses in children: to swab or not to swab. *JAMA Pediatr.* (2017) 171:798–804. doi: 10.1001/jamapediatrics.2017.0786
113. Wolthers KC, Benschop KS, Schinkel J, Molenkamp R, Bergevoet RM, Spijkerman IJ, et al. Human parechoviruses as an important viral cause of sepsislike illness and meningitis in young children. *Clin Infect Dis.* (2008) 47:358–63. doi: 10.1086/589752
114. Moe N, Pedersen B, Nordbo SA, Skanke LH, Krokstad S, Smyrnaios A, et al. Respiratory virus detection and clinical diagnosis in children attending day care. *PLoS ONE* (2016) 11:e0159196. doi: 10.1371/journal.pone.0159196
115. Martin ET, Fairchok MP, Kuypers J, Magaret A, Zerr DM, Wald A, et al. Frequent and prolonged shedding of bocavirus in young children attending daycare. *J Infect Dis.* (2010) 201:1625–32. doi: 10.1086/652405
116. Barik S. New treatments for influenza. *BMC Med.* (2012) 10:104. doi: 10.1186/1741-7015-10-104
117. Hendricks GL, Weirich KL, Viswanathan K, Li J, Shriver ZH, Ashour J, et al. Sialylneolacto-N-tetraose c (LSTc)-bearing liposomal decoys capture influenza A virus. *J Biol Chem.* (2013) 288:8061–73. doi: 10.1074/jbc.M112.437202
118. Herberg JA, Kaforou M, Wright VJ, Shailes H, Eleftherohorinou H, Hoggart CJ, et al. Diagnostic test accuracy of a 2-transcript host RNA signature for discriminating bacterial vs viral infection in febrile children. *JAMA* (2016) 316:835–45. doi: 10.1001/jama.2016.11236
119. Rivers E, Nguyen B, Havstad S, Ressler J, Muzzin A, Knoblich B, et al. Early goal-directed therapy in the treatment of severe sepsis and septic shock. *N Engl J Med.* (2001) 345:1368–77. doi: 10.1056/NEJMoa010307
120. Prkno A, Wacker C, Brunkhorst FM, Schlattmann P. Procalcitonin-guided therapy in intensive care unit patients with severe sepsis and septic shock–a systematic review and meta-analysis. *Crit Care* (2013) 17:R291. doi: 10.1186/cc13157
121. Downes KJ, Weiss SL, Gerber JS, Klieger SB, Fitzgerald JC, Balamuth F, et al. A pragmatic biomarker-driven algorithm to guide antibiotic use in the pediatric intensive care unit: The Optimizing Antibiotic Strategies in Sepsis (OASIS) study. *J Pediatric Infect Dis Soc.* (2017) 6:134–41. doi: 10.1093/jpids/piw023
122. Meisner M, Tschaikowsky K, Palmaers T, Schmidt J. Comparison of procalcitonin (PCT) and C-reactive protein (CRP) plasma concentrations at different SOFA scores during the course of sepsis and MODS. *Crit Care* (1999) 3:45–50. doi: 10.1186/cc306
123. Afshari A, Harbarth S. Procalcitonin as diagnostic biomarker of sepsis. *Lancet Infect Dis.* (2013) 13:382–4. doi: 10.1016/S1473-3099(13)70026-4
124. Wacker C, Prkno A, Brunkhorst FM, Schlattmann P. Procalcitonin as a diagnostic marker for sepsis: a systematic review and meta-analysis. *Lancet Infect Dis.* (2013) 13:426–35. doi: 10.1016/S1473-3099(12)70323-7
125. Gabay C, Kushner I. Acute-phase proteins and other systemic responses to inflammation. *N Engl J Med.* (1999) 340:448–54. doi: 10.1056/NEJM199902113400607
126. Hu X, Yu J, Crosby SD, Storch GA. Gene expression profiles in febrile children with defined viral and bacterial infection. *Proc Natl Acad Sci USA.* (2013) 110:12792–7. doi: 10.1073/pnas.1302968110
127. Woods CW, McClain MT, Chen M, Zaas AK, Nicholson BP, Varkey J, et al. A host transcriptional signature for presymptomatic detection of infection in humans exposed to influenza H1N1 or H3N2. *PLoS ONE* (2013) 8:e52198. doi: 10.1371/journal.pone.0052198
128. Zaas AK, Chen M, Varkey J, Veldman T, Hero AO III, Lucas J, et al. Gene expression signatures diagnose influenza and other symptomatic respiratory viral infections in humans. *Cell Host Microbe* (2009) 6:207–17. doi: 10.1016/j.chom.2009.07.006
129. Sampson DL, Fox BA, Yager TD, Bhide S, Cermelli S, McHugh LC, et al. A four-biomarker blood signature discriminates systemic inflammation due to viral infection versus other etiologies. *Sci Rep.* (2017) 7:2914. doi: 10.1038/s41598-017-02325-8
130. Engelmann I, Dubos F, Lobert PE, Houssin C, Degas V, Sardet A, et al. Diagnosis of viral infections using myxovirus resistance protein A (MxA). *Pediatrics* (2015) 135:e985–93. doi: 10.1542/peds.2014-1946
131. Alter SJ, Bennett JS, Koranyi K, Kreppel A, Simon R. Common childhood viral infections. *Curr Probl Pediatr Adolesc Health Care* (2015) 45:21–53. doi: 10.1016/j.cppeds.2014.12.001
132. American Academy of Pediatrics Committee on Infectious D, American Academy of Pediatrics Bronchiolitis Guidelines C. Updated guidance for palivizumab prophylaxis among infants and young children at increased risk of hospitalization for respiratory syncytial virus infection. *Pediatrics* (2014) 134:415–20. doi: 10.1542/peds.2014-1665
133. Committee on Infectious D. From the american academy of pediatrics: policy statements–modified recommendations for use of palivizumab for prevention of respiratory syncytial virus infections. *Pediatrics* (2009) 124:1694–701. doi: 10.1542/peds.2009-2345
134. Conrad DA, Christenson JC, Waner JL, Marks MI. Aerosolized ribavirin treatment of respiratory syncytial virus infection in infants hospitalized during an epidemic. *Pediatr Infect Dis J.* (1987) 6:152–8.
135. Mazur NI, Martinon-Torres F, Baraldi E, Fauroux B, Greenough A, Heikkinen T, et al. Lower respiratory tract infection caused by respiratory syncytial virus: current management and new therapeutics. *Lancet Respir Med.* (2015) 3:888–900. doi: 10.1016/S2213-2600(15)00255-6

136. DeVincenzo JP, Whitley RJ, Mackman RL, Scaglioni-Weinlich C, Harrison L, Farrell E, et al. Oral GS-5806 activity in a respiratory syncytial virus challenge study. *N Engl J Med.* (2014) 371:711–22. doi: 10.1056/NEJMoa1401184
137. Detalle L, Stohr T, Palomo C, Piedra PA, Gilbert BE, Mas V, et al. Generation and Characterization of ALX-0171, a potent novel therapeutic nanobody for the treatment of respiratory syncytial virus infection. *Antimicrob Agents Chemother.* (2016) 60:6–13. doi: 10.1128/AAC.01802-15
138. Douglas JL, Panis ML, Ho E, Lin KY, Krawczyk SH, Grant DM, et al. Small molecules VP-14637 and JNJ-2408068 inhibit respiratory syncytial virus fusion by similar mechanisms. *Antimicrob Agents Chemother.* (2005) 49:2460–6. doi: 10.1128/AAC.49.6.2460-2466.2005
139. Kim YI, Pareek R, Murphy R, Harrison L, Farrell E, Cook R, et al. The antiviral effects of RSV fusion inhibitor, MDT-637, on clinical isolates, vs its achievable concentrations in the human respiratory tract and comparison to ribavirin. *Influenza Other Respir Viruses* (2017) 11:525–30. doi: 10.1111/irv.12503
140. DeVincenzo JP, McClure MW, Symons JA, Fathi H, Westland C, Chanda S, et al. Activity of oral ALS-008176 in a respiratory syncytial virus challenge study. *N Engl J Med.* (2015) 373:2048–58. doi: 10.1056/NEJMoa1413275
141. Zamora MR, Budev M, Rolfe M, Gottlieb J, Humar A, Devincenzo J, et al. RNA interference therapy in lung transplant patients infected with respiratory syncytial virus. *Am J Respir Crit Care Med.* (2011) 183:531–8. doi: 10.1164/rccm.201003-0422OC
142. Burnett JC, Rossi JJ, Tiemann K. Current progress of siRNA/shRNA therapeutics in clinical trials. *Biotechnol J.* (2011) 6:1130–46. doi: 10.1002/biot.201100054
143. Flannery B, Reynolds SB, Blanton L, Santibanez TA, O'Halloran A, Lu PJ, et al. Influenza vaccine effectiveness against pediatric deaths: 2010-2014. *Pediatrics* (2017) 139:977–981. doi: 10.1542/peds.2016-4244
144. Malosh RE, Martin ET, Heikkinen T, Brooks WA, Whitley RJ, Monto AS. Efficacy and Safety of oseltamivir in children: systematic review and individual patient data meta-analysis of randomized controlled trials. *Clin Infect Dis.* (2018) 66:1492–500. doi: 10.1093/cid/cix1040
145. Whitley RJ, Hayden FG, Reisinger KS, Young N, Dutkowski R, Ipe D, et al. Oral oseltamivir treatment of influenza in children. *Pediatr Infect Dis J.* (2001) 20:127–33.
146. Pickering LKBC, Kimberlin DW, Long SS. *Influenza. Red Book: 2012 Report of the Committee on Infectious Diseases, American Academy of Pediatrics* (2012) pp. 439–53.
147. Zuccotti GV, Fabiano V. Influvac, a trivalent inactivated subunit influenza vaccine. *Expert Opin Biol Ther.* (2011) 11:89–98. doi: 10.1517/14712598.2011.541436
148. Herzog C, Hartmann K, Kunzi V, Kursteiner O, Mischler R, Lazar H, et al. Eleven years of Inflexal V-a virosomal adjuvanted influenza vaccine. *Vaccine* (2009) 27:4381–7. doi: 10.1016/j.vaccine.2009.05.029
149. Furuta Y, Takahashi K, Fukuda Y, Kuno M, Kamiyama T, Kozaki K, et al. *In vitro* and *in vivo* activities of anti-influenza virus compound T-705. *Antimicrob Agents Chemother.* (2002) 46:977–81. doi: 10.1128/AAC.46.4.977-981.2002
150. Hayden F. Developing new antiviral agents for influenza treatment: what does the future hold? *Clin Infect Dis.* (2009) 48 (Suppl. 1):S3–13. doi: 10.1086/591851
151. Darwish I, Mubareka S, Liles WC. Immunomodulatory therapy for severe influenza. *Expert Rev Anti Infect Ther.* (2011) 9:807–22. doi: 10.1586/eri.11.56
152. Zheng BJ, Chan KW, Lin YP, Zhao GY, Chan C, Zhang HJ, et al. Delayed antiviral plus immunomodulator treatment still reduces mortality in mice infected by high inoculum of influenza A/H5N1 virus. *Proc Natl Acad Sci USA.* (2008) 105:8091–6. doi: 10.1073/pnas.0711942105
153. Ng HH, Narasaraju T, Phoon MC, Sim MK, Seet JE, Chow VT. Doxycycline treatment attenuates acute lung injury in mice infected with virulent influenza H3N2 virus: involvement of matrix metalloproteinases. *Exp Mol Pathol.* (2012) 92:287–95. doi: 10.1016/j.yexmp.2012.03.003
154. Quispe-Laime AM, Bracco JD, Barberio PA, Campagne CG, Rolfo VE, Umberger R, et al. H1N1 influenza a virus-associated acute lung injury: response to combination oseltamivir and prolonged corticosteroid treatment. *Intensive Care Med.* (2010) 36:33–41. doi: 10.1007/s00134-009-1727-6
155. Sato K, Suga M, Akaike T, Fujii S, Muranaka H, Doi T, et al. Therapeutic effect of erythromycin on influenza virus-induced lung injury in mice. *Am J Respir Crit Care Med.* (1998) 157(3 Pt 1):853–7. doi: 10.1164/ajrccm.157.3.9703098
156. Yamaya M, Shinya K, Hatachi Y, Kubo H, Asada M, Yasuda H, et al. Clarithromycin inhibits type a seasonal influenza virus infection in human airway epithelial cells. *J Pharmacol Exp Ther.* (2010) 333:81–90. doi: 10.1124/jpet.109.162149
157. Budd A, Alleva L, Alsharifi M, Koskinen A, Smythe V, Mullbacher A, et al. Increased survival after gemfibrozil treatment of severe mouse influenza. *Antimicrob Agents Chemother.* (2007) 51:2965–8. doi: 10.1128/AAC.00219-07
158. Walsh KB, Teijaro JR, Rosen H, Oldstone MB. Quelling the storm: utilization of sphingosine-1-phosphate receptor signaling to ameliorate influenza virus-induced cytokine storm. *Immunol Res.* (2011) 51:15–25. doi: 10.1007/s12026-011-8240-z
159. Abzug MJ, Michaels MG, Wald E, Jacobs RF, Romero JR, Sanchez PJ, et al. A Randomized, double-blind, placebo-controlled trial of pleconaril for the treatment of neonates with enterovirus sepsis. *J Pediatric Infect Dis Soc.* (2016) 5:53–62. doi: 10.1093/jpids/piv015
160. Pevear DC, Hayden FG, Demenczuk TM, Barone LR, McKinlay MA, Collett MS. Relationship of pleconaril susceptibility and clinical outcomes in treatment of common colds caused by rhinoviruses. *Antimicrob Agents Chemother.* (2005) 49:4492–9. doi: 10.1128/AAC.49.11.4492-4499.2005
161. Abzug MJ, Keyserling HL, Lee ML, Levin MJ, Rotbart HA. Neonatal enterovirus infection: virology, serology, and effects of intravenous immune globulin. *Clin Infect Dis.* (1995) 20:1201–6.
162. Whitley RJ, Corey L, Arvin A, Lakeman FD, Sumaya CV, Wright PF, et al. Changing presentation of herpes simplex virus infection in neonates. *J Infect Dis.* (1988) 158:109–16.
163. Nahmias A, Josey WE, Naib ZM, Freeman MG, Fernandez RJ, Wheeler JH. Perinatal risk associated with maternal genital herpes simplex virus infection. *Am J Obstetr Gynecol.* (1971) 110:825–37. doi: 10.1016/0002-9378(71)90580-1
164. Stanberry LR, Spruance SL, Cunningham AL, Bernstein DI, Mindel A, Sacks S, et al. Glycoprotein-D-adjuvant vaccine to prevent genital herpes. *N Engl J Med.* (2002) 347:1652–61. doi: 10.1056/NEJMoa011915
165. Braig S, Luton D, Sibony O, Edlinger C, Boissinot C, Blot P, et al. Acyclovir prophylaxis in late pregnancy prevents recurrent genital herpes and viral shedding. *Eur J Obstet Gynecol Reprod Biol.* (2001) 96:55–8. doi: 10.1016/S0301-2115(00)00406-1
166. Scott LL, Sanchez PJ, Jackson GL, Zeray F, Wendel GD, Jr. Acyclovir suppression to prevent cesarean delivery after first-episode genital herpes. *Obstet Gynecol.* (1996) 87:69–73.
167. Pickering LKBC, Kimberlin DW, Long SS (editors). Herpes simplex. In: *Red Book: Report of the Committee on Infectious Diseases. 25th ed.* Elk Grove Village, IL: American Academy of Pediatrics (2000).
168. Gibb DM, Duong T, Tookey PA, Sharland M, Tudor-Williams G, Novelli V, et al. Decline in mortality, AIDS, and hospital admissions in perinatally HIV-1 infected children in the United Kingdom and Ireland. *BMJ* (2003) 327:1019. doi: 10.1136/bmj.327.7422.1019
169. Sánchez JM, Amador JTR, De Miguel SF, Tomé MIG, Conejo PR, Vivas PF, et al. Impact of highly active antiretroviral therapy on the morbidity and mortality in Spanish human immunodeficiency virus-infected children. *Pediatr Infect Disease J.* (2003) 22:863–8. doi: 10.1097/01.inf.0000091282.70253.5f
170. de Martino M, Tovo PA, Balducci M, Galli L, Gabiano C, Rezza G, et al. Reduction in mortality with availability of antiretroviral therapy for children with perinatal HIV-1 infection. Italian register for HIV infection in children and the Italian national AIDS registry. *JAMA* (2000) 284:190–7.
171. Gortmaker SL, Hughes M, Cervia J, Brady M, Johnson GM, Seage GR III, et al. Effect of combination therapy including protease inhibitors on mortality among children and adolescents infected with HIV-1. *N Engl J Med.* (2001) 345:1522–8. doi: 10.1056/NEJMoa011157
172. Hon KL, Luk MP, Fung WM, Li CY, Yeung HL, Liu PK, et al. Mortality, length of stay, bloodstream and respiratory viral infections

in a pediatric intensive care unit. *J Crit Care* (2017) 38:57–61. doi: 10.1016/j.jcrc.2016.09.019

173. Shi T, McAllister DA, O'Brien KL, Simoes EAF, Madhi SA, Gessner BD, et al. Global, regional, and national disease burden estimates of acute lower respiratory infections due to respiratory syncytial virus in young children in 2015: a systematic review and modelling study. *Lancet* (2017) 390:946–58. doi: 10.1016/S0140-6736(17)30938-8
174. Byington CL, Wilkes J, Korgenski K, Sheng X. Respiratory syncytial virus-associated mortality in hospitalized infants and young children. *Pediatrics* (2015) 135:e24–31. doi: 10.1542/peds.2014-2151
175. Dawood FS, Iuliano AD, Reed C, Meltzer MI, Shay DK, Cheng PY, et al. Estimated global mortality associated with the first 12 months of 2009 pandemic influenza A H1N1 virus circulation: a modelling study. *Lancet Infect Dis.* (2012) 12:687–95. doi: 10.1016/S1473-3099(12) 70121-4
176. Kumar A, Zarychanski R, Pinto R, Cook DJ, Marshall J, Lacroix J, et al. Critically ill patients with 2009 influenza A(H1N1) infection in Canada. *JAMA* (2009) 302:1872–9. doi: 10.1001/jama.2009.1496
177. Dominguez-Cherit G, Lapinsky SE, Macias AE, Pinto R, Espinosa-Perez L, de la Torre A, et al. Critically Ill patients with 2009 influenza A(H1N1) in Mexico. *JAMA* (2009) 302:1880–7. doi: 10.1001/jama.200 9.1536
178. Sellers SA, Hagan RS, Hayden FG, Fischer WA II. The hidden burden of influenza: a review of the extra-pulmonary complications of influenza infection. *Influenza Other Respir Viruses* (2017) 11:372–93. doi: 10.1111/irv.12470
179. Khatami A, McMullan BJ, Webber M, Stewart P, Francis S, Timmers KJ, et al. Sepsis-like disease in infants due to human parechovirus type 3 during an outbreak in Australia. *Clin Infect Dis.* (2015) 60:228–36. doi: 10.1093/cid/ciu784
180. Verboon-Maciolek MA, Groenendaal F, Hahn CD, Hellmann J, van Loon AM, Boivin G, et al. Human parechovirus causes encephalitis with white matter injury in neonates. *Ann Neurol.* (2008) 64:266–73. doi: 10.1002/ana.21445
181. Abzug MJ. Prognosis for neonates with enterovirus hepatitis and coagulopathy. *Pediatr Infect Dis J.* (2001) 20:758–63.
182. Freund MW, Kleinveld G, Krediet TG, van Loon AM, Verboon-Maciolek MA. Prognosis for neonates with enterovirus myocarditis. *Arch Dis Child Fetal Neonatal Ed.* (2010) 95:F206–12. doi: 10.1136/adc.2009.165183
183. Tebruegge M, Curtis N. Enterovirus infections in neonates. *Semin Fetal Neonatal Med.* (2009) 14:222–7. doi: 10.1016/j.siny.2009.02.002
184. Spaeder MC, Custer JW, Bembea MM, Aganga DO, Song X, Scafidi S. A multicenter outcomes analysis of children with severe viral respiratory infection due to human metapneumovirus. *Pediatr Crit Care Med.* (2013) 14:268–72. doi: 10.1097/PCC.0b013e3182720fc7
185. Spaeder MC, Fackler JC. Hospital-acquired viral infection increases mortality in children with severe viral respiratory infection. *Pediatr Crit Care Med.* (2011) 12:e317–21. doi: 10.1097/PCC.0b013e3182 230f6e
186. Sugata K, Taniguchi K, Yui A, Miyake F, Suga S, Asano Y, et al. Analysis of rotavirus antigenemia and extraintestinal manifestations in children with rotavirus gastroenteritis. *Pediatrics* (2008) 122:392–7. doi: 10.1542/peds.2007-2290
187. Dickey M, Jamison L, Michaud L, Care M, Bernstein DI, Staat MA. Rotavirus meningoencephalitis in a previously healthy child and a review of the literature. *Pediatr Infect Dis J.* (2009) 28:318–21. doi: 10.1097/INF.0b013e31818ddbe9
188. Taha TE, Graham SM, Kumwenda NI, Broadhead RL, Hoover DR, Markakis D, et al. Morbidity among human immunodeficiency virus-1-infected and -uninfected African children. *Pediatrics* (2000) 106:E77. doi: 10.1097/INF.0b013e31822cca05
189. Centers for Disease Control and Prevention. 1994 Revised classification system for human immunodeficiency virus infection in children less than 13 years of age; Official authorized addenda: human immunodeficiency virus infection codes and official guidelines for coding and reporting ICD-9-CM. Morbid. *Mortal. Week. Rep.* (1994) 43:1–10.
190. Zanone SM, Krause LK, Madhi SA, Bassat Q, Jha P, Simoes EA, et al. Challenges in estimating RSV-associated mortality rates. *Lancet Respir Med.* (2016) 4:345–7. doi: 10.1016/S2213-2600(16)30042-X
191. Leclerc F, Leteurtre S, Duhamel A, Grandbastien B, Proulx F, Martinot A, et al. Cumulative influence of organ dysfunctions and septic state on mortality of critically ill children. *Am J Respir Crit Care Med.* (2005) 171:348–53. doi: 10.1164/rccm.200405-630OC
192. Jaramillo-Bustamante JC, Marin-Agudelo A, Fernandez-Laverde M, Bareno-Silva J. Epidemiology of sepsis in pediatric intensive care units: first Colombian multicenter study. *Pediatr Crit Care Med.* (2012) 13:501–8. doi: 10.1097/PCC.0b013e3182 3c980f

13

Pediatric Vital Sign Distribution Derived from a Multi-Centered Emergency Department Database

Robert J. Sepanski[1], Sandip A. Godambe[2] and Arno L. Zaritsky[2]*

[1] Department of Quality Improvement, Children's Hospital of The King's Daughters, Norfolk, VA, United States, [2] Department of Pediatrics, Eastern Virginia Medical School, Children's Hospital of The King's Daughters, Norfolk, VA, United States

Correspondence:
Robert J. Sepanski
robert.sepanski@chkd.org

Background: We hypothesized that current vital sign thresholds used in pediatric emergency department (ED) screening tools do not reflect observed vital signs in this population. We analyzed a large multi-centered database to develop heart rate (HR) and respiratory rate centile rankings and *z*-scores that could be incorporated into electronic health record ED screening tools and we compared our derived centiles to previously published centiles and Pediatric Advanced Life Support (PALS) vital sign thresholds.

Methods: Initial HR and respiratory rate data entered into the Cerner™ electronic health record at 169 participating hospitals' ED over 5 years (2009 through 2013) as part of routine care were analyzed. Analysis was restricted to non-admitted children (0 to <18 years). Centile curves and *z*-scores were developed using generalized additive models for location, scale, and shape. A split-sample validation using two-thirds of the sample was compared with the remaining one-third. Centile values were compared with results from previous studies and guidelines.

Results: HR and RR centiles and *z*-scores were determined from ~1.2 million records. Empirical 95th centiles for HR and respiratory rate were higher than previously published results and both deviated from PALS guideline recommendations.

Conclusion: Heart and respiratory rate centiles derived from a large real-world non-hospitalized ED pediatric population can inform the modification of electronic and paper-based screening tools to stratify children by the degree of deviation from normal for age rather than dichotomizing children into groups having "normal" versus "abnormal" vital signs. Furthermore, these centiles also may be useful in paper-based screening tools and bedside alarm limits for children in areas other than the ED and may establish improved alarm limits for bedside monitors.

Keywords: heart rate, respiratory rate, infant, child, emergency service, hospital

---

Abbreviations: ED, Emergency Department; EHR, electronic health record; HR, heart rate; GAMLSS, generalized additive models for location, scale, and shape; RR, respiratory rate; TMP, temperature; BCPE, Box–Cox Power Exponential; BCT, Box–Cox "t"; PALS, Pediatric Advanced Life Support; PEARS, Pediatric Emergency Assessment, Recognition and Stabilization; CCS, Clinical Classifications Software; ICU, intensive care unit; C, Centile (percentile).

INTRODUCTION

Vital sign thresholds are incorporated into various screening tools to help identify those children at higher risk of serious medical or surgical illness (1–4). To effectively utilize vital sign data in children, however, it may be more useful to identify the magnitude of deviation from the expected vital sign distribution, considering the child's age and location of care [e.g., emergency department (ED) versus intensive care unit (ICU)], rather than determining if the vital sign value is abnormal. Since most current scoring tools consider vital signs as dichotomous variables (i.e., "normal" or "abnormal") within relatively wide age ranges, it is not surprising that most triage and scoring tools have performed poorly even though they are significantly associated with the outcome of interest (4–7).

Most screening tools use vital sign thresholds that fail to consider the physiologic stress response of a child seen in the ED. Thus, the upper "normal" vital sign thresholds observed in ED patients were higher than observed in children who were hospitalized on the ward or who were ambulatory (8–10). The value of using empirically derived ED vital sign thresholds was demonstrated in a study of a pediatric ED sepsis screening tool that incorporated temperature (TMP) adjustment for heart rate (HR) and respiratory rate (RR) (11). The tool's positive predictive value was 48.7%, almost threefold better than using the consensus systemic inflammatory response syndrome (SIRS) criteria (12), with no loss of sensitivity (11).

In sepsis, early identification of children at risk is a key recommendation for optimal management (13) since early implementation of protocol-guided sepsis care decreased sepsis-related organ dysfunction, hospital and ICU length of stay, and mortality (14–16). Clinical judgment alone misses approximately 27% of septic children seen in the ED (17). Using vital sign data with current threshold parameters is limited by the high rate of tool activation; almost 17% of febrile or hypothermic children in the ED met alert criteria, but only 2.5% of these children had severe sepsis or septic shock (17). Similarly, more than 90% of febrile children in the ED meet vital sign criteria for SIRS (5), and ~12% of all ED children triggered an alert based on tachycardia alone (4). These data suggest that current sepsis screening tools identify too many at-risk children, leading to alert fatigue (18) and reluctance to use the tool.

Recent studies empirically derived centile ranks and, in some cases, z-scores for vital sign parameters by age (9, 11). The rationale for considering the vital sign parameter's z-score or centile rank rather than "normal" versus "abnormal" is based on the enhanced statistical power of the former over the latter (19, 20).

We hypothesized that current pediatric HR and RR vital sign thresholds used in Pediatric Advanced Life Support (PALS) or derived from low-acuity ED patients do not accurately reflect empirically derived HR and RR centiles. To develop empirically derived thresholds that could be incorporated into ED screening tools and may inform monitor alarm limits, we analyzed a very large multi-institutional database to derive HR and RR centile ranks and z-scores stratified by age in children presenting to the ED. Ultimately, our goal is to derive HR and RR data that can be applied as continuous variables in electronic health record (EHR)-based tools to stratify children into risk groups or used as threshold limits in paper-based triage tools. Empirically derived vital sign distributions also may better determine alarm limits in different aged children to reduce alarm fatigue and may be useful to stratify children into risk groups for clinical trials.

MATERIALS AND METHODS

Data Source

Data in Cerner Health Facts® (21) are extracted directly from the EHR of hospitals in which Cerner has a data use agreement. All admissions, medication orders and dispensing, laboratory orders, and specimens are date and time stamped, providing a temporal relationship between treatment patterns and clinical information. Cerner Corporation has established Health Insurance Portability and Accountability Act-compliant operating policies to establish de-identification for Health Facts®.

Data Analysis

The HR and RR distributions by age were modeled using the generalized additive models for location, scale, and shape (GAMLSS) methodology and software (22, 23). GAMLSS adjusts for kurtosis and skews in the distributions and allows the generation of normalized standard centiles, or "z-scores," and smooth centile curves by age. This process requires that data are fitted to one of several mathematical distributions (24) that approximate real-world distributions of vital sign measurements. For modeling HR, the Box–Cox power exponential (BCPE) distribution was chosen based on previous work (9, 25) and goodness of fit. For modeling RR, however, BCPE was unsuitable due to the highly leptokurtic (thin, slender peaked) and heavier tailed nature of the RR distributions (as shown in **Figure 1**); therefore, an alternative distribution, the Box–Cox "t" (BCT) (26), was employed.

For modeling the distributions of RR, a natural logarithm transformation was required for model convergence. It was also necessary to introduce Gaussian statistical noise of up to ±2 breaths/min (with a mean value of 0) to overcome the reduced variation due to digit bias in the raw RR measurements (9) and so induce greater conformity to the BCT modeling distribution.

For each vital sign, our modeling process entailed a stepwise fitting procedure to calculate optimal age-specific fits for mean, SD, skew, and kurtosis, with an additive term that used "penalized B-splines" to create smooth centile curves (22). The process was repeated with patient age raised to various exponents [designated in GAMLSS literature as the "power parameter" (27)] between 0.01 and 1 to further optimize model fit. The methodology used for smoothing is necessarily subjective in that the modeler may choose between iterative methods (22, 27) that result in varying degrees of over-fitting or under-fitting of the model to the empirical data. We chose the Schwarz Bayesian Criterion for minimizing local deviation between model and data, which resulted in acceptably smooth curves that retained a good fit to the underlying vital signs data (22). A technical specification of the GAMLSS parameters that describe our centile models is found in Data Sheet S1 in Supplementary Material.

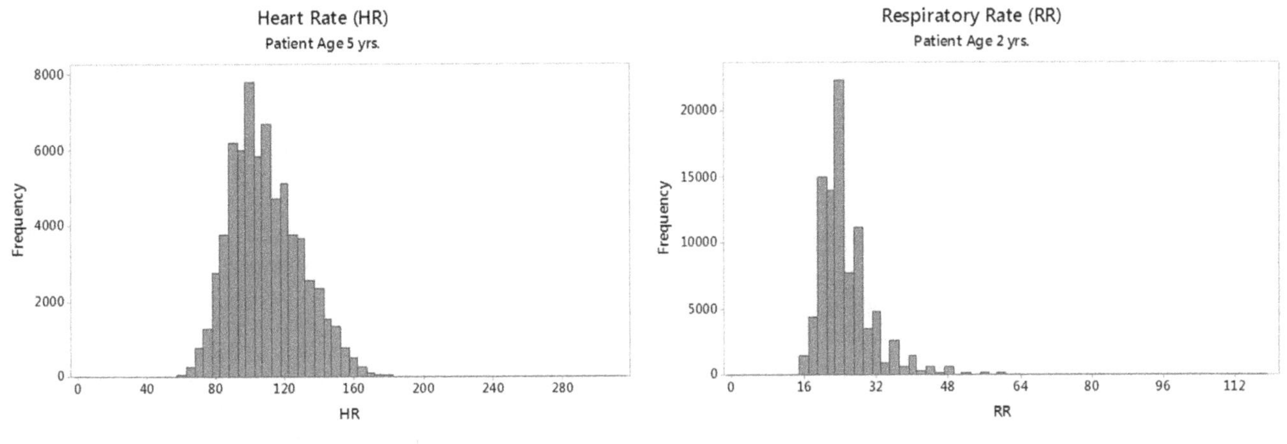

FIGURE 1 | Sample raw distributions of individual heart rate (HR) and respiratory rate (RR) parameters for a single age group.

Because our original intent was to examine both raw and TMP-corrected initial vital signs, our data capture was restricted to initial encounters having HR, RR, and TMP values taken within 15 min of one another. Encounters having two or more distinct measurements recorded for the same vital sign at the same date and time were not uncommon (comprising about 7% of the total). In such cases, we selected the average value, provided that the range of simultaneous values did not exceed 10% of the largest value for HR or RR (i.e., approximately 10–20 bpm for HR or 2–5 breaths/min for RR), or 3% of the largest value for TMP (i.e., approximately 1°C), arbitrarily chosen to exclude likely erroneous outliers; if exceeded, the encounter was excluded. Records in one or more of the following categories also were similarly excluded as likely outliers: (1) extreme (likely spurious) values of HR (<30 or >300 bpm), RR (0 or ≥120 breaths/min), or TMP (<30 or >46°C); (2) encounters classified as "Trauma Center" cases; or (3) encounters where the patient had a diagnosis of a chronic heart or respiratory condition present on admission. The latter two exclusion types (collectively ~0.4% of cases) were excluded since we did not want to include children who were more likely to have very abnormal vital signs. A summary of the selection and exclusion criteria used to determine the final data set for our study is given in Data Sheet S2 in Supplementary Material with details on specific diagnostic exclusions in Data Sheet S3 in Supplementary Material. A sensitivity analysis of the effects of these exclusions on the final modeled centile results was conducted, as described below.

Model Validation

To test model reproducibility, we performed a stratified split-sample validation whereby the full data set used for each vital sign was divided into a "training"subset consisting of two-thirds of randomly selected records from each age group, and a "test" data subset consisting of the remaining one-third of records. The training subset was modeled by GAMLSS to generate centile cutoffs, and the percentage of records with vital sign values above and below these modeled cutoffs for the 95th, 99th, 5th, and 1st centiles, respectively, were compared between the training and test data subsets using exact chi-square tests. Holm (step-down Bonferroni) (28) corrections, performed separately for HR and RR, were used to adjust for the multiple testing of each metric.

Sensitivity Analysis

To determine the effect of excluding encounters classified as "Trauma Center," or those where the patient had a diagnosis of a chronic heart or respiratory condition, the modeling of HR and RR distributions was repeated including these encounters. The resultant modeled centile values, rounded to the nearest whole number for HR and RR, were then compared between datasets of children with and without exclusions.

Comparison to Empirically Derived and Guideline-Based Vital Sign Thresholds

We graphically plotted the empirically derived 5th, 50th, and 95th centiles by age compared with the same centiles calculated by O'Leary et al. (10), derived from a large single-center ED population. We also show the upper and lower HR and RR thresholds for awake children recommended in the American Heart Association Pediatric Emergency Assessment, Recognition, and Stabilization, and PALS courses (29).

RESULTS

Data Selection

The Health Facts® data used comprises initial vital sign values and relative measurement times for HR and RR collected from ED encounters involving children (ages 0–17 years) at 169 U.S. hospitals (five were children's hospitals) for calendar years 2009 through 2013. For all encounters, only patient types classified as "Emergency" were selected, which excludes children who were hospitalized from the ED since the Health Facts database does not specifically identify those admitted patients who entered the hospital *via* the ED. Patient age was recorded as an integer age in months for children <2 years or in years for older children. Because ages were categorical rather than continuous, age was converted to represent each category by its midpoint (e.g., 0–1 month becomes 0.5 months) for modeling purposes.

Our preliminary analysis of patient TMPs taken in the ED found that TMP distributions varied according to patient age and route of measurement, making generalized TMP corrections of HR and RR problematic. Therefore, we analyzed HR and RR without TMP correction.

Characteristics of Study Subjects

A total of 1,203,042 encounters were used to study the distribution of initial HR by age, with slightly fewer (1,202,984) available for an analysis of RR. Patient information and encounters included in our study for each of the vital signs examined are presented in **Tables 1** and **2** and Data Sheet S4 and S5 in Supplementary Material. As expected, the sample sizes for age categories representing children <2 years were smaller than those for children 2 years or older due to the shorter age interval (1 month versus 1 year) represented by these categories (**Table 1**). **Table 2** lists information on patient demographics and length of stay for contributing encounters. Data Sheet S4 in Supplementary Material presents patient encounter frequencies according to the contributing hospitals' demographics. Data Sheet S5 in Supplementary Material summarizes contributing patient encounters by principal diagnosis using Clinical Classifications Software (30) categories, an Agency for Healthcare Research and Quality methodology for condensing patient ICD-9 diagnostic data into clinically meaningful groups.

Representative raw distributions (histograms) for the HR and RR (**Figure 1**) illustrate the positive skew (longer right tail) in the distributions of each vital sign, and the high kurtosis and heavy tails evident in the distribution of RR.

Centile Curves

For HR and RR (**Figures 2A,B**), the centile curves reveal a somewhat complex relationship of vital sign distributions with age for neonates and infants up to about two years of age, followed by smoothly decreasing vital sign values with age for all centiles, with values becoming nearly constant over the late adolescent age range.

Model Validation

The results of the split-sample validation of model result reproducibility (**Table 3**) for all metrics and each centile group tested showed no significant difference in the proportion of cases identified by applying the model derived cutoffs obtained from the training data subset to the empirical data in the training and test subsets, respectively, based on either the raw or Holm-adjusted chi-square P statistic.

Table 3 also shows the high general agreement between the modeled centiles and the empirical data. Ideally, the modeled centile groups ">99th" and "<1st" should each identify about 1% of the empirical data, while groups ">95th" and "<5th" should each identify about 5%. Deviations between the modeled and the empirical percentages are apparent only in the RR "<5th" and "<1st" (which identify about 3.9 and 0.7% of the respective empirical data for these groups).

Centile and *z*-Score Tables

The modeled values of HR, and RR from the 1st to 99th centiles for each age group are provided as **Tables 4** and **5**. Supplementary Material Data Sheet S6 and S7 in Supplementary Material present similarly formatted model results by age group for HR and RR as normalized standard centiles (*z*-scores) ranging from −3.0 to +3.0 SDs for HR and RR.

TABLE 1 | Number of contributing encounters by patient age group.

Age description	HR, RR[a], *N* (% of total)	Age description	HR, RR[a], *N* (% of total)
<1 month	12,860 (1.1%)	2 to <3 years	93,406 (7.8)
1 to <2 months	13,016 (1.1%)	3 to <4 years	82,813 (6.9)
2 to <3 months	13,204 (1.1%)	4 to <5 years	74,328 (6.2)
3 to <4 months	11,255 (0.9%)	5 to <6 years	68,517 (5.7)
4 to <5 months	11,846 (1.0%)	6 to <7 years	59,316 (4.9)
5 to <6 months	12,317 (1.0%)	7 to <8 years	50,664 (4.2)
6 to <7 months	12,895 (1.1%)	8 to <9 years	46,448 (3.9)
7 to <8 months	13,354 (1.1%)	9 to <10 years	44,818 (3.7)
8 to <9 months	13,580 (1.1%)	10 to <11 years	44,093 (3.7)
9 to <10 months	13,349 (1.1%)	11 to <12 years	43,225 (3.6)
10 to <11 months	13,234 (1.1%)	12 to <13 years	42,813 (3.6)
11 to <12 months	13,002 (1.1%)	13 to <14 years	45,766 (3.8)
12 to <13 months	13,016 (1.1%)	14 to <15 years	50,007 (4.2)
13 to <14 months	12,078 (1.0%)	15 to <16 years	53,940 (4.5)
14 to <15 months	11,548 (1.0%)	16 to <17 years	59,621 (5.0)
15 to <16 months	11,115 (0.9%)	17 to <18 years	65,264 (5.4)
16 to <17 months	10,805 (0.9%)		
17 to <18 months	10,351 (0.9%)		
18 to <19 months	10,012 (0.8%)		
19 to <20 months	9,476 (0.8%)		
20 to <21 months	9,085 (0.8%)		
21 to <22 months	9,011 (0.7%)		
22 to <23 months	8,878 (0.7%)		
23 to <2 years	8,716 (0.7%)		

[a]*Overall numbers for respiratory rate (RR) are slightly less than for heart rate (HR) (1,202,984 versus 1,203,042), but percentages of total for each age group as rounded are identical for HR and RR.*

TABLE 2 | Contributing encounters: patient demographics and length of stay.

Encounter characteristics	HR, RR[a]
	Mean/Median
Length of Stay (hours)	5.7/2.6
Gender	N (% of total)
Male	627,095 (52.1%)
Female	575,834 (47.9%)
Missing/Unknown/Other	113 (0.0%)
Race/ethnicity	
Caucasian	508,180 (42.2%)
African American	423,607 (35.2%)
Missing/Unknown/Other	140,270 (11.7%)
Hispanic	100,929 (8.4%)
Asian	17,524 (1.5%)
Native American	12,532 (1.0%)
Total	1,203,042[a]

[a]*Overall numbers for respiratory rate (RR) are slightly less than for heart rate (HR) (1,202,984 versus 1,203,042), but mean/median length of stay and percentages of total for each demographic characteristic as rounded are identical for HR and RR.*

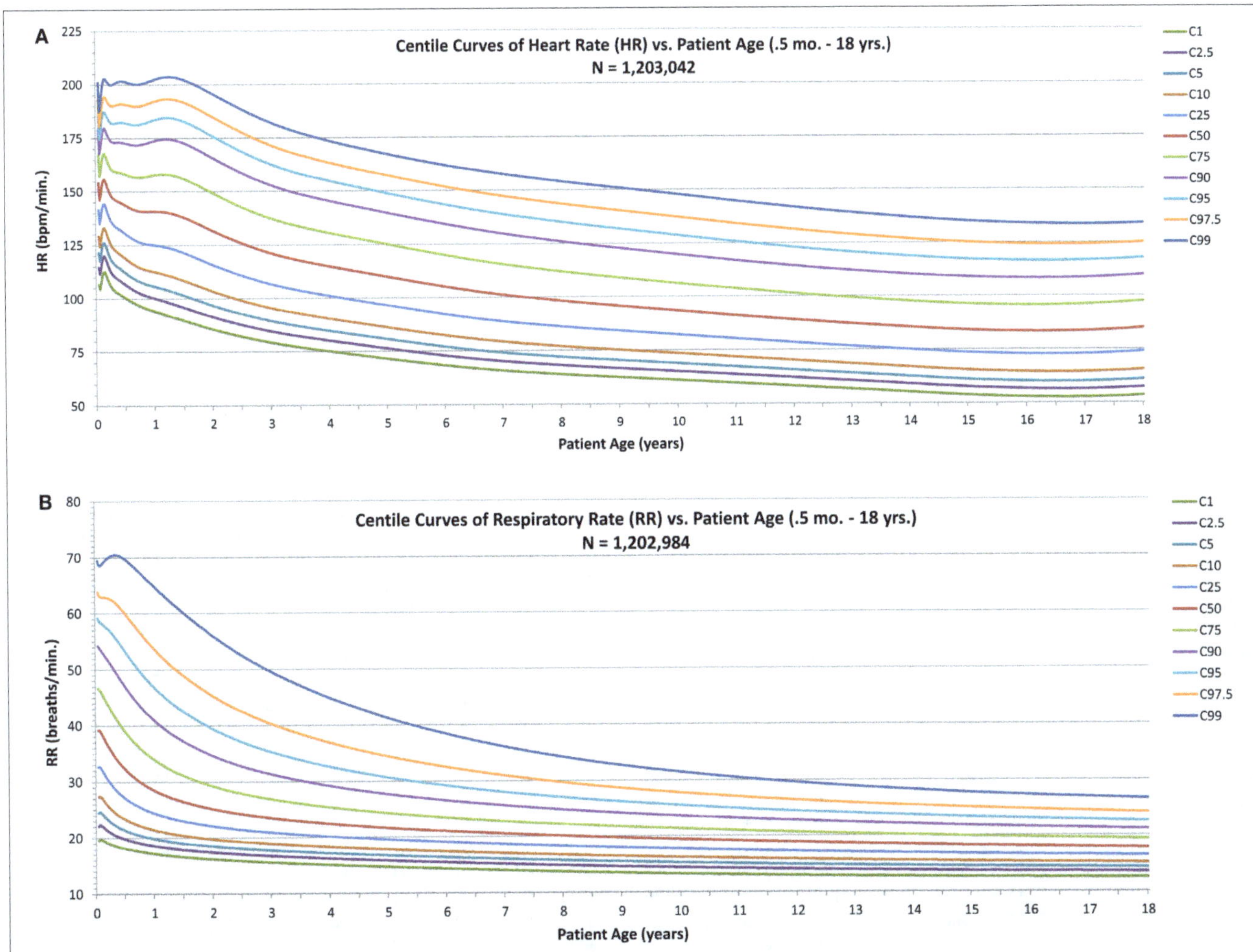

FIGURE 2 | Modeled centile curves for pediatric vital sign metrics. **(A)** The centiles from the first centile (C1) to the 99th centile (C99) for heart rate (HR) by age and **(B)** the respiratory rate (RR) centiles.

TABLE 3 | Validation of vital sign centile modeling results.

Vital sign metric	Modeled[a] centile group	Training set, *N*[b] (%)	Test set, *N*[b] (%)	Raw *P*[c]	Holm-adjusted *P*[d]
HR	>99th	6,653 (0.83)	3,325 (0.83)	0.99	1.0
HR	>95th	42,540 (5.30)	20,980 (5.23)	0.09	0.37
HR	<5th	36,890 (4.60)	18,477 (4.61)	0.85	1.0
HR	<1st	7,771 (0.97)	3,776 (0.94)	0.15	0.44
RR	>99th	7,862 (0.98)	3,961 (0.99)	0.70	0.86
RR	>95th	39,921 (4.98)	19,828 (4.94)	0.43	0.86
RR	<5th	31,091 (3.88)	15,834 (3.95)	0.06	0.22
RR	<1st	5,246 (0.65)	2,692 (0.67)	0.28	0.83

[a]*Using cutoffs obtained by modeling data in training set.*

[b]*Number of encounters with vital sign metric greater than (for 95th and 99th) or less than (for 5th and 1st) modeled cutoff.*

[c]*Comparison of cases above or below cutoff between training and test sets using exact chi-square (df = 1).*

[d]*Holm (step-down Bonferroni) corrections, performed separately for heart rate (HR) and respiratory rate (RR) were employed to adjust for multiple testing (99th, 95th, 5th, and 1st centiles) of each metric.*

Sensitivity Analysis

Each sensitivity analysis compared modeled centiles between data sets with and without predefined exclusions for 11 centile levels and 40 age categories (as presented in **Tables 4** and **5**). Our finding of only one discrepancy out of 440 combinations of centile and age for HR and four for RR—with differences of just 1 bpm for HR and 1 breath/min for each RR—shows that our choice to exclude these encounters resulted in a negligible effect on modeled centile values compared with those obtained without the exclusions.

TABLE 4 | Heart rate (HR, bpm) centiles[a] by age.

Age (years) midpoint	Age/units midpoint	Age description	C1	C2.5	C5	C10	C25	C50	C75	C90	C95	C97.5	C99
0.042	0.5 months	<1 month	106	114	121	128	140	153	165	177	184	191	198
0.125	1.5 months	1 to <2 months	112	119	126	133	144	156	168	180	187	194	202
0.208	2.5 months	2 to < 3 months	108	115	121	128	139	151	163	176	184	192	201
0.292	3.5 months	3 to <4 months	105	111	117	124	135	147	160	173	182	190	200
0.375	4.5 months	4 to <5 months	102	109	115	121	133	145	159	172	181	190	200
0.458	5.5 months	5 to <6 months	101	107	113	120	131	144	158	173	182	190	201
0.542	6.5 months	6 to <7 months	100	106	111	118	130	143	158	173	182	191	201
0.625	7.5 months	7 to <8 months	98	104	110	117	128	142	157	172	182	190	201
0.708	8.5 months	8 to <9 months	97	103	109	115	127	141	157	172	182	190	201
0.792	9.5 months	9 to <10 months	96	102	107	114	126	141	157	172	182	190	201
0.875	10.5 months	10 to <11 months	95	101	106	113	125	140	157	172	182	191	201
0.958	11.5 months	11 to <12 months	94	100	106	112	125	140	157	173	183	191	201
1.042	12.5 months	12 to <13 months	93	100	105	112	124	140	158	174	183	192	202
1.125	13.5 months	13 to <14 months	93	99	105	112	124	140	158	174	184	193	203
1.208	14.5 months	14 to <15 months	92	98	104	111	124	140	158	174	184	193	204
1.292	15.5 months	15 to <16 months	92	98	103	110	123	140	158	174	184	193	204
1.375	16.5 months	16 to <17 months	91	97	103	110	123	139	157	174	184	193	203
1.458	17.5 months	17 to <18 months	90	96	102	109	122	138	157	173	183	192	203
1.542	18.5 months	18 to <19 months	89	95	101	108	121	137	156	172	182	191	202
1.625	19.5 months	19 to <20 months	89	95	100	107	120	136	154	171	181	190	201
1.708	20.5 months	20 to <21 months	88	94	99	106	119	135	153	170	180	189	200
1.792	21.5 months	21 to <22 months	87	93	98	105	118	134	152	169	179	188	198
1.875	22.5 months	22 to <23 months	86	92	98	104	117	133	151	167	178	187	197
1.958	23.5 months	23 months to <2 years	86	92	97	104	116	132	150	166	176	185	196
2.5	2.5 years	2 to <3 years	82	88	93	99	111	126	143	159	169	178	189
3.5	3.5 years	3 to <4 years	77	82	87	93	103	118	133	149	158	167	177
4.5	4.5 years	4 to <5 years	73	78	82	88	98	112	127	142	152	160	170
5.5	5.5 years	5 to <6 years	70	75	79	84	94	107	122	137	146	154	165
6.5	6.5 years	6 to <7 years	67	71	76	81	90	103	118	132	141	149	160
7.5	7.5 years	7 to <8 years	65	69	73	78	87	99	113	128	137	145	155
8.5	8.5 years	8 to <9 years	63	67	71	76	85	97	110	124	133	141	152
9.5	9.5 years	9 to <10 years	62	66	70	74	83	94	107	121	130	138	149
10.5	10.5 years	10 to <11 years	60	64	68	73	81	92	105	118	127	136	146
11.5	11.5 years	11 to <12 years	59	63	67	71	79	90	103	116	125	133	143
12.5	12.5 years	12 to <13 years	57	61	65	69	77	88	100	113	122	130	140
13.5	13.5 years	13 to <14 years	56	59	63	67	75	86	98	111	119	127	138
14.5	14.5 years	14 to <15 years	54	58	62	66	74	84	96	109	117	125	135
15.5	15.5 years	15 to <16 years	53	57	61	65	73	84	96	108	116	124	134
16.5	16.5 years	16 to <17 years	53	57	60	65	73	83	96	108	116	124	133
17.5	17.5 years	17 to <18 years	53	57	60	65	73	84	96	109	117	124	134

[a]*Centiles abbreviated as C1 (first centile) to C99 (99th centile).*

Comparison to Current and Guideline Vital Sign Threshold

In infants, **Figure 3A** shows that the empirically derived 50th centile for HR was 9–16 bpm higher than the values determined by O'Leary et al. (10), and the 95th centiles for HR were 13–24 bpm higher than the O'Leary values, whereas the infant-aged PALS recommended upper and lower HR limits (29) were above and below the 95th and 5th centiles, respectively. The empirically derived 95th centile RR in infants (**Figure 3B**) was also higher by 7–11 breaths/min than O'Leary's data, whereas the 50th and 5th centile were similar. The PALS recommended upper RR in infants was similar to the empirically derived 95th centile range, although by 10 months of age, it steadily exceeded the empirically derived 95th centile. The lower PALS RR limit was 6–10 breaths/min above the empirically derived 5th centile and was similar to the 50th centile by 7 months of age.

In children (≥1 year), **Figure 3A** shows substantial discrepancy between the empirically derived 95th centile HR and O'Leary's (10) centile HR values up to around 10 years of age. The fifth centile for all three sets of data are similar, but the PALS upper HR limits are below the empirically derived 95th centile and are between the 50th and 75th centile for age up to ~6 years old (23–44 bpm lower from 1 through 6 years of age). Similarly, the empirically derived 95th centile RR (**Figure 3B**) is 3–6 breaths/min higher than the PALS and O'Leary values up to 4–5 years of age.

DISCUSSION

We hypothesized that empirically derived HR and RR distributions would deviate from PALS recommended distributions, and values derived from a low-acuity population of children seen in the ED. Ideally, an effective screening tool should balance high sensitivity to detect children at risk of deterioration while limiting too many false-positive patients leading to alert fatigue (5). It is important to recognize, however, that a vital sign-based screening

TABLE 5 | Respiratory rate (RR, breaths/minute) centiles[a] by age.

Age (years) midpoint	Age/units midpoint	Age description	C1	C2.5	C5	C10	C25	C50	C75	C90	C95	C97.5	C99
0.042	0.5 month	<1 month	19	22	24	27	33	39	47	54	59	64	69
0.125	1.5 months	1 to <2 month	20	22	24	27	32	38	45	53	58	63	69
0.208	2.5 months	2 to <3 month	19	21	23	26	30	37	44	52	58	63	70
0.292	3.5 months	3 to <4 month	19	21	23	25	29	35	42	51	57	63	71
0.375	4.5 months	4 to <5 month	18	20	22	24	28	34	41	49	56	62	71
0.458	5.5 months	5 to <6 month	18	20	21	23	27	33	40	48	54	61	71
0.542	6.5 months	6 to <7 month	18	20	21	23	27	32	38	46	53	60	70
0.625	7.5 months	7 to <8 month	18	19	21	23	26	31	37	45	51	58	69
0.708	8.5 months	8 to <9 month	18	19	20	22	26	30	36	44	50	57	67
0.792	9.5 months	9 to <10 month	17	19	20	22	25	30	35	43	49	56	66
0.875	10.5 months	10 to <11 month	17	19	20	22	25	29	35	42	48	55	65
0.958	11.5 months	11 to <12 month	17	19	20	21	24	29	34	41	47	54	64
1.042	12.5 months	12 to <13 month	17	18	20	21	24	28	34	40	46	53	64
1.125	13.5 months	13 to <14 month	17	18	20	21	24	28	33	40	46	52	63
1.208	14.5 months	14 to <15 month	17	18	20	21	24	28	33	39	45	51	62
1.292	15.5 months	15 to <16 month	17	18	19	21	24	27	32	39	44	51	62
1.375	16.5 months	16 to <17 month	17	18	19	21	23	27	32	38	44	50	61
1.458	17.5 months	17 to <18 month	17	18	19	21	23	27	32	38	43	50	61
1.542	18.5 months	18 to <19 month	17	18	19	20	23	27	31	37	43	49	60
1.625	19.5 months	19 to <20 month	17	18	19	20	23	26	31	37	42	48	59
1.708	20.5 months	20 to <21 month	16	18	19	20	23	26	30	36	41	48	59
1.792	21.5 months	21 to <22 month	16	18	19	20	23	26	30	36	41	47	58
1.875	22.5 months	22 to <23 month	16	18	19	20	22	26	30	35	40	47	58
1.958	23.5 months	23 month to <2 years	16	17	19	20	22	25	29	35	40	46	57
2.5	2.5 years	2 to <3 years	16	17	18	19	21	24	28	33	37	43	53
3.5	3.5 years	3 to <4 years	15	16	17	18	20	23	26	30	34	38	47
4.5	4.5 years	4 to <5 years	15	16	17	18	20	22	25	28	31	35	43
5.5	5.5 years	5 to <6 years	14	16	17	18	19	21	24	27	30	33	39
6.5	6.5 years	6 to <7 years	14	15	16	17	19	21	23	26	28	31	37
7.5	7.5 years	7 to <8 years	14	15	16	17	18	20	22	25	27	30	35
8.5	8.5 years	8 to <9 years	14	15	16	17	18	20	22	25	27	29	33
9.5	9.5 years	9 to <10 years	13	15	15	16	18	20	22	24	26	28	32
10.5	10.5 years	10 to <11 years	13	14	15	16	18	19	21	23	25	28	31
11.5	11.5 years	11 to <12 years	13	14	15	16	17	19	21	23	25	27	30
12.5	12.5 years	12 to <13 years	13	14	15	16	17	19	20	22	24	26	29
13.5	13.5 years	13 to <14 years	13	14	15	15	17	18	20	22	24	25	28
14.5	14.5 years	14 to <15 years	13	14	14	15	17	18	20	22	23	25	28
15.5	15.5 years	15 to <16 years	13	14	14	15	17	18	20	22	23	25	27
16.5	16.5 years	16 to <17 years	12	14	14	15	17	18	20	21	23	24	27
17.5	17.5 years	17 to <18 years	12	14	14	15	16	18	19	21	23	24	27

[a]*Centiles abbreviated as C1 (first centile) to C99 (99th centile).*

tool is unlikely to identify all at-risk children. Instead, recent data show that combining an EHR-based screening tool with clinician identification, timelier joint team assessments and improved escalation of care processes results in high sensitivity and specificity for identification of severe sepsis/septic shock (31).

As seen in **Figures 3A,B**, the utility of "normal" vital sign thresholds recommended by PALS (29), APLS (32), and other reference texts is limited since they group normal values into relatively wide age ranges, which encompass large physiologic ranges and thus a wide expected distribution of vital signs, and they are not empirically derived. The PALS upper HR thresholds are well below the empirically derived 95th centiles and are between the 50th and 75th centile for age up to ~6 years, leading to substantial over-identification of at-risk children.

Similarly, the empirically derived 95th centile RR (**Figure 3B**) is higher than the PALS and O'Leary values up to 4–5 years of age. The upper PALS RR limit would over-identify many adolescents, whereas the lower PALS RR values generally exceed the empirically derived value up to 12 years of age falling 2–3 breaths/min below the empirically observed fifth centile. Using PALS criteria also would overclassify up to 50% of older infants as having an abnormally low RR (**Figure 3B**).

Thus, it is not surprising that in a ward inpatient sample of over 116,000 observations, 54% of the HR and 40% of the RR vital signs observed in hospitalized children were outside textbook "normal" vital sign distributions and 38% of HR and 30% of RR observations would have resulted in increased early warning scores (9). Similarly, in an analysis of 40,356 ED visits at Colorado Children's Hospital (5), 16.3% of the children had a fever (>38.5°C) and 92.8% of these febrile children met SIRS vital sign criteria, as defined by the International Pediatric Sepsis Conference (12). Most of these children were discharged without any intervention.

Several groups have used data from EHR's to redefine the distribution of vital signs observed in children in the ED (8, 10) or hospital wards (9, 33). These analyses clearly show that the standard textbook and guideline distributions and thresholds for "abnormal" for vital signs do not reflect empirically observed distributions (9). However, our empirically derived centiles differ from centiles derived from a large (111,696) data set of children presenting to a single ED (10). Of note, this study (10) restricted its analysis to the lowest acuity children, whereas our analysis included all acuities, but excluded children seen in the ED who were subsequently admitted. This may better represent the distributions of vital signs seen in children brought to the ED, who are likely stressed by the ED environment, but who presumably are not critically or seriously ill and, thus, do not require hospitalization.

We believe our empirically derived centiles based on a very large, multi-centered database of ED visits by children provide evidence-based vital sign parameters to use in either EHR or paper-based early warning scores, to set monitor alarm limits and to risk-stratify children for clinical trials or epidemiologic studies. Rather than using dichotomous threshold values, which are often set by consensus, to define "normal" from "abnormal," we believe that these data can lead to the development of more useful objective risk stratification tools.

Although using vital sign parameter *z*-scores or centile ranks rather than "normal" versus "abnormal" is complex, EHR systems can be programmed to analyze these data to risk-stratify children, which enhances the statistical power of analyzing continuous data rather than using a dichotomous threshold (19, 20). By necessity, dichotomizing a continuous physiologic variable into two categories anticipates an unrealistic step function for risk at the threshold level. For example, if the upper limit of normal HR is set at 180 bpm, then an infant with a HR of 179 bpm is considered "normal," even though this infant is not demonstrating the same physiologic response as the same aged infant with a HR of 120 bpm.

The potential value of using risk-stratified assessment of vital signs was seen in an ED-based study of 1,750 febrile children evaluated using seven different vital sign modeling strategies to identify children with serious bacterial infections (34). The model that worked best utilized the degree of deviation of age-adjusted HR and RR from median values, with or without TMP correction.

Centile and *z*-Scores

Although we generated smooth curves for the individual vital signs, the raw vital sign distributions for RR shown in

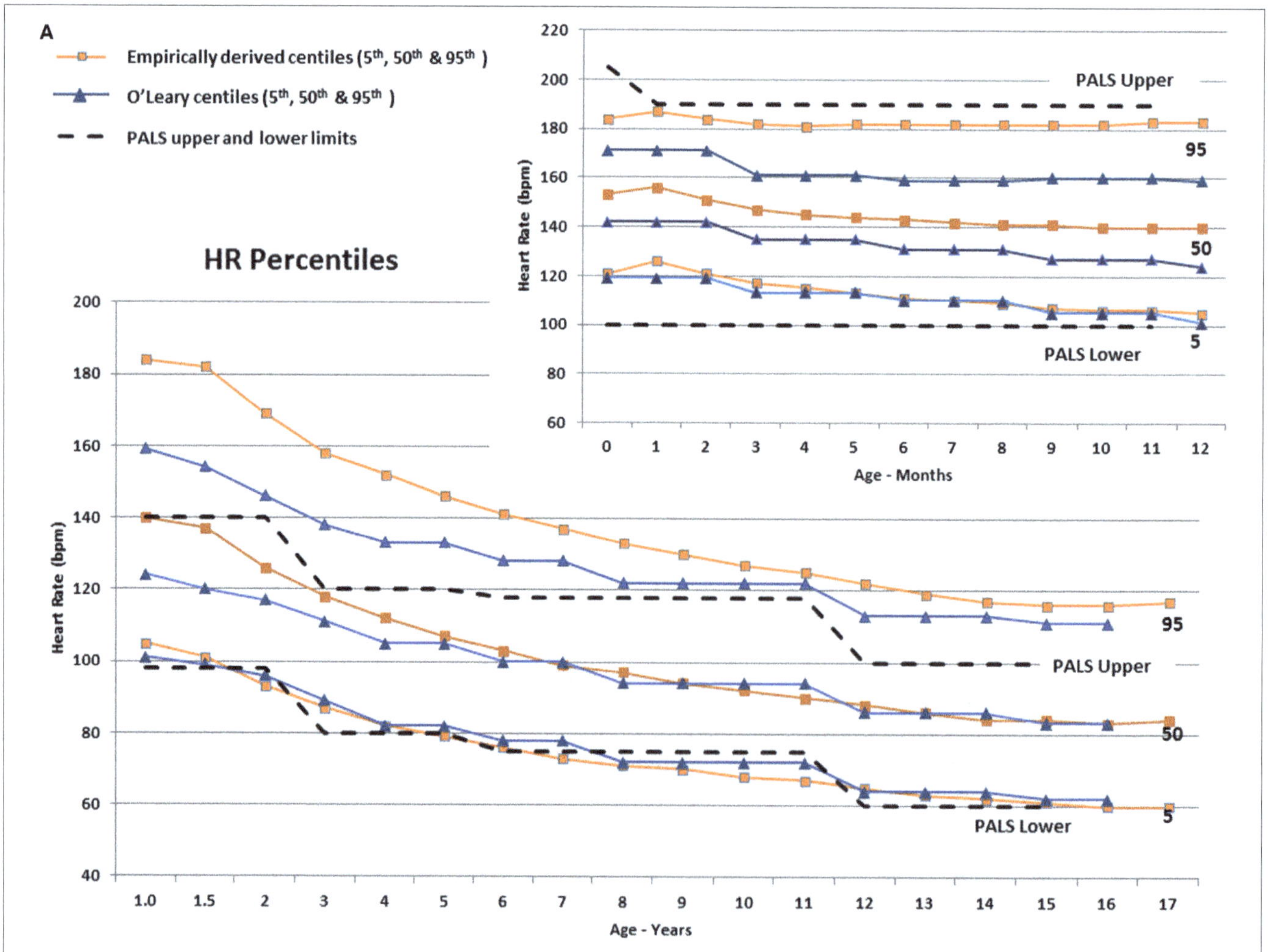

FIGURE 3 | Continued

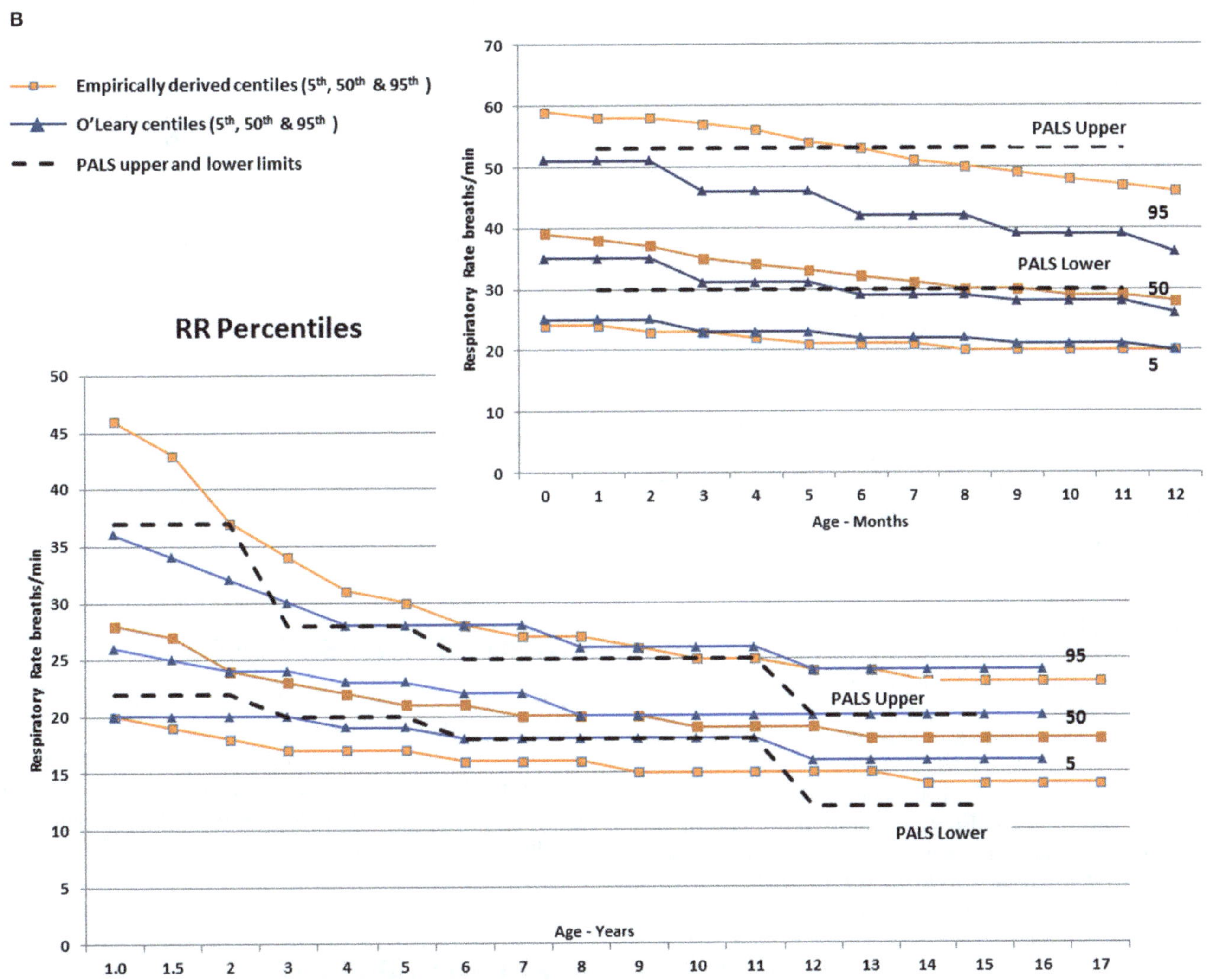

FIGURE 3 | (A) The derived 5th, 50th, and 95th HR centiles by age compared with similar centiles derived by O'Leary et al. (10) The Pediatric Advanced Life Support (PALS) (29) upper and lower HR limits are also shown (dashed lines). The smaller panel shows the centiles from 0 to 12 months of age. **(B)** The derived 5th, 50th, and 95th RR centiles by age compared with similar centiles derived by O'Leary et al. (10). The PALS (29) upper and lower RR limits are also shown (dashed lines). The smaller panel shows the centiles from 0 to 12 months of age.

Figure 1 are not Gaussian but rather show a strong kurtosis and right-tailed skew. The skewed RR may represent an increased prevalence of disease processes (i.e., respiratory conditions), which lead to more frequent elevated RR values in children presenting to the ED compared with a population of healthy, normal children.

We performed a stratified split-sample validation that showed (**Table 3**) for each vital sign metric there was no significant difference in the proportion of cases in the training versus the test subjects.

TMP-Adjusted Vital Signs

Most screening tools do not TMP adjust the HR or RR. It is well known that increased TMP increases metabolic demand, thus increasing HR and RR (33, 35, 36). Analysis of vital sign data in hospitalized children (not ICU) found a near linear increase in HR with increasing TMP of approximately 10 beats/min for each degree Centigrade increase in TMP, although the increase appears to vary by age, with the HR increasing by 15 bpm in infants per degree Centigrade versus 8 bpm in 14- to 18-year-olds (33).

We planned to analyze the effect of TMP on HR and RR, but we were not confident in adjusting oral TMP to core TMP and did not know how to correct for axillary or temporal artery TMPs. A recent systematic review of the accuracy of peripheral versus core TMPs in adults and children (37) found few studies comparing oral to core TMP in children. Axillary and infrared tympanic TMPs can vary widely from core TMP, especially in patients who have poor perfusion. Moreover, an inpatient study conducted at Cincinnati Children's Hospital and Children's Hospital of Philadelphia observed significantly different TMP histograms between the institutions, which disappeared when one of the institutions transitioned to the same thermometer used at the other hospital, showing that different thermometers can introduce additional variation in the measured TMP (33).

Limitations

Since we did not have precise ages, we used 1-month ranges (if <2 years of age) or 1-year age ranges for older children. It seems likely that the large sample size and smoothing of the data will limit the impact of including children within an entire year, especially since within any year range there is sizable normal variation based on child size and height as seen with blood pressure (38).

We chose to use extreme exclusion criteria for HR and RR. This may have resulted in the inclusion of data from children with erroneous or very abnormal vital sign values, but again the very large data set likely limits the impact of these outliers.

Further studies are needed to determine if using empirically derived vital sign thresholds would result in a lower sensitivity to identify high-risk children. Our previous analysis using empirically derived higher vital sign thresholds based on data from a single ED noted improved positive predictive value for severe sepsis/septic shock identification without affecting sensitivity (11).

CONCLUSION

In summary, the derived HR and RR centiles and z-scores from more than 1 million children seen in the ED of mostly adult hospitals were often different from currently derived centiles in children seen in the ED and from consensus-based PALS guideline vital sign thresholds. We believe our data provide a reliable representation of HR and RR distributions in stressed children seen in the ED who do not require hospitalization. These data could be used to create algorithms within EHR's to develop pragmatic risk scores that increase sensitivity and specificity and reduce alarm fatigue characteristic of dichotomous vital sign thresholds. We also believe these parameters may help establish improved alarm limits for bedside monitors and these empirically derived HR and RR thresholds may improve the performance of paper-based tools, such as those based on PALS vital sign thresholds. Finally, the data may better inform the creation of disease-specific screening tools.

AVAILABILITY OF DATA AND MATERIAL

The datasets used and analyzed during the current study are available from the corresponding author, but restrictions apply to the availability of these data since they were obtained through a written agreement with Cerner Corporation and so are not publicly available. Data may be available from the author on reasonable request and with permission of Cerner Corporation.

ETHICS STATEMENT

Since we analyzed de-identified clinical data, this is not human subjects research.

AUTHOR CONTRIBUTIONS

RS, SG, and AZ each made substantial contributions to the conception and design of the study. RS conducted the analyses and derived the centile curves and z-scores. RS and AZ jointly drafted and all three authors critically revised the manuscript for important intellectual content. All authors read and approved the final manuscript.

ACKNOWLEDGMENTS

The authors acknowledge the support of Cerner Corporation.

REFERENCES

1. Duncan H, Hutchison J, Parshuram CS. The pediatric early warning system score: a severity of illness score to predict urgent medical need in hospitalized children. *J Crit Care* (2006) 21:271–8. doi:10.1016/j.jcrc.2006.06.007
2. Parshuram CS, Duncan HP, Joffe AR, Farrell CA, Lacroix JR, Middaugh KL, et al. Multicentre validation of the bedside paediatric early warning system score: a severity of illness score to detect evolving critical illness in hospitalised children. *Crit Care* (2011) 15:R184. doi:10.1186/cc10337
3. Roukema J, Steyerberg EW, van Meurs A, Ruige M, van der Lei J, Moll HA. Validity of the Manchester Triage System in paediatric emergency care. *Emerg Med J* (2006) 23:906–10. doi:10.1136/emj.2006.038877
4. Cruz AT, Williams EA, Graf JM, Perry AM, Harbin DE, Wuestner ER, et al. Test characteristics of an automated age- and temperature-adjusted tachycardia alert in pediatric septic shock. *Pediatr Emerg Care* (2012) 28: 889–94. doi:10.1097/PEC.0b013e318267a78a
5. Scott HF, Deakyne SJ, Woods JM, Bajaj L. The prevalence and diagnostic utility of systemic inflammatory response syndrome vital signs in a pediatric emergency department. *Acad Emerg Med* (2015) 22:381–9. doi:10.1111/acem.12610
6. Ray S, Cvetkovic M, Brierley J, Lutman DH, Pathan N, Ramnarayan P, et al. Shock index values and trends in pediatric sepsis: predictors or therapeutic targets? A retrospective observational study. *Shock* (2016) 46:279–86. doi:10.1097/SHK.0000000000000634
7. Yasaka Y, Khemani RG, Markovitz BP. Is shock index associated with outcome in children with sepsis/septic shock? *Pediatr Crit Care Med* (2013) 14:e372–9. doi:10.1097/PCC.0b013e3182975eee
8. Fleming S, Thompson M, Stevens R, Heneghan C, Plüddemann A, Maconochie I, et al. Normal ranges of heart rate and respiratory rate in children from birth to 18 years of age: a systematic review of observational studies. *Lancet* (2011) 377:1011–8. doi:10.1016/S0140-6736(10)62226-X
9. Bonafide CP, Brady PW, Keren R, Conway PH, Marsolo K, Daymont C. Development of heart and respiratory rate percentile curves for hospitalized children. *Pediatrics* (2013) 131:e1150–7. doi:10.1542/peds.2012-2443
10. O'Leary F, Hayen A, Lockie F, Peat J. Defining normal ranges and centiles for heart and respiratory rates in infants and children: a cross-sectional study

of patients attending an Australian tertiary hospital paediatric emergency department. *Arch Dis Child* (2015) 100:733–7. doi:10.1136/archdischild-2014-307401
11. Sepanski RJ, Godambe SA, Mangum CD, Bovat CS, Zaritsky AL, Shah SH. Designing a pediatric severe sepsis screening tool. *Front Pediatr* (2014) 2:56. doi:10.3389/fped.2014.00056
12. Goldstein B, Giroir B, Randolph A. International pediatric sepsis consensus conference: definitions for sepsis and organ dysfunction in pediatrics. *Pediatr Crit Care Med* (2005) 6:2–8. doi:10.1097/01.PCC.0000149131.72248.E6
13. Brierley J, Carcillo JA, Choong K, Cornell T, DeCaen A, Deymann A, et al. Clinical practice parameters for hemodynamic support of pediatric and neonatal septic shock: 2007 update from the American College of Critical Care Medicine. *Crit Care Med* (2009) 37:666–88. doi:10.1097/CCM.0b013e31819323c6
14. Paul R, Neuman MI, Monuteaux MC, Melendez E. Adherence to PALS sepsis guidelines and hospital length of stay. *Pediatrics* (2012) 130:e273–80. doi:10.1542/peds.2012-0094
15. Balamuth F, Weiss SL, Fitzgerald JC, Hayes K, Centkowski S, Chilutti M, et al. Protocolized treatment is associated with decreased organ dysfunction in pediatric severe sepsis. *Pediatr Crit Care Med* (2016) 17:817–22. doi:10.1097/PCC.0000000000000858
16. Han YY, Carcillo JA, Dragotta MA, Bills DM, Watson RS, Westerman ME, et al. Early reversal of pediatric-neonatal septic shock by community physicians is associated with improved outcome. *Pediatrics* (2003) 112:793–9. doi:10.1542/peds.112.4.793
17. Balamuth F, Alpern ER, Grundmeier RW, Chilutti M, Weiss SL, Fitzgerald JC, et al. Comparison of two sepsis recognition methods in a pediatric emergency department. *Acad Emerg Med* (2015) 22:1298–306. doi:10.1111/acem.12814
18. Harrison AM, Gajic O, Pickering BW, Herasevich V. Development and implementation of Sepsis Alert Systems. *Clin Chest Med* (2016) 37:219–29. doi:10.1016/j.ccm.2016.01.004
19. Royston P, Altman DG, Sauerbrei W. Dichotomizing continuous predictors in multiple regression: a bad idea. *Stat Med* (2006) 25:127–41. doi:10.1002/sim.2331
20. Naggara O, Raymond J, Guilbert F, Roy D, Weill A, Altman DG. Analysis by categorizing or dichotomizing continuous variables is inadvisable: an example from the natural history of unruptured aneurysms. *Am J Neuroradiol* (2011) 32:437–40. doi:10.3174/ajnr.A2425
21. Cerner Corporation. *Leverage Detailed Healthcare Data: Health Facts. 2010.* Kansas City, MO: Cerner Corporation (2010).
22. Stasinopoulos M, Rigby B, Voudouris V, Heller G, De Bastiani F. *Flexible Regression and Smoothing: The GAMLSS Packages in R. GAMLSS for Statistical Modelling.* GAMLSS for Statistical Modeling (2015).
23. Stasinopoulos M, Rigby RA. Generalized additive models for location scale and shape (GAMLSS) in R. *J Stat Softw* (2007) 23:1–46. doi:10.18637/jss.v023.i07
24. Rigby B, Stasinopoulos M, Heller G, Voudouris V. *The Distribution Toolbox of GAMLSS.* GAMLSS for Statistical Modelling (2014).
25. Rigby RA, Stasinopoulos DM. Smooth centile curves for skew and kurtotic data modelled using the Box-Cox power exponential distribution. *Stat Med* (2004) 23:3053–76. doi:10.1002/sim.1861
26. Ferrari SLP, Fumes G. *Box-Cox Symmetrical Distributions and Applications to Nutritional Data.* (2016). Available from: https://arxiv.org/abs/1604.02221. Accessed October 11, 2016.
27. Rigby RA, Stasinopoulos DM. Automatic smoothing parameter selection in GAMLSS with an application to centile estimation. *Stat Methods Med Res* (2014) 23:318–32. doi:10.1177/0962280212473302
28. Aickin M, Gensler H. Adjusting for multiple testing when reporting research results: the Bonferroni vs Holm methods. *Am J Public Health* (1996) 86:726–8. doi:10.2105/AJPH.86.5.726
29. Anonymous. *Pediatric Emergency Assessment, Recognition and Stabilization.* Dallas, TX: First American Heart Association Printing (2012).
30. Agency for Healthcare Research and Quality. *Healthcare Cost and Utilization Project (HCUP). Clinical Classifications Software (CCS) for ICD-9-CM.* Rockville, MD: Agency for Healthcare Research and Quality (2016).
31. Balamuth F, Alpern ER, Abbadessa MK, Hayes K, Schast A, Lavelle J, et al. Improving recognition of pediatric severe sepsis in the emergency department: contributions of a vital sign-based electronic alert and bedside clinician identification. *Ann Emerg Med* (2017) 70:759–68. doi:10.1016/j.annemergmed.2017.03.019
32. American Academy of Pediatrics (AAP), American College of Emergency Physicians (ACEP). *APLS: The Pediatric Emergency Medicine Resource/Edition 5.* Burlington, MA: Jones & Bartlett Learning (2012).
33. Daymont C, Bonafide CP, Brady PW. Heart rates in hospitalized children by age and body temperature. *Pediatrics* (2015) 135:e1173–81. doi:10.1542/peds.2014-3738
34. Spruijt B, Vergouwe Y, Nijman RG, Thompson M, Oostenbrink R. Vital signs should be maintained as continuous variables when predicting bacterial infections in febrile children. *J Clin Epidemiol* (2013) 66:453–7. doi:10.1016/j.jclinepi.2012.09.014
35. Thompson M, Harnden A, Perera R, Mayon-White R, Smith L, McLeod D, et al. Deriving temperature and age appropriate heart rate centiles for children with acute infections. *Arch Dis Child* (2009) 94:361–5. doi:10.1136/adc.2008.145011
36. Davies P, Maconochie I. The relationship between body temperature, heart rate and respiratory rate in children. *Emerg Med J* (2009) 26:641–3. doi:10.1136/emj.2008.061598
37. Niven DJ, Laupland KB, Stelfox HT. Accuracy of peripheral thermometers for estimating temperature. *Ann Intern Med* (2016) 165:73–4. doi:10.7326/L16-0069
38. Haque IU, Zaritsky AL. Analysis of the evidence for the lower limit of systolic and mean arterial pressure in children. *Pediatr Crit Care Med* (2007) 8:138–44. doi:10.1097/01.PCC.0000257039.32593.DC

14

Autonomic Nervous System Dysfunction in Pediatric Sepsis

Colleen M. Badke[1,2], *Lauren E. Marsillio*[1,2], *Debra E. Weese-Mayer*[2,3,4] *and L. Nelson Sanchez-Pinto*[1,2,4*]

[1] Division of Critical Care Medicine, Ann & Robert H. Lurie Children's Hospital of Chicago, Chicago, IL, United States, [2] Department of Pediatrics, Northwestern University Feinberg School of Medicine, Chicago, IL, United States, [3] Center for Autonomic Medicine in Pediatrics, Ann & Robert H. Lurie Children's Hospital of Chicago, Chicago, IL, United States, [4] Stanley Manne Children's Research Institute, Chicago, IL, United States

Correspondence:
L. Nelson Sanchez-Pinto
lsanchezpinto@luriechildrens.org

The autonomic nervous system (ANS) plays a major role in maintaining homeostasis through key adaptive responses to stress, including severe infections and sepsis. The ANS-mediated processes most relevant during sepsis include regulation of cardiac output and vascular tone, control of breathing and airway resistance, inflammation and immune modulation, gastrointestinal motility and digestion, and regulation of body temperature. ANS dysfunction (ANSD) represents an imbalanced or maladaptive response to injury and is prevalent in pediatric sepsis. Most of the evidence on ANSD comes from studies of heart rate variability, which is a marker of ANS function and is inversely correlated with organ dysfunction and mortality. In addition, there is evidence that other measures of ANSD, such as respiratory rate variability, skin thermoregulation, and baroreflex and chemoreflex sensitivity, are associated with outcomes in critical illness. The relevance of understanding ANSD in the context of pediatric sepsis stems from the fact that it might play an important role in the pathophysiology of sepsis, is associated with outcomes, and can be measured continuously and noninvasively. Here we review the physiology and dysfunction of the ANS during critical illness, discuss methods for measuring ANS function in the intensive care unit, and review the diagnostic, prognostic, and therapeutic value of understanding ANSD in pediatric sepsis.

Keywords: autonomic nervous system, pediatrics, sepsis, organ dysfunction, critical care, heart rate variability, inflammation

INTRODUCTION

The autonomic nervous system (ANS) is a unique system as it regulates functions in nearly all organ systems (1). Along with immune and neuroendocrine responses, the ANS plays a major role in maintaining homeostasis when confronted with internal and external stressors, including severe infections (**Figure 1**) (2–4). The homeostatic processes in which the ANS has a primary role is extensive, but some of the most relevant during sepsis include regulation of cardiac output, vascular tone, control of breathing, airway resistance, regulation of the inflammatory response, adaptive immune modulation, gastrointestinal motility, and thermoregulation (1, 5–8).

In response to severe infections and other injuries, the central nervous system (CNS) activates the sympathetic branch of the ANS in order to make the necessary physiological and metabolic adjustments to overcome the acute physiologic stress (4). ANS dysfunction (ANSD) represents an imbalanced or maladaptive response to stress, and is often due to excessive, uncontrolled, or prolonged sympathetic activation, or inappropriate regulation by the other branch of the ANS, the parasympathetic nervous system (3). Most of the evidence on ANSD in critical care stems from research on heart rate variability (HRV), which is a marker of ANS function that is inversely correlated with organ dysfunction and mortality in both adult and pediatric patients (9–13). However, there is evidence that other markers of ANSD such as respiratory rate variability, skin thermoregulation, and baroreflex and chemoreflex sensitivity are also associated with outcomes in critically ill adults (14–16).

There are several reasons why understanding ANSD in the context of sepsis is crucial to the care of the critically ill septic child. First, sepsis is defined as a "life-threatening organ dysfunction caused by a dysregulated host response to infection" (17). Although "host response" is often equated to "immune response" in the literature, there is evidence that a dysregulated ANS response to infection is common in patients with sepsis and an early marker of organ dysfunction (18). If indeed ANSD is a central component of sepsis pathophysiology, this could have major implications in the development of new diagnostic and therapeutic strategies for sepsis. In addition, several surrogates of ANSD, including HRV and respiratory rate variability (RRV), are associated with organ dysfunction, treatment response, and outcomes in neonates, children, and adults and can be measured continuously and noninvasively (19–23). Furthermore, changes in some of these surrogates of ANSD can be detected up to 18 h before the onset of shock, which can make them effective early predictors of clinical deterioration (24).

In this paper we will review the physiology and dysfunction of the ANS during critical illness, discuss methods for measuring ANS function in the pediatric intensive care unit, and review the diagnostic and prognostic value of ANSD in pediatric sepsis.

AUTONOMIC NERVOUS SYSTEM PHYSIOLOGY AND DYSFUNCTION IN SEPSIS AND CRITICAL ILLNESS

Overview

The ANS is responsible for regulating all innervated organs (except the skeletal muscles), a remarkable task often overlooked by clinicians (1, 25, 26). It has direct effects on cardiovascular function, immunity, gastrointestinal function, thermoregulation, and other key adaptive mechanisms to stress (1, 5–8) The autonomic efferent fibers are functionally and anatomically divided into the sympathetic and parasympathetic nervous systems. Both systems can work antagonistically (e.g., in the heart, airways, and gastrointestinal tract), independently (e.g., sympathetic-mediated vascular tone), or synergistically (e.g., visual accommodation) (26). Most of the efferent response is achieved through smooth muscle constriction and relaxation, glandular secretion, cardiac muscle constriction, and cardiac cell conductivity regulation (1).

The *sympathetic nervous system* (SNS) is often characterized as the system in charge of the "fight or flight" response; however, it also carries important roles in day-to-day, non-danger situations (1, 27). Post-ganglionic sympathetic nerves travel across most of the body and secrete norepinephrine to activate the adrenergic receptors in their target organs and tissues, except in the kidney, where they secrete dopamine (**Table 1**). Chromaffin cells in the adrenal medulla also secrete catecholamines (about ~80% epinephrine and ~20% norepinephrine) into the circulation, which then travel throughout the body to activate adrenergic receptors. Additionally, the chromaffin cells secrete enkephalins which bind to opioid receptors to produce an analgesic effect (1).

The *parasympathetic nervous system* (PNS) is often referred to as the "rest and digest" system, and is in charge of energy conservation, digestion, and waste removal. The vagus nerve, which innervates most organs and tissues between the larynx and the small intestine, controls the vast majority of parasympathetic functions in the body (1, 25). Post-ganglionic parasympathetic nerves secrete acetylcholine to activate the muscarinic receptors in their target organs and tissues (**Table 1**), except in the immune system where they primarily activate nicotinic receptors (1, 5).

Cardiovascular and Respiratory Regulation

Most cardiovascular effects are mediated by the SNS, and their effects can be readily appreciated in the extremes of sympathetic dysfunction (loss of function and over-activity). Loss of function is best exemplified by spinal cord injuries, where the lack of sympathetic tone leads to orthostatic hypotension, low resting blood pressure, loss of circadian blood pressure fluctuation, and bradycardia (28). Sympathetic over-activity, seen in states of stress including critical illness, can lead to tachyarrhythmias, vasoplegia due to downregulation of adrenergic receptors, cardiac ischemia, and heart failure (3, 27, 29).

In homeostasis, heart function is tightly controlled by sympathetic activation of the ß-adrenergic receptors and parasympathetic activation of the muscarinic M_2 receptors. Sympathetic input increases SA node-mediated heart rate (chronotropy), AV node and ventricular conductivity (dromotropy), and atrial and ventricular contractility (inotropy). Parasympathetic input through the vagus nerve has a negative effect on all of these cardiac functions, except ventricular contraction, which is unaffected (1).

The baroreceptor reflex mediates the synergistic control of blood pressure by both efferent branches of the ANS. Increases in blood pressure lead to baroreceptor activation in the carotid sinuses and aortic arch, which leads to a decrease in sympathetic tone and increase in vagal tone that result in a drop in the heart rate and blood pressure. When the blood pressure is too low, a decrease in baroreceptor activity leads to the opposite effect: increased vasoconstriction, tachycardia, and cardiac contractility leading to a blood pressure increase (1, 30).

Cardio-respiratory homeostasis is primarily modulated through the chemoreceptor reflex, which is in part responsible for RRV (31). A decrease in arterial oxygen content, a rise in carbon dioxide, or a drop in pH sensed peripherally and centrally by chemoreceptors results in an increase in respiratory

Abbreviations: *PAMPs, DAMPs*, pathogen- and damage-associated molecular patterns; *TLRs*, toll-like receptors; *CRH*, corticotropin-releasing hormone; *ACTH*, adrenocorticotropic hormone; *incr.*, increased.

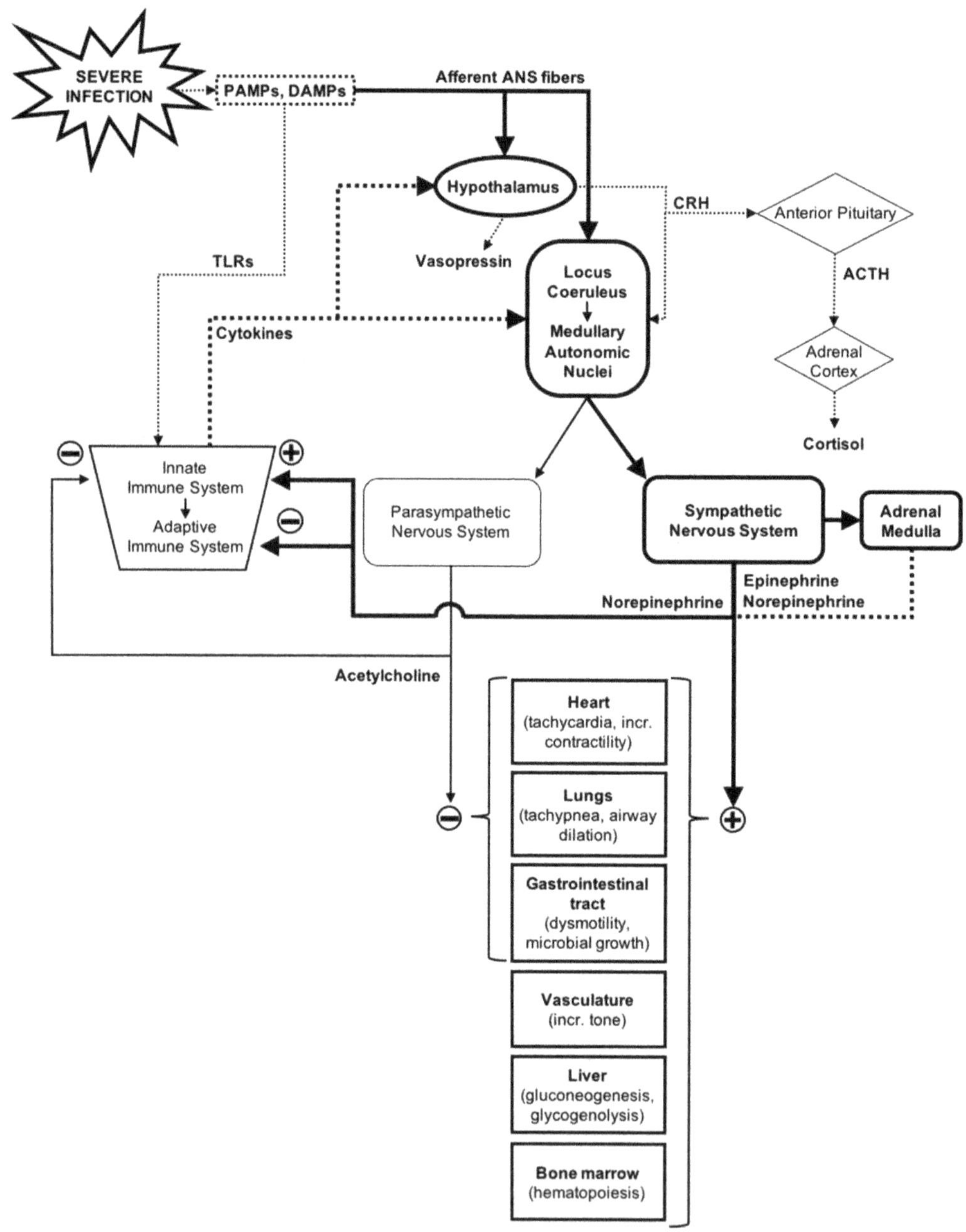

FIGURE 1 | Autonomic nervous system response to severe infections in the context of the immune and neuroendocrine response. Solid lines represent nerve pathways and dotted lines represent humoral/endocrine pathways (2–4).

rate, depth of breathing, and heart rate. Both baroreceptor and chemoreceptor sensitivity can be altered in critical illness-induced ANSD and this dysregulation is thought to be a risk factor for organ dysfunction (30).

Immune and Inflammatory Response

The influence of the ANS on the immune system is complex but extremely important, with effects on both the innate and the adaptive immune response (**Figure 1**) (7). Whereas humoral and cellular modulation may take hours or days to take effect, the response of the ANS can be instantaneous, inviting the hypothesis that the ANS may play a significant role in the early-phase immune response during sepsis (5).

The best-described ANS-immune system interaction occurs through the cholinergic anti-inflammatory pathway, which modulates the innate immune system response. Initially the CNS senses inflammation through both the humoral route (mediated by cytokines) and the neural route [mediated by the ANS afferent sensory fibers, which can sense damage- and pathogen-associated molecular patterns [DAMPs and PAMPs]] (2, 5). This leads to increased PNS output that results in acetylcholine release by the vagus nerve in the reticuloendothelial

TABLE 1 | Sympathetic Adrenergic and Parasympathetic Muscarinic Receptors: Response to Activation and Drug Effects.

Sympathetic adrenergic receptor	Response to activation	Drug effects
α_1	• Arterial and arteriolar vasoconstriction • Pupillary dilation • Decreased gastrointestinal motility and sphincter contraction • Hepatic glycogenolysis and gluconeogenesis • Pro-inflammatory cytokine production • Central nervous systems effects including anorexia	**Receptor Activation**: • Norepinephrine, epinephrine (α_1,α_2) • Phenylephrine, midodrine (α_1) • Clonidine, dexmedetomidine (α_2)
α_2	• Decreased norepinephrine release through autoreceptors (negative feedback) • Decreased acetylcholine release through parasympathetic heteroreceptors • Central nervous systems effects including sedation, analgesia, and down-regulation of sympathetic outflow (= hypotension, bradycardia) • Decreased gastrointestinal motility and gland secretion • Decreased insulin secretion • Coronary, renal, and skin vasoconstriction • Constriction of veins • Platelet aggregation • Monocyte-endothelial adhesion	**Receptor Blockade**: • Phentolamine, Phenoxybenzamine (α_1, α_2) • Doxazosin (α_1) **Norepinephrine Reuptake Inhibition**: • Cocaine, methylphenidate, amphetamines, tricyclic antidepressants.
β_1	• Increased heart rate, cardiac conductivity, and cardiac muscle contractility • Renin release from the kidney	**Receptor Activation**: • Norepinephrine, epinephrine (β_1, β_2) • Isoproterenol (β_1, β_2) • Dobutamine (β_1) • Albuterol, terbutaline (β_2)
β_2	• Bronchodilation • Decreased bronchial gland secretion • Potent coronary vasodilatation (exceeds α_2 constriction effect) • Increased heart rate, cardiac conductivity, and cardiac muscle contractility • Bladder relaxation • Skeletal muscle, pulmonary, and visceral vasodilation • Immune modulation in lymphoid tissue	**Receptor Blockade**: • Propranolol (β_1, β_2) • Atenolol, esmolol, metoprolol, nadolol, timolol ($\beta_1 > \beta_2$)
β_3	• Lypolysis and thermogenesis in adipose tissue	**Norepinephrine Reuptake Inhibition**: • Cocaine, methylphenidate, amphetamines, tricyclic antidepressants.
Parasympathetic muscarinic receptor	**Response to activation**	**Drug effects**
M_1	• Gastric acid secretion • Pancreatic amylase secretion • Cerebral vasoconstrictio	**Receptor activation**: • Acetylcholine (M_1-M_4) • Methacholine (M_1-M_4)
M_2, M_3	• Decreased heart rate, decreased cardiac conductivity • Pupillary and ciliary constriction • Lacrimal, salivary, nasopharyngeal, bronchial, and digestive gland secretion • Bronchial constriction • Increased gastrointestinal motility • Sphincter relaxation	**Receptor Blockade**: • Atropine, ipratropium, scopolamine (M_1-M_4) • Oxybutynin (M_3)
M_2, M_4	• Decreased acetylcholine release through autoreceptors (negative feedback) • Decreased norepinephrine release through sympathetic heteroreceptors	**Inhibition of Acetylcholinesterase**: • *Reversible*: Edrophonium, neostigmine, physostigmine, pyridostigmine • *Irreversible*: Organophosphates

α_1 and β_3 are activated by norepinephrine > epinephrine; α_2 and β_1 are activated by norepinephrine = epinephrine; β_2 are activated by epinephrine >> norepinephrine. Muscarinic receptors in the target organs (and the nicotinic receptors in the post-ganglionic neurons) are activated by acetylcholine (1).

system (spleen, liver, thymus, etc.). Acetylcholine activates the nicotinic receptors of tissue macrophages, which leads to a decrease in secretion of pro-inflammatory cytokines like IL-6 and TNF-α (5, 7). The importance of the vagus nerve integrity in this pathway has been established in experimental murine models, which have shown that direct electrical stimulation of the vagus nerve results in decreased TNF-α secretion, whereas vagotomy results in the opposite effect (5). Increased PNS activity, measured using HRV, has been associated with reduced pro-inflammatory cytokine levels, suggesting that the cholinergic anti-inflammatory pathway could be monitored non-invasively using HRV (32).

The SNS has effects on both the adaptive and the innate immune systems. Epinephrine and norepinephrine activation of α_1-adrenergic receptors in reticuloendothelial macrophages can lead to pro-inflammatory cytokine release, although in prolonged septic states, epinephrine down-regulates IL-6 and TNF-α production (33). In parallel, norepinephrine activation of ß$_2$-adrenergic receptors in helper T cells in the lymphatic tissue can lead to an immunosuppressive Th2 polarization, particularly in the setting of sepsis (7, 33).

Neuroendocrine Response

Neuroendocrine physiology is closely linked to autonomic regulation (**Figure 1**) (1). In response to perturbation, like inflammation and tissue damage in sepsis, the CNS activates both ANS and neuroendocrine pathways (i.e., the hypothalamic-pituitary-adrenal [HPA] axis, the hypothalamic-pituitary-thyroid axis, and the hypothalamic-neurohypophyseal axis) (4). Sensing can occur through cytokine-mediated central activation, or through ANS sensory fiber input, which can sense pathogens and tissue damage via receptors for DAMPs and PAMPs (2). In the case of hypothalamic-neurohypophyseal axis, the ANS baro- and chemoreceptors can also stimulate the release of vasopressin (4, 29).

Activation of the HPA axis results in cortisol release from the adrenal cortex, while activation of the SNS leads to a release of catecholamines from the adrenal medulla. The net effect of these pathways leads to increased glucose production and availability, which is an adaptive response to stress designed to enhance energy availability to vital organs (2). Cortisol can also enhance the response to catecholamines and has anti-inflammatory effects that can ultimately modulate ANS activation (34). Adrenal insufficiency, characterized by low cortisol levels, often develops in sepsis and is associated with poor outcomes (2). Observational studies have shown that adrenal insufficiency is associated with reduced HRV, and that response to hydrocortisone therapy is associated with recovery of normal HRV, further illustrating the close interactions between the ANS and the neuroendocrine response (23).

Gastrointestinal Function

The enteric nervous system branch of the ANS plays a key role in the modulation of gastrointestinal motility and digestion (6). The vagus nerve and the sacral parasympathetic nerves promote motility, sphincter relaxation, and digestive gland secretion (including salivary, gastric, pancreatic glands). On the other hand, sympathetic stimulation of α-adrenergic receptors decrease gastrointestinal motility and sphincter constriction (1). During critical illness, parasympathetic suppression or excessive sympathetic activity can lead to functional ileus, digestive dysfunction, and feeding intolerance (6).

The ANS appears to also have a direct effect on the gut microbiome. For example, microbes are capable of responding to neuroendocrine hormones. Specifically, catecholamines may induce microbial change to more pathogenic phenotypes, and these microbes may have exponential growth in response to host stress within hours of sensing higher catecholamine levels (35, 36). In addition, the afferent sensory fibers of the vagus nerve are activated by microbes in the gut and appear to distinguish between pathogenic and non-pathogenic organisms. Further research is needed to determine the role of this sensing in the cholinergic anti-inflammatory pathway activity and the immunomodulatory effects of gut bacteria (37).

Thermoregulation

Core body temperature is tightly regulated by the CNS via behavioral and autonomic responses. The behavioral responses (e.g., putting on or removing clothing) are by far the most powerful strategies, but many critically ill patients lack the ability to implement behavioral responses and thus depend heavily on autonomic defenses such as sweating and pre-capillary vasodilation in response to heat, and arteriovenous (AV) shunt constriction and shivering in response to cold (8). The AV shunts are short connections between arterioles and veins that primarily exist in the distal extremities, and can carry about 10,000 times more flow than capillaries of the same length (8, 38). As such, these AV shunts, which are heavily innervated by sympathetic fibers, can significantly change the peripheral blood flow resistance. When open, lower resistance allows for significant flow to the extremities so that heat dissipates; closed they increase the resistance and reduce flow to the extremities, keeping the body-generated heat in the core (8, 38). Despite their limited distribution in the body, AV shunts have a profound effect on core temperature, and are the most commonly activated thermoregulatory defense in cool environments.

When hyperthermic, skin vasodilation can have significant impact on hemodynamics given that skin blood flow can increase up to the equivalent of 60% of the cardiac output (38). In homeostasis, autonomic responses work in concert, and sympathetic input to the heart will often match the cardiac output demands, but this may not be the case in some critical care situations.

MEASURES OF AUTONOMIC NERVOUS SYSTEM FUNCTION IN THE INTENSIVE CARE UNIT

General Considerations

Potential confounders that could affect the measurement of ANS function in the pediatric intensive care unit include age, mechanical ventilation, neuromuscular blockade, the administration of catecholamines and sedatives, and pre-existing autonomic dysregulation. Some studies in critically ill adults suggest that mechanical ventilation and catecholamines do not affect HRV or baroreflex and chemoreflex sensitivity (13, 39). Sedation, on the other hand, appears to affect HRV and RRV mostly in patients with low organ dysfunction burden, but it does not appear to significantly affect HRV in more critically ill patients (13, 40, 41).

Heart Rate Variability

Cardiovascular homeostasis requires continuously varying levels of sympathetic and parasympathetic inputs to the heart, resulting in a continuously changing heart rate, even during normal resting conditions (12). HRV is defined as the fluctuation in time between consecutive heart beats that is present in normal physiologic conditions (42). ANSD may result in an imbalance between sympathetic and parasympathetic inputs, usually resulting in a reduced HRV (12).

There are several examples of successful evaluations of real-time analysis of HRV in the intensive care unit (19, 22, 43–45). Nemati et al. recently described a real-time sepsis prediction tool for critically ill adult patients, which included, amongst multiple measures, heart rate entropy, a measure of HRV. This observational study showed that electronic health record data can predict sepsis 4 to 12 h earlier than SOFA scores or clinical suspicion of sepsis, with a areas under the receiver operating characteristic curve of 0.83–0.85 (44). Moorman et al. evaluated a real-time heart rate characteristic scoring tool for sepsis prediction in premature neonates, which was associated with a significantly decreased risk of mortality in a multi-center study, with a number needed to monitor of 48 neonates to prevent one death (19). These studies demonstrate the feasibility of incorporation of HRV evaluation into routine clinical care with the potential benefit of identifying disease trajectory and response to therapy in patients with sepsis.

Respiratory Rate Variability

Similar to HRV, the ANS regulates variability in the respiratory rate with input from chemoreceptors and baroreceptors (46). Dysregulated RRV can be seen in many disease states. For example, altered RRV has been associated with extubation failure in adults (15, 16, 47). In addition, one study showed that lower RRV was associated with increased mortality in mechanically-ventilated patients, even when controlling for neuromuscular blockade (14). While there is some confounding of RRV by sedatives, measurement of this variability has been found to be reliable in adult ICUs (21, 40). Research studies are lacking in pediatrics and in the sepsis population, however, given the importance of autonomic control over breathing, it is likely that dysregulated RRV is common in sepsis.

Baroreflex Sensitivity

The baroreflex sensitivity measures the ability of the ANS to modulate the vagal and sympathetic tone with changes in blood pressure (30). Invasive methods like the phenylephrine bolus technique to evaluate lengthening of the heart beat interval after increasing the systolic blood pressure has been used in the clinical setting, but other non-invasive measures of baroreflex sensitivity, based on the effects of unprovoked fluctuations of blood pressures on heart rate, also exist (12). Decreased baroreflex sensitivity has been documented in critically ill adults with organ dysfunction and in animal models of sepsis (13, 48).

Chemoreflex Sensitivity

Stimulation of the peripheral and central chemoreceptors by decreases in arterial oxygen levels and/or pH or increases in arterial carbon dioxide produce an increase in respiratory rate and sympathetic tone. In the ICU, chemoreflex sensitivity can be calculated as the regression slope of arterial oxygen tension to heart rate interval duration (12). Decreased sensitivity has been associated with organ dysfunction in critically ill patients, including in those with sepsis (13).

AUTONOMIC NERVOUS SYSTEM DYSFUNCTION IN PEDIATRIC SEPSIS: CURRENT STATE AND FUTURE DIRECTIONS

As a key component of the host response to infection, dysregulation of the ANS response is likely an important contributing factor to organ dysfunction in patients with sepsis (18). ANSD, typically measured using HRV, is prevalent in pediatric sepsis and correlates with disease severity and trajectory (10, 49). Recognition of ANSD may lead to earlier diagnosis of sepsis, which could have therapeutic and prognostic implications for patients, including earlier initiation of therapies, shorter duration of organ dysfunction, and decreased mortality (44). For example, using bedside HRV monitoring as a predictive tool of sepsis in premature neonates has been associated with decreased risk of mortality (19, 50–52). The limited use of non-invasive monitoring of ANS function in the ICU is in part due to technological complexities, particularly in children, although the digitalization of the healthcare system is facilitating the implementation of the systems and algorithms necessary to do so (53, 54). In addition, HRV varies with patient factors such as age, gender, medications, and mechanical ventilation, which creates challenges for its use and interpretation at the bedside. Further research is necessary to determine the individual and additive effect of these factors on HRV and its usefulness as a predictor. In addition, novel measures of ANS function, such as continuous temperature monitoring, automated pupillometry, and non-invasive baroreflex and chemoreflex sensitivity have shown promise in the monitoring of ANSD in other populations and could potentially have application as effective biomarkers in pediatric sepsis, but further study is necessary. (12, 55–57).

Advanced understanding of ANSD pathophysiology in pediatric sepsis could also help identify potential therapeutic targets. Sympathetic over-activity, which is common in sepsis and other critical illnesses, can lead to tachyarrhythmias, diastolic dysfunction, inflammation, immune suppression, platelet aggregation, and gastrointestinal dysmotility (3, 5, 6, 27, 33). Additionally, excessive sympathetic outflow has been postulated to cause catecholamine-resistant vasoplegia via α-adrenergic receptor desensitization (29). Similarly, suppressed vagal tone has been associated with chronic inflammation and functional ileus, which can also hinder recovery from sepsis (5, 6). Whether modulating sympathetic and parasympathetic activity could lead to improved outcomes in pediatric sepsis remains to be studied. However, some human and animal studies show promise. For example, sympathetic suppression with α_2 agonists like dexmedetomidine and β_1-blockade with esmolol has been associated with improvement in vasoplegia in shock states (29). Statins can reduce sympathetic outflow and preserve parasympathetic tone, and have been associated with reduced inflammation and lower likelihood of developing sepsis in adult patients (12, 58). And vagal nerve stimulation has been associated with reduced inflammation and improved gut and lung epithelial integrity in animal and human studies, although its role in sepsis has not been explored (5, 7, 59).

CONCLUSION

The ANS plays a major role in maintaining homeostasis in response to infections and other types of stress. ANSD represents an imbalanced or maladaptive response and is prevalent in pediatric sepsis. Better understanding of ANSD in pediatric sepsis could have significant diagnostic, prognostic, and therapeutic implications.

AUTHOR CONTRIBUTIONS

LS-P and CB designed the review. All four authors made substantial contributions to drafting and final approval of the manuscript.

REFERENCES

1. Wehrwein EA, Orer HS, Barman SM. Overview of the anatomy, physiology, and pharmacology of the autonomic nervous system. *Compr Physiol.* (2016). 6:1239–78. doi: 10.1002/cphy.c150037
2. Annane D, Pastores SM, Arlt W, Balk RA, Beishuizen A, Briegel J, et al. Critical illness-related corticosteroid insufficiency (CIRCI): a narrative review from a Multispecialty Task Force of the Society of Critical Care Medicine (SCCM) and the European Society of Intensive Care Medicine (ESICM). *Intensive Care Med.* (2017) 43:1781–92. doi: 10.1007/s00134-017-4914-x
3. Dünser MW, Hasibeder WR. Sympathetic overstimulation during critical illness: adverse effects of adrenergic stress. *J Intensive Care Med.* (2009) 24:293–316. doi: 10.1177/0885066609340519
4. Sharshar T, Hopkinson NS, Orlikowski D, Annane D. Science review: the brain in sepsis–culprit and victim. *Crit Care.* (2005) 9:37–44. doi: 10.1186/cc2951
5. Czura C, Tracey K. Autonomic neural regulation of immunity. *J Int Med.* (2005) 257:156–66. doi: 10.1111/j.1365-2796.2004.01442.x
6. Fruhwald S, Holzer P, Metzler H. Gastrointestinal motility in acute illness. *Wien Klin Wochenschr.* (2008) 120:6–17. doi: 10.1007/s00508-007-0920-2
7. Marvar PJ, Harrison DG. Inflammation, immunity and the autonomic nervous system. *Primer Auton. Nerv. Syst.* 2012:325–9. doi: 10.1016/B978-0-12-386525-0.00067-6
8. Sessler DI. Thermoregulatory defense mechanisms. *Crit Care Med.* (2009) 37(7 Suppl.):S203–10. doi: 10.1097/CCM.0b013e3181aa5568
9. Papaioannou VE, Maglaveras N, Houvarda I, Antoniadou E, Vretzakis G. Investigation of altered heart rate variability, nonlinear properties of heart rate signals, and organ dysfunction longitudinally over time in intensive care unit patients. *J Crit Care* (2006) 21:95–103. discussion: 4. doi: 10.1016/j.jcrc.2005.12.007
10. Ellenby MS, McNames J, Lai S, McDonald BA, Krieger D, Sclabassi RJ, et al. Uncoupling and recoupling of autonomic regulation of the heart beat in pediatric septic shock. *Shock* (2001) 16:274–7. doi: 10.1097/00024382-200116040-00007
11. Goldstein B, Fiser DH, Kelly MM, Mickelsen D, Ruttimann U, Pollack MM. Decomplexification in critical illness and injury: relationship between heart rate variability, severity of illness, and outcome. *Crit Care Med.* (1998) 26:352–7. doi: 10.1097/00003246-199802000-00040
12. Schmidt H, Hoyer D, Wilhelm J, Soffker G, Heinroth K, Hottenrott K, et al. The alteration of autonomic function in multiple organ dysfunction syndrome. *Crit Care Clin.* (2008) 24:149–63. doi: 10.1016/j.ccc.2007.10.003
13. Schmidt H, Muller-Werdan U, Hoffmann T, Francis DP, Piepoli MF, Rauchhaus M, et al. Autonomic dysfunction predicts mortality in patients with multiple organ dysfunction syndrome of different age groups. *Crit Care Med.* (2005) 33:1994–2002. doi: 10.1097/01.CCM.0000178181.91250.99
14. Gutierrez G, Das A, Ballarino G, Beyzaei-Arani A, Turkan H, Wulf-Gutierrez M, et al. Decreased respiratory rate variability during mechanical ventilation is associated with increased mortality. *Intensive Care Med.* (2013) 39:1359–67. doi: 10.1007/s00134-013-2937-5
15. Seely AJ, Bravi A, Herry C, Green G, Longtin A, Ramsay T, et al. Do heart and respiratory rate variability improve prediction of extubation outcomes in critically ill patients? *Crit Care.* (2014) 18:R65. doi: 10.1186/cc13822
16. Bien MY, Hseu SS, Yien HW, Kuo BI, Lin YT, Wang JH, et al. Breathing pattern variability: a weaning predictor in postoperative patients recovering from systemic inflammatory response syndrome. *Intensive Care Med.* (2004) 30:241–7. doi: 10.1007/s00134-003-2073-8
17. Singer M, Deutschman CS, Seymour CW, Shankar-Hari M, Annane D, Bauer M, et al. The third international consensus definitions for sepsis and septic shock (Sepsis-3). *J Am Med Assoc.* (2016) 315:801–10. doi: 10.1001/jama.2016.0287
18. Pontet J, Contreras P, Curbelo A, Medina J, Noveri S, Bentancourt S, et al. Heart rate variability as early marker of multiple organ dysfunction syndrome in septic patients. *J Crit Care.* (2003) 18:156–63. doi: 10.1016/j.jcrc.2003.08.005
19. Moorman JR, Carlo WA, Kattwinkel J, Schelonka RL, Porcelli PJ, Navarrete CT, et al. Mortality reduction by heart rate characteristic monitoring in very low birth weight neonates: a randomized trial. *J Pediatr.* (2011) 159:900-6 e1. doi: 10.1016/j.jpeds.2011.06.044
20. Mayampurath A, Volchenboum S, Sanchez-Pinto L. Using photoplethysmography data to estimate heart rate variability and its association with organ dysfunction in pediatric oncology patients. *npj Digit Med.* (2018) 1:29. doi: 10.1038/s41746-018-0038-0
21. Bradley B, Green GC, Batkin I, Seely AJ. Feasibility of continuous multiorgan variability analysis in the intensive care unit. *J Crit Care.* (2012) 27:218.e9–20. doi: 10.1016/j.jcrc.2011.09.009
22. Kasaoka S, Nakahara T, Kawamura Y, Tsuruta R, Maekawa T. Real-time monitoring of heart rate variability in critically ill patients. *J Crit Care* (2010) 25:313–6. doi: 10.1016/j.jcrc.2009.06.047
23. Morris JA, Jr., Norris PR, Waitman LR, Ozdas A, Guillamondegui OD, Jenkins JM. Adrenal insufficiency, heart rate variability, and complex biologic systems: a study of 1,871 critically ill trauma patients. *J Am Coll Surg.* (2007) 204:885–92. Discussion: 92–3. doi: 10.1016/j.jamcollsurg.2007.01.019
24. Green GC, Bradley B, Bravi A, Seely AJ. Continuous multiorgan variability analysis to track severity of organ failure in critically ill patients. *J Crit Care* (2013) 28:879 e1-11. doi: 10.1016/j.jcrc.2013.04.001
25. Mathias CJ, Iodice V, Low D. Autonomic dysfunction: recognition, diagnosis, investigation, management, and autonomic neurorehabilitation. *Handb Clin Neurol.* (2013) 110:239–53. doi: 10.1016/B978-0-444-52901-5.00020-4
26. Rees CA. Lost among the trees? The autonomic nervous system and paediatrics. *Arch Dis Child.* (2014) 99:552–62. doi: 10.1136/archdischild-2012-301863
27. Malpas SC. Sympathetic nervous system overactivity and its role in the development of cardiovascular disease. *Physiol Rev.* (2010) 90:513–57. doi: 10.1152/physrev.00007.2009
28. Teasell RW, Arnold JM, Krassioukov A, Delaney GA. Cardiovascular consequences of loss of supraspinal control of the sympathetic nervous system after spinal cord injury. *Arch Phys Med Rehabil.* (2000) 81:506–16. doi: 10.1053/mr.2000.3848
29. Levy B, Fritz C, Tahon E, Jacquot A, Auchet T, Kimmoun A. Vasoplegia treatments: the past, the present, and the future. *Crit Care* (2018) 22:52. doi: 10.1186/s13054-018-1967-3
30. Schmidt HB, Werdan K, Müller-Werdan U. Autonomic dysfunction in the ICU patient. *Curr Opin Crit Care.* (2001) 7:314–22. doi: 10.1097/00075198-200110000-00002

31. Prabhakar NR. Oxygen Sensing. *Primer Auton. Nerv. Syst.* 2012:331–3. doi: 10.1016/b978-0-12-386525-0.00068-8
32. Cooper TM, McKinley PS, Seeman TE, Choo TH, Lee S, Sloan RP. Heart rate variability predicts levels of inflammatory markers: evidence for the vagal anti-inflammatory pathway. *Brain Behav Immun.* (2015) 49:94–100. doi: 10.1016/j.bbi.2014.12.017
33. Hartmann C, Radermacher P, Wepler M, Nussbaum B. Non-hemodynamic effects of catecholamines. *Shock* (2017) 48:390–400. doi: 10.1097/SHK.0000000000000879
34. Boonen E, Van den Berghe G. Endocrine responses to critical illness: novel insights and therapeutic implications. *J Clin Endocrinol Metab.* (2014) 99:1569–82. doi: 10.1210/jc.2013-4115
35. Lyte M. The effect of stress on microbial growth. *Anim Health Res. Rev.* (2014) 15:172–4. doi: 10.1017/S146625231400019X
36. Belay T, Sonnenfeld G. Differential effects of catecholamines on *in vitro* growth of pathogenic bacteria. *Life Sci.* (2002) 71:447–56. doi: 10.1016/S0024-3205(02)01683-1
37. Forsythe P, Bienenstock J, Kunze WA. Vagal pathways for microbiome-brain-gut axis communication. *Adv Exp Med Biol.* (2014) 817:115–33. doi: 10.1007/978-1-4939-0897-4_5
38. Charkoudian N. Skin blood flow in adult human thermoregulation: how it works, when it does not, and why. *Mayo Clin Proc.* (2003). 78:603–12. doi: 10.4065/78.5.603
39. Korach M, Sharshar T, Jarrin I, Fouillot J-P, Raphaël J-C, Gajdos P, et al. Cardiac variability in critically ill adults: influence of sepsis. *Crit. Care Med.* (2001) 29:1380–5. doi: 10.1097/00003246-200107000-00013
40. Bradley BD, Green G, Ramsay T, Seely AJ. Impact of sedation and organ failure on continuous heart and respiratory rate variability monitoring in critically ill patients: a pilot study. *Crit Care Med.* (2013) 41:433–44. doi: 10.1097/CCM.0b013e31826a47de
41. Nagaraj SB, McClain LM, Zhou DW, Biswal S, Rosenthal ES, Purdon PL, et al. Automatic classification of sedation levels in ICU patients using heart rate variability. *Crit Care Med.* (2016) 44:e782–9. doi: 10.1097/CCM.0000000000001708
42. Heart rate variability: standards of measurement, physiological interpretation and clinical use. Task force of the european society of cardiology and the North American Society of pacing and electrophysiology. *Circulation.* (1996) 93:1043–65.
43. Ahmad S, Ramsay T, Huebsch L, Flanagan S, McDiarmid S, Batkin I, et al. Continuous multi-parameter heart rate variability analysis heralds onset of sepsis in adults. *PLoS One.* (2009) 4:e6642. doi: 10.1371/journal.pone.0006642
44. Nemati S, Holder A, Razmi F, Stanley MD, Clifford GD, Buchman TG. An interpretable machine learning model for accurate prediction of sepsis in the ICU. *Crit Care Med.* (2018) 46:547–53. doi: 10.1097/CCM.0000000000002936
45. Yokota Y, Kawamura Y, Matsumaru N, Shirai K. Septic Shock Prediction by Real Time Monitoring of Heart Rate Variability. In: Jobbágy Á, editor. *5th European Conference of the International Federation for Medical and Biological Engineering. IFMBE Proceedings. 37*: Springer Berlin Heidelberg (2012). p. 195–8.
46. Cutsforth-Gregory JK, Benarroch EE. Nucleus of the solitary tract, medullary reflexes, and clinical implications. *Neurology.* (2017) 88:1187–96. doi: 10.1212/WNL.0000000000003751
47. Bien MY, Shui Lin Y, Shih CH, Yang YL, Lin HW, Bai KJ, et al. Comparisons of predictive performance of breathing pattern variability measured during T-piece, automatic tube compensation, and pressure support ventilation for weaning intensive care unit patients from mechanical ventilation. *Crit Care Med.* (2011) 39:2253–62. doi: 10.1097/CCM.0b013e31822279ed
48. Pancoto JA, Correa PB, Oliveira-Pelegrin GR, Rocha MJ. Autonomic dysfunction in experimental sepsis induced by cecal ligation and puncture. *Auton Neurosci.* (2008) 138:57–63. doi: 10.1016/j.autneu.2007.10.006
49. Toweill D, Sonnenthal K, Kimberly B, Lai S, Goldstein B. Linear and nonlinear analysis of hemodynamic signals during sepsis and septic shock. *Crit Care Med.* (2000) 28:2051–7. doi: 10.1097/00003246-200006000-00063
50. Fairchild KD. Predictive monitoring for early detection of sepsis in neonatal ICU patients. *Curr Opin Pediatr.* (2013) 25:172–9. doi: 10.1097/MOP.0b013e32835e8fe6
51. Griffin MP, Lake DE, O'Shea TM, Moorman JR. Heart rate characteristics and clinical signs in neonatal sepsis. *Pediatr Res.* (2007) 61:222–7. doi: 10.1203/01.pdr.0000252438.65759.af
52. Griffin MP, O'Shea TM, Bissonette EA, Harrell FE, Jr., Lake DE, Moorman JR. Abnormal heart rate characteristics preceding neonatal sepsis and sepsis-like illness. *Pediatr Res.* (2003) 53:920–6. doi: 10.1203/01.PDR.0000064904.05313.D2
53. Sanchez-Pinto LN, Luo Y, Churpek MM. Big data and data science in critical care. *Chest.* (2018). doi: 10.1016/j.chest.2018.04.037. [Epub ahead of print].
54. Typpo KV, Wong HR, Finley SD, Daniels RC, Seely AJ, Lacroix J. Monitoring severity of multiple organ dysfunction syndrome: new technologies. *Pediatr Crit Care Med.* (2017) 18(3 Suppl. 1):S24–S31. doi: 10.1097/PCC.0000000000001050
55. Patwari PP, Stewart TM, Rand CM, Carroll MS, Kuntz NL, Kenny AS, et al. Pupillometry in congenital central hypoventilation syndrome (CCHS): quantitative evidence of autonomic nervous system dysregulation. *Pediatr Res.* (2012) 71:280–5. doi: 10.1038/pr.2011.38
56. Saiyed R, Rand CM, Carroll MS, Koliboski CM, Stewart TM, Brogadir CD, et al. Congenital central hypoventilation syndrome (CCHS): Circadian temperature variation. *Pediatr Pulmonol.* (2016) 51:300–7. doi: 10.1002/ppul.23236
57. Muppidi S, Adams-Huet B, Tajzoy E, Scribner M, Blazek P, Spaeth EB, et al. Dynamic pupillometry as an autonomic testing tool. *Clin Auton Res.* (2013) 23:297–303. doi: 10.1007/s10286-013-0209-7
58. Millar PJ, Floras JS. Statins and the autonomic nervous system. *Clin Sci.* (2014) 126:401–15. doi: 10.1042/CS20130332
59. Levy G, Fishman JE, Xu DZ, Dong W, Palange D, Vida G, et al. Vagal nerve stimulation modulates gut injury and lung permeability in trauma-hemorrhagic shock. *J Trauma Acute Care Surg.* (2012) 73:338–42. Discussion: 42 doi: 10.1097/TA.0b013e31825debd3

15

Sepsis: Changing Definitions, Unchanging Treatment

Nchafatso Gikenyi Obonyo [1,2,3,4*], *Luregn Jan Schlapbach* [5,6,7,8] *and John Francis Fraser* [3,8,9]

[1] Initiative to Develop African Research Leaders (IDeAL-DELTAS), Kilifi, Kenya, [2] KEMRI-Wellcome Trust Research Programme, CGMRC, Kilifi, Kenya, [3] Critical Care Research Group, The Prince Charles Hospital, Chermside, QLD, Australia, [4] Wellcome Trust Centre for Global Health Research, Imperial College London, London, United Kingdom, [5] Paediatric Critical Care Research Group, Child Health Research Centre, The University of Queensland, South Brisbane, QLD, Australia, [6] Paediatric Intensive Care Unit, Queensland Children's Hospital, South Brisbane, QLD, Australia, [7] Department of Pediatrics, Inselspital Universitätsspital Bern, Bern, Switzerland, [8] Faculty of Medicine, The University of Queensland, Herston, QLD, Australia, [9] School of Medicine, Griffith University, Gold Coast, QLD, Australia

Correspondence:
Nchafatso Gikenyi Obonyo
nobonyo@kemri-wellcome.org

The recently revised Sepsis-3 definitions were based on criteria that were derived and validated in adult patient databases from high income countries. Both sepsis and septic shock continue to account for a substantial proportion of mortality globally, especially amongst children in low-and-middle income country settings. It is therefore urgent to develop and validate standardized criteria for sepsis that can be applied to pediatric populations in different settings, including in- and outside intensive care, both in high- and low/middle- income countries. This will be a pre-requisite to evaluate the impact of sepsis treatment strategies to improve clinical outcomes.

Keywords: sepsis, septic shock, definitions, pediatric populations, treatment bundles

BACKGROUND

In 2016, the International Sepsis Definition Taskforce convened by the Society of Critical Care Medicine, and the European Society of Intensive Care Medicine, updated definitions and clinical criteria for sepsis. These should facilitate recognition, targeted management of patients with sepsis and also improve accurate characterization of the global sepsis burden (1). Sepsis-3 defines sepsis as life-threatening organ dysfunction caused by a dysregulated host response to infection, while the concept of septic shock incorporates profound circulatory, cellular and metabolic abnormalities associated with a greater risk of mortality (1). These new Sepsis-3 criteria reflect advances made in the understanding of the pathobiology, epidemiology, and management of sepsis. While the concept underlying the new sepsis definition can be applied to all age groups, the operationalization of definition was derived and validated in adult cohorts only.

In May, 2017, the World Health Assembly (WHA), the World Health Organization's (WHO) decision-making body, adopted a resolution recognizing the need to improve the prevention, diagnosis, and management of sepsis as a priority (2). It is currently estimated that 30 million cases and 6 million sepsis-related deaths occur worldwide each year including 3 million newborns and 1.2 million children who suffer from sepsis globally on an annual basis (3). Translating the WHO resolution at national and international level into actions leading to improved outcomes for children will require addressing the unique features characterizing epidemiology, host responses, and outcomes (4) to ensure accurate definition, and targeted treatment.

DEFINITIONS OF PEDIATRIC SEPSIS

The Sepsis-3 criteria were based on systematic reviews, Delphi processes, and stringent methodology to develop and validate robust criteria for sepsis (1, 5, 6), and the merit in this data-driven approach is widely recognized. Yet, validity remains restricted to the adult populations in which the criteria were developed and tested, and a gap exists in relation to pediatric sepsis. Several studies have demonstrated that the application of Sepsis-3 derived criteria to children in intensive care settings in high income countries performs reasonably well (7, 8). However, a number of challenges remain to be addressed to translate these to settings outside intensive care, including emergency departments, and in particular low-and-middle income (LMIC) settings (3). In the global context, pediatric sepsis burden occurs disproportionately in LMICs with a devastating impact on neonatal and childhood mortality (2). However, robust data on the burden of pediatric sepsis in LMICs remain scarce (3). Currently, there is no definition of pediatric sepsis that is harmonized with Sepsis-3, a shortcoming recognized by the 2016 Sepsis International Consensus Taskforce which acknowledged the need to develop similar definitions for pediatric populations, incorporating clinical criteria that take age-dependent variation into account (9). Presently used clinical criteria for diagnosing sepsis in children in LMICs include the 2005 Pediatric Sepsis Consensus Conference (PSCC) (10, 11) and the World Health Organization's Integrated Management of Childhood Illnesses (WHO-IMCI) (12). Further criteria facilitating assessment of septic shock in neonates and children were proposed by the American College of Critical Care Medicine (ACCM) in 2002 and subsequently updated in 2007 (13) and 2014 (14). These have also been applied in LMICs settings but to varied extents due to limitations in ability to implement criteria such as inotrope therapy as well as intensive care hemodynamic monitoring and support. **Box 1** below compares and contrasts different criteria used to identify pediatric sepsis. Of note, subtle but substantial differences exist in some of the cut-off values for various variables used in defining sepsis when comparing the PSCC, WHO-IMCI, and ACCM criteria (**Table 1**).

CHANGING DEFINITIONS, UNCHANGING TREATMENT

The Surviving Sepsis Campaign (SSC) guidelines focus on antibiotics, fluids, and inotropes as key elements of initial resuscitation (16). In the 2018 update of the adult Surviving Sepsis Campaign (SSC) bundle, a 1 h sepsis bundle for immediate management of sepsis is described, combining elements from previous 3 and 6 h bundles (17). The 1 h sepsis bundle makes a strong recommendation of administering 30 ml/kg bolus of crystalloid for resuscitation of adults with hypotension or lactate ≥4 mmol/L but further grades this recommendation as low quality given the available supporting evidence (17). In children, the recent ACCM recommendations advocate for administration of appropriate antibiotics, fluid boluses of up to 60 ml/kg, followed by initiation of inotropic support all within <60 min, ideally within as little as 15 min, in children with septic shock (14). While there is supportive retrospective evidence for the recommendations of the 1 h sepsis bundle in children highlighting the need for early sepsis recognition,

BOX 1 | Criteria to recognize sepsis and septic shock in children.

Pediatric Sepsis Consensus Conference definitions

The 2005 pediatric Sepsis Consensus Conference, PSCC, definition of sepsis is systemic inflammatory response syndrome (SIRS) in the presence of, or as a result of, suspected or proven infection, whereby SIRS comprises temperature dysregulation (defined as core body temperature >38.5 or <36°C); tachycardia (defined as a mean heart rate >2 SD above normal for age in the absence of external stimulus chronic drugs, or painful stimuli; or otherwise unexplained persistent elevation over a 0.5–4 h time period or for children <1 year old); bradycardia (defined as a mean heart rate <10th percentile for age in the absence of external vagal stimulus, βeta-blocker drugs, or congenital heart disease; or otherwise unexplained persistent depression over a 0.5 h time period); respiratory rate dysregulation (defined as a mean respiratory rate >2 SD above normal for age or mechanical ventilation for an acute process not related to underlying neuromuscular disease or the receipt of general anesthesia); leucocyte count elevated or depressed for age, or >10% immature neutrophils, but not secondary to chemotherapy-induced leukopenia (10, 11). Septic shock was defined as presence of sepsis and cardiovascular organ dysfunction in the PSCC definition (10, 11).

World Health Organization definitions

In the World Health Organization-Integrated Management of Childhood Illnesses, WHO-IMCI, sepsis is a diagnosis of exclusion, defined as presence of acute fever (>39°C) and severe illness when no other cause is found (12), while septic shock includes cold hands with poor peripheral perfusion; increased capillary refill time (>3 s); fast and weak pulse volume; hypotension; and decreased mental status (lethargy) (12).

American College of Critical Care Medicine clinical practice parameters for hemodynamic support of pediatric and neonatal septic shock (2017 update)

The American College of Critical Care Medicine defines sepsis as presence of hypothermia or hyperthermia plus clinical signs of inadequate tissue perfusion including any of the following: decreased or altered mental status; capillary refill time >2 s, diminished pulses, mottled cool extremities (cold shock); flash capillary refill, bounding peripheral pulses, wide pulse pressure (warm shock); urine output <1 ml/kg/h. Hypotension is not necessary for clinical diagnosis of septic shock, but its presence in a child with clinical suspicion of infection is confirmatory (14).

Fluid Expansion as Supportive Therapy definitions

The Fluid Expansion As Supportive Therapy, FEAST, trial recruitment criteria required presence of the following: 1) fever (axillary body temperature >37.5 or <36°C); 2) impaired consciousness (prostration or coma) and/or respiratory distress (increased work of breathing); 3) impaired perfusion (evidenced by one or more of the following criteria: capillary refill time of 3 or more seconds, lower limb temperature gradient, weak radial pulse volume, or severe tachycardia >180 beats per minute in children younger than 12 months of age, >160 beats per minute in children 1–5 years of age, or >140 beats per minute in children older than 5 years of age) (15).

TABLE 1 | Selected age-specific variables are compared between different criteria to recognize sepsis and septic shock in children.

Variable		Cut-off values (per age-group)				
		Heart rate (beats/min)		Respiratory rate (breaths/min)	Leucocyte count (WBC X 10^9/L)	Systolic Blood Pressure (mm Hg)
Age-group classification	**Age**	**Tachycardia**	**Bradycardia**	**Tachypnoea**	**Leucocytosis or leucopenia**	**Hypotension (11)**
(A) Pediatric Sepsis Consensus Conference 2005 (PSCC) Criteria (10).						
• Newborns	0 days–1 week	>180	<100	>50	>34	<59
• Neonates	1 week–1 month	>180	<100	>40	>19.5 or <5	<79
• Infant	1 month–1 year	>180	<90	>34	>17.5 or <5	<75
• Toddler and pre-school	2–5 years	>140	N/A	>22	>15.5 or <6	<74
• School age child	6–12 years	>130	N/A	>18	>13.5 or <4.5	<83
• Adolescent and young adult	13 < 18 years	>110	N/A	>14	>11 or < 4.5	<90
Temperature** (hyper- or hypothermia)	> 38.5 or < 36.0 °C					
Prolonged capillary refill time	> 5 s					

Variable	Cut-off values (per age-group)
(B) American College of Critical Care Medicine (ACCM) ## (13, 14).	
Temperature (hyper- or hypothermia)	No cut-off values described
Urine output	<1 ml/kg/h
Mental status	Decreased or altered mental status
Capillary refill time	Prolonged >2 s (cold shock) or flash capillary refill (warm shock)
Pulses	Diminished pulses and mottled cool extremities (cold shock) or bounding peripheral pulses with wide pulse pressure (warm shock)

Variable		Cut-off values (per age-group)				
		Heart rate (beats/min)		Systolic BP (mm Hg)	Respiratory rate (breaths/min)$$	
Age-group classification	**Age**	**Tachycardia**	**Bradycardia**	**Hypotension**	**Tachypnoea**	**Bradypnoea**
(C) World Health Organization-Integrated Management of Childhood Illnesses (WHO-IMCI) criteria (12).						
	0 ≤ 1 year	>160	<100	<60	≥60	<20
	> 1 year ≤ 3 years	>150	<90	<70	≥50	<20
	> 3 years ≤ 6 years	>140	<80	<75	≥40	<20
Temperature (hyperthermia)	>39.0°C					
Prolonged capillary refill time	>3 s					
Hypoxia (SPO_2)	<90%					

*** Temperature cut-off values apply for all ages and are based on core temperature measured by rectal, bladder, oral, or central catheter probe. ## Clinical diagnosis of shock based on ACCCM criteria requires suspected infection manifested by hypothermia or hyperthermia, and any of the above-listed clinical signs of inadequate tissue perfusion. $$ Respiratory rate criteria based on slightly different age-group classification cut-off values (i.e., < 2months, 2–11 months and 1–5 years).*

sampling for blood cultures, and administration of broad spectrum antibiotics (18), several components of the recognition and resuscitation bundles are based on expert opinion rather than evidence. Administration of rapid fluid boluses remains a cornerstone of treatment of shock, but the potential for harm related to large volume fluid administration is increasingly considered.

In 2011, the Fluid Expansion As Supportive Therapy (FEAST) multi-center randomized clinical trial (15) used pragmatic clinical and age-specific criteria for pediatric sepsis. These criteria in the FEAST trial were designed to generate practical, evidence-based data for management of children with severe febrile illness and impaired perfusion in resource-poor settings in sub-Saharan Africa and included over 3,000 patients (15). The landmark FEAST trial demonstrated that fluid boluses significantly increased 48 h mortality in acutely ill children with impaired perfusion in the resource-limited settings in South Saharan Africa (15, 19). A recent animal model of hyperdynamic endotoxaemic shock (20) reported paradoxical higher vasopressor requirement to maintain mean arterial blood pressure (MAP) following fluid bolus resuscitation which may account for some of the pathophysiology underlying findings in the FEAST study (21). More recently, the use of fluid boluses in septic shock in both pediatric (22) and adult populations (23, 24) is undergoing evaluation in several randomized controlled trials (Restrictive Intravenous Fluids Trial in Sepsis, RIFTS;

Crystalloid Liberal or Vasopressors Early Resuscitation in Sepsis, CLOVERS).

In the 2016 update of the WHO pediatric emergency triage, assessment and treatment (ETAT) guideline, despite a search of 1,600 references, including 3 randomized controlled trials (RCTs), only the FEAST trial met the inclusion criteria for consideration regarding pediatric sepsis and septic shock (25).

Post hoc and pre-specified sub-group analyses of the FEAST trial suggested that the excess mortality observed with fluid bolus therapy was not attributable to factors such as under-recognition of fluid overload, high prevalence of malaria (57%) and severe anemia (hemoglobin levels below 5 g/dL in 32%) in the study population; indeed fluid boluses were associated with adverse outcomes in all sub-groups analyzed (19, 26).

In contrast to adults, where large trials were performed on key interventions such as the use of hydrocortisone in septic shock (27), or on the use of norepinephrine and dopamine in septic shock (28), there are no comparably powered pediatric trials published or ongoing. Currently, to the best of our knowledge there are no large randomized controlled trials ongoing which compare fluid bolus therapy with alternative interventions such as vasopressors, or steroids in pediatric patients with septic shock (29), resulting in ongoing controversy around best practice.

In the past decade, outside the FEAST trial, only a relatively small number of interventional trials in pediatric sepsis were conducted, the majority of those with <100 included patients (30–33). In 2008, Santhanam et al. found no differences in mortality or resolution of shock when comparing resuscitation of 147 children with septic shock using 40 mls/kg fluid over 15 min followed by dopamine vs. 20 mls/kg fluid over 20 min up to a maximum of 60 mls/kg/h followed by dopamine (34). Oliveira et al. observed reduced mortality when using superior vena cava oxygenation as an end-point in goal-directed therapy in children with septic shock (35). A more recent trial from the United Kingdom highlighted challenges pertinent to feasibility of trials investigating the volume of fluid resuscitation in sepsis (22).

Future research on optimal hemodynamic support in sepsis and septic shock should consider assessing the role of volume, type (balanced crystalloids vs. normal saline) (36, 37), rate, and temperature of fluids and evaluate fluid-sparing strategies such as early vasoactive and inotrope support. Studies should include sites in resource-limited settings *inter alia* (26), as well as addressing and adjusting for variations attributable to different settings pertinent to host and pathogen characteristics all of which are likely to affect susceptibility, response, and outcomes (38).

In conclusion, it is urgent that the pediatric community collaborates across the globe to address the need for meaningful, pertinent and harmonized sepsis criteria that can be applied to children in different settings, including in- and outside intensive care, both in high-income countries and LMIC. This will allow the rigorous evaluation of the impact of sepsis bundles. Robust criteria will facilitate design and recruitment into novel trials to improve the evidence for currently recommended treatments to result in improved outcomes for children with sepsis.

AUTHOR CONTRIBUTIONS

All authors listed have made a substantial, direct and intellectual contribution to the work, and approved it for publication.

REFERENCES

1. Singer M, Deutschman CS, Seymour CW, Shankar-Hari M, Annane D, Bauer M, et al. The third International Consensus Definitions for Sepsis and Septic Shock (Sepsis-3). *J Am Med Assoc.* (2016) 315:801–10. doi: 10.1001/jama.2016.0287
2. Kissoon N, Reinhart K, Daniels R, Machado MFR, Schachter RD, Finfer S. Sepsis in children: global implications of the world health assembly resolution on sepsis. *Pediatr Crit Care Med.* (2017) 18:e625–7. doi: 10.1097/PCC.0000000000001340
3. Fleischmann-Struzek C, Goldfarb DM, Schlattmann P, Schlapbach LJ, Reinhart K, Kissoon N. The global burden of paediatric and neonatal sepsis: a systematic review. *Lancet Respir Med.* (2018) 6:223–30. doi: 10.1016/S2213-2600(18)30063-8
4. Schlapbach LJ, Straney L, Alexander J, MacLaren G, Festa M, Schibler A, et al. Mortality related to invasive infections, sepsis, and septic shock in critically ill children in Australia and New Zealand, 2002-13: a multicentre retrospective cohort study. *Lancet Infect Dis.* (2015) 15:46–54. doi: 10.1016/S1473-3099(14)71003-5
5. Shankar-Hari M, Phillips GS, Levy ML, Seymour CW, Liu VX, Deutschman CS, et al. Developing a new definition and assessing new clinical criteria for septic shock: for the third international consensus definitions for sepsis and septic shock (Sepsis-3). *J Am Med Assoc.* (2016) 315:775–87. doi: 10.1001/jama.2016.0289
6. Seymour CW, Liu VX, Iwashyna TJ, Brunkhorst FM, Rea TD, Scherag A, et al. Assessment of clinical criteria for sepsis: for the Third International Consensus Definitions for sepsis and septic shock (Sepsis-3). *J Am Med Assoc.* (2016) 315:762–74. doi: 10.1001/jama.2016.0288
7. Schlapbach LJ, Straney L, Bellomo R, MacLaren G, Pilcher D. Prognostic accuracy of age-adapted SOFA, SIRS, PELOD-2, and qSOFA for in-hospital mortality among children with suspected infection admitted to the intensive care unit. *Intensive Care Med.* (2018) 44:179–88. doi: 10.1007/s00134-017-5021-8
8. Matics TJ, Sanchez-Pinto LN. Adaptation and validation of a pediatric sequential organ failure assessment score and evaluation of the Sepsis-3 definitions in critically Ill children. *JAMA Pediatr.* (2017) 171:e172352. doi: 10.1001/jamapediatrics.2017.2352
9. Raith EP, Udy AA, Bailey M, McGloughlin S, MacIsaac C, Bellomo R, et al. Prognostic accuracy of the SOFA Score, SIRS Criteria, and qSOFA score for in-hospital mortality among adults with suspected infection admitted to the intensive care unit. *J Am Med Assoc.* (2017) 317:290–300. doi: 10.1001/jama.2016.20328
10. Goldstein B, Giroir B, Randolph A. International Consensus Conference on Pediatric S. International pediatric sepsis consensus conference: definitions for sepsis and organ dysfunction in pediatrics. *Pediatr Crit Care Med.* (2005) 6:2–8. doi: 10.1097/01.PCC.0000149131.72248.E6
11. Goldstein B, Giroir B, Randolph A. Values for systolic blood pressure. *Pediatr*

Crit Care Med. (2005) 6:500–1. doi: 10.1097/01.PCC.0000167568.79952.92
12. Pocket Book of Hospital Care for Children. *Guidelines for the Management of Common Childhood Illnesses*. Geneva: WHO Guidelines Approved by the Guidelines Review Committee (2013).
13. Brierley J, Carcillo JA, Choong K, Cornell T, Decaen A, Deymann A, et al. Clinical practice parameters for hemodynamic support of pediatric and neonatal septic shock: 2007 update from the American College of Critical Care Medicine. *Crit Care Med.* (2009) 37:666–88. doi: 10.1097/CCM.0b013e31819323c6
14. Davis AL, Carcillo JA, Aneja RK, Deymann AJ, Lin JC, Nguyen TC, et al. American College of Critical Care Medicine Clinical Practice Parameters for Hemodynamic Support of Pediatric and Neonatal Septic Shock. *Crit Care Med.* (2017) 45:1061–93. doi: 10.1097/CCM.0000000000002425
15. Maitland K, Kiguli S, Opoka RO, Engoru C, Olupot-Olupot P, Akech SO, et al. Mortality after fluid bolus in African children with severe infection. *N Engl J Med.* (2011) 364:2483–95. doi: 10.1056/NEJMoa1101549
16. Rhodes A, Evans LE, Alhazzani W, Levy MM, Antonelli M, Ferrer R, et al. Surviving Sepsis Campaign: International Guidelines for Management of Sepsis and Septic Shock: 2016. *Intensive Care Med.* (2017) 43:304–77. doi: 10.1007/s00134-017-4683-6
17. Levy MM, Evans LE, Rhodes A. The surviving sepsis campaign bundle: 2018 update. *Crit Care Med.* (2018) 46:997–1000. doi: 10.1097/CCM.0000000000003119
18. Evans IVR, Phillips GS, Alpern ER, Angus DC, Friedrich ME, Kissoon N, et al. Association Between the New York Sepsis Care Mandate and In-Hospital Mortality for Pediatric Sepsis. *J Am Med Assoc.* (2018) 320:358–67. doi: 10.1001/jama.2018.9071
19. Maitland K, George EC, Evans JA, Kiguli S, Olupot-Olupot P, Akech SO, et al. Exploring mechanisms of excess mortality with early fluid resuscitation: insights from the FEAST trial. *BMC Med.* (2013) 11:68. doi: 10.1186/1741-7015-11-68
20. Byrne L, Obonyo NG, Diab S, Dunster K, Passmore M, Boon AC, et al. An ovine model of hyperdynamic endotoxemia and vital organ metabolism. *Shock* (2018) 49:99–107. doi: 10.1097/SHK.0000000000000904
21. Byrne L, Obonyo NG, Diab SD, Dunster KR, Passmore MR, Boon AC, et al. Unintended consequences: fluid resuscitation worsens shock in an ovine model of endotoxemia. *Am J Respir Crit Care Med.* (2018) 198:1043–54. doi: 10.1164/rccm.201801-0064OC
22. Inwald DP, Canter R, Woolfall K, Mouncey P, Zenasni Z, O'Hara C, et al. Restricted fluid bolus volume in early septic shock: results of the fluids in shock pilot trial. *Arch Dis Child.* (2018) 1–6. doi: 10.1136/archdischild-2018-314924
23. Andrews B, Semler MW, Muchemwa L, Kelly P, Lakhi S, Heimburger DC, et al. Effect of an early resuscitation protocol on in-hospital mortality among adults with sepsis and hypotension: a randomized clinical trial. *J Am Med Assoc.* (2017) 318:1233–40. doi: 10.1001/jama.2017.10913
24. Hjortrup PB, Haase N, Bundgaard H, Thomsen SL, Winding R, Pettila V, et al. Restricting volumes of resuscitation fluid in adults with septic shock after initial management: the CLASSIC randomised, parallel-group, multicentre feasibility trial. *Intensive Care Med.* (2016) 42:1695–705. doi: 10.1007/s00134-016-4500-7
25. *Guideline: Updates on Paediatric Emergency Triage, Assessment and Treatment: Care of Critically-Ill Children.* Geneva: WHO Guidelines Approved by the Guidelines Review Committee (2016).
26. Kawasaki T. Update on pediatric sepsis: a review. *J Intensive Care* (2017) 5:47. doi: 10.1186/s40560-017-0240-1
27. Venkatesh B, Finfer S, Cohen J, Rajbhandari D, Arabi Y, Bellomo R, et al. Adjunctive glucocorticoid therapy in patients with septic shock. *N Engl J Med.* (2018) 378:797–808. doi: 10.1056/NEJMoa1705835
28. De Backer D, Aldecoa C, Njimi H, Vincent JL. Dopamine versus norepinephrine in the treatment of septic shock: a meta-analysis*. *Critical Care Med.* (2012) 40:725–30. doi: 10.1097/CCM.0b013e31823778ee
29. Gelbart B, Glassford NJ, Bellomo R. Fluid bolus therapy-based resuscitation for severe sepsis in hospitalized children: a systematic review. *Pediatric Crit Care Med.* (2015) 16:e297-307. doi: 10.1097/PCC.0000000000000507
30. Upadhyay M, Singhi S, Murlidharan J, Kaur N, Majumdar S. Randomized evaluation of fluid resuscitation with crystalloid (saline) and colloid (polymer from degraded gelatin in saline) in pediatric septic shock. *Indian Pediatr.* (2005) 42:223–31.
31. Ventura AM, Shieh HH, Bousso A, Goes PF, de Cassia FOFI, de Souza DC, et al. Double-blind prospective randomized controlled trial of dopamine versus epinephrine as first-line vasoactive drugs in pediatric septic shock. *Crit Care Med.* (2015) 43:2292–302. doi: 10.1097/CCM.0000000000001260
32. Ramaswamy KN, Singhi S, Jayashree M, Bansal A, Nallasamy K. Double-blind randomized clinical trial comparing dopamine and epinephrine in pediatric fluid-refractory hypotensive septic shock. *Pediatr Crit Care Med.* (2016) 17:e502–12. doi: 10.1097/PCC.0000000000000954
33. Sankar J, Ismail J, Sankar MJ, C PS, Meena RS. Fluid Bolus Over 15-20 versus 5-10 minutes each in the first hour of resuscitation in children with septic shock: a randomized controlled trial. *Pediatr Crit Care Med.* (2017) 18:e435–5. doi: 10.1097/PCC.0000000000001269
34. Santhanam I, Sangareddi S, Venkataraman S, Kissoon N, Thiruvengadamudayan V, Kasthuri RK. A prospective randomized controlled study of two fluid regimens in the initial management of septic shock in the emergency department. *Pediatr Emerg Care* (2008) 24:647–55. doi: 10.1097/PEC.0b013e31818844cf
35. de Oliveira CF, de Oliveira DS, Gottschald AF, Moura JD, Costa GA, Ventura AC, et al. ACCM/PALS haemodynamic support guidelines for paediatric septic shock: an outcomes comparison with and without monitoring central venous oxygen saturation. *Intensive Care Med.* (2008) 34:1065–75. doi: 10.1007/s00134-008-1085-9
36. Semler MW, Self WH, Wanderer JP, Ehrenfeld JM, Wang L, Byrne DW, et al. Balanced crystalloids versus saline in critically ill adults. *N Engl J Med.* (2018) 378:829–39. doi: 10.1056/NEJMoa1711584
37. Weiss SL, Babl FE, Dalziel SR, Balamuth F. Is chloride worth its salt? *Intensive Care Med.* (2018) 17:150. doi: 10.1007/s00134-018-5477-1
38. Giuliano JS Jr, Markovitz BP, Brierley J, Levin R, Williams G, Lum LC, et al. Comparison of pediatric severe sepsis managed in U.S. and European ICUs. *Pediatr Crit Care Med.* (2016) 17:522–30. doi: 10.1097/PCC.0000000000000760

16

Neonatal Ventilator Associated Pneumonia: A Quality Improvement Initiative Focusing on Antimicrobial Stewardship

Anouk Goerens[1], Dirk Lehnick[2], Michael Büttcher[1,3], Karin Daetwyler[1,4], Matteo Fontana[1,4], Petra Genet[1,4], Marco Lurà[1,5], Davide Morgillo[1,4], Sina Pilgrim[1,4], Katharina Schwendener-Scholl[1,4], Nicolas Regamey[1,5], Thomas J. Neuhaus[1] and Martin Stocker[1,4]*

[1] Department of Pediatrics, Children's Hospital Lucerne, Lucerne, Switzerland, [2] Clinical Trial Unit, University of Lucerne, Lucerne, Switzerland, [3] Infectious Diseases Unit, Children's Hospital Lucerne, Lucerne, Switzerland, [4] Pediatric and Neonatal Intensive Care Unit, Children's Hospital Lucerne, Lucerne, Switzerland, [5] Pediatric Pulmonology Unit, Children's Hospital Lucerne, Lucerne, Switzerland

***Correspondence:**
Martin Stocker
martin.stocker@luks.ch

Background and Aims: Neonatal ventilator associated pneumonia (VAP) is a common nosocomial infection and a frequent reason for empirical antibiotic therapy in NICUs. Nonetheless, there is no international consensus regarding diagnostic criteria and management. In a first step, we analyzed the used diagnostic criteria, risk factors and therapeutic management of neonatal VAP by a literature review. In a second step, we aimed to compare suspected vs. confirmed neonatal VAP episodes in our unit according to different published criteria and to analyze interrater-reliability of chest x-rays. Additionally, we aimed to evaluate the development of VAP incidence and antibiotic use after implementation of multifaceted quality improvement changes regarding antimicrobial stewardship and infection control (VAP-prevention-bundle, early-extubation policy, antimicrobial stewardship rounds).

Methods: Neonates until 44 weeks of gestation with suspected VAP, hospitalized at our level-III NICU in Lucerne from September 2014 to December 2017 were enrolled. VAP episodes were analyzed according to 4 diagnostic frameworks. Agreement regarding chest x-ray interpretation done by 10 senior physicians was assessed. Annual incidence of suspected and confirmed neonatal VAP episodes and antibiotic days were calculated and compared for the years 2015, 2016, and 2017.

Results: 17 studies were identified in our literature review. Overall, CDC-guidelines or similar criteria, requesting radiographic changes as main criteria, are mostly used. Comparison of suspected vs. confirmed neonatal VAP episodes showed a great variance (20.4 vs. 4.5/1,000 ventilator-days). The interrater-reliability of x-ray interpretation was poor (intra-class correlation 0.25). Implemented changes resulted in a gradual decline in annual VAP incidence and antibiotic days from 2015 compared with 2017 (28.8 vs. 7.4 suspected episodes/1,000 ventilator-days, 5.5 vs. 0 confirmed episodes/1,000 ventilator-days and 211 vs. 34.7 antibiotic days/1,000 ventilation-days, respectively).

Conclusion: The incidence of suspected VAP and concomitant antibiotic use is much higher than for confirmed VAP, therefore inclusion of suspected episodes should be considered for accurate evaluation. There is a high diagnostic inconsistency and a low reliability of interpretation of chest x-rays regarding VAP. Implementation of combined antimicrobial stewardship and infection control measures may lead to an effective decrease in VAP incidence and antibiotic use.

Keywords: neonatal ventilator associated pneumonia, diagnostic criteria, quality improvement, antibiotic stewardship, infection control, risk factors

BACKGROUND AND AIMS

Ventilator associated pneumonia (VAP) is defined as a nosocomial lower airway infection, i.e. pneumonia, in intubated patients with onset after 48 h or more of invasive mechanical ventilation[1] (1). VAP is usually caused by airway colonization by potential pathogens, which disseminate due to inadequate immune response of the newborn's immature innate immune system. The immaturity of the immune system is especially significant in premature and growth restricted newborns (2). Sources of airway colonization can be the patient's own flora, i.e., bacterial overgrowth in oral secretions, reflux and aspiration of gastric fluid or the patient's environment with its caretakers and equipment (2, 3).

VAP is one of the most frequently diagnosed nosocomial infections (4) and, after suspected early onset sepsis, second most reason for antibiotic intervention in NICUs (5, 6). There is no international consensus on definition of VAP regarding the neonatal population (3, 7). In most recommendations radiographic changes are considered as one of the main crireria. However, underlying lung disease may complicate the interpretation of radiographic changes in this population. Reported frequency of neonatal VAP show a large range (2.7–10.9 cases per 1,000 ventilator days) in developed countries (3). VAP incidence can be reduced by infection control measures such as VAP-prevention-bundles (8–10). Epidemiologic studies demonstrated that quality improvement initiatives, not the introduction of new therapies or research approaches, resulted in a decline of mortality of neonates in the last decade (11).

Antibiotics are among the most frequently used medications in neonatal intensive care (12). There is a high variance of antibiotic use when comparing different NICUs. This observation suggests relevant overuse and underlines the need for implementation of antibiotic stewardship (13, 14). Prompt antibiotic therapy for possible infections in this vulnerable population is crucial for good outcome (15). On the other hand, inadequate antibiotic use results in increasing occurrence of multidrug resistant bacteria (16). In addition, recently published studies underline that antibiotic treatment in early life has an impact on the individual's microbiome with potential consequences for future health (17–20). Prolonged duration of antibiotic use in preterm infants is also associated with higher mortality and morbidity such as chronic lung disease, retinopathy of prematurity, periventricular leukomalacia and necrotizing enterocolitis (16, 21). Neonatologists and pediatricians should be aware that starting antibiotics may be in some circumstances more harmful than beneficial. The mind-set of antibiotic treatment just for safety reasons is no longer justified (20).

Aim of this study was to perform a review of the current literature to present an overview of the most commonly used diagnostic criteria, risk factors and therapeutic management for neonatal VAP. Secondly to analyze all suspected neonatal VAP episodes in our unit within the study period according to various predefined diagnostic criteria[1] (22, 23). We hypothesized that a high variance in incidence between clinically suspected and confirmed neonatal VAP would exist. Additionally, because interpretation of chest x-rays is a corner stone of VAP diagnosis, we wanted to analyze the interrater-reliability of all chest x-rays done for suspected neonatal VAP episodes, hypothesizing that interrater-reliability would be modest to low. Last, we aimed to describe and compare annual incidence of neonatal VAP and antibiotic use for neonatal VAP in our NICU during a quality improvement initiative with implementation of multifaceted changes focused both on antimicrobial stewardship and infection control. We hypothesized that implementation of these changes decreases incidence of, as well as antibiotic use for neonatal VAP.

METHODS

Literature Review

The literature review was done applying the approach of the PRISMA-statement for systematic reviews (24). PubMed was searched using the following search terms: "diagnosis + neonatal ventilator associated pneumonia," "antibiotic therapy + neonatal ventilator associated pneumonia," and "neonatal ventilator associated pneumonia" sorted by best match, with restriction to available full text in English or German. The first search was run in December 2017, the last search was run in March 2018. In addition, further studies were identified

Abbreviations: CDC, Center for Diseases Control and Prevention; CLABSI, Central line associated blood stream infections; CPAP, Continuous positive airway pressure; CRIB, Clinical risk index for babies; CRP, C-reactive protein; ECDC, European Centre for Disease Prevention and Control; ETA, Endotracheal aspirate; ETT, Endotracheal tube; I:T ratio, Immature neutrophils to total neutrophils; ICC, Intra-class correlation coefficient; LUS, Lung ultrasound; NICU, Neonatal intensive care unit; VAP, Ventilator associated pneumonia; WBC, White blood cell count.

[1] *0512-TED-PPS-HAI-antimicrobial-use-protocol.* Available online at: https://ecdc.europa.eu/sites/portal/files/media/en/publications/Publications/0512-TED-PPS-HAI-antimicrobial-use-protocol.pdf (Accessed September 16, 2017).

reviewing references in found publications. Inclusion was based on the described population (only neonatal population) and the content of the study (diagnostic criteria and/or risk factors and/or management of VAP).

Study Setting

For our study, approval of the national ethics committee was obtained (Project-ID 2017-01842). The patients' parents/guardians were informed beforehand and gave consent for the study. Recordings of suspected neonatal VAP episodes as well as the single-center quality improvement initiative were undertaken at our level-III NICU in Lucerne. The Children's Hospital Lucerne is a teaching hospital for Pediatrics and Neonatology and the unit is a referral level III NICU (perinatal center) with all pediatric specialties including neonatal surgery, but without cardiac surgery (except surgical closure of persistent ductus arteriosus). The NICU is part of the Swiss neonatal collaboration with regular quality assessment and center-to-center comparison (25).

For this study, neonatal VAP was defined as VAP occurring in neonates below 44 weeks of corrected gestational age. Therefore, the study population consists of neonates with a corrected gestational age between 23 0/7 and 43 6/7 weeks hospitalized during the study period of September 1st, 2014 to December 31st, 2017. September 1st, 2014 data collection was started with implementation of a prospective surveillance program assessing VAP, central line associated blood stream infections (CLABSI) and use of antibiotics on the NICU. Every morning between 6 and 8 a.m. the on-site physician recorded patients with suspected VAP, CLABSI and patients on antibiotic treatment. The recordings were verified and entered into the NICU's surveillance database by the NICU's data manager.

Definitions of Suspected and Confirmed Neonatal VAP

Suspected VAP was defined according to the following criteria: ventilation for more than 48 h and new start or change of antibiotic therapy due to worsening of ventilation conditions and/or clinical deterioration and/or radiological changes compatible with pneumonia and/or changes of tracheal secretions and/or abnormal laboratory parameters (CRP > 20 mg/l, leukocytosis/-penia, I:T ratio > 0.2).

To compare the variance between clinically suspected (all episodes in our study population) and confirmed neonatal VAP, four different frameworks for diagnosis of VAP were applied on all suspected VAP episodes of our study population retrospectively. Patients fulfilling the diagnostic criteria of at least one of the frameworks were defined as confirmed VAP. Suspected episodes not fulfilling any criteria were addressed as non-confirmed VAP. The frameworks we used for further diagnosis were: 1. Center for Diseases Control and Prevention (CDC): Criteria for defining nosocomial pneumonia for infants $\leq$1 year old (22); 2. European Centre for Disease Prevention and Control (ECDC)[1]; 3. Diagnostic criteria for laboratory confirmed VAP according to a surveillance study with definition for infection specifically adapted for neonates from a Dutch NICU (23); 4. Diagnostic criteria for clinical VAP according to a surveillance study with definition for infection specifically adapted for neonates from a Dutch NICU (23). **Table 1** shows a listing of all used definitions.

Interrater-Reliability of Chest-X-Ray Interpretation

Chest x-rays for suspected VAP episodes were ordered according to the physician in charge. The primary evaluation was done by the radiologist in charge and used for evaluation of confirmed neonatal VAP. For analysis of interrater-reliability, all chest x-rays ordered for suspected neonatal VAP were reviewed separately by all board approved neonatologists, pediatric pulmonologists and pediatric infectious disease specialists of the children's hospital of Lucerne (total of 10 senior physicians: 7 board approved neonatologists, 2 board approved pediatric pulmonologists and 1 board approved specialist for pediatric infectious diseases). They all reported if radiographic changes caused by neonatal VAP were present with a 4-point Likert scale (yes, possibly yes, possibly no, no). All x-rays were anonymized and all raters were blinded for the written interpretation by the radiologist.

Quality Improvement Initiative

Within our quality improvement initiative we analyzed prospectively all episodes of suspected neonatal VAP and antibiotic use during and after implementation of multifaceted changes regarding infection control and antimicrobial stewardship in our NICU. The prospective surveillance program started in September 2014. The staff of the NICU was aware of the quality improvement initiative focused on antimicrobial stewardship, but was not informed regarding details of the ongoing analyzes for the study.

Since 2007, prescription of antibiotics in our unit is standardized by use of a web based guideline (www.idosecalc.ch) specifying drug, dose and duration of therapy (7–10 days of therapy recommended for hospital acquired pneumonia). Starting December 2015, the following multifaceted quality improvement changes were introduced over 2 years (**Table 2**): Firstly, a new policy for early-extubation minimizing duration of invasive ventilation was introduced in December 2015. Secondly, since December 2015, infectious disease specialists have been involved in the NICU every week for an antimicrobial stewardship round. Thirdly, a care bundle was implemented in our neonatal and pediatric ICU in December 2016, including the following measures: strict hand hygiene before and after patient contact and handling respiratory equipment, wearing gloves when in contact with secretions, ventilator circuit changes every 14 days or when visibly soiled, oral care every 2–4 h, head of bed elevation, draining ventilator condensate before repositioning of the patient, using endotracheal tube (ETT) with cuff when possible (usually not applicable for preterm neonates), choosing size of the ETT carefully to reduce numbers of reintubation.

Data Sources

Clinical signs, oxygen requirement, ventilation requirements and further physical measurements as required according to the criteria for VAP were extracted from patient files. Antibiotic

TABLE 1 | Used definitions for diagnosing neonatal VAP.

Suspected neonatal VAP (NICU Lucerne) (Study population)	Neonates below 44 weeks of corrected gestational age Ventilation for more than 48 hours AND new start or change of antibiotic therapy due to: - worsening of ventilation conditions (increased oxygen requirements, worsening pCO_2, increased ventilator demand) - AND/OR clinical deterioration (T > 38.0°C or <36.5°C, P > 170/min or <100/min, apnea >20%) - AND/OR radiological changes compatible with pneumonia - AND/OR changes of tracheal secretions - AND/OR abnormal laboratory parameters (CRP > 20mg/l, leukocytosis/-penia, I:T ratio > 0.2)
CDC Criteria for Infants < 1 year old (Group 1)	Patients without underlying diseases have ≥1 chest x-ray; Patients with underlying diseases have ≥2 chest x-rays with one of the following (new and persistent OR progressive and persistent): - Infiltrate - Consolidation - Cavitation - Pneumatoceles AND: - Worsening gas exchange (e.g., O_2 desaturations, increased oxygen requirements, or increased ventilator demand) AND three of the following: - Temperature instability - Leukopenia (≤4000 WBC/mm^3) or leukocytosis (>15,000 WBC/mm^3) and left shift (>10% band forms) - New onset of purulent sputum or change in character of sputum or increased respiratory secretions or increased suctioning requirements - Apnea, tachypnea, nasal flaring with retraction of chest wall or grunting - Wheezing, rales or rhonchi - Cough - Bradycardia (<100 beats/min) or tachycardia (>170 beats/min)
European Centre for Disease Prevention and Control (ECDC) (Group 2)	Invasive respiratory device present (even intermittently) in the 48 preceding the onset of infection AND: - respiratory compromise AND: - new infiltrate, consolidation or pleural effusion on chest x-ray AND at least four of: - temperature >38°C or < 36.5°C or temperature instability - tachycardia or bradycardia - tachypnoea or apnoea - dyspnoea - increased respiratory secretions - new onset of purulent sputum - isolation of a pathogen from respiratory secretions - C-reactive protein > 2.0 mg/dL - I/T ratio > 0.2
Diagnostic criteria for laboratory confirmed VAP according to a surveillance study with definition for infection specifically adapted for neonates from a Dutch NICU (Group 3)	One of the following: - purulent sputum - changes in sputum characteristics - deterioration of ventilation conditions AND new emergence or progression of one of the following: - Infiltration - Consolidation - Pleural adhesion - Pleural effusion AND: - Isolation of a pathogenic microorganism or detection of a bacterial/viral antigen in the tracheal aspirate, bronchial secretion or sputum
Diagnostic criteria for clinical VAP according to a surveillance study with definition for infection specifically adapted for neonates from a Dutch NICU (Group 4)	One of the following: - purulent sputum - changes in sputum characteristics - deterioration of ventilation conditions AND new emergence or progression of one of the following: - Infiltration - Consolidation - Pleural adhesion - Pleural effusion AND: - No isolation of a pathogenic microorganism or detection of a bacterial/viral antigen in the tracheal aspirate, bronchial secretion or sputum - Administration of relevant antimicrobial therapy for at least seven days

TABLE 2 | Implemented quality improvement changes in our NICU.

	Standardized subscription of antibiotic therapies (start 2007)	Prospective surveillance program (start 09/2014)	Policy for early-extubation (start 12/2015)	Antibiotic stewardship rounds (start 12/2015)	New VAP-prevention-bundle (start 12/2016)
2015	Yes	Yes			
2016	Yes	Yes	Yes	Yes	
2017	Yes	Yes	Yes	Yes	Yes

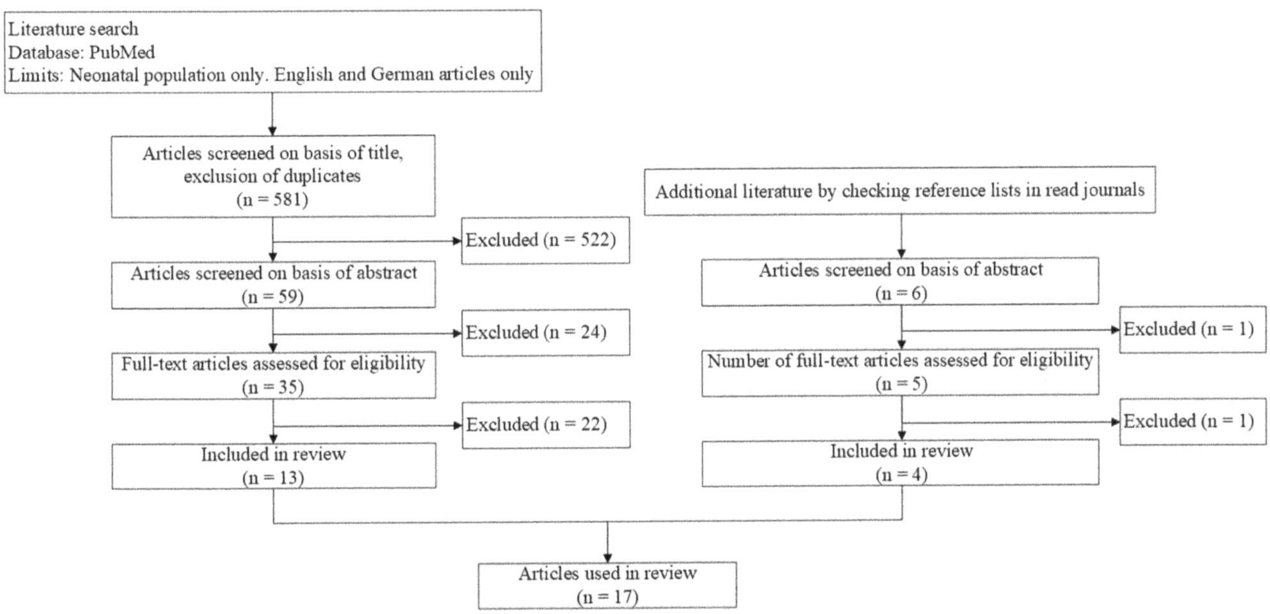

FIGURE 1 | Flow-chart showing literature research.

days and laboratory results were obtained from electronic patient files and reports of hospitalization. All laboratory measurements were ordered according to the request of the physician in charge and the unit's policy to use full white blood count (WBC), I:T ratio and C-reactive protein (CRP) for evaluation of suspected infection and guidance of duration of antibiotic therapy. According to the unit's policy, blood cultures and cultures of tracheal aspirates ought to be obtained before start or change of antibiotic therapy. Results were obtained from electronic patient files. Tracheal aspirates were examined microscopically with a semi-quantitative analysis of leukocytes. Purulent tracheal aspirates were defined as leucocytes ≥ 2 within the scale from 0 to 3.

Statistical Analyses

All data were anonymized before statistical analysis. Data collection in our NICU is generally performed for the period of a whole year (January to December), therefore annual calculations of suspected and confirmed VAP episodes and antibiotic use could only be done for the 3 complete years of the study: 2015, 2016, and 2017. The episodes in 2014 were not included in calculations as the observational period started in September.

Incidence of suspected and confirmed neonatal VAP episodes, as well as incidence of all separate groups (1–4) were calculated for the period of January 2015–December 2017 and extrapolated for 1,000 ventilator-days. Comparison of agreement between the four different diagnostic criteria was calculated using intra-class correlation coefficients (ICC). Risk factors such as gestational age, birth weight and duration of mechanical ventilation were compared between the two groups of non-confirmed and confirmed neonatal VAP. Agreement between raters for the evaluation of the chest x-rays with the 4-point Likert scale was assessed utilizing intra-class correlation coefficients (ICC). All raters evaluated all chest x-rays (fully crossed design). An ICC > 0.8 was considered as excellent, >0.6 as good agreement between raters. Annual incidence of suspected and confirmed VAP episodes and antibiotic days were calculated for 1,000 ventilator-days. To assess the existence of a possible trend regarding annual incidence of suspected VAP episodes, duration of antibiotic therapy per suspected episode and antibiotic days for suspected episodes, the nonparametric test for trend proposed by Cuzick was used (Wilcoxon-type test for trend) as the approximation works for small sample sizes (26).

TABLE 3 | Systematic review: Overview of incidence, diagnostic criteria, risk factors and treatment.

Source	Study design, (No of patients)	Neonatal VAP incidence	Diagnostic criteria	Risk factors	Treatment
Afjeh et al. (27) Iran	Prospective cohort study (81 patients)	11.6 VAP/1,000 ventilator-days	CDC guidelines for infants ≤1 year old	Independent risk factors: Purulent sputum, longer duration of mechanical ventilation, antacid therapy	Not specified
Apisarnthanarak et al. (28) USA	Prospective cohort study (229 patients)	4–6.5 VAP/1,000 ventilator-days	CDC guidelines for infants ≤1 year old	Independent risk factors: Prior bloodstream infection, longer duration of mechanical ventilation (marginally significant)	Not specified
Azab et al. (8) Egypt	Prospective cohort study (143 patients)	73 VAP episodes	Foglia et al. (29)	Not specified	Not specified
Badr et al. (30) Egypt	Prospective observational study (56 patients)	32 VAP episodes	CPIS (clinical pulmonary infection score)	Longer duration of mechanical ventilation, low gestational age, low birth weight	Not specified
Cernada et al. (1) Spain	Prospective observational study (198 patients)	10.9 VAP/1,000 ventilator-days	CDC guidelines for infants ≤1 year old + positive BAL (BAL with blind protected catheter to diminish contamination)	Independent risk factor: Days of mechanical ventilation Others: Days of oxygen, times of reintubations, numbers of transfusions, previous bloodstream infection, enteral feeding, low gestational age, low birth weight, female sex	Not specified
Deng et al.(31) China	Case-control study (349 patients)	25.6 VAP/1,000 ventilator-days	At least 3 of the following: temperature instability OR new onset of purulent sputum, change in character of sputum, increased respiratory secretions, increased suctioning OR leukocytes >10x10E9 cells/l,<3x10E9 cells/l OR two or more abnormal chest X-rays OR apnea, tachypnea, nasal flaring, grunting [Adapted Foglia et al.(29)]	Independent risk factors: Low birth weight, neonate respiratory distress syndrome, parenteral alimentation, reintubation (>3x), mechanical ventilation ≥ 7 days Others: Age < 3d, gestational age <37 weeks, Bronchopulmonary dysplasia, previous blood stream infection, hypoxic ischemic encephalopathy, frequent drawing of blood, bronchoscopy	Cephalosporin 61.2%, Penicillin derivatives 45.5%, Aminoglycosides 13.4%, Metronidazole 20.1%, Macrolides 11.2%, Quinolones 17.8%, Vancomycin 11.6%, Sulfa derivatives 8.1%, Antifungal agents 8.9%, Antiviral agents 8.6% Duration: 5.4 ± 3.2 days
Fallahi et al. (32) Iran	Prospective cross-sectional study (66 patients)	22 VAP episodes	Modified CDC guidelines for infants ≤1 year old	Lower gestational age, lower birth weight, longer duration of hospital stay, prolonged ventilator need	Not specified
Katayama et al. (33) Japan	Prospective study	49 VAP episodes	Increased ventilator demand with increased amount of endotracheal aspirate + microorganisms and polymorphonuclear leukocytes in gram-stained smears of aspirates + increased CRP and/or intracellular bacteria on gram-stained smears	Not specified	Immediate gram-staining and examination of sputum aspirates by a neonatal physician: - Gram-negative bacilli: Piperacillin or Piperacillin + Amikacin - Gram-positive cocci: Vancomycin
Kawanishi et al. (34) Japan	Retrospective observational study (71 patients)	14 VAP episodes	Foglia et al. (29)	Low birth weight (esp. <626g), times of ventilator tube changes, longer duration of mechanical ventilation	Not specified

(Continued)

TABLE 3 | Continued

Source	Study design, (No of patients)	Neonatal VAP incidence	Diagnostic criteria	Risk factors	Treatment
Khattab et al. (35) Egypt	Not specified (85 patients)	47 VAP episodes (55.2%)	CDC guidelines	Prematurity, low birth weight, longer duration of mechanical ventilation	Not specified
Lee et al. (36) Taiwan	Retrospective observational study (114 patients)	7.1 VAP/1,000 ventilator-days	CDC guidelines for infants ≤1 year old	Longer duration of mechanical ventilation, longer parenteral nutrition, low gestational age, low birth weight	Not specified
Murila et al. (37) Australia	Retrospective study (124 patients)	74 positive ETA cultures, 58 VAP episodes	Positive culture of endotracheal secretion + overall condition + change in respiratory status (increased FiO2, increased ventilator support, new infiltrate on Chest X-ray)	Not specified	Treatment: Vancomycin + Imipenem
Petdachai (38) Thailand	Prospective observational study (170 patients)	70.3 VAP/1,000 ventilator-days	Modified CDC guidelines for infants ≤1 year old	Independent risk factors: Umbilical catheterization, respiratory distress syndrome, orogastric tube Others: Lower birth weight, longer duration of mechanical ventilation, longer hospital stay	Not specified
Thatrimontrichai et al. (39) Thailand	Prospective cohort study (128 patients)	10.1 VAP/1,000 ventilator-days	CDC guidelines for infants ≤1 year old	Independent risk factors: Birth weight <750g, sedative medication Others: Reintubation rate, antihistamine use	Not specified
Tripathi et al. (40) India	Prospective observational study (98 patients)	37.2 VAP/1,000 ventilator-days	CDC guidelines for pediatric patients	Independent risk factors: Longer duration of mechanical ventilation, very low birth weight Others: Prematurity, numbers of reintubation, length of NICU stay	Not specified
Yuan et al. (41) China	Retrospective cohort study (259 patients)	52 VAP episodes	New and persistent radiographic evidence of focal infiltrate Plus 2 of the following: fever >38°C, leukocytes >12x10E9 cells/l, purulent sputum No hyaline membrane disease, meconium aspiration, atelectasis as possible diagnosis	Independent risk factors: Reintubation, longer duration of mechanical ventilation, treatment with opiates, endotracheal suctioning Others: transfusion, parenteral nutrition	Not specified
Van der Zwet et al. (23) The Netherlands	Retrospective surveillance study (742 patients)	5.8 - 19.7 (mean 11.8) VAP/1,000 ventilator days (depending on birth weight)	Modified CDC guidelines for infants ≤1 year old	Mechanical ventilation, low birthweight	Not specified

RESULTS

Literature Review

A total of 17 studies were included in the review. The flow chart in **Figure 1** shows the process of selecting studies for inclusion in the literature review. **Table 3** is a listing of these recent studies, giving an overview of the used diagnostic criteria, the most important risk factors and the used therapeutic management for VAP in newborns. The CDC guidelines for infants ≤1 year old were the most often applied criteria followed by similar and adapted criteria. Except for the criteria used in the study by Katayama et al. (33), all request abnormal chest x-rays as part of their criteria. Longer duration of mechanical ventilation, low birth weight, low gestational age and numbers of reintubation were the prevalent risk factors for VAP. Long duration of mechanical ventilation was the most important risk factor. Even though the database was reviewed for studies regarding antibiotic therapy, only three studies (31, 33, 37) discussed the treatment of VAP.

TABLE 4 | Incidence of suspected and confirmed neonatal VAP (in total and for groups 1 – 4).

	Total n	VAP episodes/1,000 ventilator-days (2015–2017)
Suspected neonatal VAP episodes	36	20.4
Confirmed neonatal VAP episodes (fulfilling diagnostic criteria for at least one out of the 4 groups)	10	4.5
Group 1 (CDC Criteria for Infants < 1 year old)	3	1.9
Group 2 (European Centre for Disease Prevention and Control (ECDC)	4	2.6
Group 3 (Diagnostic criteria for laboratory confirmed VAP according to Dutch NICU)	9	3.8
Group 4 (Diagnostic criteria for clinical VAP according to Dutch NICU)	8	3.8

Suspected vs. Confirmed Neonatal VAP

Comparison of suspected with confirmed neonatal VAP episodes showed a great variance over the whole study period: 20.4 vs. 4.5/1,000 ventilator-days. The particular incidence of confirmed neonatal VAP after applying the 4 different diagnostic criteria (groups 1–4) is shown in **Table 4**. Comparison of agreement between the different diagnostic criteria showed an ICC of 0.55, thus showing a moderate agreement.

The age of neonates in our study population (n=36) ranged between 24 3/7 and 41 1/7 (median 28 4/7) gestational weeks at the time of diagnosis. They weighed between 345 and 3,770 g (median 650 g). The 26 neonates with non-confirmed VAP were between 24 3/7 and 41 1/7 (median 27 6/7) gestational weeks old and weighed between 345 and 3,770 g (median 630 g). Duration of mechanical ventilation varied between 3 to 103 days (median 12.5 days). The 10 neonates with confirmed VAP episodes were between 26 5/7 and 40 0/7 (median 29 1/7) weeks and had a birth weight between 345 and 3,690 g (median 670 g). They were intubated between 10 and 37 days (median 26 days) at time of diagnosis. **Figure 2** shows a comparison of the patients' gestational age, birth weight and duration of intubation between the non-confirmed and confirmed neonatal VAP cases.

Thirty-one out of the 36 analyzed tracheal aspirates showed bacterial growth (**Table 5**). Thirteen of the 31 culture positive tracheal aspirates also showed a purulent sputum. Among the 10 neonates with confirmed VAP, 8 had culture positive tracheal aspirates, thereof 4 presented with purulent sputum. **Table 5** shows a listing of these results and of all isolated pathogens. In 13 cases only cultures of tracheal aspirates without blood cultures were taken. Of the 23 analyzed blood cultures only one showed bacterial growth (Staphylococcus aureus). This patient also showed growth of Staphylococcus aureus in the tracheal aspirate but was not diagnosed as a confirmed VAP according to our applied criteria.

Comparison of agreement in rating all chest x-rays done for suspected neonatal VAP episodes showed an ICC of 0.25, thus showing a poor agreement between the 10 raters.

Quality Improvement Initiative

Characteristics of the NICU's patient population for 2015 - 2017 are shown in **Table 6**. There were no relevant differences except a reduction in mean ventilation days per patient from 2015 to 2017. Implemented changes resulted in a gradual decline in annual neonatal VAP incidence and antibiotic days. The annual neonatal VAP incidence for 2015 vs. 2017 was 28.8 vs. 7.4 suspected episodes/1,000 ventilator-days and 5.5 vs. 0 confirmed episodes/1,000 ventilator-days (**Table 7**). Antibiotic days declined from 211 in 2015 to 34.7 antibiotic days/1,000 ventilator-days in 2017 for suspected episodes and from 52 in 2015 to 0 antibiotic days/1,000 ventilator-days in 2017 for confirmed episodes. Duration of antibiotic treatment of suspected VAP episodes also declined over the years with a median duration of 8 (7–10) days in 2014 vs. 5 (2–7) days in 2017 (**Figure 3**). Cuzick's nonparametric test for trend showed a statistically significant trend for decreasing annual incidence of suspected VAP episodes, decreasing duration of antibiotic therapy per suspected VAP episode as well as decreasing annual antibiotic days for suspected VAP episodes from 2015 to 2017 (**Table 7**).

DISCUSSION

Our literature review showed that CDC guidelines for infants ≤1 year old or similar criteria to diagnose neonatal VAP were most often applied. These criteria are not especially adapted for the neonate or premature born population. The diagnostic criteria in 16 out of the 17 studies in our literature review requested abnormal chest x-rays. Evaluation of all chest x-rays done for suspected VAP episodes in our NICU showed a poor agreement between 10 senior physicians. This is in line with published studies describing the challenges of interpreting radiographic changes in patients with underlying lung diseases (29, 42, 43). An alternative diagnostic tool for lung pathologies is lung ultrasound (LUS). Different studies described the usefulness and accuracy of lung ultrasound for diagnosis of pneumonia in children (44, 45).

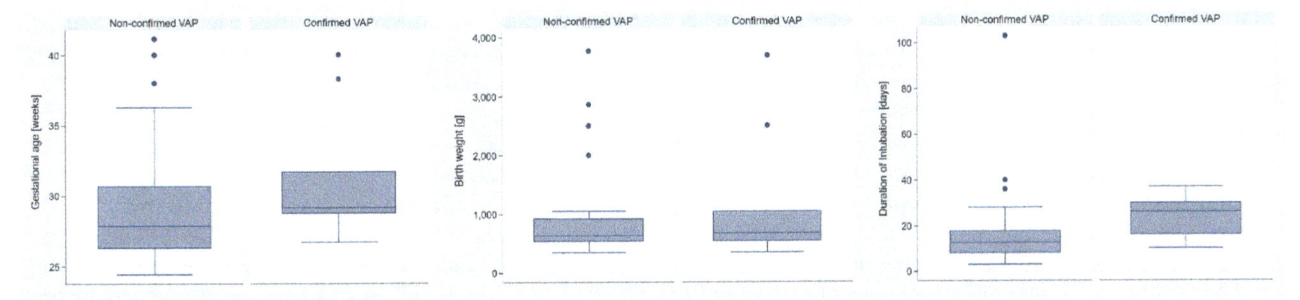

FIGURE 2 | Comparison of gestational age, birth weight and duration of intubation; non-confirmed ($n = 26$) vs. confirmed ($n = 10$) neonatal VAP episodes.

TABLE 5 | Results of analyzed tracheal aspirates.

	Purulent sputum (n)	Positive tracheal aspirate culture (*n*)	Multiple bacterial growth (*n*)	Pathogens
Suspected VAP	13/36	31/36	8/36	
Non-confirmed VAP	9/26	23/26	7/26	15x gram-positive bacteria: 6x Staphylococcus epidermidis, 4x Entero-coccus faecalis, 4x Staphylococcus aureus, 1x Staphylococcus haemolyticus 12x gram-negative bacteria: 3x Escherichia coli, 2x Acinetobacter, 1x Enterobacter aerogenes, 1x Enterobacter cloacae, 1x Pseudomonas aeruginosa, 1x Klebsiella pneumoniae, 1x Klebsiella oxytoca, 1x Stenotrophomonas maltophilia, 1x Serratia marcescens Other: 2x Ureaplasma urealyticum1x Candida albicans 3x no bacterial growth
Confirmed VAP	4/10	8/10	1/10	4x gram-positive bacteria: 1x Staphylococcus aureus, 1x Staphylococcus haemolyticus, 1x Enterococcus faecalis, 1x Bacillus cereus 5x gram-negative bacteria: 3x Escherichia coli, 1x Pseudomonas aeruginosa, 1x Stenotrophomonas maltophilia 2x no bacterial growth

Also, LUS has shown to be highly accurate for diagnosis of neonatal respiratory distress syndrome (46–48). LUS has been shown to be equivalent to chest x-rays in these studies. Hiles et al. (47) even described less intra-observer discrepancy in identification of small pneumonias. Further studies concerning sonographic diagnosis of pneumonia in the neonatal population are needed.

Additionally, unspecific clinical and laboratory findings challenge further the correct diagnosis of neonatal VAP (3, 49). Existence of purulent sputum is part of most used diagnostic criteria for VAP[1] (22, 23). Only 4/10 of our confirmed neonatal VAP episodes showed purulent sputum. On the other hand, 31 out of all 36 neonates and 23 of the 26 non-confirmed VAP episodes showed bacterial growth in the analyzed tracheal aspirate. This might be caused by a high rate of colonization without clinical relevance. Cultures of tracheal aspirates are routinely taken if VAP is suspected although they are not part of most diagnostic criteria (37). Other authors described the frequent occurance of colonized tracheal aspirates (37, 50). A study by Ruiz et al. (51) showed no significant difference in diagnostic accuracy between noninvasive (tracheobronchial aspiration) vs. invasive (fiberoptic bronchoscopy with protected specimen brush and bronchoalveolar lavage) investigation techniques regarding VAP, thus not supporting more invasive procedures with more side effects. A study comparing treated vs. untreated episodes of culture-positive endotracheal aspirates showed that treated episodes also showed worse ventilation conditions, clinical symptoms and laboratory parameters (37), highlighting the limited usefulness of one diagnostic parameter by itself.

The moderate correlation for diagnosis of VAP according to 4 different frameworks in our study underlines the diagnostic problem. Incidence of VAP is often used as quality indicator and the discussed insecurity regarding diagnosis is a potential bias (49). Our findings, consistent with the published literature regarding the difficulty to diagnose neonatal VAP, demand an adaption of current diagnostic criteria for the neonatal population. On the other hand, due to the critical illness of neonates on the ventilator, early start of empiric antibiotic therapy for suspected VAP is mandatory. The challenge is to reevaluate empiric therapy after 24 to 36 hours combining clinical, laboratory and cultural findings. **Figure 4** shows a possible algorithm to approach suspected VAP.

Comparison of incidence between suspected and confirmed neonatal VAP episodes in our NICU showed a 4.5 times higher rate for suspected vs. confirmed VAP episodes/1,000 ventilator-days (20.4 vs. 4.5). Our rate of 4.5 confirmed VAP episodes/1,000 ventilator-days over the whole study period is in line with the published incidence in the studies in our systematic review (2.7–11.8 in developed countries). Prompt antibiotic therapy for possible infections is important for optimal outcome in the neonate population (15) and newborns with suspected VAP are often treated empirically without reviewing defined criteria for VAP (6). Median duration of antibiotic treatment for suspected and confirmed VAP episodes in our cohort was 7 (2–18) and 7.5 (5–18) days, respectively. Also, Cantey et al. recently reported a wide range of antibiotic treatment duration for culture-negative neonatal pneumonia from 5 to 14 days (median 7 days) (5). Taking into account antibiotic treatment for all episodes of suspected neonatal VAP, overall antibiotic use is much higher than reported for confirmed VAP. Our results show a 3.5 times higher number in antibiotic days when including all suspected VAP episodes. We conclude that an inclusion of suspected VAP episodes should be considered for accurate assessment and quality control of VAP incidence and antibiotic use in the neonatal population.

Implementation of multifaceted changes regarding antimicrobial stewardship as well as infection control in our NICU resulted in an annual decrease of suspected and confirmed VAP episodes. Infection control measures are aimed at the prevention of nosocomial or healthcare-associated infections (52). Methods used for infection control include hand hygiene, isolation guidelines, handling and disinfection of patient care equipment, instruments and devices and use of personnel protective equipment (53). Introduction of VAP-care-bundles to prevent infections has already been done in different units showing a potential significant reduction of VAP episodes after implementation (8, 9). Furthermore, our changes resulted in an important annual decline in overall antibiotic days and treatment days per VAP episode. Antimicrobial stewardship aims to reduce inappropriate antibiotic therapy by improving selection, duration, dosage and application route of drugs (54). A systematic review by Kaki et al. (54) showed that implementation of antimicrobial stewardship interventions in different hospitals resulted in reduction of overall antibiotic use, inappropriate therapy, duration of therapy and adverse events toward antibiotics. A recently published antibiotic stewardship study by Cantey et al. (5) reported a safe reduction of antibiotic use for pneumonia in a NICU population. The implemented changes in our unit not only reduced confirmed neonatal VAP episodes, but also the numbers of suspected episodes. This resulted in a 6-fold reduction of at least partly unnecessary antibiotic days per 1,000 ventilator-days (211 vs. 34.7/1,000 ventilator-days for 2015 vs. 2017) and a statistically significant trend for decreasing duration of antibiotic therapy and antibiotic days in total over time from 2015 to 2017. Both, reduction of antibiotic days as well as declining VAP incidences resulted in this trend, with reduction of VAP episodes statistically being the more important composite. As several changes were initiated at various time points, it is not possible to distinguish the impact of a single measure. We assume that both, infection control and

TABLE 6 | Annual comparison of clinical characteristics of the patient population in our NICU.

	2015	2016	2017
Newborns n	302	299	291
Preterm infants <32 weeks of gestation n (%)	63 (20.9%)	76 (25.4%)	82 (28.2%)
Preterm infants <28 weeks of gestation n (%)	22 (7.3%)	23 (7.7%)	26 (8.9%)
Mechanically ventilated newborns n (%)	97 (32.1%)	82 (27.4%)	82 (28.2%)
Ventilation days n	730	436	404
Duration (days) of mechanical ventilation (mean)	7.5	5.3	4.9
Newborns with CPAP n (%)	185 (61.3%)	199 (66.6%)	244 (83.8%)
CRIB II - Score	6.5 (±2.8)	6 (±2.8)	5.7 (±2.5)
Hospitalization days n	1,968	1,622	1,622
Mortality newborns n (%)	10 (3.3%)	6 (2%)	5 (1.7%)
Mortality preterm infants <32 weeks of gestation, n (%)	6 (9.5%)	3 (3.9%)	3 (3.7%)
Mortality preterm infants <28 weeks of gestation, n (%)	5 (22.7%)	3 (13%)	3 (11.5%)

TABLE 7 | Incidence of suspected and confirmed neonatal VAP and antibiotic use.

	2014 (only 09-12/14)	2015	2016	2017	Total
Suspected VAP episodes n	4	21	8	3	36
Suspected VAP episodes n/1,000 ventilator-days*		28.8	18.3	7.4	20.4
Antibiotic days for suspected episodes n/1,000 ventilator-days*		211	107.8	34.7	136.9
Duration of antibiotic treatment/suspected VAP episode median in days (min – max)**	8 (7–10)	7 (2–18)	6.5 (3–9)	5 (2–7)	7 (2–18)
Confirmed VAP episodes n	3	4	3	0	10
Confirmed VAP episodes n/1,000 ventilator-days		5.5	6.9	0	4.5
Antibiotic days for confirmed episodes n/1,000 ventilator-days		52.1	50.5		38.2
Duration of antibiotic treatment/confirmed VAP episode median in days (min – max)	9 (7–10)	7.5 (5–18)	7 (6–9)		7.5 (5–18)

*Cuzick's nonparametric test for trend $p < 0.001$.

** Cuzick's nonparametric test for trend $p = 0.005$.

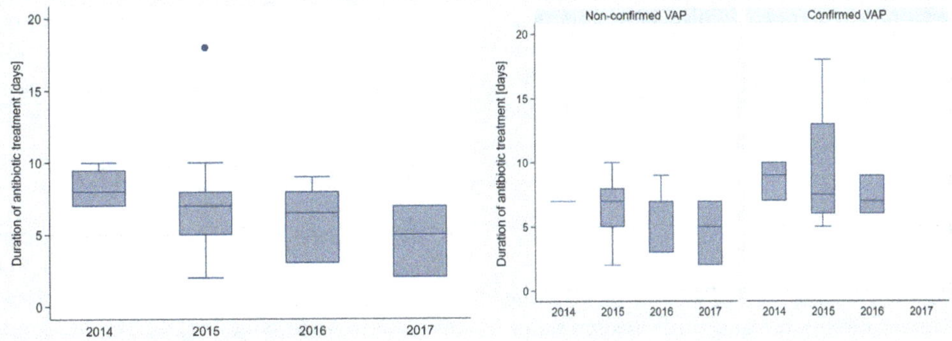

FIGURE 3 | Comparison of duration of antibiotic treatment (antibiotic days/VAP episode) according to year. Left: all episodes ($n = 36$), right: non-confirmed ($n = 26$) vs. confirmed ($n = 10$) neonatal VAP.

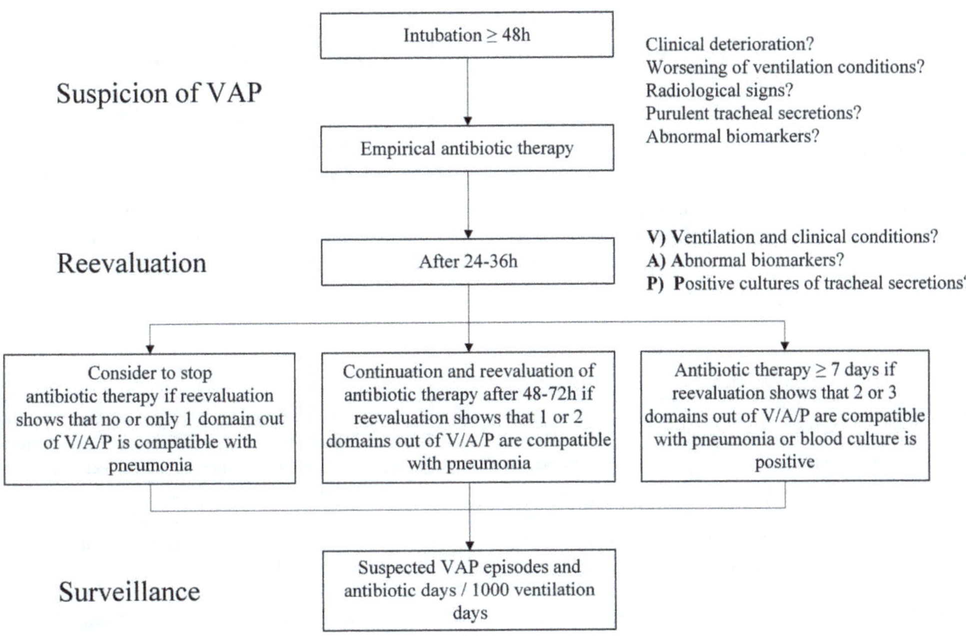

FIGURE 4 | Possible algorithm to approach suspected VAP.

antibiotic stewardship measures together had an impact on the observed reduction in incidence of neonatal VAP and antibiotic use: antimicrobial stewardship measures by increasing awareness toward antibiotic therapy, and infection control measures by reducing VAP episodes and thus antibiotic therapy. A position paper published by the Association for Professionals in Infection Control and Epidemiology (APIC), the Society for Healthcare Epidemiology of America (SHEA), and the Society of Infectious Disease Pharmacists (SIDP) stated the importance of joining antimicrobial stewardship and infection control measures, as implementation of a combination of both is more effective than one measure by itself (10).

All studies in our systematic review state long duration of mechanical ventilation as a risk factor for developing neonatal VAP. Comparing patient population of non-confirmed vs. confirmed VAP episodes, confirmed episodes in our NICU were also associated with longer duration of mechanical ventilation. Studies by Hentschel et al. (55) and Geffers et al. (56) showed lower pneumonia rates in patients ventilated with CPAP-devices compared to intubated patients. These studies support the strategy toward early extubation. Implementation of our early-extubation policy in our unit resulted in a decrease of duration of invasive ventilation without increase of mortality.

There are several limitations to our study: Firstly and most important, this is not an intervention study with a control group aiming to prove the causative benefit of the implemented changes. Nevertheless, the reduction of incidence and antibiotic use for neonatal VAP is remarkable. The NICU's patient population did not change remarkably over the three years and there were no other changes over the study period applied. Therefore, we could not determine any other apparent reason for the decline in numbers. Secondly, the sample size of VAP episodes is small and therefore it was not possible to further analyze and compare more risk factors or clinical indicators. Also numbers for confirmed VAP episodes are only descriptive as no further statistical calculations were done due to the even smaller sample size. Thirdly, whereas all VAP episodes were collected prospectively, diagnostic analyzes according to the 4 frameworks were done in retrospect.

CONCLUSIONS

Diagnosis and confirmation of neonatal VAP is difficult, resulting in a great variance between suspected and confirmed episodes. An adaption of current diagnostic criteria for the neonate population might be helpful for more consistency. Inclusion of both confirmed and suspected episodes should be considered for accurate evaluation and comparison of VAP incidence and antibiotic use in the neonatal population as quality indicators. Implementation of combined antimicrobial stewardship and infection control measures may lead to an effective decrease in both VAP incidence and antibiotic use.

ETHICS STATEMENT

The study was carried out in accordance with the recommendations of the national ethics committee (Ethikkommission Nordwest- und Zentralschweiz EKNZ: Project-ID 2017-01842) with informed consent from patients' parents/guardians. The EKNZ exempt to have a written consent due to the fully anonymized data and the quality improvement focus of the study without need of additional information than obtained from patient files.

AUTHOR CONTRIBUTIONS

MS devised the project, details of implementation were discussed between MS and AG. Data collection and writing of the manuscript was done by AG, closely revised by MS. Statistical calculations were done by DL. The literature review was done by AG. Interpretation of chest-x-rays was done by NR, MB, ML, KD, KS-S, SP, PG, DM, MF, and MS. Critical revising of the work was done by TN, NR, MB, ML, KS-S, SP, PG, DM, MF, and KD. All authors read and approved the submitted version of this manuscript.

ACKNOWLEDGMENTS

Special thanks to Barbara Imboden, the NICU's data manager for all the work she has put in this beforehand and of course the indispensable nursing team of our NICU. Special thanks as well to Evelyne Eichenberger and Luzia Vetter being part of the interprofessional working group for development and implementation of the VAP-prevention-bundle.

REFERENCES

1. Cernada M, Aguar M, Brugada M, Gutiérrez A, López JL, Castell M, et al. Ventilator-associated pneumonia in newborn infants diagnosed with an invasive bronchoalveolar lavage technique: a prospective observational study. *Pediatr Crit Care Med.* (2013) 14:55–61. doi: 10.1097/PCC.0b013e318253ca31
2. Hooven TA, Polin RA. Pneumonia. *Semin Fetal Neonatal Med.* (2017) 22:206–13. doi: 10.1016/j.siny.2017.03.002
3. Cernada M, Brugada M, Golombek S, Vento M. Ventilator-associated pneumonia in neonatal patients: an update. *Neonatology* (2014) 105:98–107. doi: 10.1159/000355539
4. Willson DF, Hoot M, Khemani R, Carrol C, Kirby A, Schwarz A, et al. Pediatric ventilator-associated infections: the ventilator-associated infection study. *Pediatr Crit Care Med.* (2017) 18:e24–34. doi: 10.1097/PCC.0000000000001001
5. Cantey JB, Wozniak PS, Pruszynski JE, Sánchez PJ. Reducing unnecessary antibiotic use in the neonatal intensive care unit (SCOUT): a prospective interrupted time-series study. *Lancet Infect Dis.* (2016) 16:1178–84. doi: 10.1016/S1473-3099(16)30205-5
6. Cantey JB, Wozniak PS, Sánchez PJ. Prospective surveillance of antibiotic use in the neonatal intensive care unit: results from the SCOUT study. *Pediatr Infect Dis J.* (2015) 34:267–72. doi: 10.1097/INF.0000000000000542
7. Bradley JS. Considerations unique to pediatrics for clinical trial design in hospital-acquired pneumonia and ventilator-associated pneumonia. *Clin Infect Dis.* (2010) 51(Suppl. 1):S136–43. doi: 10.1086/653063
8. Azab SFA, Sherbiny HS, Saleh SH, Elsaeed WF, Elshafiey MM, Siam AG, et al. Reducing ventilator-associated pneumonia in neonatal intensive care unit using "VAP prevention Bundle": a cohort study. *BMC Infect Dis.* (2015) 15:314. doi: 10.1186/s12879-015-1062-1
9. Weber CD. Applying adult ventilator-associated pneumonia bundle evidence to the ventilated neonate. *Adv Neonatal Care* (2016) 16:178–90. doi: 10.1097/ANC.0000000000000276
10. Manning ML, Septimus EJ, Ashley ESD, Cosgrove SE, Fakih MG, Schweon SJ, et al. Antimicrobial stewardship and infection prevention—leveraging the synergy: a position paper update. *Infect Control Hosp Epidemiol.* (2018) 39:467–72. doi: 10.1017/ice.2018.33
11. Spitzer AR. Has quality improvement really improved outcomes for babies in the neonatal intensive care unit? *Clin Perinatol.* (2017) 44:469–83. doi: 10.1016/j.clp.2017.04.005
12. Clark RH, Bloom BT, Spitzer AR, Gerstmann DR. Reported medication use in the neonatal intensive care unit: data from a large national data set. *Pediatrics* (2006) 117:1979–87. doi: 10.1542/peds.2005-1707
13. Schulman J, Dimand RJ, Lee HC, Duenas GV, Bennett MV, Gould JB. Neonatal intensive care unit antibiotic use. *Pediatrics* (2015) 135:826–33. doi: 10.1542/peds.2014-3409
14. Liem TBY, Krediet TG, Fleer A, Egberts TCG, Rademaker CMA. Variation in antibiotic use in neonatal intensive care units in the Netherlands. *J Antimicrob Chemother.* (2010) 65:1270–5. doi: 10.1093/jac/dkq107
15. Weiss SL, Fitzgerald JC, Balamuth F, Alpern ER, Lavelle J, Chilutti M, et al. Delayed antimicrobial therapy increases mortality and organ dysfunction duration in pediatric sepsis. *Crit Care Med.* (2014) 42:2409–17. doi: 10.1097/CCM.0000000000000509
16. Cantey JB, Patel SJ. Antimicrobial stewardship in the NICU. *Infect Dis Clin North Am.* (2014) 28:247–61. doi: 10.1016/j.idc.2014.01.005
17. Jernberg C, Löfmark S, Edlund C, Jansson JK. Long-term impacts of antibiotic exposure on the human intestinal microbiota. *Microbiol Read Engl.* (2010) 156:3216–23. doi: 10.1099/mic.0.040618-0
18. Schulfer A, Blaser MJ. Risks of antibiotic exposures early in life on the developing microbiome. *PLoS Pathog* (2015) 11:e1004903. doi: 10.1371/journal.ppat.1004903
19. Gensollen T, Iyer SS, Kasper DL, Blumberg RS. How colonization by microbiota in early life shapes the immune system. *Science* (2016) 352:539–44. doi: 10.1126/science.aad9378

20. Mukhopadhyay S, Puopolo KM. Antibiotic use and mortality among premature infants without confirmed infection-perpetrator or innocent bystander? *JAMA Pediatr.* (2016) 170:1144–6. doi: 10.1001/jamapediatrics.2016.2836
21. Ting JY, Synnes A, Roberts A, Deshpandey A, Dow K, Yoon EW, et al. Association between antibiotic use and neonatal mortality and morbidities in very low-birth-weight infants without culture-proven sepsis or necrotizing enterocolitis. *JAMA Pediatr.* (2016) 170:1181–7. doi: 10.1001/jamapediatrics.2016.2132
22. 6pscvapcurrent.pdf. Available online at: https://www.cdc.gov/nhsn/pdfs/pscmanual/6pscvapcurrent.pdf (Accessed September 16, 2017).
23. van der Zwet WC, Kaiser AM, van Elburg RM, Berkhof J, Fetter WPF, Parlevliet GA, et al. Nosocomial infections in a Dutch neonatal intensive care unit: surveillance study with definitions for infection specifically adapted for neonates. *J Hosp Infect.* (2005) 61:300–11. doi: 10.1016/j.jhin.2005.03.014
24. Liberati A, Altman DG, Tetzlaff J, Mulrow C, Gotzsche PC, Ioannidis JPA, et al. The PRISMA statement for reporting systematic reviews and meta-analyses of studies that evaluate healthcare interventions: explanation and elaboration. *BMJ* (2009) 339:b2700. doi: 10.1136/bmj.b2700
25. Berger TM, Steurer MA, Woerner A, Meyer-Schiffer P, Adams M, Swiss Neonatal Network. Trends and centre-to-centre variability in survival rates of very preterm infants (<32 weeks) over a 10-year-period in Switzerland. *Arch Dis Child Fetal Neonatal Ed.* (2012) 97:F323–8. doi: 10.1136/fetalneonatal-2011-301008
26. Cuzick J. A wilcoxon-type test for trend. *Stat Med.* (1985) 4:87–90. doi: 10.1002/sim.4780040112
27. Afjeh SA, Sabzehei MK, Karimi A, Shiva F, Shamshiri AR. Surveillance of ventilator-associated pneumonia in a neonatal intensive care unit: characteristics, risk factors, and outcome. *Arch Iran Med.* (2012) 15:567–71. doi: 012159/AIM.0012
28. Apisarnthanarak A, Holzmann-Pazgal G, Hamvas A, Olsen MA, Fraser VJ. Ventilator-associated pneumonia in extremely preterm neonates in a neonatal intensive care unit: characteristics, risk factors, and outcomes. *Pediatrics* (2003) 112:1283–9. doi: 10.1542/peds.112.6.1283
29. Foglia E, Meier MD, Elward A. Ventilator-associated pneumonia in neonatal and pediatric intensive care unit patients. *Clin Microbiol Rev.* (2007) 20:409–25, table of contents. doi: 10.1128/CMR.00041-06
30. Badr MA, Ali YF, Albanna EAM, Beshir MR, Amr GE. Ventilator associated pneumonia in critically-ill neonates admitted to neonatal intensive care unit, zagazig university hospitals. *Iran J Pediatr.* (2011) 21:418–24.
31. Deng C, Li X, Zou Y, Wang J, Wang J, Namba F, et al. Risk factors and pathogen profile of ventilator-associated pneumonia in a neonatal intensive care unit in China. *Pediatr Int.* (2011) 53:332–7. doi: 10.1111/j.1442-200X.2011.03382.x
32. 20272-pdf.pdf. Available online at: http://cdn.neoscriber.org/cdn/serve/313ea/c85402d4f1abb36c538a084940e4815755ccd005/20272-pdf.pdf (Accessed March 2, 2018).
33. Katayama Y, Minami H, Enomoto M, Takano T, Hayashi S, Lee YK. Usefulness of Gram staining of tracheal aspirates in initial therapy for ventilator-associated pneumonia in extremely preterm neonates. *J Perinatol.* (2010) 30:270–4. doi: 10.1038/jp.2009.144
34. Kawanishi F, Yoshinaga M, Morita M, Shibata Y, Yamada T, Ooi Y, et al. Risk factors for ventilator-associated pneumonia in neonatal intensive care unit patients. *J Infect Chemother.* (2014) 20:627–30. doi: 10.1016/j.jiac.2014.06.006
35. Khattab AA, El-Lahony DM, Soliman WF. Ventilator-associated pneumonia in the neonatal intensive care unit. *Menoufia Med J.* (2014) 27:73–7. doi: 10.4103/1110-2098.132753
36. Lee P-L, Lee W-T, Chen H-L. Ventilator-associated pneumonia in low birth weight neonates at a neonatal intensive care unit: a retrospective observational study. *Pediatr Neonatol.* (2017) 58:16–21. doi: 10.1016/j.pedneo.2015.10.014
37. Murila F, Francis JV, Bland A, Kumbla S, Doherty R, Sehgal A. Interpreting positive cultures of endotracheal aspirates: factors associated with treatment decisions in ventilated neonates. *J Paediatr Child Health* (2011) 47:728–33. doi: 10.1111/j.1440-1754.2011.02041.x
38. Petdachai W. Ventilator-associated pneumonia in a newborn intensive care unit. *Southeast Asian J Trop Med Public Health* (2004) 35:724–9.
39. Thatrimontrichai A, Rujeerapaiboon N, Janjindamai W, Dissaneevate S, Maneenil G, Kritsaneepaiboon S, et al. Outcomes and risk factors of ventilator-associated pneumonia in neonates. *World J Pediatr.* (2017) 13:328–34. doi: 10.1007/s12519-017-0010-0
40. Paper02_Jan2010_.pdf. Available online at: http://www.akspublication.com/Paper02_Jan2010_.pdf?B1=Full$+$Text$+$PDF (Accessed March 2, 2018).
41. Yuan T-M, Chen L-H, Yu H-M. Risk factors and outcomes for ventilator-associated pneumonia in neonatal intensive care unit patients. *J Perinat Med.* (2007) 35:334–8. doi: 10.1515/JPM.2007.065
42. Klompas M. Interobserver variability in ventilator-associated pneumonia surveillance. *Am J Infect Control.* (2010) 38:237–9. doi: 10.1016/j.ajic.2009.10.003
43. Morrow BM, Argent AC. Filling the gaps in neonatal VAP. *Pediatr Crit Care Med.* (2013) 14:105–6. doi: 10.1097/PCC.0b013e31825b8648
44. Copetti R, Cattarossi L. Ultrasound diagnosis of pneumonia in children. *Radiol Med.* (2008) 113:190–8. doi: 10.1007/s11547-008-0247-8
45. Reali F, Sferrazza Papa GF, Carlucci P, Fracasso P, Di Marco F, Mandelli M, et al. Can lung ultrasound replace chest radiography for the diagnosis of pneumonia in hospitalized children? *Respiration* (2014) 88:112–5. doi: 10.1159/000362692
46. Lovrenski J. Lung ultrasonography of pulmonary complications in preterm infants with respiratory distress syndrome. *Ups J Med Sci.* (2012) 117:10–7. doi: 10.3109/03009734.2011.643510
47. Hiles M, Culpan A-M, Watts C, Munyombwe T, Wolstenhulme S. Neonatal respiratory distress syndrome: chest X-ray or lung ultrasound? a systematic review. *Ultrasound* (2017) 25:80–91. doi: 10.1177/1742271X16689374
48. Vergine M, Copetti R, Brusa G, Cattarossi L. Lung ultrasound accuracy in respiratory distress syndrome and transient tachypnea of the newborn. *Neonatology* (2014) 106:87–93. doi: 10.1159/000358227
49. Cordero L, Ayers LW, Miller RR, Seguin JH, Coley BD. Surveillance of ventilator-associated pneumonia in very-low-birth-weight infants. *Am J Infect Control* (2002) 30:32–9. doi: 10.1067/mic.2002.119995
50. Gibbs K, Holzman IR. Endotracheal tube: friend or foe? bacteria, the endotracheal tube, and the impact of colonization and infection. *Semin Perinatol.* (2012) 36:454–61. doi: 10.1053/j.semperi.2012.06.008
51. Ruiz M, Torres A, Ewig S, Marcos MA, Alcón A, Lledó R, et al. Noninvasive versus invasive microbial investigation in ventilator-associated pneumonia. *Am J Respir Crit Care Med.* (2000) 162:119–25. doi: 10.1164/ajrccm.162.1.9907090
52. WHO-HIS-SDS-2016.10-eng.pdf. Available online at: http://apps.who.int/iris/bitstream/handle/10665/246235/WHO-HIS-SDS-2016.10-eng.pdf;jsessionid=6C5077BF50A066B4F577CA5882023273?sequence=1 (Accessed April 15, 2018).
53. *Infection Control Basics. Infection Control CDC.* Available online at: https://www.cdc.gov/infectioncontrol/basics/index.html (Accessed April 15, 2018).
54. Kaki R, Elligsen M, Walker S, Simor A, Palmay L, Daneman N. Impact of antimicrobial stewardship in critical care: a systematic review. *J Antimicrob Chemother.* (2011) 66:1223–30. doi: 10.1093/jac/dkr137
55. Hentschel J, Brüngger B, Stüdi K, Mühlemann K. Prospective surveillance of nosocomial infections in a Swiss NICU: low risk of pneumonia on nasal continuous positive airway pressure? *Infection* (2005) 33:350–5. doi: 10.1007/s15010-005-5052-x
56. Geffers C, Baerwolff S, Schwab F, Gastmeier P. Incidence of healthcare-associated infections in high-risk neonates: results from the German surveillance system for very-low-birthweight infants. *J Hosp Infect.* (2008) 68:214–21. doi: 10.1016/j.jhin.2008.01.016

17

The Role of Parental Concerns in the Recognition of Sepsis in Children

Amanda Harley[1,2,3]*, Jos M. Latour*[4] *and Luregn J. Schlapbach*[1,2,5]*

[1] Paediatric Critical Care Research Group, Child Health Research Centre and Faculty of Medicine, The University of Queensland, Brisbane, QLD, Australia, [2] Paediatric Intensive Care Unit, Queensland Children's Hospital, Children's Health Queensland, Brisbane, QLD, Australia, [3] School of Nursing, The University of Queensland, Brisbane, QLD, Australia, [4] Faculty of Health and Human Sciences, School of Nursing and Midwifery, University of Plymouth, Plymouth, United Kingdom, [5] Department of Paediatrics, Bern University Hospital, Inselspital, University of Bern, Bern, Switzerland

***Correspondence:**
Luregn J. Schlapbach
l.schlapbach@uq.edu.au*

Background: Sepsis is a time critical disease and outcomes strongly depend on time to initiation of appropriate treatment in hospital. A range of studies have assessed sepsis recognition in hospital settings, whereas little is known about sepsis recognition in the community. The decision-making of parents in seeking medical care may substantially impact survival of children with sepsis. An improved understanding of the parental perspective in recognizing sepsis is urgently needed to inform the design of education campaigns and consideration of using parental concerns as a trigger in sepsis screening tools.

Aim: To review the literature on parental concerns in the diagnosis of sepsis in children.

Methods: A literature review on parental concerns in pediatric sepsis was performed accessing publications in PubMed, CINAHL and Medline published between 1990 and 2018. In addition, we compared guidelines and online institutional sepsis recognition tools and assessed whether parental concerns were used for screening.

Results: Out of 188 articles reviewed, 11 met the criteria. One article was found prospectively assessing the diagnostic performance of parental concern in children evaluated for infection, indicating high positive (16.4) and negative likelihood ratio (0.23) for sepsis/meningitis in presence of parental concerns. The role of parental concern was listed as a sign assisting recognition of sepsis in four studies reporting original data, and six reviews commented on parental concern listed as a factor upon diagnosis of sepsis. When comparing selected examples of institutional sepsis pathways available online, parental concern was variably listed as a criterion to prompt evaluation for sepsis.

Conclusions: Despite some guidelines emphasizing the role of parental concern in recognizing sepsis, there is a paucity of data in the field. An improved understanding of whether parental concerns adds diagnostic value to sepsis recognition at acceptable sensitivity and specificity is urgently needed. Future prospective studies should assess whether including parental concerns in sepsis screening tools benefits the assessment resulting in early diagnosis and treatment of children with sepsis.

Keywords: child, concern, diagnosis, infection, parent, recognition, sepsis, septic shock

INTRODUCTION

Sepsis represents a leading cause of global childhood mortality (1–3). In response to the recent resolution by the World Health Organization recognizing sepsis as a priority in healthcare(4, 5), several national and regional healthcare systems have implemented sepsis pathways to improve recognition and early treatment of sepsis in hospital settings (6). Sepsis in children remains a time critical disease and the majority of deaths and multi-organ dysfunction occur within the first 48 h of admission (7–10), highlighting the relevance of timely intervention. While interventional trials in children and adults have failed to result in reduced mortality (11–13), observational studies have consistently indicated that time to sepsis treatment strongly impacts on sepsis survival (14–18).

Physiologic criteria, early warning tools, and electronic health-record based trigger tools have been reported to improve the recognition of children with severe bacterial infections, and sepsis (19–23). Currently used sepsis recognition tools yield high sensitivity but mostly at the expense of poor specificity, given that most infectious illnesses in children manifest with fever, tachycardia, and tachypnea (24, 25). Inaccurate sepsis diagnosis may lead to unnecessary antibiotic therapy, hospitalization, and missed alternative diagnoses. The importance of balancing the need for rapid sepsis recognition vs. potential adverse effects on patients, healthcare resource use and antimicrobial resistance related to overtreatment is becoming increasingly recognized (26, 27) implicating an urgent need for rigorous studies on sepsis recognition.

Importantly, sepsis starts most commonly in the community and the decision and timing of parents in seeking medical care for children is likely to contribute to severity upon presentation and sepsis-related outcomes. Root cause analyses after fatal sepsis outcomes in children often report on recurrent presentations to hospital (16) and anecdotal data reveals parents in such cases often indicated concerns that "this disease is different" suggesting parents may have sensed the potential severity of the disease prior to the recognition of sepsis by clinicians. Increasing parental education has been demonstrated to reduce infant mortality due to infections in low income settings (28, 29). Yet the potential value of including parental assessment in discriminating children with mild infections from sepsis has received little attention. The capacity of parents to assess whether a disease presents differently to previous common febrile illnesses could potentially result in improved diagnostic accuracy of sepsis assessment.

We therefore aimed to review the literature on parental concerns in recognizing sepsis in children, with particular focus on studies reporting on diagnostic accuracy. In addition, we searched whether online available institutional sepsis screening tools include parental concern as a trigger for recognition or escalation.

METHODS

Objectives

To review the literature on parental concern in the diagnosis of sepsis in children.

Eligibility Criteria

The Population-Intervention-Control-Outcome-Study design (PICOS) approach was applied and guided the literature review focusing on: (P) pediatric age groups of <18 years of age; with (I) parental concern utilized as an assessment tool; (C) control consisting of standard diagnostic approach without including parental concern as a diagnostic tool; (O) diagnosis of sepsis and diagnostic accuracy of sepsis diagnosis as outcomes; and (S) both quantitative and qualitative original research, case reports, editorials/viewpoints, guidelines, and reviews included.

Search Strategy

Three strategies for data collection were utilized: First, a comprehensive search for published literature through international databases was performed. Second, we manually searched reference lists from articles identified through the database search. Third, we considered additional articles identified as relevant by the authors. Publications were accessed in three literature databases: MEDLINE, CINAHL and PUBMED. Search terms used included: "Concern" OR "worry" OR "fear," AND "infant" OR "pediatric" OR "pediatric" OR "child" OR "neonate" OR "childhood," AND "sepsis" OR "septic" OR "severe sepsis" OR "septic shock" OR "bacteremia" OR "severe infection" OR "systemic inflammatory response syndrome," AND "parent" OR "family" OR "caregiver" OR "mother" OR "father" (**Supplementary Table 1**).

Studies were considered if they were published as full text in the English language between January 1st 1990 and September 1st 2018. Duplicate references were removed manually. Original research, case reports, editorials/viewpoints, guidelines, and reviews were considered. The initial title and abstract screen for further review was conducted by two authors (AH, LS). Articles for full text review were selected by applying the search terms to the titles and abstracts of articles.

We then performed a two-stage review of full text articles. In the first stage, we searched articles that provided original data on parental concerns in pediatric sepsis. We considered publications that defined sepsis, including septic shock and severe sepsis, according to the 2005 International Pediatric Sepsis Definition Conference (30), the American College of Chest Physicians (31), or adaptations from the recent Sepsis-3 criteria (24, 32). We included articles which reported on parental concern for children below 18 years as part of diagnostic assessment for patients presenting with sepsis or severe infection. Given the low yield of only one article meeting the PICOS criteria, we included studies reporting on severe infections, and bacteraemia. In the second stage, we searched full-text articles that reported on the use or importance of parental concerns in pediatric sepsis without providing original data.

Articles were excluded if full text was unavailable in English was unavailable. All full text articles identified underwent review by two independent investigators (AH, LJS). Clarification for inclusion was resolved by discussion. Due to the paucity of data reporting on diagnostic accuracy, sensitivity, specificity, and negative and positive predictive value in relation to parental concern, a meta-analysis could not be performed.

Inclusion of Parental Concerns in Pediatric Sepsis Pathways

In order to compare examples of pediatric sepsis pathways in relation to utilization of parental concern, we selected published or online accessible pediatric sepsis pathways available in English language which were published in the past 5 years (date of updated search September 1st 2018). We limited the search to published international pediatric sepsis guidelines, and to pathways of jurisdictions which had previously reported on state- or nationwide sepsis campaigns (14, 33–35). This resulted in examples of pathways from three continents (North America, Europe and Oceania). These examples were selected to show different approaches to the recognition of sepsis in children. Pathways were then searched for the presence of a field listing parental concern as a risk factor or warning sign for sepsis. We considered terms such as "concern" (OR "worry" OR "fear"), and "parent" (OR "family" OR "caregiver" OR "mother/maternal" OR "father/paternal").

RESULTS

Study Selection

The search of the databases yielded 219 results and an additional four articles through other sources. After exclusion of duplicates and records in languages other than English, 188 remained (**Figure 1**). Abstract review by two assessors excluded 156 articles as the records were not reporting on sepsis diagnosis pertinent to parental concerns and children. Reference chaining identified a further 19 articles. In total, 51 Articles were selected for full-text review by two assessors. Of these, a further 40 were excluded because of one study in non-English language (36), and 39 because they did not report on parental concern in relation to recognition of sepsis. We included 11 articles in the review, of which five reported original data, out of which one only reported on diagnostic accuracy. Six articles were reviews reporting on parental concern without original data.

Study Characteristics

Only one study reported original data on diagnostic accuracy of parental assessment in relation to sepsis (**Table 1**). Van den Bruel performed a prospective multicenter study in primary care settings including 3981 children which presented to 121 physicians (General practitioners, pediatricians, and emergency physicians) (37). The study was designed to assess diagnostic accuracy of several clinical features including physiological variables, clinician perception that "something is wrong," and parental concern. Parental concern was defined as the parental perception or statement that the "disease is different." Classification and regression tree analysis was performed to define the best performing criteria and criteria combination for clinical practice. Out of the 3981 included children (mean age 5.0 years, range = 0.02–16.9 years), 31 (0.78%) had a serious bacterial infection and 9 (0.22%) were diagnosed with sepsis and/or meningitis. Presence of parental concern that the disease is different was associated with an odds ratio (OR) of 70.5 (95%-CI 14.5 to 341.4) for sepsis/meningitis in the decision tree model, and a sensitivity of 77.8%, specificity of 95.1%, positive predictive value (PPV) of 3.6%, negative predictive value (NPV) of 100%, positive likelihood ratio (PLR) of 16.4, and negative likelihood ratio (NLR) of 0.23. In comparison, the assessment by the treating physician that "something is wrong" was associated with sepsis with an OR of 268 (33–2,163) and a sensitivity of 88.9% and specificity of 97.1%. The sensitivity of parental concern to capture any serious bacterial infection was 46.4%, and the according specificity was 96.8%, PPV 9.5%, NPV 99.6%, PLR 14.35 and NLR 0.55, respectively.

Four further studies reported original data, however none of these reported on diagnostic accuracy (**Table 2**). A secondary analysis of the 2007 Van den Bruel study investigated the role of clinician's gut feeling that something is wrong in the patients. Parental concern was identified as the strongest factor increasing the likelihood of clinician's gut feeling that something is wrong (univariate OR 26.93; 9.02 to 80.41, multivariate OR 36.26; 12.28 to 107.07) (38). However, the secondary analysis did not comment on the predictive accuracy of parental concern in relation to serious bacterial infection. Another study by Van den Bruel et al. (39) performed qualitative interviews with families and practitioners of 18 children hospitalized for severe bacterial infection with a mean age of 2.5 years (range 14 days to 11 years). Parents reported findings such as "*The moment he was sitting on my lap and suddenly collapsed, I was really frightened and came here immediately. At that moment I just knew it was more than just a cold.*" Van den Bruel et al. (39) referring to a 2-year-old child with sepsis. The authors concluded that parents have a high accuracy in describing the behavior of their children and to assess how the current behavior compares with normal behavior, and with behavior during previous illnesses. Another study performed qualitative interviews with General Practitioners to assess their attitudes in relation to recognizing children with meningitis and meningococcal septicemia (40). No patient data was assessed. Parental concern, and maternal "instinct" that the child was not right were mentioned as sometimes representing the only clues to a severe disease. Another study interviewed 95 parents from primary care inner city settings and performed focus groups to explore parental concerns about acute pediatric illness (41). Fever, cough and risk of meningitis emerged as key areas of concern. Sepsis was not specifically mentioned, however parents reported their fear that they may fail to recognize a life-threatening condition.

Six review articles were included which reported on parental concern in diagnosis of sepsis (**Table 3**). Two systematic reviews analyzed the findings from 36, and 35 articles, respectively, including 30 articles reporting on clinical features in relation to diagnosis of serious infection in children in developed countries (43, 47). The original study of Van den Bruel was the only study in both reviews which reported on parental concern to assist in the diagnosis of serious infection in children (37). While clinician's gut feeling that something was wrong performed better than parental concerns, the diagnostic accuracy of both parental concern and clinician's gut feeling outperformed most routinely used physiological or observational data in other studies. Four further non-systematic reviews and narratives were identified which listed parental concerns as a feature of children presenting with life-threatening infections or sepsis (42, 44–46). These

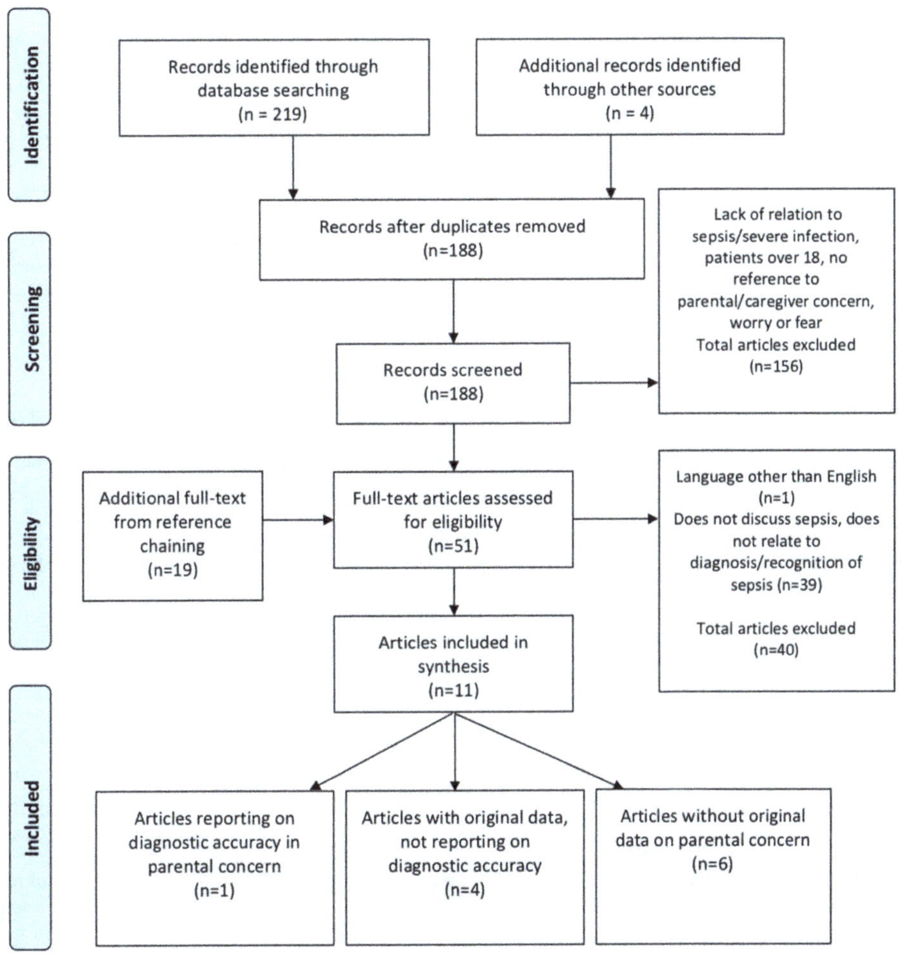

FIGURE 1 | PRISMA flow diagram.

articles did not use any original data to justify this but rather commented on the value of parental concern in the perspective by the authors.

Examples of Use of Parental Concern in Guidelines and Institutional Pathways

We assessed published and online available international pediatric sepsis guidelines pathways and guidelines in relation to the role of parental concern in the recognition of sepsis. In addition, we selected examples of published and online available institutional pathways designed for the recognition of sepsis in children (**Table 4**). The selection was limited to jurisdictions which has previously published on the state- or nation-wide implementation of sepsis bundles, specifically the United Kingdom, New York State in the United States, and New South Wales in Australia (14, 33–35).

Two recent international guidelines pertinent to pediatric age groups, the American College of Critical Care Medicine Guidelines 2017 (48), and the 2013 Surviving Sepsis Campaign (49) guidelines, recommend that institutions implement sepsis screening tools. Parental concerns are not featured in these two guidelines. In contrast, the National Institute for Health and Care Excellence (NICE) (https://www.nice.org.uk/guidance/ng51/resources) and Sepsis Trust (Sepsis 6) (https://sepsistrust.org/professional-resources/clinical/) guidelines in the U.K. Both list parental concern as a feature of sepsis recognition. Two examples of institutional pathways from New York State, United States (http://pediatrics.aappublications.org/content/pediatrics/137/3/e20144082.full.pdf), and New South Wales, Australia (http://www.cec.health.nsw.gov.au/__data/assets/pdf_file/0008/343475/Pediatric-Sepsis-Pathway-Sept-2016-with-watermark.pdf), further illustrate that the utilization of parental concern varies in these pathways. Some list parental concern specifically as a feature that should support clinicians to think "Could this be sepsis," others list it as one of several criteria prompting treatment, and some do not mention parental concern specifically.

DISCUSSION

In this literature review on parental concerns as a tool to assist in the recognition of sepsis, we identified a paucity of

TABLE 1 | Original studies reporting on diagnostic accuracy of parental concern in diagnosis of severe infection and sepsis.

References and country of enrolment	Study design	Patients	Inclusion criteria	Outcomes in relation to parental concern	Comments
Van den Bruel et al. (37), Belgium	Prospective observational multicentre study	3981, of which 31 (0.78%) had a serious infection; of which 9/3981 had sepsis (0.22%)	Children presenting to General practitioner, pediatrician or the emergency department with acute illness	Serious bacterial infection: Pneumonia, meningitis, sepsis, pyelonephritis, osteomyelitis, bacterial gastroenteritis	Parental concern was described as "different illness" with the definition of a "statement by the parents that this illness was different from previous illnesses." Presence of parental concern was associated with odds ratio for sepsis/meningitis of 70.5 (14.5–341.4); Sensitivity 77.8%, specificity 95.3%.

TABLE 2 | Original studies reporting on parental concern as diagnostic measure of sepsis, not reporting on diagnostic accuracy of parental concern.

References and country of enrolment	Study design	*N* patients	Inclusion criteria	Outcomes in relation to parental concern	Comments
Van den Bruel et al. (38), Belgium	Prospective observational multicentre study (121 physicians)	3980, of which 21 (0.53%) had a serious infection; of which 1/3980 had sepsis (0.02%)	Children presenting to General Practitioner, pediatrician or the emergency department with acute illness <5 day	Serious bacterial infection requiring hospital admission for >24 h: Pneumonia, meningitis, sepsis, pyelonephritis, osteomyelitis, bacterial gastroenteritis	Secondary analysis of the same dataset as published in Van den Bruel et al. (37) (**Table 1**). Parental concern was the strongest factor associated with a clinician's gut feeling that something was wrong OR 26.9, 9.0 to 80.4).
Van den Bruel et al. (39), Belgium	Single-site qualitative study. Interviews with parents and clinicians	No patients; Parents of 18 cases and 9 of the respective general practitioners interviewed	Families of children diagnosed with severe bacterial infection	N/A	Parental assessment that the disease is different from other diseases is highlighted.
Brennan et al. (40), United Kingdom	Qualitative prospective multi centre study. Semi-structured interviews.	26 General Practitioners	General practitioners of the area	N/A	General practitioners were interviewed to identify diagnostic approach in children with meningitis. Maternal intuition that "the child isn't quite right" and parental concern were stated as factors influencing medical decision making about the seriousness of infection.
Kai et al. (41), United Kingdom	Qualitative prospective study. Focus groups and interviews	95 parents	Parents registered at a General practitioner practice, at regional care facilities, and from parent groups	N/A	The concerns of parents related to lack of personal control and perceived threat by a serious illness (which may result in meningitis, disability, or death). Cough and fever were key concerns, and did not necessarily relate to severity. Parents were worried about failing to recognize a serious problem, and may struggle to define the severity of illness.

evidence to guide best practice. Only one study was found which assessed diagnostic accuracy of parental concerns in serious infections, suggesting superior performance of parental concern in comparison to routine physiological-based criteria. Several reviews highlighted the potential of parental concerns in recognizing children with life-threatening infections. Despite the fact that sepsis starts most commonly at home, the role of recognition of sepsis by parents to improve accuracy of early sepsis diagnosis represents a neglected field. Yet, several institutional and national sepsis quality improvement tools have embedded assessment for parental concerns as part of standardized sepsis screening. Our findings indicate an urgent need for well-designed diagnostic accuracy studies to define the value of assessing parental concerns in sepsis recognition in acute care settings. To the best of our knowledge this is the first review providing a comprehensive overview in the field.

The study by Van den Bruel prospectively assessed parental concerns, defined as a parental perception that the disease was different from previous illnesses (37). Despite the sample size of this well-designed study including 3982 visits to

TABLE 3 | Reviews reporting on parental concern in relation to diagnosis of sepsis.

References	Scope of review	Study design	*N* studies	Inclusion criteria	Outcomes	Comments:
Van den Bruel et al. (41)	Until June 2009	Meta analysis/review	30 studies included	Diagnostic accuracy studies on children to predict serious infection	Serious infection	1 study commenting on parental concern (37): High odds ratio for serious bacterial infection in presence of parental concern, and in presence of clinician instinct that something different
Niehues (42)	2009–29 Aug 2013	Narrative review	N/A	Pediatric fever management	N/A	Review on febrile infections in children. "Degree of parental concern" listed as a strong red flag
Thompson et al. (43)	Oct 2008. Update June 2009	Systematic review and validation of prediction rules	35 studies included in review	Prediction rules to identify children with serious infections in Emergency settings	Serious infection	1 study commenting on parental concern (37): Parental concern that the illness is different from previous illnesses (Likelihood ratio + 14) and the clinician's gut feeling that something is wrong (Likelihood ratio + 23)
Long (44)	N/A	Narrative review	N/A	N/A	N/A	Review on family stressors and perception during sepsis. Role of parents in recognizing altered behavior mentioned.
Printz (45)	N/A	Narrative review	N/A	N/A	N/A	Review on management of febrile illness. States that clinicians should listen to parental concerns as indicators of serious illness. Parents as experts of their child.
Yung (46)	N/A	Narrative review	N/A	N/A	N/A	Review on recognition of menincoccemia. Concerns of parents, relatives or friends are listed as clues for early recognition. Parents as best judges of the health of their children. Note of worry of relatives/friends which seems more extreme than presenting signs.

General Practitioners, Pediatricians, and Emergency Settings, the prevalence of serious infections was very low, and very few of the serious infections were reported as sepsis, hence resulting in low power for sepsis as an outcome. Despite these limitations, the performance of parental concern was clearly superior to routinely used physiological markers. The authors assessed as well the diagnostic value of clinician's gut feeling with serious infections and identified both parental and healthcare worker concerns as good predictors (38). Yet these findings may not necessarily reflect diagnostic performance in Emergency Department settings where patient acuity is higher. In addition, in larger Emergency Departments, a majority of parents already has gone through a selection process by community physicians and parental concern potentially may be less discriminative, restricting the generalizability of the findings by Van den Bruel.

Qualitative studies have shown that parents of children presenting with severe infections report on changes in their child's observed behavior ranging from altered crying or mentation, to moaning or inconsolability (43, 47), highlighting the role of parents as experts of their child's behavior. The value of parental involvement in healthcare decision-making and provision has been increasingly recognized in areas other than sepsis, building up on the unique position of parents being experts of their child. Structured parental education on early recognition of severe infections has become standard in the management of oncologic children and children discharged with indwelling medical devices (50, 51). While the setting fever and neutropenia may allow easier operationalization than the more vague concept of sepsis, parents of immunosuppressed children are empowered to raise concerns and are often considered part of the experts in making informed decisions about best care to their children. Importantly, in resource poor settings, maternal education has been demonstrated to lead to reduced infection-related mortality during childhood (28), likely through improved prevention and faster recognition of disease leading to earlier treatment.

At present, several campaigns incorporate parental education and empowerment on sepsis, for example the Sepsis Assessment and Management (SAM) tool in the United Kingdom (http://www.southdevonandtorbayccg.nhs.uk/your-health/Documents/sam-sepsis-leaflet.pdf). The Public Health England and the UK Sepsis Trust jointly lead a campaign to improve parental awareness and knowledge of sepsis (http://www.independent.co.uk/life-style/health-and-families/health-news/sepsis-campaign-

TABLE 4 | Selected examples of online available guidelines and pathways on pediatric sepsis recognition.

Owner/institution/ publication date	Website	Type	Target group	Location	Mention of parental concern	Role/utilization of parental concern
American College of Critical Care Medicine, 2017	https://www.ncbi.nlm.nih.gov/pubmed/28509730	Guideline	Neonatal and pediatric	Endorsed by multiple national and international societies	Not mentioned	N/A
Surviving Sepsis Campaign, 2013	http://www.ncbi.nlm.nih.gov/pubmed/23361625	Guideline	Adult and pediatric	ED, PICU, and inpatient unit; Endorsed by multiple national and international societies	Not mentioned	N/A
National Institute for Health and Care Excellence (NICE), 2017	https://www.nice.org.uk/guidance/ng51/resources	Guideline and institutional pathway	Adult, pediatric, and neonate	ED, PICU, and inpatient unit; United Kingdom	Yes. –" Pay particular attention to concerns expressed by the person and their family or carer" –"Parental or carer concern is important and should be acknowledged" –"Parent or carer concern that child is behaving differently from usual"	Used as screening "Could this be sepsis?" and as moderate-to-high risk criterium
United Kingdom Sepsis Trust, 2018	https://sepsistrust.org/professional-resources/clinical/	Pathway	Pediatric	ED, United Kingdom	Yes. - In <5 year and 5 to 12 year age groups: "Parents very worried"	Used as Amber Flag criterium
Department of Pediatrics, New York University, 2016	http://pediatrics.aappublications.org/content/pediatrics/137/3/e20144082.full.pdf	Pathway	Pediatric	Inpatient Unit, New York, United States	Not mentioned	N/A
Sepsis Kills, Clinical Excellence Commission, 2016	http://www.cec.health.nsw.gov.au/__data/assets/pdf_file/0008/343475/Pediatric-Sepsis-Pathway-Sept-2016-with-watermark.pdf	Pathway	Adult and Pediatric	ED, and inpatient unit, New South Wales, Australia	Yes -"High level parental concern "	Used as screening "Are you concerned your patient could have sepsis?"

Current pediatric sepsis guidelines and selected examples of pathways from the United Kingdom, United States, and Australia are shown in reference to whether parental concern in sepsis recognition is mentioned.

nhs-jeremy-hunt-children-condition-what-are-symptoms-signs-child-health-a7476426.html. In New York State, education of children on sepsis has become mandatory as part of the Rory Staunton regulations (http://www.nysed.gov/curriculum-instruction/sepsis). Kerkhof et al analyzed data from over 6,000 children and assessed the predictive performance of NICE criteria and suggested future iterations should consider parental concern (52). The more recent NICE guidelines on the recognition of sepsis in children include parental concerns.

Several challenges may arise when including parental concerns as a tool to recognize sepsis: First, the prevalence of sepsis is very low across most pediatric Emergency Departments where hundreds of children present daily with non-septic febrile infections. At the same time, most parents of children with acute infections attending Emergency Departments (rather than General Practitioners) may have substantial concerns. Second, the parental understanding on the possible life-threatening nature of a disease is likely influenced by common belief ("cough" or "fever" is dangerous) rather than specific features of disease. Yet, the paternalistic approach assuming that medical practitioners and Early Warning Tools (19, 53, 54) perform superior to parents may falls short of daily challenges in the provision of medical care: the level of experience of many doctors involved in initial patient assessment may be low, and during busy periods medical staff may not always have sufficient time to assess all patients thoroughly.

Third, the need for, and the benefit of antimicrobial stewardship may not be directly evident to parents who present with a child with a mild disease yet are concerned this could be sepsis—some parents may request antibiotic therapy to prevent or treat potential progression to a severe disease (25). Indeed, a cluster randomized controlled factorial trial evaluated a brief intervention to elicit parental concern combined with safety net advice and found increased antibiotic prescribing in children allocated to this arm (55). The study findings imply that over-prescription of antibiotics needs to be considered as a balancing measure when designing interventions focusing on parental concern. Forth, a study in east Africa (56) investigated the educational background of parents in relation to presentations for pediatric illness and demonstrated that the majority of the parents had very limited knowledge of their children's health problems as assessed in the study. This illustrates the considerable cultural and educational challenges in applying parental concern-based approaches in low income settings. Finally, individual parents may have different perceptions and approaches to risks related to infectious diseases and treatment (57).

Future studies should prospectively assess the diagnostic accuracy of parental assessment of infectious disease severity across low, middle, and high income settings with particular focus on sepsis and septic shock. Further information is needed to specifically analyze the benefit of providing targeted sepsis education to parents. Given the unique role of parents as experts of their child, such interventions have in principle a substantial potential to enhance the diagnostic performance of screening for sepsis as part of a rule-in approach. Yet, such approaches needs to be balanced against the risk that creating community awareness of sepsis may lead to excessive consumption of healthcare resources for children with mild infections, and lead to unnecessary treatment. Hence, while it may be beneficial for clinicians to include questions pertinent to the level of parental concern in their assessment of the acutely ill child evaluated for infection, clinicians should be empowered to consider diagnoses other than sepsis and make an informed decision to rule-out sepsis if such is considered unlikely (25). Parents should be considered key partners in safety netting of such children where sepsis was ruled out—ongoing observation at home with the availability for prompt representation to reassess may potentially reduce adverse outcomes from late sepsis presentations.

Limitations

Several limitations of this review need to be considered. First, only one original study was identified reporting on the diagnostic accuracy of parental concerns in the recognition of sepsis, with a very small number of children meeting the outcome, and a meta-analysis could not be performed. Second, the design and quality of included articles was variable, ranging from original quantitative studies, original qualitative studies, and high quality systematic reviews to non-systematic narratives. In view of the lack of data, the review was extended to include original studies not reporting on diagnostic accuracy and reviews referring to parental concern in children with sepsis. Third, only abstracts leading to full text publications in English were considered, and this may have further reduced the yield of the search. Finally, the overview of institutional sepsis pathways represents a selection pertinent to recently published international sepsis guidelines, and jurisdictions who have reported on sepsis pathway implementation.

CONCLUSION

In conclusion, this review identified a paucity of data analyzing the role of parental concerns in recognizing sepsis. Several guidelines and institutional protocols emphasize the importance of listening to parents and utilize parental concerns as one of the trigger criteria for sepsis recognition. Parental concern needs to be considered to improve accuracy in recognizing life-threatening infections in children. Education on utilizing parental concerns to recognize sepsis has the potential to lead to better outcomes in paediatric sepsis. However, understanding parental perceptions of sepsis, and parental decision-making in seeking advice is urgently needed to inform on optimal design of education campaigns, and to assist in the design of sepsis recognition bundles. Prospective studies are needed testing the sensitivity, specificity, and negative and positive predictive value of parental concerns in sepsis in various settings, while assessing the potential impact on antibiotic and health care resource use.

AUTHOR CONTRIBUTIONS

AH and LS designed the study. All abstracts were checked by AH and LS. AH and LS went through each of the full texts. JL assisted in study design, review of results, and manuscript writing. LS and AH wrote the first draft of the manuscript. All authors contributed to manuscript revision and approved the final version.

ACKNOWLEDGMENTS

We thank Kate McEnery, Pediatric Critical Care Research Group, Brisbane, for critical comments on the topic which have informed the design of this project, and the librarians at the Gold Coast University Hospital, Southport, Australia, for help in database searches.

REFERENCES

1. Fleischmann-Struzek C, Goldfarb DM, Schlattmann P, Schlapbach LJ, Reinhart K, Kissoon N. The global burden of paediatric and neonatal sepsis: a systematic review. *Lancet Respir Med.* (2018) 6:223–30. doi: 10.1016/S2213-2600(18)30063-8
2. Schlapbach LJ, Straney L, Alexander J, MacLaren G, Festa M, Schibler A, et al. Mortality related to invasive infections, sepsis, and septic

shock in critically ill children in Australia and New Zealand, 2002-13: a multicentre retrospective cohort study. *Lancet Infect Dis.* (2015) 15:46–54. doi: 10.1016/S1473-3099(14)71003-5

3. Ruth A, McCracken CE, Fortenberry JD, Hall M, Simon HK, Hebbar KB. Pediatric severe sepsis: current trends and outcomes from the pediatric Health Information Systems database. *Pediatr Crit Care Med.* (2014) 15:828–38. doi: 10.1097/PCC.0000000000000254
4. Reinhart K, Daniels R, Kissoon N, Machado FR, Schachter RD, Finfer S. Recognizing sepsis as a global health priority - A WHO resolution. *N Engl J Med.* (2017) 377:414–7. doi: 10.1056/NEJMp1707170
5. Kissoon N, Reinhart K, Daniels R, Machado FR, Schachter RD, Finfer S. Sepsis in children: global implications of the world health assembly resolution on sepsis. *Pediatr Crit Care Med.* (2017) 18:e625–7. doi: 10.1097/PCC.0000000000001340
6. Rhodes A, Evans LE, Alhazzani W, Levy MM, Antonelli M, Ferrer R, et al. Surviving sepsis campaign: international guidelines for management of sepsis and septic shock: 2016. *Intensive Care Med.* (2017) 43:304–77. doi: 10.1007/s00134-017-4683-6
7. Schlapbach LJ, MacLaren G, Festa M, Alexander J, Erickson S, Beca J, et al. New Zealand intensive care society centre for, E. resource, Australian, and G. New Zealand Intensive Care Society Paediatric Study, Prediction of pediatric sepsis mortality within 1 h of intensive care admission. *Intensive Care Med.* (2017) 43:1085–96. doi: 10.1007/s00134-017-4701-8
8. Agyeman KA, Schlapbach LJ, Giannoni E, Stocker M, Posfay-Barbe KM, Heininger U, et al. Swiss pediatric sepsis, epidemiology of blood culture-proven bacterial sepsis in children in Switzerland: a population-based cohort study. *Lancet Child Adolesc Health.* (2017) 1:124–33. doi: 10.1016/S2352-4642(17)30010-X
9. Cvetkovic M, Lutman D, Ramnarayan P, Pathan N, Inwald DP, Peters MJ. Timing of death in children referred for intensive care with severe sepsis: implications for interventional studies. *Pediatr Crit Care Med.* (2015) 16:410–7. doi: 10.1097/PCC.0000000000000385
10. Weiss SL, Balamuth F, Hensley J, Fitzgerald JC, Bush J, Nadkarni VM, et al. The epidemiology of hospital death following pediatric severe sepsis: when, why, and how children with sepsis die. *Pediatr Crit Care Med.* (2017) 18:823–30. doi: 10.1097/PCC.0000000000001222
11. Maitland K, Kiguli S, Opoka RO, Engoru C, Olupot-Olupot P, Akech SO, et al. Mortality after fluid bolus in African children with severe infection. *N Engl J Med.* (2011) 364:2483–95. doi: 10.1056/NEJMoa1101549
12. Nadel S, Goldstein B, Williams MD, Dalton H, Peters M, Macias WL, et al. R.E.s. Sepsis, and g. Organ dysfunction in children: a gLobal perspective study, Drotrecogin alfa (activated) in children with severe sepsis: a multicentre phase III randomised controlled trial. *Lancet.* (2007) 369:836–43. doi: 10.1016/S0140-6736(07)60411-5
13. Angus DC, Barnato AE, Bell D, Bellomo R, Chong CR, Coats TJ, et al. A systematic review and meta-analysis of early goal-directed therapy for septic shock: the ARISE, ProCESS and ProMISe Investigators. *Intensive Care Med.* (2015) 41:1549–60. doi: 10.1007/s00134-015-3822-1
14. Evans IVR, Phillips GS, Alpern ER, Angus DC, Friedrich ME, Kissoon N, et al. Association between the new york sepsis care mandate and in-hospital mortality for pediatric sepsis. *JAMA.* (2018) 320:358–67. doi: 10.1001/jama.2018.9071
15. Weiss SL, Fitzgerald JC, Balamuth F, Alpern ER, Lavelle J, Chilutti M, et al. Delayed antimicrobial therapy increases mortality and organ dysfunction duration in pediatric sepsis. *Crit Care Med.* (2014) 42:2409–17. doi: 10.1097/CCM.0000000000000509
16. Launay E, Gras-Le Guen C, Martinot A, Assathiany R, Martin E, Blanchais T, et al. Why children with severe bacterial infection die: a population-based study of determinants and consequences of suboptimal care with a special emphasis on methodological issues. *PLoS ONE.* (2014) 9:e107286. doi: 10.1371/journal.pone.0107286
17. Kumar A, Roberts D, Wood KE, Light B, Parrillo JE, Sharma S, et al. Duration of hypotension before initiation of effective antimicrobial therapy is the critical determinant of survival in human septic shock. *Crit Care Med.* (2006) 34:1589–96. doi: 10.1097/01.CCM.0000217961.75225.E9
18. Seymour CW, Gesten F, Prescott HC, Friedrich ME, Iwashyna TJ, Phillips GS, et al. Time to treatment and mortality during mandated emergency care for sepsis. *N Engl J Med.* (2017) 376:2235–44. doi: 10.1056/NEJMoa1703058
19. Balamuth F, Alpern ER, Abbadessa MK, Hayes K, Schast A, Lavelle J, et al. Improving recognition of pediatric severe sepsis in the emergency department: contributions of a vital sign-based electronic alert and bedside clinician identification. *Ann Emerg Med.* (2017) 70:759–768.e2. doi: 10.1016/j.annemergmed.2017.03.019
20. Irwin AD, Grant A, Williams R, Kolamunnage-Dona R, Drew RJ, Paulus S, et al. Predicting risk of serious bacterial infections in febrile children in the emergency department. *Pediatrics.* (2017) 140:e20162853. doi: 10.1542/peds.2016-2853
21. Lane RD, Funai T, Reeder R, Larsen GY. High reliability pediatric septic shock quality improvement initiative and decreasing mortality. *Pediatrics.* (2016) 138:e20154153. doi: 10.1542/peds.2015-4153
22. Verbakel JY, Lemiengre MB, De Burghgraeve T, De Sutter A, Aertgeerts B, Bullens DM, et al. Validating a decision tree for serious infection: diagnostic accuracy in acutely ill children in ambulatory care. *BMJ Open.* (2015) 5:e008657. doi: 10.1136/bmjopen-2015-008657
23. Geldsetzer P, Williams TC, Kirolos A, Mitchell S, Ratcliffe LA, Kohli-Lynch MK, et al. The recognition of and care seeking behaviour for childhood illness in developing countries: a systematic review. *PLoS ONE.* (2014) 9:e93427. doi: 10.1371/journal.pone.0093427
24. Schlapbach LJ, Kissoon N. Defining Pediatric Sepsis. *JAMA Pediatr.* (2018) 172:312–4. doi: 10.1001/jamapediatrics.2017.5208
25. Schlapbach LJ, Weiss SL, Wolf J. Reducing collateral damage from mandates for time to antibiotics in pediatric sepsis-primum non nocere. *JAMA Pediatr.* (2019). doi: 10.1001/jamapediatrics.2019.0174. [Epub ahead of print].
26. Klompas M, Calandra T, Singer M. Antibiotics for sepsis-finding the equilibrium. *JAMA.* (2018) 320:1433–4. doi: 10.1001/jama.2018.12179
27. Singer M. Antibiotics for sepsis: does each hour really count, or is it incestuous amplification? *Am J Respir Crit Care Med.* (2017) 196:800–2. doi: 10.1164/rccm.201703-0621ED
28. Gakidou E, Cowling K, Lozano R, Murray CJ. Increased educational attainment and its effect on child mortality in 175 countries between 1970 and 2009: a systematic analysis. *Lancet.* (2010) 376:959–74. doi: 10.1016/S0140-6736(10)61257-3
29. Schlapbach LJ, Ostrowski JA, MacLaren G. The excess burden of severe sepsis in Indigenous Australian children: can anything be done? *Med J Aust.* (2017) 207:45–6. doi: 10.5694/mja17.00464
30. Goldstein B, Giroir B, Randolph A. International pediatric sepsis consensus conference: definitions for sepsis and organ dysfunction in pediatrics. *Pediatr Crit Care Med.* (2005) 6:2–8. doi: 10.1097/01.PCC.0000149131.72248.E6
31. Levy MM, Fink MP, Marshall JC, Abraham E, Angus D, Cook D, et al. 2001 SCCM/ESICM/ACCP/ATS/SIS international sepsis definitions conference. *Crit Care Med.* (2003) 31:1250–6. doi: 10.1097/01.CCM.0000050454.01978.3B
32. Singer M, Deutschman CS, Seymour CW, Shankar-Hari M, Annane D, Bauer M, et al. The third international consensus definitions for sepsis and septic shock (Sepsis-3). *JAMA.* (2016) 315:801–10. doi: 10.1001/jama.2016.0287
33. Burrell AR, McLaws ML, Fullick M, Sullivan RB, Sindhusake D. SEPSIS KILLS: early intervention saves lives. *Med J Aust.* (2016) 204:73.e1–7. doi: 10.5694/mja15.00657
34. Daniels R, Nutbeam T, McNamara G, Galvin C. The sepsis six and the severe sepsis resuscitation bundle: a prospective observational cohort study. *Emerg Med J.* (2011) 28:507–12. doi: 10.1136/emj.2010.095067
35. McMenamin L, Murch N, Daniels R. Severe sepsis, social media and the #Sepsis 6: 'Tweeting' national innovations. *Acute Med.* (2013) 12:83–8.
36. Oostenbrink R, de Groot R, Moll HA. Fever of unknown origin in a young child: diagnosis and treatment. *Nederlands Tijdschrift Voor Geneeskunde.* (1999) 143:185–90.
37. Van den Bruel A, Aertgeerts B, Bruyninckx R, Aerts M, Buntinx F. Signs and symptoms for diagnosis of serious infections in children: a prospective study in primary care. *Br J Gene Pract.* (2007) 57:538–46.
38. Van den Bruel A, Thompson M, Buntinx F, Mant D. Clinicians' gut feeling about serious infections in children: observational study. *BMJ.* (2012) 345:e6144. doi: 10.1136/bmj.e6144
39. Van den Bruel A, Bruyninckx R, Vermeire E, Aerssens P, Aertgeerts B, Buntinx F. Signs and symptoms in children with a serious infection: a qualitative study. *BMC Family Pract.* (2005) 6:36. doi: 10.1186/1471-2296-6-36

40. Brennan CA, Somerset M, Granier SK, Fahey TP, Heyderman RS. Management of diagnostic uncertainty in children with possible meningitis: a qualitative study. *Br J Gene Pract.* (2003) 53:626–31.
41. Kai J. What worries parents when their preschool children are acutely ill, and why: a qualitative study. *BMJ.* (1996) 313:983–6.
42. Niehues T. The febrile child: diagnosis and treatment. *Deutsches Aerzteblatt Int.* (2013) 110:764–74. doi: 10.3238/arztebl.2013.0764
43. Thompson M, Van den Bruel A, Verbakel J, Lakhanpaul M, Haj-Hassan T, Stevens R, et al. Systematic review and validation of prediction rules for identifying children with serious infections in emergency departments and urgent-access primary care. *Health Technol Assess.* (2012) 16:1–100. doi: 10.3310/hta16150
44. Long LE. Stress in families of children with sepsis. *Crit Care Nurs Clin N Am.* (2003) 15:47–53. doi: 10.1016/S0899-5885(02)00041-2
45. Printz V, Hobbs AM-E, Teuten P, Prosad Paul S. Clinical update: assessment and management of febrile children. *Commun Pract.* (2016) 89:32–7.
46. Yung AP, McDonald MI. Early clinical clues to meningococcaemia. *Med J Aust.* (2003) 178:134–7. doi: 10.5694/j.1326-5377.2003.tb05106.x
47. Van den Bruel A, Haj-Hassan T, Thompson M, Buntinx F, Mant D. Diagnostic value of clinical features at presentation to identify serious infection in children in developed countries: a systematic review. *Lancet.* (2010) 375:834–45. doi: 10.1016/S0140-6736(09)62000-6
48. Davis AL, Carcillo JA, Aneja RK, Deymann AJ, Lin JC, Nguyen TC, et al. American college of critical care medicine clinical practice parameters for hemodynamic support of pediatric and neonatal septic shock. *Crit Care Med.* (2017) 45:1061–93. doi: 10.1097/CCM.0000000000002425
49. Dellinger RP, Levy MM, Rhodes A, Annane D, Gerlach H, Opal SM, et al. Surviving Sepsis Campaign: international guidelines for management of severe sepsis and septic shock, 2012. *Inten Care Med.* (2013) 39:165–228. doi: 10.1007/s00134-012-2769-8
50. Ku BC, Bailey C, Balamuth F. Neutropenia in the febrile child. *Pediatr Emerg Care.* (2016) 32:329–34. doi: 10.1097/PEC.0000000000000809
51. Ammann RA, Hirt A, Luthy AR, Aebi C. Predicting bacteremia in children with fever and chemotherapy-induced neutropenia. *Pediatr Infect Dis J.* (2004) 23:61–7. doi: 10.1097/01.inf.0000106782.30100.4f
52. Kerkhof E, Lakhanpaul M, Ray S, Verbakel JY, Van den Bruel A, Thompson M, et al. The predictive value of the NICE "red traffic lights" in acutely ill children. *PLoS ONE.* (2014) 9:e90847. doi: 10.1371/journal.pone.0090847
53. Chapman SM, Wray J, Oulton K, Pagel C, Ray S, Peters MJ. 'The Score Matters': wide variations in predictive performance of 18 paediatric track and trigger systems. *Arch Dis Child.* (2017) 102:487–95. doi: 10.1136/archdischild-2016-311088
54. Balamuth F, Alpern ER, Grundmeier RW, Chilutti M, Weiss SL, Fitzgerald JC, et al. Comparison of two sepsis recognition methods in a pediatric emergency department. *Acad Emerg Med.* (2015) 22:1298–306. doi: 10.1111/acem.12814
55. Lemiengre MB, Verbakel JY, Colman R, De Burghgraeve T, Buntinx F, Aertgeerts B, et al. Reducing inappropriate antibiotic prescribing for children in primary care: a cluster randomised controlled trial of two interventions. *Br J Gene Pract.* (2018) 68:e204–e210. doi: 10.3399/bjgp18X695033
56. Makworo D, Laving AM. Acute medical conditions in under five year old children at a public hospital in Kenya. *East Afr Med J.* (2010) 87:340–4.
57. Madsen KA, Bennett JE, Downs SM. The role of parental preferences in the management of fever without source among 3- to 36-month-old children: a decision analysis. *Pediatrics.* (2006) 117:1067–76. doi: 10.1542/peds.2005-1865

18

Effects of Probiotic Supplementation on the Gut Microbiota and Antibiotic Resistome Development in Preterm Infants

Eirin Esaiassen[1,2], Erik Hjerde[3], Jorunn Pauline Cavanagh[1,2], Tanja Pedersen[4], Jannicke H. Andresen[5], Siren I. Rettedal[6], Ragnhild Støen[7,8], Britt Nakstad[9,10], Nils P. Willassen[3] and Claus Klingenberg[1,2]*

[1] Paediatric Research Group, Department of Clinical Medicine, UiT The Arctic University of Norway, Tromsø, Norway, [2] Department of Paediatrics, University Hospital of North Norway, Tromsø, Norway, [3] Department of Chemistry, Norstruct, UiT The Arctic University of Norway, Tromsø, Norway, [4] Department of Paediatrics, Haukeland University Hospital, Bergen, Norway, [5] Department of Neonatal Intensive Care, Oslo University Hospital, Oslo, Norway, [6] Department of Paediatrics, Stavanger University Hospital, Stavanger, Norway, [7] Department of Paediatrics, St. Olavs University Hospital, Trondheim, Norway, [8] Department of Laboratory Medicine, Children's and Women's Health, University of Science and Technology, Trondheim, Norway, [9] Department of Paediatric and Adolescents Medicine, Akershus University Hospital, Nordbyhagen, Norway, [10] Institute of Clinical Medicine, Faculty of Medicine, University of Oslo, Oslo, Norway

***Correspondence:**
Claus Klingenberg
claus.klingenberg@unn.no

Objectives: In 2014 probiotic supplementation (*Lactobacillus acidophilus* and *Bifidobacterium longum* subspecies *infantis;* Infloran®) was introduced as standard of care to prevent necrotizing enterocolitis (NEC) in extremely preterm infants in Norway. We aimed to evaluate the influence of probiotics and antibiotic therapy on the developing gut microbiota and antibiotic resistome in extremely preterm infants, and to compare with very preterm infants and term infants not given probiotics.

Study design: A prospective, observational multicenter study in six tertiary-care neonatal units. We enrolled 76 infants; 31 probiotic-supplemented extremely preterm infants <28 weeks gestation, 35 very preterm infants 28–31 weeks gestation not given probiotics and 10 healthy full-term control infants. Taxonomic composition and collection of antibiotic resistance genes (resistome) in fecal samples, collected at 7 and 28 days and 4 months age, were analyzed using shotgun-metagenome sequencing.

Results: Median (IQR) birth weight was 835 (680–945) g and 1,290 (1,150–1,445) g in preterm infants exposed and not exposed to probiotics, respectively. Two extremely preterm infants receiving probiotic developed NEC requiring surgery. At 7 days of age we found higher median relative abundance of *Bifidobacterium* in probiotic supplemented infants (64.7%) compared to non-supplemented preterm infants (0.0%) and term control infants (43.9%). *Lactobacillus* was only detected in small amounts in all groups, but the relative abundance increased up to 4 months. Extremely preterm infants receiving probiotics had also much higher antibiotic exposure, still overall microbial diversity and resistome was not different than in more mature infants at 4 weeks and 4 months.

Conclusion: Probiotic supplementation may induce colonization resistance and alleviate harmful effects of antibiotics on the gut microbiota and antibiotic resistome.

Clinical Trial Registration: Clinicaltrials.gov: NCT02197468. https://clinicaltrials.gov/ct2/show/NCT02197468

Keywords: gut microbiota, preterm infant, shotgun metagenome sequencing, taxonomy, bifidobacteria, lactobacilli, colonization resistance

INTRODUCTION

Preterm infants experience unique challenges in establishing their gut microbiota. Cesarean deliveries, extensive antenatal, and neonatal antibiotic exposure, parenteral nutrition and residing for long periods in a neonatal intensive care unit (NICU), may cause unpredictable perturbations of the gut microbiota development (1). Gut microbiota dysbiosis in the first weeks of life is associated with perturbations of the developing immune system (2), and an increased risk of necrotizing enterocolitis (NEC) (3). Probiotic supplementation aims to restore the gut microbiota, and thereby preventing NEC and other complications (4–6). Meta-analyses of randomized and observational trials show that probiotic supplementation, mainly with bifidobacteria and/or lactobacilli, reduce rates of NEC (4, 5, 7, 8). The effects seem to be strain-specific (5) and not all products are efficacious (9). Still, based on recent evidence (4, 10) and expert opinion (11), many NICUs in Europe, Australia, and Canada have implemented routine probiotic-supplementation to preterm infants. Probiotics are infrequently used in preterm infants in the USA (12). Risks of probiotic sepsis and contaminations of probiotic products may explain skepticism (13–16). Some experts recommend waiting for additional studies to confirm the safety and efficacy of an available and reliable product (17). Moreover, there is a paucity of in-depth knowledge on microbiological effects and effective dose of probiotic therapy.

Antibiotics are the most commonly prescribed medications in the NICU (18), and prolonged therapy increases the risk of NEC (19, 20). Antibiotics may influence both the physiological gut microbiota composition and the collection of antibiotic resistance genes (ARGs) in the gut, defined as the gut antibiotic resistome (21, 22). However, there is limited knowledge on how probiotic supplementation and antibiotic therapy influence the gut antibiotic resistome in extremely preterm infants.

In Norway probiotic supplementation was implemented as standard of care for extremely preterm infants in 2014. In a longitudinal multi-center study, using shotgun-metagenomic sequencing, we set out to evaluate the influence of probiotics and antibiotic therapy on the developing gut microbiota and antibiotic resistome in extremely preterm infants supplemented with probiotics. We also compared these results to very preterm infants not supplemented with probiotics and a group of healthy, full-term infants.

Abbreviations: ARG, Antibiotic resistance genes; CARD, Comprehensive antibiotic resistance database; CFU, Colony forming units; FDR, False discovery rate; FTC, Full-term control; NEC, Necrotizing enterocolitis; NICU, Neonatal intensive care unit; NMDS, Non-metrical multidimensional scaling; NVPVP, Non-probiotic very preterm; PEP, Probiotic extremely preterm.

MATERIALS AND METHODS

Study Patients and Sampling Procedure

We prospectively planned to include two convenient groups of preterm infants from six Norwegian NICUs; one group of extremely preterm infants (gestational age 25–27 weeks) supplemented with probiotics, and one group of very preterm infants (gestational age 28–31 weeks) not supplemented with probiotics. Exclusion criteria were gestation below 25 weeks and/or an early, life threatening condition leading to high risk of not surviving the first weeks of life. We included a control group of 10 healthy, vaginally delivered full-term control (FTC) infants born at the University Hospital of Northern Norway. Sample size calculation for studies assessing gut microbiota taxonomic composition can be performed by assessing matrices of pairwise distances between groups (23). We expected that around 30 infants in each group of preterm infants would afford 90% statistical power to detect differences in gut microbiota composition that were smaller than effects previously observed in microbiota studies of antibiotic exposure (23). The sample size was also adapted to cover the high expenses for shotgun-metagenome sequencing. The original protocol (24) focused on taxonomic composition. We decided post hoc to add a resistome analysis.

After careful instructions, fecal samples were collected by a nurse in the NICU at around seven and 28 days of age, and by the parents at home at around 4 months of age. We used a commercially available sampling kit (OMNIgen GUT kit, DNA Genotek, Ottawa, Canada) allowing storage of samples at ambient temperatures for up to 14 days before DNA extraction (25). We obtained routine clinical data including details on antibiotic exposure. NEC was defined as Bell's stage 2–3 (26).

DNA Extraction, Library Preparation, and Sequencing

Total metagenomic DNA was extracted using the NorDiag Arrow Stool DNA Extraction kit (NorDiag, Oslo, Norway). An extra beadbeating step was added to facilitate cell lysis as studies have shown that this can increase extraction of DNA from Gram-positive bacteria. DNA was quantified using the Nanodrop 1000 and Qubit® 2.0 Fluorometer (Invitrogen, Carlsbad, CA, USA) along with the Qubit® dsDNA HR assay kit (Thermo Fisher Scientific, Waltham, MA, USA). DNA was then stored at −70°C. The indexed paired-end libraries were prepared for whole genome sequencing using the Nextera XT Kit (Illumina, San Diego, CA, USA), according to the manufacturer's instructions. Fifty nanograms of genomic DNA was tagmented at 55°C for 10 min. The tagmented DNA was amplified with two primers from Nextera DNA sample preparation Index Kit. PCR products were cleaned using Agencourt AMPure XP beads (Beckman Coulter, Indiana, USA). Purified PCR products were quantified using the Qubit® 2.0 (Invitrogen, Carlsbad, CA, USA), along with the Qubit® dsDNA HS assay kit (Thermo Fisher Scientific, Waltham, MA, USA). The fragment size distribution (500–1,000 bp) was analyzed using the Agilent 2100 Bioanalyzer System (Agilent Technologies, Waldbronn, Germany). The samples were pooled at concentration of 4 nM per sample. Eight to twelve samples were pooled per each sequencing run. Pooled samples was denatured with 0.2 N NaOH, then diluted to 10 pM with hybridization buffer. Subsequently, samples were submitted for v3 reagents with 2 × 300 cycles paired-end sequencing using the Illumina Miseq platform, according to the manufacturer's instructions. In total, 184 samples were sequenced to an average (range) sequence depth of 4.8 (1.8–12.6) million reads per sample for microbiota and functional analysis. Prior to all downstream data analysis, the sequence quality was calculated using FastQC (v0.11.3). All samples were screened for human contamination using Deconseq with default parameters and build up 38 of the human genome as reference. Quality filtering of the read was performed using Trimmomatic v0.36 with LEADING:3, TRAILING:3, MINLEN:75 as parameter settings. Assemblies were performed on the trimmed reads using MEGAHIT. Functional annotation was added using an in-house genome annotation pipeline, the META-pipe (Department of Chemistry, University of Tromsø, Norway [https://arxiv.org/abs/1604.04103]). The sequences are deposited in the European Nucleotide Archive (www.ebi.ac.uk/ena); study accession nr. PRJEB29052.

Taxonomic Profiling

The relative abundance of bacteria at genus level was calculated from the trimmed reads using MetaPhlAn 2.0 (27). Relative abundance tables for each individual sample were merged. To calculate longitudinal changes, sequences were reconstructed using the Lowest Common Ancestor (LCA) classifier.

The Gut Antibiotic Resistome

The prediction of genes presumed to confer antibiotic resistance was performed on the assembled metagenomes using Abricate [https://github.com/tseemann/abricate] against the resistance gene identifier in the Comprehensive Antibiotic Resistance Database (CARD; version 1.1.1; Dept. of Biochemistry and Biomedical Science, McMaster University, Canada, https://card.mcmaster.ca/home]) (25–28) with the minimum identity threshold set to 75% (28). Because of the fragmented nature of the metagenome assemblies, and therefore presence of fragmented genes, multiple hits against the same antibiotic resistance gene (ARG) were regarded as one hit. Data are presented as distribution of ARG classes among the three different groups of infants at three time points. Classes of antibiotic resistance genes in the CARD database and the specific genes included in each class are listed below

- Beta lactamase: *blaMIR, blaZ, blaACT, blaTEM, blaCMY, blaLEN, blaADC, blaACI, blaOXA, blaOXY, blaSHV, blaDHA, blaOKP, blaACC, blaSED, blaMOR, blaCMG, blaCFE, cfiA, cepA, cfxA*
- Methicillin resistance: *mecA*
- Aminoglycosides: *aac(6′)-aph(2), aac(6′)-Ic, aac(6′)-Im, aadA, aadB, aadD, aadE, ant(6)-Ia, aph(2)-Ib, aph(3)-Ia, aph(3)-III, spc, str, strA,strB*
- Tetracyclines: *tet(A), tet(B), tet(M), tet(K), tet(X), tet(O), tet(L), tet(U), tet(Q), tet(W), tet(S), tet(32), tet(34), tet(35), tet(37), tet(40), tet(41), Otr(A)*
- Fluoroquinolones: *QnrB, QnrD*
- MLS: Macrolide: *erm(A), erm(B), erm(C), erm(F),erm(G), erm(T), erm(X), mph(A), mph(C); Lincosamide: lnu(B), lnu(C); Streptogranin: vat(B), vat(F)*
- ABC efflux: *lsa(A),lsa(B), lsa(C), msr(A), mrs(C), msr(D), ole(B), car(A)*
- RND efflux pumps: *oqxA*
- Efflux pumps: *vga(A), mef(A)*
- Multidrug efflux pumps: *norA*
- Chloramphenicol: *cat, catA, catB, catS, cmlA, cml*
- Fosfomycin: *fos(A)*
- Sulfonamides: *sul1, sul2*
- Antibiotic target: *dfrA, dfrG*
- Vancomycin: *VanC, VanS, VanT, VanR, VanY*
- Metronidazole: *nimB*

In order to obtain quantitative measures of the putative ARGs in each sample, the quality trimmed reads were analyzed using Short, Better Representative Extract Dataset (ShortBRED) (29) against a formatted CARD database and normalized per total reads in each sample. Data are presented as abundance of ARGs among the three different groups of infants at three time points. Using ShortBRED we identified the antibiotic resistance gene classes and genes listed below:

- Class A Beta lactamase
- Class C Beta lactamase
- Aminoglycoside acetyltransferase
- Aminoglycoside phosphotransferase
- Aminoglycoside nucleotidyltransferase
- Tetracycline efflux
- Tetracycline ribosomal protection
- Quinolone resistance
- Macrolide/MLS resistance
- Adenosine triphosphate (ATP)-binding cassette (ABC) efflux pump
- Resistance/nodulation/division (RND) antibiotic efflux
- Major facilitator superfamily (MFS) antibiotic efflux
- Multidrug efflux pump activity
- Multidrug resistance efflux pump
- Genes modulating antibiotic efflux: *norA, baeR, marA, phoQ, ramA, soxR*
- Small multidrug resistance (SMR) antibiotic efflux

- Chloramphenicol acetyltransferase
- Antibiotic target
- Genes modulating resistance: *WblE, WhiB*
- rRNA methyltransferase
- Other ARG: *bacA*

Probiotic Supplementation

A consensus-based protocol for probiotic supplementation was implemented in Norway in 2014 (30). Extremely preterm infants, contributing to around 90% of NEC cases in Norway, were considered as the target group for probiotic prophylaxis. At this time, probiotics was not used routinely for more mature preterm infants (≥28 weeks gestation) in any Norwegian neonatal unit. After considering the safety profile, a widely used probiotic combination product was selected (Infloran®) (31). One capsule Infloran contained 10^9 colony forming units (CFU) *Lactobacillus acidophilus* (ATCC 4356) and 10^9 CFU *B. longum* subspecies *infantis* (ATCC 15697). One-half capsule once daily was initiated on day 3–4 and increased to one capsule daily after 4–7 days. One capsule was opened and the content was diluted in 2 ml of breast milk, or formula. It was thereafter administered enteral via a nasogastric tube, either 1 ml (1/2 capsule) or 2 ml (one capsule).

Influence of Antibiotic Therapy

To quantify changes in the gut microbiota composition and resistome after antibiotic exposure, we stratified four different categories of antibiotic exposure: (i) antenatal exposure, (ii) short (≤72 h) vs. prolonged (>72 h) exposure in the first week of life (19, 22), (iii) any exposure after first week of life (yes/no), and (iv) narrow- vs. broad-spectrum exposure after first week of life. Potential effects of antenatal exposure and short vs. prolonged therapy after birth were only investigated at 7 days of age. We defined regimens including third-generation cephalosporins or carbapenems as a broad-spectrum regimens when compared to regimens containing aminoglycosides for coverage against Gram-negative bacteria. This definition was based on the fact that neonatal empiric treatment using a third-generation cephalosporin for Gram-negative coverage induce significantly higher antibiotic resistance rates among colonizing bacteria than a regimen containing an aminoglycoside (32).

Ethics, Trial Registration, and Statistical Analysis

The study was approved by the Norwegian Regional Ethical Committee (2014/930/REK nord) and registered in Clinicaltrials.gov (https://clinicaltrials.gov/ct2/show/NCT02197468). Informed written consent was obtained from all parents.

Data were analyzed using IBM-SPSS version 22 (IBM, Armonk NY, USA) statistical software, the R statistical framework (version 3.2.4; http://www.r-project.org/), and Statistical Analysis of Metagenomic Profiles (STAMP) software package (33). We used Mann–Whitney *U*-test or a Kruskal-Wallis test for comparisons between two or multiple independent groups. We used a Poisson generalized linear model to calculate trends in the relative abundance of genera and ARGs in the gut microbiota. Corrections based on multiple comparisons were performed by the Benjamini–Hochberg false discovery rate (FDR) (34). A FDR $Q \leq 0.10$ was considered significant for any analyses with multiple comparisons. A standard $P \leq 0.05$ was considered significant for all other analyses.

Alpha diversity was assessed by calculating the Shannon Diversity index (MEGAN, v5.10.6) (35). To detect changes in alpha diversity over time, we first performed a normality test and found that the residuals were normally distributed. Therefore, differences in alpha diversity over time between the three different groups were calculated using linear mixed models. The same model was used to calculate the influence of antibiotic exposure on alpha diversity. Multiple beta diversity metrics of samples was performed using non-metrical multidimensional scaling (NMDS) based on a matrix of Bray-Curtis distances calculated using the vegan R package. Differences between groups were tested using permutational multivariate analysis on beta diversity matrices.

RESULTS

Study Population and Antibiotic Exposure

Figure 1 shows study flow. We enrolled 66 preterm infants and 10 healthy full-term control (FTC) infants between February and October 2015. The six study sites had different admission numbers, and recruited each between 7 and 24 preterm infants (**Figure 1**). Clinical characteristics, antibiotic and probiotic exposure, duration of parenteral nutrition and enteral nutrition data are reported in **Table 1**. The "probiotic extremely preterm (PEP)" infants received much more antibiotics than the "non-probiotic very preterm (NPVP)" infants after first week of life. Two infants in the PEP-group were operated for NEC, both survived.

Taxonomic Composition

On day 7, we found higher relative abundance of *Bifidobacterium* and *Lactobacillus* in PEP-infants compared to NPVP-infants (**Figure 2A**, **Table 2**). FTC infants had higher abundance of some genera (*Streptococcus, Veilonella,* and *Haemophilus*) that were only sparsely present in the two preterm infant groups (**Figure 2A**). Mode of delivery did not lead to detectable differences in the microbiota composition within the preterm groups on day 7 (data not shown).

On day 28, there was a striking increase in relative abundance of *Escherichia* in the PEP-infants and a similar striking increase in relative abundance of *Bifidobacterium* in NPVP-infants. FTC infants had significantly higher relative abundance of *Lactobacillus* than NPVP-infants. Overall, at 28 days of age the FTC- and NPVP-infants had higher abundance of *Veilonella* and *Streptococcus* than PEP-infants, while both preterm groups had higher relative abundance of *Staphylococcus* and *Enterococcus* than FTC-infants (**Figure 2B**).

By 4 months of age, there were no significant differences in taxonomic profile between PEP- and FTC-infants. The NPVP-infants had more *Prevotella* than PEP-infants, but otherwise all three groups were similar (**Figure 2C**). Duration of parenteral nutrition did not lead to detectable differences in

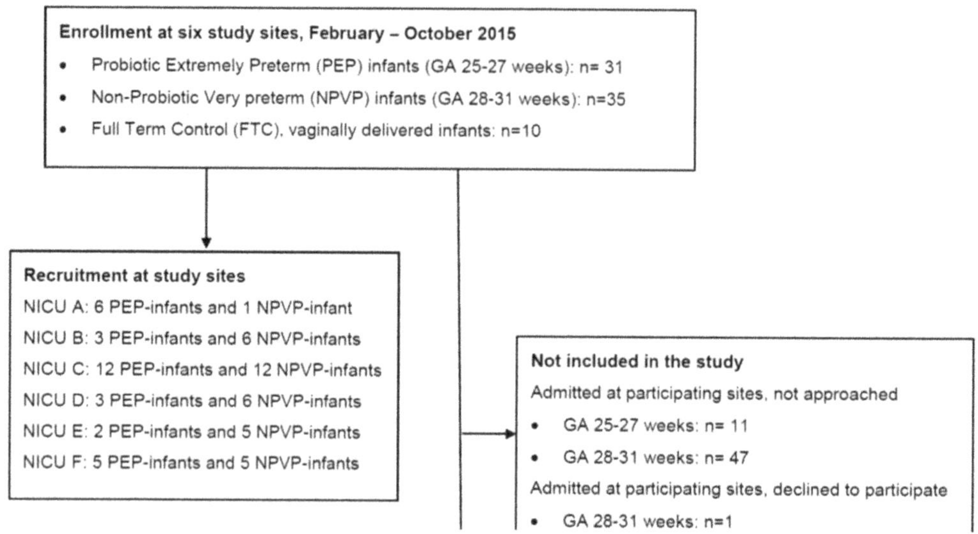

FIGURE 1 | CONSORT study flow diagram. PEP, probiotic extremely preterm; NPVP, non-probiotic very preterm; FTC, full term control; NICU, Neonatal Intensive care Unit.

TABLE 1 | Clinical background data.

	Probiotic extremely preterm (PEP) infants (*n* = 31)	**Non-probiotic very preterm (NPVP) infants** (*n* = 35)	**Full term control (FTC) infants** (*n* = 10)
Birth weight [grams], median (IQR)	835 (680–945)	1,290 (1,150–1,445)	3,613 (3,394–3,733)
Gestational age [weeks], median (IQR)	26 (26–27)	30 (29–30)	40 (40–41)
Gender			
Male, *n* (%)	13 (42%)	20 (57%)	3 (30)
Female, *n* (%)	18 (58%)	15 (43%)	7 (70)
Route of delivery			
Cesarean, *n* (%)	21 (68%)	20 (57%)	0 (0)
Vaginal, *n* (%)	10 (32%)	15 (43%)	10 (100)
CRIB score, mean (SD)	11 (2)	5 (2)	–
Any antenatal antibiotic exposure, *n* (%)	8 (26%)	12 (34%)	0 (0)
Any antibiotic exposure first week of life*, *n* (%)	30 (97%)	27 (77%)	–
Median (IQR) days—antibiotics exposed infants	6 (4–7)	4 (3–5)	–
Any antibiotic exposure after first week of life, *n* (%)	22 (71%)	5 (14%)	–
Narrow spectrum regimen after first week of life, *n* (%)	14 (45%)	3 (9%)	–
Broad-spectrum** regimen after first week of life, *n* (%)	8 (26%)	2 (5%)	–
Median (IQR) days antibiotics in exposed infants	6.5 (3–13)	10 (5.5–14)	
Total days antibiotics, median (IQR); antibiotics exposed infants, *n*	9.5 (6–18) *n* = 30	4 (3–6) *n* = 27	–
Total days of probiotic supplementation, median (IQR)	46 (40–57)	–	–
Parenteral nutrition, *n* (%)	31 (100%)	16 (46%)	–
Median (IQR) days parenteral nutrition	9 (6–13)	5 (3–8)	–
Exclusive human milk nutrition until discharge	17 (55%)	16 (46%)	10 (100)

CRIB, Clinical Risk Index for Babies; IQR, interquartile range.
**Only ampicillin or penicillin + gentamicin were used in all preterm infants in first week of life.*
***We defined regimens including third-generation cephalosporins or carbapenems as a broad-spectrum regimen.*

the microbial composition between the preterm group(s) on 28 days and at 4 months of age (data not shown). We found no differences in abundance of bifidobacteria and or lactobacilli between hospitals at any time point.

Influence of Antibiotic Exposure on Taxonomic Composition

We found no significant influence of antenatal antibiotic exposure on the gut microbiota composition on day 7. However,

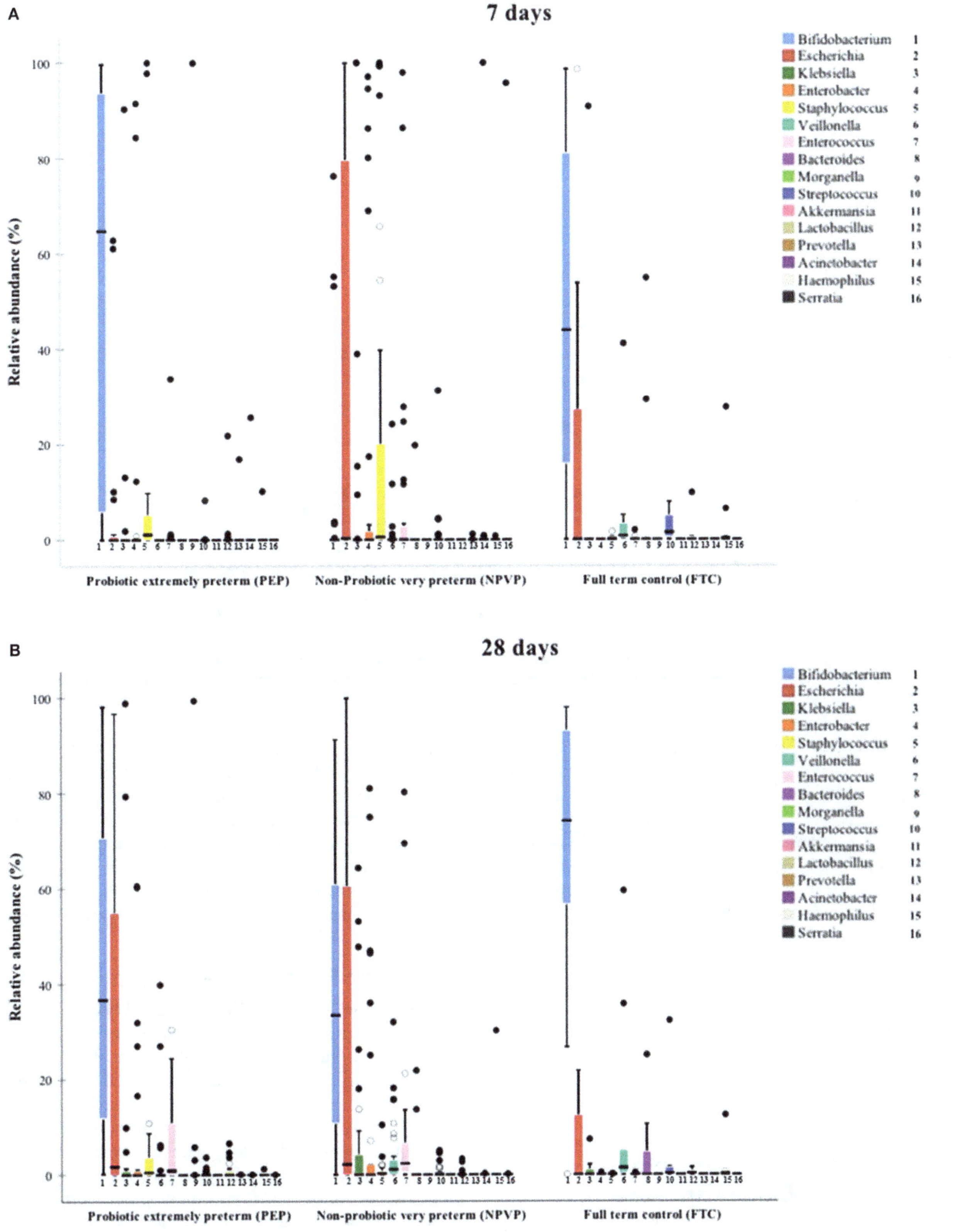

FIGURE 2 | Continued

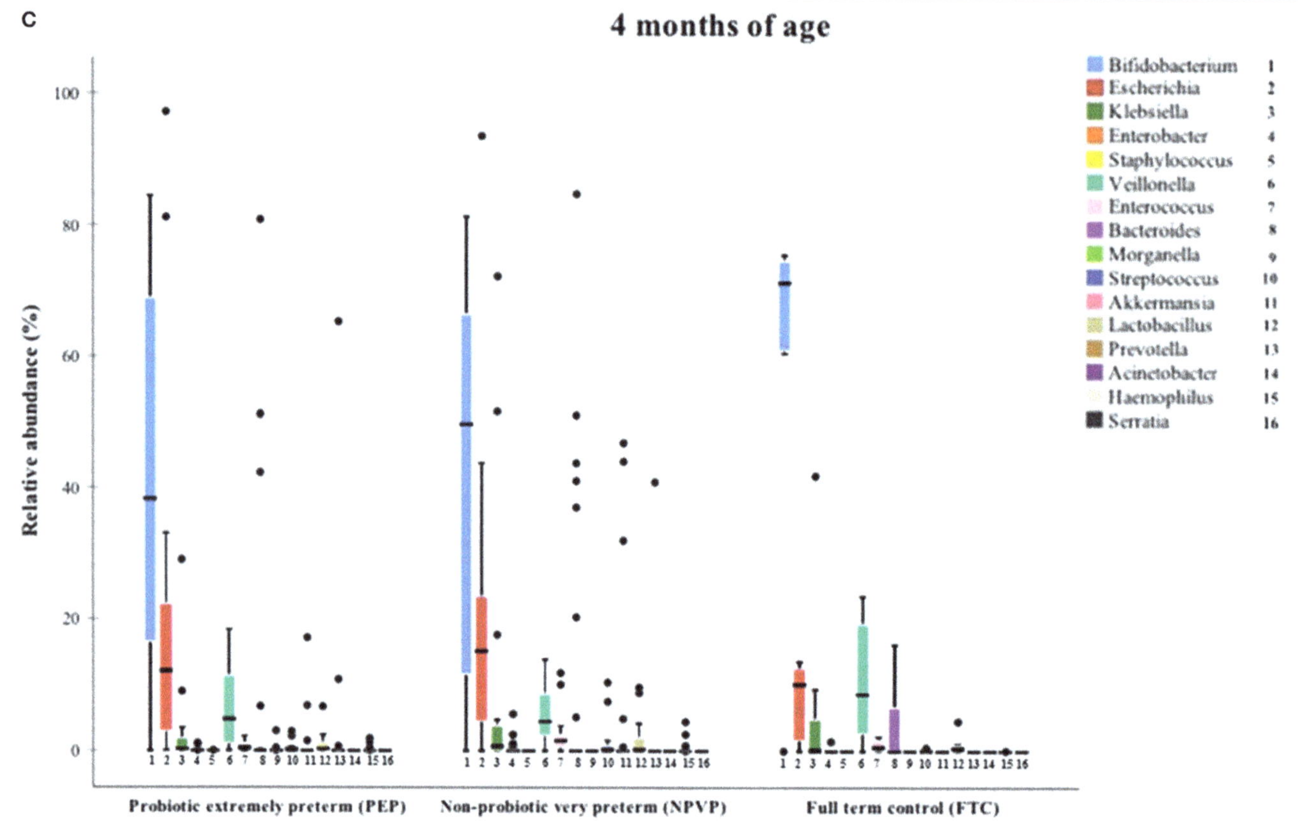

FIGURE 2 | (A–C) Median relative abundance of dominant taxa at genus level. Box plot diagram where the inside bar represent median, the outer horizontal line of the box represents the 25th and the 75th percentile. **(A)** Median relative abundance at 7 days. **(B)** Median relative abundance at 28 days. **(C)** Median relative abundance at 4 months.

57/66 (86%) preterm infants also received antibiotic therapy (ampicillin or penicillin + gentamicin) during the first week of life (**Table 1**), limiting the possibility to detect isolated effects of antenatal exposure. There was no difference in the gut microbiota between those exposed to a short (≤72 h) compared to a prolonged (>72 h) course during first week of life. Broad-spectrum antibiotic therapy after the first week of life was mainly given to PEP-infants. Only one child in the NPVP-group received third generation cephalosporins after first week of life. At 4 months of age there was reduced relative abundance of *Lactobacillus* and *Veilonella* in those exposed to broad-spectrum antibiotics compared to infants exposed to narrow-spectrum therapy (**Tables 3**, **4**). Moreover, there was a non-significant trend toward reduced relative abundance of *Bifidobacterium* and increased relative abundance of *Escherichia* among all preterm infants exposed to broad-spectrum antibiotics at both 28 days and 4 months of age (**Tables 3**, **4**).

Diversity of the Gut Microbiota and Influence of Antibiotic Exposure

We found large intra-individual differences in the gut microbiota composition, in particular at 7 and 28 days of age (**Figures 2A–C**). The alpha diversity increased significantly with age in both preterm infant groups, but not in FTC-infants (**Figure 3A**). FTC-infants had significant higher diversity compared to PEP infants at 7 days of age. On day 28 and at 4 months of age, there were no significant differences in alpha diversity between any groups. Significant overall community (beta diversity) differences using Bray-Curtis dissimilarity were detected comparing the three groups on infants (PEP, NPVP, and FTC) at 7 days of age ($P = 0.001$) and 28 days of age ($P = 0.003$) (**Figures 3B–D**). However, we found no difference in alpha or beta diversity between different categories of antibiotic exposure at the three sampling time points.

Antibiotic Resistome–Distribution of ARG Classes and Abundance of ARGs

In all three groups, we identified putative ARGs conferring resistance to nine different classes of antibiotics, including beta lactams, aminoglycosides, tetracyclines, fosfomycine, sulphonamides, vancomycin, and the macrolide-lincosamide-streptogramin B group. Genes conferring resistance to fluoroquinolones and chloramphenicol were only detected in PEP- and NPVP-infants. Several genes encoding efflux pumps were also identified at all three sampling time points. In total 99 unique ARGs were identified, of which 28 (28%) were located on mobile genetic elements, and these latter were found in more than 80% of all infants (**Table 5**).

We found 21 different genes encoding beta-lactamases, including broad-spectrum and extended-spectrum beta

TABLE 2 | Median relative abundance (%) of dominant genera in infant gut microbiota at 7, 28 days, and 4 months of age.

Genus	7 days ($n = 60$ fecal samples)					28 days ($n = 64$ fecal samples)					4 months ($n = 60$ fecal samples)				
	PEP ($n = 20$)	**NPVP ($n = 30$)**	**FTC ($n = 10$)**	***P*-value**	**FDR Q**	**PEP ($n = 24$)**	**NPVP ($n = 31$)**	**FTC ($n = 9$)**	***P*-value**	**FDR Q**	**PEP ($n = 24$)**	**NPVP ($n = 29$)**	**FTC ($n = 7$)**	***P*-value**	**FDR Q**
Bifidobacterium	64.7	0.00***	43.9	**<0.001**	**<0.001**	36.7	33.5	74.1	0.088	0.156	38.3	49.6	71.2	0.243	0.555
Escherichia	0.00	0.27	0.02	0.107	0.245	1.76	2.10	0.00	0.351	0.511	12.1	15.2	10.10	0.377	0.754
Klebsiella	0.00	0.00	0.00	0.737	0.786	0.00	0.00	0.00	0.663	0.816	0.25	0.67	0.11	0.738	1.0
Enterobacter	0.00	0.00	0.00	0.125	0.222	0.00	0.00	0.00	0.225	0.360	0.00	0.00	0.00	0.110	0.440
Staphylococcus†	1.10	0.54	0.05	0.230	0.368	0.51	0.23	0.01*	**0.038**	**0.076**	0.00	0.00	0.00	0.472	0.839
Veilonella†	0.00	0.00*	0.75***	**<0.001**	**<0.001**	0.00	1.09*	1.38*	**0.018**	**0.072**	4.75	4.44	8.59	0.812	1.0
Enterococcus†	0.00	0.01	0.00	0.118	0.236	0.90	2.35	0.00*	**0.003**	**0.016**	0.39	1.53**	0.58	0.019	0.152
Bacteroides†	0.00	0.00	0.00	**0.005**	**0.013**	0.00	0.00	0.00	**0.001**	**0.008**	0.00	0.00	0.00	0.996	1.0
Morganella	0.00	0.00	0.00	0.368	0.535	0.00	0.00*	0.00	**0.030**	**0.069**	0.00	0.00	0.00	0.098	0.523
Streptococcus	0.00	0.00	1.45***	**<0.001**	**<0.001**	0.00	0.06*	0.26*	**0.018**	**0.058**	0.15	0.14	0.06	0.149	0.477
Akkermansia	0.00	0.00	0.00	1.0	1.0	0.00	0.00	0.00	1.00	1.0	0.00	0.00	0.00	0.171	0.456
Lactobacillus	0.00	0.00*	0.23	**0.004**	**0.013**	0.00	0.00	0.23	**0.019**	**0.051**	0.26	0.18	0.42	0.682	1.0
Prevotella†	0.00	0.00	0.00	0.716	0.818	0.00	0.00	0.00	0.435	0.580	0.00	0.00**	0.00	**0.001**	**0.016**
Acinetobacter	0.00	0.00	0.00	0.525	0.70	0.00	0.00	0.00	0.834	0.953	0.00	0.00	0.00	1.000	1.0
Haemophilus	0.00	0.00	0.14*	**<0.001**	**<0.001**	0.00	0.00	0.07**	**<0.001**	**<0.001**	0.00	0.00	0.00	0.996	1.0
Serratia	0.00	0.00	0.00	0.607	0.747	0.00	0.00	0.00	0.834	0.890	0.00	0.00	0.00	1.000	1.0

PEP, probiotic extremely preterm; NPVP, non-probiotic very preterm; FTC, full term control; FDR, false discovery rate.

Dominant genera have an overall median relative abundance > 0.5% at 7 days, 28 days, and 4 months of age.

*Overall comparison of all three treatment groups at each time point by non-parametric Kruskal–Wallis test. Post-hoc comparisons by non-parametric Mann–Whitney U–test (NPVP or FTC vs. PEP) (***$P < 0.001$, **$P < 0.01$, *$P < 0.05$).*

†Comparison between the three different time points was by a generalized linear model with a Poisson family (†$P < 0.05$).

Bold indicates significant differences in median relative abundance of bacterial genera between the three groups (P- and Q-value).

TABLE 3 | Influence of antibiotic exposure (broad* vs. narrow) on taxonomic composition in all preterm infants (both PEP- and NPVP-infants) with fecal samples and who received antibiotics after first week of life.

Antibiotic regimen	Microbiota at 28 days Median relative abundance			Microbiota at 4 months Median relative abundance			FDR Q
	Broad* (*n* = 7**)	Narrow (*n* = 15**)	*P*	Broad* (*n* = 9**)	Narrow (*n* = 13**)	*P*	
BACTERIAL GENERA							
Bifidobacterium	14.4	28.9	0.783	14.3	41.5	0.096	0.512
Escherichia	44.5	1.40	0.368	17.4	9.9	0.209	0.669
Klebsiella	0.00	0.00	0.680	0.25	0.57	0.845	0.623
Enterobacter	0.00	0.45	0.123	0.00	0.00	0.235	0.627
Staphylococcus	0.42	0.08	0.783	0.00	0.00	1.00	1.00
Veilonella	0.00	0.00	0.945	1.25	6.01	**0.001**	**0.016**
Enterococcus	2.73	0.68	0.783	0.64	0.39	0.647	1.00
Streptococcus	0.00	0.00	0.630	0.07	0.18	0.126	0.504
Lactobacillus	0.00	0.00	0.891	0.00	0.87	0.071	0.568

*PEP, probiotic extremely preterm; NPVP, non-probiotic very preterm. *We defined regimens including third-generation cephalosporins or carbapenems as a broad-spectrum regimen.*
***Number of fecal samples included in these analyses.*
Median relative abundance of Bacteroides, Morganella, Akkermansia, Prevotella, Acinetobacter, Haemophilus, and Serratia were <0.001 at 28 days and 4 months of age and there were no statistical difference between groups.
Bold indicate significant difference between broad- and narrow-spectrum antibiotic exposure.
FDR, false discovery rate; only calculated for comparisons with P < 0.05.

TABLE 4 | Influence of antibiotic exposure (broad* vs. narrow) on taxonomic composition in only the PEP-infants with fecal samples and who received antibiotics after first week of life.

Antibiotic regimen	Microbiota at 28 days Median relative abundance			Microbiota at 4 months Median relative abundance			FDR Q
	Broad* (*n* = 5**)	Narrow (*n* = 12**)	*P*	Broad* (*n* = 7**)	Narrow (*n* = 11**)	*P*	
BACTERIAL GENERA							
Bifidobacterium	14.39	32.50	0.574	14.31	45.96	0.035	0.187
Escherichia	44.54	0.69	0.160	33.06	9.88	0.179	0.477
Klebsiella	0.00	0.00	0.721	0.26	0.57	1.000	1.00
Enterobacter	0.00	0.52	0.195	0.00	0.00	0.143	0.572
Staphylococcus	0.42	0.36	0.879	0.00	0.00	1.000	1.000
Veilonella	0.00	0.00	0.506	0.96	6.01	**0.004**	**0.064**
Enterococcus	2.73	0.15	0.506	0.33	0.40	0.536	0.858
Streptococcus	0.54	0.00	0.442	0.07	0.14	0.285	0.651
Lactobacillus	0.00	0.00	0.959	0.00	1.21	**0.004**	**0.032**

*PEP, probiotic extremely preterm. *We defined regimens including third-generation cephalosporins or carbapenems as a broad-spectrum regimen.*
***Number of fecal samples included in these analyses.*
Median relative abundance of Bacteroides, Morganella, Akkermansia, Prevotella, Acinetobacter, Haemophilus, and Serratia were <0.001 at 28 days and 4 months of age and there were no statistical difference between groups.
Bold indicate significant difference between broad- and narrow-spectrum antibiotic exposure.
FDR, false discovery rate; only calculated for comparisons with P < 0.05.

lactamases (ESBLs). ESBL-genes were represented at all three time points in NPVP- and FTC-infants, but not detected in PEP-infants. The methicillin resistance gene (*mecA*) was identified at 7 and 28 days of age in 11/35 NPVP-infants and 13/31 PEP-infants, but not at 4 months of age. Only one PEP-infant and four NPVP-infants were persistent fecal carriers of *mecA* at days 7 and 28. Vancomycin ARGs were identified at 4 months of age in 16 infants, but only four of these had received vancomycin. Many of the ARGs identified, encoded resistance to other antibiotics than those used in the NICUs.

On day 7 NPVP-infants had higher abundance of ARGs from four different ARG classes and PEP-infants higher abundance of ARGs from two other ARG classes (**Table 6**). Only 24% of

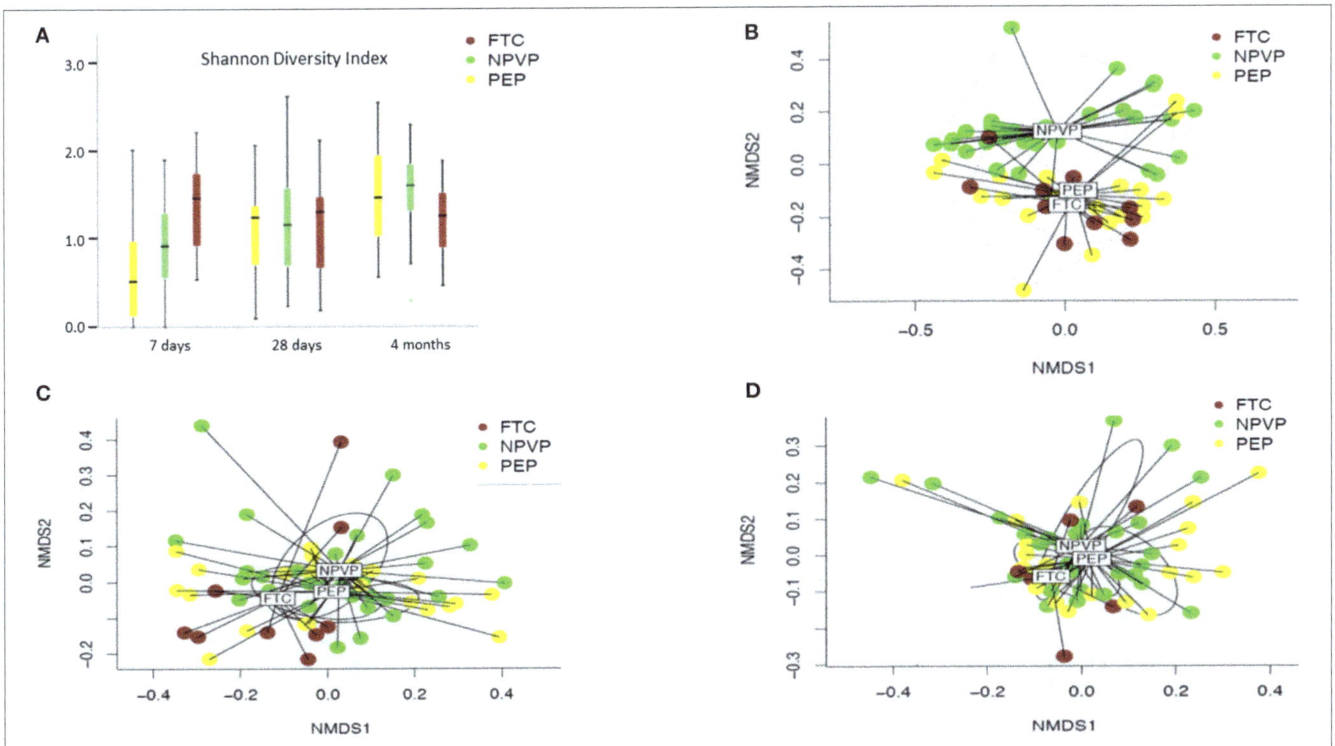

FIGURE 3 | (A–D) Alpha diversity calculated by Shannon diversity index and beta diversity between PEP, NPVP, and FTC infants calculated by non-metrical multidimensional scaling (NMDS). Box plot diagram where the inside bar represent median, the outer horizontal line of the box represents the 25th and the 75th percentile. Error bars represent the standard error. Differences between groups at a given time point and at different time points were tested with linear mixed model. **(A)** Shannon diversity index of three groups of infants at three sampling points. **(B)** Beta diversity (NMDS) at 7 days. **(C)** Beta diversity (NMDS) at 28 days. **(D)** Beta diversity (NMDS) at 4 months.

TABLE 5 | Distribution of classes of antibiotic resistance genes among infants in each group.

Antibiotic group or resistance mechanism**	7 days			28 days			4 months		
	PEP *n* = 20*	NPVP *n* = 30*	FTC *n* = 10*	PEP *n* = 24*	NPVP *n* = 31*	FTC *n* = 9*	PEP *n* = 24*	NPVP *n* = 29*	FTC *n* = 7*
Beta lactamases	10/20	24/30	3/10	19/24	22/31	6/9	18/24	25/29	4/7
MecA gene	9/20	11/30	–	5/24	5/31	–	–	–	–
Aminoglycoside	8/20	14/30	3/10	11/24	16/31	2/9	12/24	16/29	2/7
Tetracycline	9/20	22/30	8/10	17/24	30/31	9/9	23/24	29/29	7/7
Fluoroquinolones	–	1/30	–	1/24	–	–	3/24	4/29	–
Macrolides	7/20	5/30	2/10	6/24	2/31	–	2/24	–	–
MLS	3/20	9/30	3/10	4/24	11/31	3/9	8/24	15/29	4/7
ABC efflux pumps	6/20	7/30	–	16/24	24/31	4/9	17/24	23/29	7/7
RND efflux pumps	7/20	12/30	2/10	12/24	18/24	4/9	12/24	19/24	5/7
Efflux pumps	3/20	3/30	8/10	2/24	4/31	2/9	6/24	8/24	3/7
Multidrug Efflux pump	9/20	14/30	1/10	11/24	7/31	1/9	–	–	–
Chloramphenicol	3/30	9/30	–	6/24	7/31	–	9/24	3/29	–
Fosfomycine	18/20	21/30	3/10	22/24	25/31	5/9	20/24	27/29	4/7
Sulfonamides	2/20	3/30	–	6/24	7/31	–	10/24	9/29	2/7
Antibiotic target	1/20	1/30	–	4/24	4/31	–	6/24	3/29	3/7
Antibiotic inactivation	–	2/30	1/10	1/24	1/31	–	6/24	7/29	2/7
Vancomycin	–	–	–	–	–	–	5/24	8/29	3/7
Metronidazole	–	–	–	–	–	–	–	1/29	–

PEP, probiotic extremely preterm; NPVP, non-probiotic very preterm; FTC, full term control.
**Number of fecal samples included in these analyses.*
***See Methods for further explanation of which antibiotic resistance genes that are included in these groups.*

TABLE 6 | Median abundance of antibiotic resistance genes among infants in each group.

Antibiotic resistance genes (ARG) encoding	7 days (n = 60 fecal samples)					28 days (n = 64 fecal samples)					4 months (n = 60 fecal samples)				
Classes of ARG	PEP (n = 20)	NPVP (n = 30)	FTC (n = 10)	*P*	FDR Q	PEP (n = 24)	NPVP (n = 31)	FTC (n = 9)	*P*	FDR Q	PEP (n = 24)	NPVP (n = 29)	FTC (n = 7)	*P*	*FDR Q*
Class A Beta lactamase	0.61	4.2*	0.00*	**0.001**	**0.020**	0.00	0.00	0.00	0.080	0.586	1.43	1.0	0.00	0.443	1.327
Class C Beta lactamase	0.00	0.00	0.20	0.126	0.229	0.98	0.22	0.00	0.492	0.812	9.1	12.7	9.5	0.605	1.134
Aminoglycoside acetyltransferase	0.00	0.00	0.00	0.202	0.311	–	–	–	–	–	–	–	–	–	–
Aminoglycoside phosphotransferase	0.00	0.00	0.00	0.590	0.653	0.00	0.16	0.00	0.114	0.497	–	–	–	–	–
Aminoglycoside nucleotidyltransferase	0.00	0.00	0.00	0.765	0.765	0.00	0.00	0.00	0.296	0.426	0.00	0.00	0.00	0.584	0.814
Tetracycline efflux	0.00	0.00*	0.00	**0.015**	**0.050**	0.00	0.00	0.00	0.173	0.423	0.00	0.00	0.00	0.174	1.949
Tetracycline ribosomal protection	0.00	0.26	4.4*	**0.047**	0.118	0.52	3.7	1.77	0.397	0.615	6.4	23.4	23.4	0.407	1.041
Quinolone resistance†	9.0	21.6	5.3	0.062	0.138	9.81	7.6	0.77	0.133	0.470	9.2	9.4	7.1	0.501	1.186
Macrolide/MLS resistance	0.00	0.00	0.00	0.757	0.797	–	–	–	–	–	–	–	–	–	–
ABC efflux pump†	0.13	1.15	0.25	0.206	0.294	1.06	1.35	0.06*	0.013	0.414	0.70	0.96	0.83	0.766	0.887
RND antibiotic efflux	5.2	41.9*	38.4	**0.034**	**0.097**	37.7	53.7	4.1	0.170	0.683	94.0	116.7	90.3	0.674	0.936
MFS antibiotic efflux	1.16	113.3	29.0	0.339	0.342	85.8	119.1	16.0	0.056	0.489	105.2	119.5	84.7	0.614	0.839
Multidrug efflux pump activity	0.00	24.6	1.92	0.337	0.449	20.9	21.7	4.9	0.346	0.478	10.0	14.0	8.1	0.616	1.552
Multidrug resistance efflux pump	0.00	0.00	0.00	0.668	0.742	0.00	0.00	0.00	0.603	0.678	0.18	0.00	0.60	0.496	0.819
Gene modulating antibiotic efflux	5.6	41.0**	0.76	**0.012**	**0.060**	14.7	20.1	0.34	0.163	0.376	19.7	27.7	27.5	0.645	0.871
SMR antibiotic efflux	–	1.2	–	–	–	0.00	0.00	0.00	0.914	0.932	–	–	–	–	–
Chloramphenicol acetyltransferase	0.00	0.00	0.00	**0.071**	0.142	–	–	–	–	–	–	–	–	–	–
Antibiotic target†	0.48	0.00	0.00**	**0.013**	**0.052**	0.00	0.00	0.00	0.266	0.396	0.00	0.00	0.00	0.720	0.768
Gene modulating resistance	53.5	8.1**	39.2	**0.003**	**0.030**	37.6	27.8	44.6	0.419	0.419	37.5	45.8	46.2	0.678	1.286
rRNA methyltransferase†	0.00	10.6	10.6	0.128	0.213	6.0	8.8	1.72	0.008	0.464	4.1	5.4	4.4	0.665	0.887
Other ARG†	5.3	16.7**	2.02	**0.011**	**0.073**	7.3	8.4	0.26	0.132	0.413	7.2	10.5	6.3	0.613	

Numbers are presented as median total reads normalized by the total number of reads in each fecal sample.
Antibiotic resistance genes analyzed using ShortBRED.
PEP, probiotic extremely preterm infants; NPVP, non-probiotic very preterm infants; FTC, full-term control; FDR, false discovery rate.
Comparisons between all three treatment groups by nonparametric Kruskal–Wallis test.
*Post-hoc comparisons by non-parametric Mann–Whitney U-test (vs. PEP) (**$P < 0.01$, *$P < 0.05$).*
Comparison between different time points by generalized linear model with a Poisson family ($^{\dagger}P < 0.05$).
Genes modulating antibiotic efflux: norA, baeR, marA, phoQ, ramA, soxR. Genes modulating resistance: WblE, WhiB. Other ARG: bacA.
Bold indicates significant differences in median abundance of antibiotic resistance genes between the three groups (P- and Q-value).

TABLE 7 | Influence of antibiotic exposure (broad vs. narrow spectrum regimen after first week of life) on abundance of antibiotic resistance genes (ARGs) in all preterm infants.

Antibiotic resistance gene (ARG) classes***	ARGs at 28 days Absolute counts/total abundance				ARGs at 4 months Absolute counts/total abundance			
	Broad* (n = 7**)	Narrow (n = 15**)	*P*	FDR *Q*	Broad* (n = 9**)	Narrow (n = 13**)	*P*	FDR *Q*
Class A Beta lactamase	0.00	0.00	0.447	0.731	5.00	3.01	0.324	0.864
Class C Beta lactamase	44.96	0.00	**0.021**	**0.095**	9.11	8.16	0.235	0.752
Aminoglycoside phosphotransferase	6.14	0.00	0.078	0.281	–	–	–	–
Aminoglycoside nucleotidyltransferase	0.93	0.00	**0.008**	**0.072**	0.00	0.00	0.794	0.851
Tetracycline efflux	52.29	0.00	**0.014**	**0.084**	7.92	0.00	0.235	0.94
Tetracycline ribosomal protection	5.97	0.00	0.210	0.540	11.68	2.17	0.393	0.886
Quinolone resistance	29.75	9.43	0.298	0.671	9.40	8.34	0.357	0.816
ABC efflux pump	3.23	1.07	0.392	0.784	0.70	0.64	0.471	0.814
RND antibiotic efflux	312.10	37.73	0.875	0.875	94.00	84.96	0.393	0.63
MFS antibiotic efflux	272.36	117.02	0.490	0.68	119.50	107.51	0.404	0.59
Multidrug efflux pump activity	22.08	26.53	0.581	0.70	19.08	13.63	0.647	0.69
Multidrug resistance efflux pump	0.00	0.00	0.162	0.486	3.02	0.00	0.017	0.272
Gene modulating antibiotic efflux	75.30	15.53	0.490	0.73	19.65	20.86	0.393	0.63
SMR antibiotic efflux	0.00	0.00	0.447	0.805	–	–	–	–
Antibiotic target	1.70	0.00	**0.002**	**0.030**	2.36	0.00	0.096	0.512
Gene modulating resistance	16.25	22.83	0.535	0.69	9.68	39.10	0.043	0.344
rRNA methyltransferase	8.59	9.07	0.581	0.65	8.41	5.56	0.601	0.67
Other ARG	24.40	12.15	0.680	0.72	7.21	7.36	0.601	0.74

**We defined regimens including third-generation cephalosporins or carbapenems as a broad-spectrum regimen.*
***Number of fecal samples included in these analyses.*
****See Materials and Methods section for further explanation of which antibiotic resistance genes that are included in these groups.*
FDR, false discovery rate.
Bold indicates significant differences in abundance of antibiotic resistance genes between broad- and narrow-spectrum regimens (P- and Q-value).

ARG-classes changed significantly their abundance during the three sampling points ($P < 0.05$) (**Table 6**).

On day 7 and at 4 months of age, different antibiotic exposure did not result in significant difference in total abundance of ARGs. However, on day 28, we detected significantly higher abundances of four classes of ARGs, including genes encoding beta-lactam and aminoglycoside resistance, in preterm infants exposed to broad-spectrum antibiotics compared to infants treated with narrow-spectrum regimens (**Table 7**). For the subset of preterm infants given probiotics there were no significant differences in abundance of ARGs at 4 weeks and 4 months (**Table 8**).

DISCUSSION

The main aim of this explorative, observational multi-center study was to obtain in-depth knowledge on how probiotics and antibiotic therapy influenced the developing gut microbiota and antibiotic resistome of preterm infants. Previous studies have shown that the gut microbiota in preterm infants differs from term infants with limited diversity and delayed acquisition of a stable profile (36–38). However, most studies have assessed the gut microbiota composition collapsed at higher taxonomic rank levels (above species-genera level) by sequencing of the 16S ribosomal RNA gene (31, 39). There is limited data (21) on the association between use of probiotics, antibiotics and gut resistome development using shotgun-metagenomic sequencing.

Bifidobacteria strongly dominated the gut microbiota in extremely preterm infants only few days after commencing probiotic supplementation, in sharp contrast to very preterm infants not receiving probiotics who predominantly had *Escherichia*. High levels of probiotic bacteria are not necessarily indicative of colonization, but may represent the passage of DNA from the administered probiotic species through the host (40). Still, early dominance of bifidobacteria may theoretically enhance the risk of translocation to the blood stream, in particular during first weeks of life in extremely preterm infants when enteral nutrition with "fuel for bifidobacteria" is not yet fully established (13, 14). However, bifidobacterial infections are usually mild (14, 41), in contrast to sepsis caused by Gram-negative bacteria (*Proteobacteria*), which in preterm infants are the first colonizers of the intestinal tract. Previous studies have shown that the gut microbiota of preterm infants shortly after birth have a high proportion of *Proteobacteria* and that a bloom of *Bifidobacterium* occurs first around 33 weeks of age, in line with our findings in NPVP-infants at 7 and 28 days of age (42, 43).

Lactobacillus was only detected in small amounts in all groups, but relative abundance increased up to 4 months of age in all three groups. High levels of *Bifidobacterium* and barely detectable levels of *Lactobacillus* have been reported earlier in infants

TABLE 8 | Influence of antibiotic exposure (broad vs. narrow after first week of life) on abundance of antibiotic resistance genes (ARGs) in probiotic supplemented extremely preterm (PEP) infants.

Antibiotic resistance genes (ARGs) classes***	ARGs at 28 days Absolute counts/total abundance				ARGs at 4 months Absolute counts/total abundance			
	Broad* (*n* = 5**)	Narrow (*n* = 12**)	*P*	FDR Q	Broad* (*n* = 7**)	Narrow (*n* = 11**)	*P*	FDR Q
Class A Beta lactamase	0.00	0.00	0.799	0.846	1.43	3.01	0.596	0.867
Class C Beta lactamase	45.96	0.00	0.009	0.162	9.11	9.52	0.328	0.875
Aminoglycoside phosphotransferase	6.14	0.00	0.082	0.369	–	–	–	–
Aminoglycoside nucleotidyltransferase	0.93	0.00	0.104	0.312	0.00	0.00	0.860	
Tetracycline efflux	29.55	0.00	0.019	0.171	7.92	7.92	0.375	0.857
Tetracycline ribosomal protection	6.49	0.00	0.082	0.369	11.68	28.48	0.246	0.787
Quinolone resistance	29.75	7.08	0.506	0.828	9.40	9.40	0.425	0.85
ABC efflux pump	3.23	0.43	0.279	0.628	0.70	1.10	0.479	0.852
RND antibiotic efflux	312.10	19.81	0.799	0.900	94.00	93.09	0.536	0.858
MFS antibiotic efflux	272.36	79.67	0.506	0.759	70.92	111.28	0.860	0.917
Multidrug efflux pump activity	22.08	24.71	0.879	0.879	19.08	6.55	0.647	0.863
Multidrug resistance efflux pump	0.00	0.00	0.234	0.602	3.02	3.02	0.069	0.368
Gene modulating antibiotic efflux	75.30	13.81	0.328	0.656	19.65	24.88	0.008	0.128
SMR antibiotic efflux	0.00	0.00	0.506	0.759	–	–	–	–
Antibiotic target	1.70	0.00	0.064	0.030	2.36	0.00	0.151	0.604
Gene modulating resistance	16.25	33.15	0.442	0.756	9.68	60.81	0.043	0.344
rRNA methyltransferase	5.15	6.23	0.799	0.846	8.41	2.85	0.930	0.930
Other ARG	24.40	7.31	0.506	0.700	7.21	7.21	0.724	0.891

**We defined regimens including third-generation cephalosporins or carbapenems as a broad-spectrum regimen.*
***Number of fecal samples included in these analyses.*
****See Materials and Methods section for further explanation of which antibiotic resistance genes that are included in these groups.*
FDR, false discovery rate. Aminoglycoside acetyltransferase, Macrolide resistance genes, Chloramphenicol acetyltransferase were only present at 7 days of age.

supplemented with equal doses of a probiotic combination of bifidobacteria and lactobacilli (31). A possible explanation for this observation is the spatial organization of intestinal bacteria, where lactobacilli are found in intestinal crypts, thus less accessible when collecting luminal contents (44). Indeed, a recent study in adults showed marked differences between the small intestine microbiota compared to the colonic microbiota (45), indicating the scientific limitations with fecal samples when aiming to understand the entire human intestinal ecosystem.

There is no consensus on the optimal dose of probiotics. One study from India compared standard and high-dose probiotic regimens and found no difference in proportion of infants colonized or quantitative colonization rates with probiotic species (46). Most large randomized trial have used daily doses of 1 × 10^8-10^9 CFU (40, 47, 48). Some authors suggest that at least 1 × 10^9 CFU is required to achieve a beneficial effect, in line with the doses used in our study (49). We observed an early and high relative abundance of *Bifidobacterium* in PEP-infants. However, we did not use traditional microbiological methods to assess the overall bacterial abundance in the gut. Some authors have suggested that a gradual increase in probiotic supplementation concomitantly with increased enteral nutrition may replicate the physiological gut microbiota development, and secure gut growth, digestive maturation and an appropriate response to bacterial colonization (50, 51). Our study does not allow us to draw any conclusions on dosing. A recent study reported that a daily dose of the same probiotic used in our study (Infloran®) leads to significantly higher levels of *Bifidobacterium* when compared to dosing bi-weekly or weekly (52).

A lower relative abundance of *Bifidobacterium, Lactobacillus, and Veilonella*, and a higher relative abundance of *Escherichia*, were observed at day 28 and 4 months of age among infants treated with broad-spectrum compared to narrow-spectrum antibiotic regimens. Reduced abundance of protective anaerobe commensals and higher abundance of *Enterobacteriaceae* after antibiotic exposure has also previously been reported (53, 54). When comparing presence and absence of antibiotic exposure after the first week of life, no differences in diversity or taxonomic composition were found. Previous studies on alpha diversity and influence of antibiotic treatment have shown inconsistent results (55). However, infants who were most heavily exposed to antibiotic treatment in our study were also supplemented with probiotics. In animals, probiotics may alleviate the potential loss of microbial diversity created by antibiotic treatment (56). This may explain why PEP-infants, exposed to massive antibiotic pressure, did not have reduced microbial gut diversity compared to other groups. Thus, probiotic supplementation may offer a protective effect partly compensating harmful effects of antibiotics in preterm infants. However, the early low number of taxa in preterm infant stools places constraints on interpreting diversity changes as diversity in a non-complex population may reflect changes in only one taxon.

In line with others, we found that the gut antibiotic resistome of preterm and term infants is established early, independent of antibiotic exposure (21, 57–59). We detected significant higher abundance of ARGs in infants receiving broad-spectrum antibiotics compared to narrow-spectrum regimens. Gibson and co-workers also showed that broad-spectrum antibiotic therapy in preterm infants, was associated with enrichment of specific ARGs (21). We aimed to investigate how probiotic supplementation can influence the gut antibiotic resistome. Overall, there were no differences in distribution of ARG-classes or abundance of ARGs at 28 days and 4 months of age between PEP-infants, exposed to massive antibiotic therapy, and the two other groups with limited or no antibiotic exposure. One possible mechanism for this finding is that probiotic bacteria can produce bacteriocins that improve mucosal integrity and thereby reduces the pathogenic bacterial population and antibiotic resistance (60).

Strengths and Limitations

At the time of this study, probiotic supplementation to extremely preterm infants was considered "standard of care" in Norway. We were therefore beyond equipoise to perform a randomized study comparing probiotic to no probiotic supplementation in this population. The NPVP-infant group has limitations as a control group due to maturational differences and the difference in antibiotic exposure compared to the PEP-infants. However, more antibiotic exposure in the PEP-infants would most likely have led to less diversity and higher abundance of ARGs. Still, we found few differences between the two preterm groups at 28 days and 4 months of age, suggesting a protective effect of probiotics in the PEP-infant group. The gut microbiota composition of preterm infants may differ between hospitals (61), but our multi-center approach intended to average local differences and strengthen generalizability. Infants harbor a much lower gut microbial diversity compared to adults. Any variation in the gut microbiota composition caused by storage may thus theoretically have a proportionally greater effect on the composition (25). We chose a standardized sampling technique in order to avoid potential biases due to freezing of samples at different time points and temperature variation during transport to the laboratory. However, in the most immature infants the DNA content in the early fecal samples was very low, and we were only able to obtain sequence data from 20/31 samples at 1 week of age.

CONCLUSION

Probiotic-supplemented extremely preterm (PEP) infants had a high relative abundance of *Bifidobacterium* at 1 week of age, only few days after start of probiotic supplementation. PEP-infants were also exposed to much more antibiotics, but overall microbial diversity and resistome was not different than in more mature infants at 4 weeks and 4 months. We speculate that probiotic supplementation may induce colonization resistance and thereby partly alleviate harmful effects of antibiotics on gut microbiota composition and the antibiotic resistome development.

AUTHOR CONTRIBUTIONS

EE organized all phases of the study, analyzed data, wrote the first version of the manuscript, and revised the manuscript. She had full access to all of the data in the study and takes responsibility for the integrity of the data and the accuracy of the data analysis. TP, JA, SR, RS, and BN were responsible for inclusion of patients at participating centers, data retrieval, and revised the manuscript. JC, EH, and NW took part in study design, were responsible for microbiological (JC) and bioinformatic (EH, NW) analyses and revised the manuscript. CK conceptualized and designed the study, directed all phases of the study, and revised the final manuscript. He had full access to all of the data in the study and takes responsibility for the integrity of the data and the accuracy of the data analysis. All authors approved the final manuscript as submitted and agree to be accountable for all aspects of the work.

ACKNOWLEDGMENTS

We thank the parents of the infants participating in this study and the nurses at the participating centers for helping collect fecal samples.

REFERENCES

1. Groer MW, Luciano AA, Dishaw LJ, Ashmeade TL, Miller E, Gilbert JA. Development of the preterm infant gut microbiome: a research priority. *Microbiome* (2014) 2:38. doi: 10.1186/2049-2618-2-38
2. Olin A, Henckel E, Chen Y, Lakshmikanth T, Pou C, Mikes J, et al. Stereotypic immune system development in newborn children. *Cell* (2018) 5:1277–92.e14. doi: 10.1016/j.cell.2018.06.045
3. Pammi M, Cope J, Tarr PI, Warner BB, Morrow AL, Mai V, et al. Intestinal dysbiosis in preterm infants preceding necrotizing enterocolitis: a systematic review and meta-analysis. *Microbiome* (2017) 1:31. doi: 10.1186/s40168-017-0248-8
4. AlFaleh K, Anabrees J. Probiotics for prevention of necrotizing enterocolitis in preterm infants. *Cochrane Database Syst Rev.* (2014) 10:CD005496. doi: 10.1002/14651858.CD005496.pub4

5. Aceti A, Gori D, Barone G, Callegari ML, Di Mauro A, Fantini MP, et al. Probiotics for prevention of necrotizing enterocolitis in preterm infants: systematic review and meta-analysis. *Ital J Pediatr*. (2015) 41:89. doi: 10.1186/s13052-015-0199-2
6. Sawh SC, Deshpande S, Jansen S, Reynaert CJ, Jones PM. Prevention of necrotizing enterocolitis with probiotics: a systematic review and meta-analysis. *PeerJ*. (2016) 4:e2429. doi: 10.7717/peerj.2429
7. Lau CS, Chamberlain RS. Probiotic administration can prevent necrotizing enterocolitis in preterm infants: a meta-analysis. *J Pediatr Surg*. (2015) 8:1405–12. doi: 10.1016/j.jpedsurg.2015.05.008
8. Olsen R, Greisen G, Schroder M, Brok J. Prophylactic probiotics for preterm infants: a systematic review and meta-analysis of observational studies. *Neonatology* (2016) 2:105–12. doi: 10.1159/000441274
9. Costeloe K, Bowler U, Brocklehurst P, Hardy P, Heal P, Juszczak E, et al. A randomised controlled trial of the probiotic Bifidobacterium breve BBG-001 in preterm babies to prevent sepsis, necrotising enterocolitis and death: the Probiotics in Preterm infantS (PiPS) trial. *Health Technol Assess*. (2016) 66:1–194. doi: 10.3310/hta20660.
10. Denkel LA, Schwab F, Garten L, Geffers C, Gastmeier P, Piening B. Protective effect of dual-strain probiotics in preterm infants: a multi-center time series analysis. *PLoS ONE* (2016) 6:e0158136. doi: 10.1371/journal.pone.0158136
11. Tarnow-Mordi W, Soll RF. Probiotic supplementation in preterm infants: it is time to change practice. *J Pediatr*. (2014) 5:959–60. doi: 10.1016/j.jpeds.2013.12.050
12. Viswanathan S, Lau C, Akbari H, Hoyen C, Walsh MC. Survey and evidence based review of probiotics used in very low birth weight preterm infants within the United States. *J Perinatol*. (2016) 12:1106–11. doi: 10.1038/jp.2016.144.
13. Esaiassen E, Cavanagh P, Hjerde E, Simonsen GS, Stoen R, Klingenberg C. Bifidobacterium longum subspecies infantis bacteremia in 3 extremely preterm infants receiving probiotics. *Emerg Infect Dis*. (2016) 9:1664–6. doi: 10.3201/eid2209.160033
14. Zbinden A, Zbinden R, Berger C, Arlettaz R. Case series of Bifidobacterium longum bacteremia in three preterm infants on probiotic therapy. *Neonatology* (2015) 1:56–9. doi: 10.1159/000367985
15. Kolacek S, Hojsak I, Berni Canani R, Guarino A, Indrio F, et al. Commercial probiotic products: a call for improved quality control. a position paper by the ESPGHAN working group for probiotics and prebiotics. *J Pediatr Gastroenterol Nutr*. (2017) 1:117–24. doi: 10.1097/mpg.0000000000001603
16. Vallabhaneni S, Walker TA, Lockhart SR, Ng D, Chiller T, Melchreit R, et al. Notes from the field: fatal gastrointestinal mucormycosis in a premature infant associated with a contaminated dietary supplement–Connecticut, 2014. *MMWR Morb Mortal Wkly Rep*. (2015) 6:155–6.
17. Frost BL, Modi BP, Jaksic T, Caplan MS. New medical and surgical insights into neonatal necrotizing enterocolitis: a review. *JAMA Pediatr*. (2017) 1:83–8. doi: 10.1001/jamapediatrics.2016.2708
18. Hsieh EM, Hornik CP, Clark RH, Laughon MM, Benjamin DK Jr, Smith PB. Medication use in the neonatal intensive care unit. *Am J Perinatol*. (2014) 9:811–21. doi: 10.1055/s-0033-1361933.
19. Esaiassen E, Fjalstad JW, Juvet LK, van den Anker JN, Klingenberg C. Antibiotic exposure in neonates and early adverse outcomes: a systematic review and meta-analysis. *J Antimicrob Chemother*. (2017) 72:1858–70. doi: 10.1093/jac/dkx088
20. Cotten CM, Taylor S, Stoll B, Goldberg RN, Hansen NI, Sanchez PJ, et al. Prolonged duration of initial empirical antibiotic treatment is associated with increased rates of necrotizing enterocolitis and death for extremely low birth weight infants. *Pediatrics* (2009) 1:58–66. doi: 10.1542/peds.2007-3423
21. Gibson MK, Wang B, Ahmadi S, Burnham CA, Tarr PI, Warner BB, et al. Developmental dynamics of the preterm infant gut microbiota and antibiotic resistome. *Nat Microbiol*. (2016) 1:16024. doi: 10.1038/nmicrobiol.2016.24
22. Fjalstad JW, Esaiassen E, Juvet LK, van den Anker JN, Klingenberg C. Antibiotic therapy in neonates and impact on gut microbiota and antibiotic resistance development: a systematic review. *J Antimicrob Chemother*. (2017) 73:569–80. doi: 10.1093/jac/dkx426
23. Kelly BJ, Gross R, Bittinger K, Sherrill-Mix S, Lewis JD, Collman RG, et al. Power and sample-size estimation for microbiome studies using pairwise distances and PERMANOV. *Bioinformatics* (2015) 15:2461–8. doi: 10.1093/bioinformatics/btv183
24. Klingenberg C. *Preterm Infant Gut (PINGU) - a Norwegian Multi Centre Study (PINGU)*. Available online at: https://clinicaltrials.gov/ct2/show/NCT02197468
25. Hill CJ, Brown JR, Lynch DB, Jeffery IB, Ryan CA, Ross RP, et al. Effect of room temperature transport vials on DNA quality and phylogenetic composition of faecal microbiota of elderly adults and infants. *Microbiome* (2016) 1:19. doi: 10.1186/s40168-016-0164-3
26. Neu J, Walker WA. Necrotizing enterocolitis. *N Engl J Med*. (2011) 3:255–64. doi: 10.1056/NEJMra1005408
27. Truong DT, Franzosa EA, Tickle TL, Scholz M, Weingart G, Pasolli E, et al. MetaPhlAn2 for enhanced metagenomic taxonomic profiling. *Nat Methods* (2015) 10:902–3. doi: 10.1038/nmeth.3589
28. McArthur AG, Waglechner N, Nizam F, Yan A, Azad MA, Baylay AJ, et al. The comprehensive antibiotic resistance database. *Antimicrob Agents Chemother*. (2013) 7:3348–57. doi: 10.1128/aac.00419-13
29. Kaminski J, Gibson MK, Franzosa EA, Segata N, Dantas G, Huttenhower C. High-specificity targeted functional profiling in microbial communities with shortBRED. *PLoS Comput Biol*. (2015) 12:e1004557. doi: 10.1371/journal.pcbi.1004557
30. Klingenberg C. *Manual of Neonatal Medicine*. 5th Edn. Tromsø: Paediatric Deptartment, University Hospital of Northern Norway (2017).
31. Abdulkadir B, Nelson A, Skeath T, Marrs EC, Perry JD, Cummings SP, et al. Routine use of probiotics in preterm infants: longitudinal impact on the microbiome and metabolome. *Neonatology* (2016) 4:239–47. doi: 10.1159/000442936
32. de Man P, Verhoeven BA, Verbrugh HA, Vos MC, van den Anker JN. An antibiotic policy to prevent emergence of resistant bacilli. *Lancet* (2000) 9208:973–8. doi: 10.1016/S0140-6736(00)90015-1
33. Parks DH, Tyson GW, Hugenholtz P, Beiko RG. STAMP: statistical analysis of taxonomic and functional profiles. *Bioinformatics* (2014) 21:3123–4. doi: 10.1093/bioinformatics/btu494
34. Benjamini Y, Hochberg Y. Controlling the false discovery rate: a practical and powerful approach to multiple testing. *J R Stat Soc Series B* (1995) 57:289–300.
35. Huson DH, Auch AF, Qi J, Schuster SC. MEGAN analysis of metagenomic data. *Genome Res*. (2007) 3:377–86. doi: 10.1101/gr.5969107
36. Weng M, Walker WA. The role of gut microbiota in programming the immune phenotype. *J Dev Orig Health Dis*. (2013) 3:203–14. doi: 10.1017/s2040174412000712
37. Hill CJ, Lynch DB, Murphy K, Ulaszewska M, Jeffery IB, O'Shea CA, et al. Evolution of gut microbiota composition from birth to 24 weeks in the INFANTMET Cohort. *Microbiome* (2017) 1:4. doi: 10.1186/s40168-016-0213-y
38. Arboleya S, Binetti A, Salazar N, Fernandez N, Solis G, Hernandez-Barranco A, et al. Establishment and development of intestinal microbiota in preterm neonates. *FEMS Microbiol Ecol*. (2012) 3:763–72. doi: 10.1111/j.1574-6941.2011.01261.x
39. Stewart CJ, Embleton ND, Marrs EC, Smith DP, Nelson A, Abdulkadir B, et al. Temporal bacterial and metabolic development of the preterm gut reveals specific signatures in health and disease. *Microbiome* (2016) 1:67. doi: 10.1186/s40168-016-0216-8
40. Jacobs SE, Tobin JM, Opie GF, Donath S, Tabrizi SN, Pirotta M, et al. Probiotic effects on late-onset sepsis in very preterm infants: a randomized controlled trial. *Pediatrics* (2013) 6:1055–62. doi: 10.1542/peds.2013-1339
41. Bertelli C, Pillonel T, Torregrossa A, Prod'hom G, Fischer CJ, Greub G, et al. Bifidobacterium longum bacteremia in preterm infants receiving probiotics. *Clin Infect Dis*. (2015) 6:924–7. doi: 10.1093/cid/ciu946
42. Wang Y, Hoenig JD, Malin KJ, Qamar S, Petrof EO, Sun J, et al. 16S rRNA gene-based analysis of fecal microbiota from preterm infants with and without necrotizing enterocolitis. *ISME J*. (2009) 8:944–54. doi: 10.1038/ismej.2009.37
43. Butel MJ, Suau A, Campeotto F, Magne F, Aires J, Ferraris L, et al. Conditions of bifidobacterial colonization in preterm infants: a prospective analysis. *J Pediatr Gastroenterol Nutr*. (2007) 5:577–82. doi: 10.1097/MPG.0b013e3180406b20
44. Swidsinski A, Loening-Baucke V, Lochs H, Hale LP. Spatial organization of bacterial flora in normal and inflamed intestine: a fluorescence *in situ* hybridization study in mice. *World J Gastroenterol*. (2005) 8:1131–40. doi: 10.3748/wjg.v11.i8.1131

45. Villmones HC, Haug ES, Ulvestad E, Grude N, Stenstad T, Halland A, et al. Species level description of the human ileal bacterial microbiota. *Sci Rep.* (2018) 1:4736. doi: 10.1038/s41598-018-23198-5
46. Dutta S, Ray P, Narang A. Comparison of stool colonization in premature infants by three dose regimes of a probiotic combination: a randomized controlled trial. *Am J Perinatol.* (2015) 8:733–40. doi: 10.1055/s-0034-1395473
47. Costeloe K, Hardy P, Juszczak E, Wilks M, Millar MR. Bifidobacterium breve BBG-001 in very preterm infants: a randomised controlled phase 3 trial. *Lancet* (2016) 10019:649–60. doi: 10.1016/s0140-6736(15)01027-2
48. Gritz EC, Bhandari V. The human neonatal gut microbiome: a brief review. *Front Pediatr.* (2015) 3:17. doi: 10.3389/fped.2015.00017
49. Deshpande GC, Rao SC, Keil AD, Patole SK. Evidence-based guidelines for use of probiotics in preterm neonates. *BMC Med.* (2011) 9:92. doi: 10.1186/1741-7015-9-92
50. Siggers RH, Siggers J, Thymann T, Boye M, Sangild PT. Nutritional modulation of the gut microbiota and immune system in preterm neonates susceptible to necrotizing enterocolitis. *J Nutr Biochem.* (2011) 6:511–21. doi: 10.1016/j.jnutbio.2010.08.002
51. Cilieborg MS, Boye M, Sangild PT. Bacterial colonization and gut development in preterm neonates. *Early Hum Dev.* (2012) 88:S41–9. doi: 10.1016/j.earlhumdev.2011.12.027
52. Watkins C, Murphy K, Dempsey EM, O'Shea CA, Murphy BP, O'Toole PW, et al. Dose-interval study of a dual probiotic in preterm infants. *Arch Dis Child Fetal Neonatal Ed.* (2018) 20:313468. doi: 10.1136/archdischild-2017-313468
53. Hall MA, Cole CB, Smith SL, Fuller, Rolles CJ. Factors influencing the presence of faecal lactobacilli in early infancy. *Arch Dis Childhood* (1990) 2:185–88.
54. Fouhy F, Guinane CM, Hussey S, Wall R, Ryan CA, Dempsey EM, et al. High-throughput sequencing reveals the incomplete, short-term recovery of infant gut microbiota following parenteral antibiotic treatment with ampicillin and gentamicin. *Antimicrob Agents Chemother.* (2012) 11:5811–20. doi: 10.1128/aac.00789-12
55. Rose G, Shaw AG, Sim K, Wooldridge DJ, Li MS, Gharbia S, et al. Antibiotic resistance potential of the healthy preterm infant gut microbiome. *PeerJ.* (2017) 5:e2928. doi: 10.7717/peerj.2928
56. Grazul H, Kanda LL, Gondek D. Impact of probiotic supplements on microbiome diversity following antibiotic treatment of mice. *Gut Microbes* (2016) 2:101–14. doi: 10.1080/19490976.2016.1138197
57. Fouhy F, Ogilvie LA, Jones B, Ross RP, Ryan AC, Dempsey EM, et al. Identification of aminoglycoside and beta-lactam resistance genes from within an infant gut functional metagenomic library. *PLoS ONE* (2014) 9:e108016. doi: 10.1371/journal.pone.0108016
58. von Wintersdorff CJ, Wolffs PF, Savelkoul PH, Nijsen RR, Lau S, Gerhold K, et al. The gut resistome is highly dynamic during the first months of life. *Future Microbiol.* (2016) 4:501–10. doi: 10.2217/fmb.15.154
59. Moore AM, Patel S, Forsberg KJ, Wang B, Bentley G, Razia Y, et al. Pediatric fecal microbiota harbor diverse and novel antibiotic resistance genes. *PLoS ONE* (2013) 11:e78822. doi: 10.1371/journal.pone.0078822
60. Pamer EG. Resurrecting the intestinal microbiota to combat antibiotic-resistant pathogens. *Science* (2016) 6285:535–8. doi: 10.1126/science.aad9382
61. Ravi A, Estensmo ELF, Abee-Lund TML, Foley SL, Allgaier B, Martin CR, et al. Association of the gut microbiota mobilome with hospital location and birth weight in preterm infants. *Pediatr Res.* (2017) 82:829–838. doi: 10.1038/pr.2017.146

19

Continuous-Infusion Vancomycin in Neonates: Assessment of a Dosing Regimen and Therapeutic Proposal

Manon Tauzin [1], Robert Cohen [2,3,4,5,6], Xavier Durrmeyer [1,3,7], Gilles Dassieu [1], Jérôme Barre [4,8] and Laurence Caeymaex [1,4,9]*

[1] Neonatal Intensive Care Unit, Centre Hospitalier Intercommunal de Créteil, Créteil, France, [2] ACTIV, Association Clinique et Thérapeutique Infantile du Val de Marne, Saint-Maur des Fossés, France, [3] Université Paris Est, IMRB- GRC GEMINI, Créteil, France, [4] Clinical Research Center, Centre Hospitalier Intercommunal de Créteil, Créteil, France, [5] Groupe de Pathologie Infectieuse Pédiatrique, Paris, France, [6] Unité Court Séjour, Petits Nourrissons, Service de Néonatologie, Centre Hospitalier Intercommunal de Créteil, Créteil, France, [7] Inserm, U1153, Obstetrical, Perinatal and Pediatric Epidemiology Team, Epidemiology and Biostatistics Sorbonne, Paris Descartes University, Paris, France, [8] Department of Pharmacology, Centre Hospitalier Intercommunal de Créteil, Créteil, France, [9] Department of Research in Ethics EA1610 Studies on Science and Technics, Paris Est University, Créteil, France

***Correspondence:**
Manon Tauzin
manon.tauzin@gmail.com

Introduction: Vancomycin remains the reference antibiotic in neonates for care-related infections caused by ß-lactam–resistant Gram-positive bacteria. Achieving the optimal serum vancomycin level is challenging because of high inter-individual variability and the drug's narrow therapeutic window. Continuous infusion might offer pharmacokinetic and practical advantages, but we lack consensus on the dosing regimen. The aim was to determine the proportion of neonates achieving an optimal therapeutic vancomycin level at the first vancomycin concentration assay and which dosing regimen is the most suitable for neonates.

Methods: All neonates receiving continuous-infusion vancomycin (loading dose 15 mg/kg and maintenance dose 30 mg/kg/d) in a neonatal intensive care unit were retrospectively analyzed. The proportion of neonates reaching the target serum vancomycin level was calculated. After reviewing the literature to identify all published articles proposing a dosing regimen for continuous-infusion vancomycin for neonates, regimens were theoretically applied to our population by using maintenance doses according to covariate(s) proposed in the original publication.

Results: Between January 2013 and December 2014, 75 neonates received 91 vancomycin courses by continuous infusion. Median gestational age, birth weight, and postnatal age were 27 weeks (interquartile range 26–30.5), 815 g (685–1,240), and 15 days (9–33). At the first assay, only 28/91 (30.8%) courses resulted in vancomycin levels between 20 and 30 mg/L (target level), 23/91 (25.3%) >30 mg/L and 40/91 (43.9%) <20 mg/L. We applied six published dosing regimens to our patients. One of these dosing regimens based on corrected gestational age (CGA) and serum creatinine level (SCR) would have allowed us to prescribe lower doses to neonates with high vancomycin levels and higher doses to neonates with low levels.

Conclusions: A simplified dosing regimen of continuous-infusion vancomycin did not achieve therapeutic ranges in neonates; a patient-tailored dosing regimen taking into account CGA and SCR level or an individualized pharmacokinetic model can help to anticipate the inter-individual variability in neonates and would have been more suitable.

Keywords: vancomycin, continuous-infusion, neonates, dosing, pharmacokinetics

INTRODUCTION

Vancomycin is a glycopeptide antibiotic frequently prescribed for neonatal care-related infections caused by Gram-positive bacteria such as coagulase-negative Staphylococci (CoNS), methicillin-resistant *Staphylococcus aureus* (MRSA), and Enterococci species (1). Because of the narrow therapeutic window and the lack of consensus on a toxicity threshold, determining the optimal dosing regimen for vancomycin is difficult, particularly for premature neonates, including those born before 28 weeks' gestation.

Vancomycin is a time-dependant antibiotic. It is sensitive to high inoculum effect and inhibited by biofilms (2). Its pharmacokinetics are characterized by an unbound fraction higher in neonates (about 90%) than adults and children (3), a nearly total renal clearance correlated with creatinine clearance and a half life of 3.5 to 10 h (2, 4). Vancomycin is administered intravenously because of its very low oral bioavailability. At all ages and even more so in neonates, the serum levels of vancomycin achieved feature high inter-individual variability (4). Covariates reported to influence its clearance are weight, gestational age (GA), corrected gestational age (CGA), post-natal age (PNA), co-medication with non-steroidal anti-inflammatory drugs, and serum creatinine (SCR) level, which could be interrelated (4, 5).

A ratio of 24-h area under the curve (AUC_{0-24h}) to minimum inhibitory concentration (MIC) >400 mg.h/L for total vancomycin is considered predictive of optimal antibacterial efficiency against MRSA in adults (6). This AUC_{0-24h}/MIC ratio is based on studies of adults using discontinuous infusion of vancomycin with a target trough level of 15 to 20 mg/L (7). In clinical practice, the AUC_{0-24h}/MIC ratio is difficult to estimate during discontinuous infusion (8) but is easy to estimate with steady-state levels during continuous infusion with the assumption that the level is relatively stable during infusion. For instance, for *S. aureus* infection [modal MIC 1 mg/L, MIC breakpoint 2 mg/L (9)], a steady-state level of vancomycin ≥17 mg/L corresponds to an AUC_{0-24h}/MIC ratio ≥400 mg.h/L. Concerning CoNS infection, consistent data for neonates in an experimental animal model suggested an optimal efficacy of vancomycin and a decrease in induced resistance with an AUC_{0-24h}/MIC ratio >400 mg.h/L (10). These data have not been validated in human neonates. For CoNS [modal MIC 2 mg/L, MIC breakpoint 4 mg/L (9)], a steady-state level of 33 mg/L would be necessary to achieve an AUC_{0-24h}/MIC ratio >400 mg.h/L.

Because of the lack of consensus on efficacy and toxicity thresholds and an optimal dosing regimen, vancomycin dosing regimens between centers exhibit large heterogeneity (11). Continuous administration is controversal, notably in neonates, and data are mostly extrapolated from adult studies (12). Continuous administration requires a continuous availability of line but neonates, especially preterm neonates, often have a central catheter. Furthermore, vancomycin is stable for at least 48 h and compatible with parenteral nutrition (13) and the only one practical limitation can be drug incompatibilities. However, the major advantage of continuous infusion in neonates concomitant to parenteral nutrition is practical: preventing numerous catheter manipulations could decrease the risk of catheter-related infection (14). Therapeutic levels are achieved faster with continuous infusion, without clinical superiority as compared with discontinuous infusion (15, 16). Furthermore, with continuous infusion, fewer blood samples are required to adjust the optimal dosing regimen, possibly because therapeutic levels are achieved faster (17, 18). A steady-state level can be sampled at any time, for example, concomitant to a scheduled blood test, and is easier to interpret than trough levels (17, 19).

Few data are available on continuous infusion in neonates, particularly for premature infants born before 28 weeks' gestation (5). Different dosing regimens and different target levels have been proposed; with this heterogeneity, choosing an optimal dosing strategy in neonatology is difficult. Pharmacokinetics studies tend to develop individualized pharmacokinetic models with patient-tailored dosing regimens (8, 20).

The aim of this study was to assess the efficiency of a simplified dosing regimen of continuous-infusion vancomycin (loading dose 15 mg/kg and maintenance dose 30 mg/kg/d) in a neonatal intensive care unit (NICU) in neonates with suspected care-related infections caused by ß-lactam–resistant Gram-positive bacteria. We assessed the proportion of neonates with serum vancomycin level achieving the chosen target with a first therapeutic drug monitoring. We then determined which dosing regimen, among those published, would have been the most adequate in our population.

MATERIAL AND METHODS

Population and Collected Data

We included all neonates receiving vancomycin with at least one serum vancomycin concentration assay between January

Abbreviations: CoNS, coagulase-negative staphylococci; MRSA, methicillin-resistant *Staphylococcus aureus*; GA, gestational age; CGA, corrected gestational age; PNA, post-natal age; SCR, serum creatinine; AUC_{0-24h}, 24-h area under the curve; MIC, minimum inhibitory concentration; NICU, neonatal intensive care unit; IUGR, intra-uterine growth restriction; EUCAST, European Committee on Antimicrobial Susceptibility Testing.

2013 and December 2014 in the NICU of Center Hospitalier Intercommunal de Créteil (France). The following data were retrospectively collected from patient charts: GA in weeks (wks) based on the best obstetrical estimate, birth weight (g), intra-uterine growth restriction (IUGR, birth weight <10th percentile for gestational age), sex, PNA in days (d), corrected gestational age (wks), current weight (g), SCR level (μmol/L) before treatment (quantified by the Jaffe method, Roche diagnostics, Indianapolis, IN, USA), serum vancomycin level (mg/L), delay between loading dose and blood sample (h), and microbiological data (results of blood cultures). No other consent than consent to usual standard care from parents was requested because the studied treatment was a standard of care. The local ethics committee of Créteil hospital approved the anonymous collection of data and their publication.

Vancomycin Dosing Regimen

Vancomycin was administered by continuous infusion via a central or peripheral catheter starting with a loading dose of 15 mg/kg over 1 h followed by a maintenance dose of 30 mg/kg/d (21). A blood sample was drawn at least 18 h after the loading dose to reach the steady state (20). Serum vancomycin level was determined by the immunoturbidimetric technique (QMS system of Vancomycin, Seradyn Inc., Indianapolis, IN, USA). If the target level was not reached in the first sample, the maintenance dose was adjusted according to clinicians' choice and a new vancomycin assay was performed at least 24 h after dose adjustment until the target level of 20 to 30 mg/L was achieved.

Assessed Outcomes

Our first goal was to determine the proportion of neonates reaching the target serum vancomycin level and to identify independent covariates associated with low or high therapeutic levels. The target level used was 20 to 30 mg/L (19).

Our second objective was to assess different continuous-infusion regimens proposed in the literature as applied to our population. We determined whether each proposed regimen would have resulted in a significantly higher, equal or lower vancomycin dose within each subgroup of our population: infants with a first therapeutic drug monitoring <20 mg/L (underdose), 20 to 30 mg/L (appropriate dose), and >30 mg/L (overdose). For each patient, we used the covariate(s) proposed in the original publication.

Literature Search

MEDLINE was searched via PubMed to identify all published articles proposing a dosing regimen for continuous-infusion vancomycin for neonates. The search was conducted in August 2018 with the following terms: neonates AND vancomycin AND (dosing OR continuous). We selected English-language articles that proposed a detailed dosing regimen for continuous infusion of vancomycin in neonates that could be reproduced in our population.

Statistical Analysis

The association between vancomycin levels and variables (GA, birth weight, PNA, CGA, current weight, IUGR, sex, timing of assay, and SCR level) was analyzed by using R 3.3.2 (http://www.R-project.org). To facilitate results' interpretation for clinicians, continuous variables were separated into dichotomous variables with cut-offs set according to the literature and commonly used categories: GA < or ≥ 28 weeks (22), CGA < or ≥ 32 weeks (22), neonate weight ≤ or > 1,000 g (23), PNA ≤ or > 14 days (24, 25), timing of assay ≤ 24 h or > 24 h (20), and SCR level < or ≥ 70 μmol/L (20, 21). Descriptive data are described with median and interquartile range (IQR) or mean (SD). Chi-square or Fisher exact test was used to determine covariates with significantly different distribution among vancomycin level subgroups (low level, target level, and high level). $P \leq 0.05$ was considered statistically significant. Covariates with $p < 0.1$ on univariate analysis were included in a multivariate analysis. We used multinomial logistic regression to determine covariates independently related to low and high levels as compared with the target level ($p < 0.05$), estimating adjusted odds ratios (aOR) and 95% confidence intervals (CIs).

TABLE 1 | Demographic and clinical characteristics of neonates ($n = 75$) under continuous infusion with vancomycin ($n = 91$ therapy episodes) for care-related infections caused by ß-lactam–resistant Gram-positive bacteria.

	N (%)	Median [IQR]
Gestational age (weeks)		27 [26–30.5]
<28	40 (53.3)	
≥28	35 (46.7)	
Birth weight (g)		815 [685–1,240]
≤1,000	41 (54.7)	
>1,000	34 (45.3)	
Intrauterine growth restriction	33 (44)	
Sex		
Male	43 (57.3)	
Female	32 (42.7)	
Postnatal age (d)		15 [9–33]
≤14	42 (46.2)	
>14	49 (53.8)	
Corrected gestational age (weeks)		30 [28–34.5]
<32	52 (57.2)	
≥32	39 (42.8)	
Current weight (g)		1,230 [940–1,790]
≤1,000	30 (33)	
>1,000	61 (67)	
Serum creatinine level before treatment (μmol/L) ($n = 68$)		52 [26.5–70]
>70	17 (25)	
≤70	51 (75)	
First vancomycin level (mg/L)		21.1 [16.3–29.7]
Number of samples per treatment		2 [1–2.5]
Time of first sampling (h)		25.5 [23.9–33.3]
Treatment duration (d)		4 [3–7]

To compare doses proposed by each dosing regimen reported in the literature with actual doses given to our patients, we used Student *t*-test and report mean differences and 95% CIs.

RESULTS

Population

From January 2013 to December 2014, 75 neonates received 99 vancomycin courses by continuous infusion. Eight treatments were excluded because the neonates did not receive the dosing regimen evaluated. Patient characteristics are summarized in **Table 1**. Median gestational age and birth weight were 27 weeks (IQR 26–30.5) and 815 g (IQR 685–1,240); 40/75 neonates (53.3%) were born before 28 weeks' GA. Overall, 184 serum vancomycin samples were assayed, with a median of 2 (IQR 1–2.5) determinations per patient. A first blood sample was taken 18.5 to 93.5 h after the loading dose. SCR level before treatment was available for 68 patients and ranged from 15 to 116 μmol/L; for 17/68 (25%) neonates, the SCR level was >70 μmol/L.

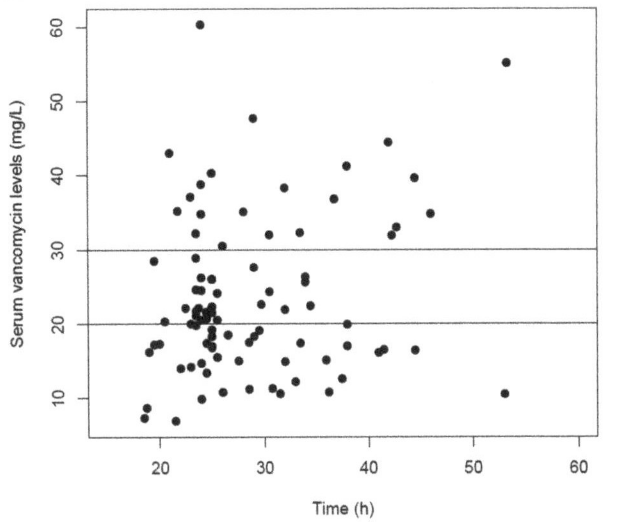

FIGURE 1 | Serum vancomycin level (mg/L) on time (h). Horizontal lines represent the target level of 20 to 30 mg/L.

Microbiological Data

For 24/91 (26.4%) courses, at least one blood culture was positive: 17/91 only one positive blood culture and 7/91 (7.7%) at least two positive blood cultures. Most (67/91; 73.6%) had negative blood cultures. Bacterial species found were CoNS (17/91; 18.7%), *S. aureus* (3/91; 3.3%) with one MRSA, *Streptococcus sp.* (2/91; 2.2%), *Escherichia coli* (1/91; 1%), and *Streptococcus pneumoniae* (1/91; 1.1%). The distribution of CoNS was *S. epidermidis* ($n = 10$), *S. haemoliticus* ($n = 2$), and *S. capitis* ($n = 5$).

Serum Vancomycin Levels

Vancomycin serum levels ranged from 6.9 to 60.3 mg/L. For 28/91 (30.8%) courses, a level of 20 to 30 mg/L was achieved in the first assay; 40/91 (43.9%) had low therapeutic levels, <20 mg/L, and 23/91 (25.3%) had levels >30 mg/L. For seven (7.7%), the level was >40 mg/L. Vancomycin levels on time are displayed in **Figure 1**. A total of 49 neonates had a second sample assayed and for 18/49 (36.7%), serum levels were at the chosen target; three retained a level >40 mg/L. At the first assay or after dose titration, for 56/91 (61.5%) courses, the therapeutic level between 20 and 30 mg/L was reached. For those neonates, the median time to achieving a therapeutic level was 34 h (IQR 24.5–74.5).

Covariates Analysis

On univariate analysis, we identified five covariates significantly related to vancomycin serum levels: PNA ($p = 0.001$), sex ($p = 0.05$), CGA ($p = 0.004$), current weight ($p = 0.04$), and SCR level ($p < 0.0001$) (**Table 2**). On multivariate analysis, only three of these covariates remained significantly associated with serum vancomycin level: PNA > 14 days (aOR = 25.6, 95% CI [3.2–201.5], $p = 0.002$) and CGA ≥ 32 weeks were related to low level (aOR = 48.2, 95% CI [7.0–334.6], $p < 0.001$) and SCR level > 70 μmol/L was associated with high level (aOR = 33.0, 95% CI [4.0–272.6], $p = 0.001$). There was no association between timing of vancomycin assay and vancomycin serum levels ($p = 0.4$) (**Table 2** and **Figure 1**).

Literature Search

The search algorithm identified 146 studies in Pubmed (144 after removal of duplicates): 51 referred to discontinuous infusion of vancomycin; 29 did not propose a detailed dosing schedule of vancomycin; 40 did not address our subject; 10 were not in English; six proposed a dosing schedule for neonates on extracorporeal life support or intraventricular injection; and two presented a preventive dosing regimen. Finally, six studies detailed different dosing regimens of continuous-infusion vancomycin for neonates (**Table 3**). Five studies agreed on a loading dose of 7 to 20 mg/kg to quickly reach target levels (15, 20, 21, 26, 28). Maintenance doses ranged from 10 to 60 mg/kg/d, with a unique dose of 30 mg/kg/d (21) or a dose adjusted to SCR level, CGA, birth weight, current body weight, and/or PNA (15, 20, 26–28). The proportion of patients achieving the chosen target level of 10 to 30 mg/L (21, 26), 10 to 25 mg/L (27) or 15 to 25 mg/L (15, 20) were 70.7% (20), 75% (27), 77% (15), 88% (26), 89.2% (21), respectively.

Dosing Regimen From the Literature Applied to Our Population

We compared mean doses and mean differences between our maintenance dose (30 mg/kg/d) and maintenance dose proposed by each dosing regimen from the literature (**Table 4**).

Three dosing regimen from the literature would have proposed significantly higher vancomycin doses to neonates with a low vancomycin level, <20 mg/L: mean dose (SD) of 36.4 (8.1) mg/kg/d (27), 38.5 (9.5) mg/kg/d (15), and 48.5 (20) mg/kg/d (20). Two dosing regimens would have proposed the same dose: mean dose (SD) of 30 (0) mg/kg/d (21, 27). One dosing regimen would have proposed lower doses to neonates with low vancomycin level: mean dose (SD) of 20.6 (6.5) mg/kg/d (26) (**Table 4**).

TABLE 2 | Distribution of covariates by vancomycin level.

Covariates	Vancomycin level (mg/L)			
	<20	20–30	>30	*p*-value
Gestational age (wks)				
<28	19	17	16	0.16
≥28	21	12	6	
Birth weight (g)				
≤1,000	24	17	12	0.9
>1,000	16	12	10	
Intra-uterine growth restriction				
Absence	18	16	13	0.5
Presence	22	13	9	
Sex				
Male	18	16	17	0.05
Female	22	13	5	
Postnatal age (d)				
≤14	10	17	15	0.001
>14	30	12	7	
Corrected gestational age (wks)				
<32	21	21	15	0.004
≥32	8	8	25	
Current weight (g)				
≤1,000	8	11	11	0.04
>1,000	32	18	11	
Serum creatinine level (μmol/L)				
≤70	25	20	6	<0.0001
>70	2	3	12	
Time of first sampling (h)				0.4
≤24	11	12	7	
>24	29	16	15	

For patients with a vancomycin level in the target range (20–30 mg/L), four dosing regimens would have proposed similar doses as the actual dose given to our patients: mean dose (SD) of 30 (0) (21, 27), 30.8 (8.1) (20), and 31.4 (8.3) (15) mg/kg/d. One would have proposed significantly lower doses: mean dose (SD) of 16.1 (4.6) mg/kg/d (26) and one significantly higher doses: mean dose (SD) of 32.2 (5.6) mg/kg/d (28) (**Table 4**).

For patients with a high vancomycin level, >30 mg/L, three dosing regimens would have proposed significantly lower doses: mean dose (SD) of 22.6 (7.3) (15), 15.7 (6.8) (26), and 24.4 (5.1) (27) mg/kg/d. Two would have proposed similar doses [25.4 (12.8) (20), and 30 (0) mg/kg/d (21)] and one significantly higher doses [33.8 (6.4) mg/kg/d (28)] (**Table 4**).

Finally, one dosing algorithm (15) would have proposed lower doses to patients with high levels, similar doses to those with levels in the target range and higher doses to those with low levels (**Table 4**).

DISCUSSION

This study presents a cohort of premature neonates receiving continuous infusion of vancomycin and is the first study comparing the six dosing regimens reported in the literature for neonates. We evaluated the proportion of patients reaching the therapeutic vancomycin range. With the dosing regimen used in our department (loading dose of 15 mg/kg and maintenance dose of 30 mg/kg/d), only 30.8% of neonates achieved target vancomycin levels of 20 to 30 mg/L, 43.9% had low therapeutic levels and 25.3% had levels >30 mg/L. These disappointing results confirm that a simplified regimen does not fit a population of neonates characterized by high inter-individual variability and the important pharmacokinetic changes in the first weeks of life (kidney maturation and changes in volume of distribution) (4).

After comparing dosing regimens proposed in the literature, the dosing regimen proposed by Patel et al. seemed the most adequate for our population. This model is easy to apply and includes cofactors of variability such as SCR level and CGA. Applied to our neonates with a target level of 20 to 30 mg/L, the model proposed significantly lower doses to neonates with high vancomycin levels and higher doses to those with low therapeutic levels. The individualized pharmacokinetic model proposed by Zhao et al. would also propose more appropriate doses to a large proportion of neonates. Indeed, it proposed significantly higher doses to neonates with low levels and lower doses to those with high levels (even if not significant, $p = 0.13$). This model can be adjusted to the chosen target level, which is an advantage when the clinician wants to adjust the target level to the MIC. In a previous study, a prospective validation of this model with 190 neonates showed that 72% reached the target level (15–25 mg/L) at the first therapeutic drug monitoring (29). The other evaluated dosing regimens proposed lower doses, even for patients with already low therapeutic levels (26), or higher doses, even for patients with already high levels (28). Those dosing regimen do not fit our population. An explanation could be the differences between vancomycin and serum creatinine measurement methods as demonstrated in some studies (30).

Concerns have been raised about the efficacy threshold of target concentrations because of increased vancomycin MICs with CoNS infection (4) and toxicity issues. According to the European Committee on Antimicrobial Susceptibility Testing (9), the modal MIC is 2 mg/L for CoNS and 1 mg/L for *S. aureus* infections. To reach the AUC_{0-24h}/MIC ratio >400 mg.h/L as advised, a steady-state level >33 mg/L for CoNS infection and >17 mg/L for *S. aureus* infection would be needed to reach optimal efficiency and limit resistance (2, 18, 21). *S. aureus* infections are characterized by severe clinical presentation and metastatic risk (31). CoNS infections, with central line catheters, are rarely metastatic and have less severe clinical and biological presentations, but therapeutic failure can be attributed in part to biofilms produced (32). Moreover, the AUC_{0-24h}/MIC target >400 mg.h/L was developed for MRSA infections, so a CoNS-specific pharmacodynamic target should be established, especially for neonates (33). Hence, for CoNS, an initial level < 30 mg/L could be sufficient despite a high MIC.

Concerning the upper threshold of the target concentration, a study of adults showed an AUC_{0-24h} >1,300 mg.h/L, corresponding to a steady-state level >55 mg/L, associated with increased risk of nephrotoxicity (34). Adult and pediatric studies suggest that without reaching such high levels, an upper

TABLE 3 | Proposed dosing regimens from the literature.

References	Population	Loading dose (mg/kg)	Maintenance dose (mg/kg/d)	Covariates
Pawlotsky et al. (26)	Patients, 29 GA: 30.5 (3.7) weeks[a] CGA: 33.9 (4.8) weeks [a]	7		CGA (wks)
			10	25–26
			12	27–28
			15	29–30
			18	31–32
			20	33–34
			23	35–36
			26	37–38
			29	39–40
			31	41–42
			34	43–44
			40	>45
Plan et al. (27)	Patients, 72 GA <34 weeks	0	30	SCR level < 90 μmol/L
			20	SCR level > 90 μmol/L
Oudin et al. (21)	Patients, 47 GA 29 (23–41) weeks[b] CGA 32.7 (27–47) weeks [b]	20	30	
Zhao et al. (20)	Patients, 116 CGA 33.8 (5.3) weeks[a]	= Target concentration × Vd (in mg)	= Target concentration × CL × 24 h (in mg/24 h)	$Vd = 0.791 \times (cW/1{,}416)^{0.898}$ $CL = 0.0571 \times (cW/1{,}416)^{0.513} \times (bW/1{,}010)^{0.599} \times (1+0.282 \times (PNA/17)) \times (1/(SCR/42)^{0.525})$
Patel et al. (15)	Patients, 60 GA 29 (24–41) weeks[b] CGA 36 (26–62) weeks [b]	15	50	SCR level < 40 μmol/L and CGA > 40 weeks
			40	SCR level < 40 μmol/L and CGA < 40 weeks
			30	SCR level 40–60 μmol/L
			20	SCR level > 60 μmol/L
Janssen et al. (28)	Patients, 464 GA 32 (24–41) weeks[b] CGA 34 (25–44) weeks [b]	10.5 to 13	25	PNA ≤ 7 days + bW ≤ 1,000 g
				PNA 8–14 days + bW ≤ 700 g
			27	PNA ≤ 7 days + bW 1,000–1,500 g
			30	PNA ≤ 7 days + bW 1,500–2,500 g
				PNA 14–28 days + bW ≤ 700 g
			32	PNA 8–14 days + bW 700–1,000 g
				PNA >28 days + cW < 2.5 kg
			36	PNA ≤7 days + bW > 2,500 g
				PNA 8–14 days + bW 1,000–1,500 g
			40	PNA 8–14 days + bW 1,500–2,500 g
				PNA > 28 days + cW 2.5–5 kg
			42	PNA 14–28 days + bW 700–1,000 g
			45	PNA 14–28 days + bW 1,000–1,500 g
			48	PNA 8–14 days + bW > 2,500 g
			52	PNA 14–28 d + bW 1,500–2,500 g
				PNA >28 days + cW 5–10 kg
			60	PNA 14–28 days + bW > 2,500 g
				PNA > 28 days + cW > 10 kg

GA, gestational age; CGA, corrected gestational age; SCR, serum creatinine; Vd, volume of distribution; CL, clearance; cW, current weight; bW, birth weight; PNA, post natal age.
[a]*Mean (SD).*
[b]*Median (range).*

TABLE 4 | Mean doses and mean differences (95% CIs) proposed by the six dosing regimens evaluated for each group of patients (low, target and high vancomycin levels).

Dosing regimen		**Low level (<20 mg/L) (*n* = 40)**	**Target level (20–30 mg/L) (*n* = 28)**	**High level (>30 mg/L) (*n* = 23)**
Our dosing regimen	Mean dose (SD)	30 (0)	30 (0)	30 (0)
	Mean difference (95% CI)	–	–	–
	P-value[a]	–	–	–
Pawlotsky et al.(26)	Mean dose (SD)	20.6 (6.5)	16.1 (4.6)	15.7 (6.8)
	Mean difference (95% CI)	−9.4 (−11.5 to −7.4)	−13.9 (−15.6 to −12.1)	−14.3 (−11.4 to −17.2)
	P-value[a]	<0.001	<0.001	<0.001
Plan et al. (27)	Mean dose (SD)	30 (0)	30 (0)	24.4 (5.1)
	Mean difference (95% CI)	0	0	−5.6 (−8.3 to −2.9)
	P-value[a]	–	–	<0.001
Oudin et al. (21)	Mean dose (SD)	30 (0)	30 (0)	30 (0)
	Mean difference (95% CI)	0	0	0
	P-value[a]	–	–	–
Zhao et al. (20)	Mean dose (SD)	48.5 (20)	30.8 (8.1)	25.4 (12.8)
	Mean difference (95% CI)	18.5 (10.7 to 26.4)	0.8 (−2.8 to 4.4)	−4.6 (−10.7 to 1.5)
	P-value[a]	<0.001	0.63	0.13
Patel et al. (15)	Mean dose (SD)	38.5 (9.5)	31.4 (8.3)	22.6 (7.3)
	Mean difference (95% CI)	8.5 (4.8 to 12.3)	1.4 (−2.3 to 5.1)	−7.4 (−10.9 to −3.8)
	P-value[a]	<0.001	0.45	<0.001
Janssen et al. (28)	Mean dose (SD)	36.4 (8.1)	32.2 (5.6)	33.8 (6.4)
	Mean difference (95% CI)	6.4 (3.8 to 9.0)	2.2 (0.1 to 4.4)	3.8 (1.0 to 6.6)
	P-value[a]	<0.001	0.04	0.009

[a] *Student t-test comparing mean dose of our dosing algorithm with mean dose of each dosing regimen.*
95% CI, 95% confidence interval.

threshold might be about 30 mg/L (35) (AUC_{0-24h} 700 mg.h/L), which might be increased to 37.5 mg/L (AUC_{0-24h} 900 mg.h/L), an adequate threshold in terms of risk for bacteria with a MIC of 2 mg/L (36, 37). In our study, for two neonates, the SCR level was higher after than before treatment, but linking the accountability to vancomycin was difficult (one neonate in a context of perinatal asphyxia and the other with multiorgan failure in a context of extreme prematurity). Studies of vancomycin-associated nephrotoxicity in neonatology conclude that the condition is rare and reversible and proof of a dose–toxicity relationship is lacking, even with levels >30 mg/L or associated with an aminoglycoside (38). However, careful monitoring should be carried out especially in high-risk neonates with nephrotoxic comedication (non-steroidal anti-inflammatory drugs, diuretics), with low birth weight or with severe illness (sepsis, patent ductus arteriosus).

CGA and high SCR level have been linked to interindividual variability in vancomycin levels, along with other covariates such as weight, PNA, GA, ventilation type, and co-treatments (4). However, residual variability remains despite accounting for these factors. Thus, therapeutic drug monitoring still seems necessary. The usual timing for vancomycin drug monitoring is at least 18 to 24 h after the initation or modification of treatment (20). Dosing adjustment was not satisfactory in our study, with 63% of levels in secondary samples remaining outside of the target. A method based on a linear relationship between the maintenance dose and steady-state level has been proposed: adjusted dose = maintenance dose × target level/last vancomycin level (19, 20).

Our study has several limitations. First, it was a retrospective study that can imply imprecision in recorded data. Second, SCR level was available before treatment for only three-quarters of the neonates, which prevented us from applying published dosing regimens to all our patients. Following this study, creatinine measurement became mandatory to manage vancomycin treatment in our department. Another limitation is the lack of documentation of MICs of bacteria, with 74% of blood cultures remaining negative. Therefore, we could not evaluate the proportion of MICs >1 mg/L that would require higher vancomycin levels. Finally, even if other studies already described the use of continuous infusion vancomycin in neonates, our cohort mainly contained extremely premature neonates <28 weeks' GA, a very challenging population.

CONCLUSIONS

Continuous-infusion vancomycin for neonates offers a practical and pharmacokinetic interest. The use of a dosing regimen taking into account CGA and SCR level or an individualized pharmacokinetic model can help to anticipate the inter-individual variability in neonates and seems more adapted than a simplified dosing regimen. Validation of a dosing regimen in a controlled trial with a large number of patients would allow to evaluate performances in achieving target levels and for better assessment of short- and long-term toxicity. Despite a patient-tailored dosing regimen, therapeutic drug monitoring still seems necessary.

ETHICS STATEMENT

The local ethics committee of Créteil hospital approved the anonymous collection of data and their publication.

AUTHOR CONTRIBUTIONS

MT and RC designed and conducted the study. MT collected and analyzed patient data. MT, RC, XD, and LC interpreted results. MT wrote the manuscript with major contributions by RC and reviewing by LC, XD, GD, and JB. All authors read and approved the final manuscript.

ACKNOWLEDGMENTS

We thank Stéphane Bechet and Dr. Corinne Levy (ACTIV) for technical support and Dr. Claude Danan and Dr. Fabrice Decobert for advice.

REFERENCES

1. Lutsar I, Chazallon C, Carducci FIC, Trafojer U, Abdelkader B, de Cabre VM, et al. Current management of late onset neonatal bacterial sepsis in five European countries. *Eur J Pediatr.* (2014) 173:997–1004. doi: 10.1007/s00431-014-2279-5
2. Vandecasteele SJ, De Vriese AS, Tacconelli E. The pharmacokinetics and pharmacodynamics of vancomycin in clinical practice: evidence and uncertainties. *J Antimicrob Chemother.* (2013) 68:743–8. doi: 10.1093/jac/dks495
3. Smits A, Pauwels S, Oyaert M, Peersman N, Spriet I, Saegeman V, et al. Factors impacting unbound vancomycin concentrations in neonates and young infants. *Eur J Clin Microbiol Infect Dis.* (2018) 37:1503–10. doi: 10.1007/s10096-018-3277-8
4. de Hoog M, Mouton JW, van den Anker JN. Vancomycin: pharmacokinetics and administration regimens in neonates. *Clin Pharmacokinet.* (2004) 43:417–40. doi: 10.2165/00003088-200443070-00001
5. Pacifici GM, Allegaert K. Clinical pharmacokinetics of vancomycin in the neonate: a review. *Clin São Paulo Braz.* (2012) 67:831–7. doi: 10.6061/clinics/2012(07)21
6. Frymoyer A, Hersh AL, El-Komy MH, Gaskari S, Su F, Drover DR, et al. Association between vancomycin trough concentration and area under the concentration-time curve in neonates. *Antimicrob Agents Chemother.* (2014) 58:6454–61. doi: 10.1128/AAC.03620-14
7. Liu C, Bayer A, Cosgrove SE, Daum RS, Fridkin SK, Gorwitz RJ, et al. Clinical practice guidelines by the infectious diseases society of America for the treatment of methicillin-resistant *Staphylococcus aureus* infections in adults and children: executive summary. *Clin Infect Dis Off Publ Infect Dis Soc Am.* (2011) 52:285–92. doi: 10.1093/cid/cir034
8. Jacqz-Aigrain E, Leroux S, Zhao W, van den Anker JN, Sharland M. How to use vancomycin optimally in neonates: remaining questions. *Expert Rev Clin Pharmacol.* (2015) 8:635–48. doi: 10.1586/17512433.2015.1060124
9. *European Committee on Antimicrobial Susceptibility Testing (EUCAST).* (2017). Available online at: http://mic.eucast.org/consultéenseptembre; http://www.eucast.org/mic_distributions_and_ecoffs/
10. Ramos-Martín V, Johnson A, Livermore J, McEntee L, Goodwin J, Whalley S. Pharmacodynamics of vancomycin for CoNS infection: experimental basis for optimal use of vancomycin in neonates. *J Antimicrob Chemother.* (2016) 71:992–1002. doi: 10.1093/jac/dkv451
11. Leroux S, Zhao W, Biran V, Jacqz-Aigrain E. Posologie des antibiotiques chez le nouveau-né : variations des pratiques et comment y remédier e *Arch Pédiatr.* (2016) 23:966–73. doi: 10.1016/j.arcped.2016.06.002
12. Ward RM, Allegaert K, de Groot R, van den Anker JN. Commentary: continuous infusion of vancomycin in neonates: to use or not to use remains the question. *Pediatr Infect Dis J.* (2014) 33:606–7. doi: 10.1097/INF.0000000000000244
13. Raverdy V, Ampe E, Hecq J-D, Tulkens PM. Stability and compatibility of vancomycin for administration by continuous infusion. *J Antimicrob Chemother.* (2013) 68:1179–82. doi: 10.1093/jac/dks510
14. Stevens TP, Schulman J. Evidence-based approach to preventing central line-associated bloodstream infection in the NICU: evidence-based approach to preventing NICU CLABSI. *Acta Paediatr.* (2012) 101:11–6. doi: 10.1111/j.1651-2227.2011.02547.x
15. Patel AD, Anand D, Lucas C, Thomson AH. Continuous infusion of vancomycin in neonates. *Arch Dis Child.* (2013) 98:478–9. doi: 10.1136/archdischild-2012-303197
16. Kim J, Walker SAN, Iaboni DC, Walker SE, Elligsen M, Dunn MS, et al. Determination of vancomycin pharmacokinetics in neonates to develop practical initial dosing recommendations. *Antimicrob Agents Chemother.* (2014) 58:2830–40. doi: 10.1128/AAC.01718-13
17. Saugel B, Nowack MCM, Hapfelmeier A, Umgelter A, Schultheiss C, Thies P, et al. Continuous intravenous administration of vancomycin in medical intensive care unit patients. *J Crit Care.* (2013) 28:9–13. doi: 10.1016/j.jcrc.2012.02.003
18. Wysocki M, Delatour F, Faurisson F, Rauss A, Pean Y, Misset B, et al. Continuous versus intermittent infusion of vancomycin in severe staphylococcal infections: prospective multicenter randomized study. *Antimicrob Agents Chemother.* (2001) 45:2460–7. doi: 10.1128/AAC.45.9.2460-2467.2001
19. Waineo MF, Kuhn TC, Brown DL. The pharmacokinetic/pharmacodynamic rationale for administering vancomycin via continuous infusion. *J Clin Pharm Ther.* (2015) 40:259–65. doi: 10.1111/jcpt.12270
20. Zhao W, Lopez E, Biran V, Durrmeyer X, Fakhoury M, Jacqz-Aigrain E. Vancomycin continuous infusion in neonates: dosing optimisation and therapeutic drug monitoring. *Arch Dis Child.* (2013) 98:449–53. doi: 10.1136/archdischild-2012-302765
21. Oudin C, Vialet R, Boulamery A, Martin C, Simon N. Vancomycin prescription in neonates and young infants: toward a simplified dosage. *Arch Dis Child Fetal Neonatal Ed.* (2011) 96:F365–70. doi: 10.1136/adc.2010.196402
22. Blencowe H, Cousens S, Oestergaard MZ, Chou D, Moller A-B, Narwal R, et al. National, regional, and worldwide estimates of preterm birth rates in the year 2010 with time trends since 1990 for selected countries: a systematic analysis and implications. *Lancet Lond Engl.* (2012) 379:2162–72. doi: 10.1016/S0140-6736(12)60820-4
23. Gross JR, Kaplan SL, Kramer WG, Mason EO. Vancomycin pharmacokinetics in premature infants. *Pediatr Pharmacol N Y N.* (1985) 5:17–22.
24. Dersch-Mills D, Bengry T, Akierman A, Alshaikh B, Yusuf K. Assessment of initial vancomycin dosing in neonates. *Paediatr Child Health.* (2014) 19:e30–34.
25. Pottel H, Vrydags N, Mahieu B, Vandewynckele E, Croes K, Martens F. Establishing age/sex related serum creatinine reference intervals from hospital laboratory data based on different statistical methods. *Clin Chim Acta.* (2008) 396:49–55. doi: 10.1016/j.cca.2008.06.017
26. Pawlotsky F, Thomas A, Kergueris MF, Debillon T, Roze JC. Constant rate infusion of vancomycin in premature neonates: a new dosage schedule. *Br J Clin Pharmacol.* (1998) 46:163–7.
27. Plan O, Cambonie G, Barbotte E, Meyer P, Devine C, Milesi C, et al. Continuous-infusion vancomycin therapy for preterm neonates with

suspected or documented Gram-positive infections: a new dosage schedule. *Arch Dis Child Fetal Neonatal Ed.* (2008) 93:F418–21. doi: 10.1136/adc.2007.128280

28. Janssen EJH, Välitalo PAJ, Allegaert K, de Cock RFW, Simons SHP, Sherwin CMT, et al. Towards rational dosing algorithms for vancomycin in neonates and infants based on population pharmacokinetic modeling. *Antimicrob Agents Chemother.* (2016) 60:1013–21. doi: 10.1128/AAC.01968-15
29. Leroux S, Jacqz-Aigrain E, Biran V, Lopez E, Madeleneau D, Wallon C, et al. Clinical utility and safety of a model-based patient-tailored dose of vancomycin in neonates. *Antimicrob Agents Chemother.* (2016) 60:2039–42. doi: 10.1128/AAC.02214-15
30. Zhao W, Kaguelidou F, Biran V, Zhang D, Allegaert K, Capparelli EV, et al. External evaluation of population pharmacokinetic models of vancomycin in neonates: transferability of published vancomycin population pharmacokinetic models in neonates. *Br J Clin Pharmacol.* (2013) 75:1068–80. doi: 10.1111/j.1365-2125.2012.04406.x
31. Qiao Y, Ning X, Chen Q, Zhao R, Song W, Zheng Y, et al. Clinical and molecular characteristics of invasive community-acquired *Staphylococcus aureus* infections in Chinese children. *BMC Infect Dis.* (2014) 14:582. doi: 10.1186/s12879-014-0582-4
32. Healy CM. Features of invasive staphylococcal disease in neonates. *Pediatrics.* (2004) 114:953–61. doi: 10.1542/peds.2004-0043
33. Padari H, Oselin K, Tasa T, Metsvaht T, Lõivukene K, Lutsar I. Coagulase negative *Staphylococcal sepsis* in neonates: do we need to adapt vancomycin dose or target? *BMC Pediatr.* (2016) 16:206. doi: 10.1186/s12887-016-0753-0
34. Lodise TP, Patel N, Lomaestro BM, Rodvold KA, Drusano GL. Relationship between initial vancomycin concentration-time profile and nephrotoxicity among hospitalized patients. *Clin Infect Dis.* (2009) 49:507–14. doi: 10.1086/600884
35. Ingram PR, Lye DC, Tambyah PA, Goh WP, Tam VH, Fisher DA. Risk factors for nephrotoxicity associated with continuous vancomycin infusion in outpatient parenteral antibiotic therapy. *J Antimicrob Chemother.* (2008) 62:168–71. doi: 10.1093/jac/dkn080
36. Le J, Bradley JS, Murray W, Romanowski GL, Tran TT, Nguyen N, et al. Improved vancomycin dosing in children using area under the curve exposure. *Pediatr Infect Dis J.* (2013) 32:e155–63. doi: 10.1097/INF.0b013e318286378e
37. Neely MN, Youn G, Jones B, Jelliffe RW, Drusano GL, Rodvold KA, et al. Are vancomycin trough concentrations adequate for optimal dosing? *Antimicrob Agents Chemother.* (2014) 58:309–16. doi: 10.1128/AAC.01653-13
38. Lestner JM, Hill LF, Heath PT, Sharland M. Vancomycin toxicity in neonates: a review of the evidence. *Curr Opin Infect Dis.* (2016) 29:237–47. doi: 10.1097/QCO.0000000000000263

20

Key Components for Antibiotic Dose Optimization of Sepsis in Neonates and Infants

Tamara van Donge[1], *Julia A. Bielicki*[1,2], *John van den Anker*[1,3,4] *and Marc Pfister*[1,5*]

[1] *Paediatric Pharmacology and Pharmacometrics, University Children's Hospital Basel, University of Basel, Basel, Switzerland,* [2] *Paediatric Infectious Diseases Research Group, Institute for Infection and Immunity, St George's, University of London, London, United Kingdom,* [3] *Intensive Care and Department of Paediatric Surgery, Erasmus MC-Sophia Children's Hospital, Rotterdam, Netherlands,* [4] *Division of Clinical Pharmacology, Children's National Health System, Washington, DC, United States,* [5] *Certara LP, Princeton, NJ, United States*

Correspondence:
Marc Pfister
marc.pfister@ukbb.ch

Sepsis in neonates and infants remains a major cause of death despite a decline in child mortality and morbidity over the last decades. A key factor in further reducing poor clinical outcomes is the optimal use of antibiotics in sepsis management. Developmental changes such as maturation of organ function and capacity of drug metabolizing enzymes can affect the pharmacokinetic profile and therefore the antibiotic exposure and response in neonates and infants. Optimal antibiotic treatment of sepsis in neonates and young infants is dependent on several key components such as the determination of treatment phase, the administered dose and the resulted drug exposure and microbiological response. During the initial phase of suspected sepsis, the primary focus of empirical treatment is to assure efficacy. Once bacterial infection as the cause of sepsis is confirmed the focus shifts toward a targeted treatment, ensuring an optimal balance between efficacy and safety. Interpretation of antibiotic exposure and microbiological response in neonates and infants is multifaceted. The response or treatment effect can be determined by the microbiological parameters (MIC) together with the characteristics of the pathogen (time- or concentration dependent). The antibiotic response is influenced by the properties of the causative pathogen and the unique characteristics of the vulnerable patient population such as reduced humoral response or reduced skin barrier function. Therapeutic drug monitoring (TDM) of antibiotics may be used to increase effectiveness while maximizing safety and minimizing the toxicity, but requires expertise in different fields and requires collaborations between physicians, lab technicians, and quantitative clinical pharmacologists. Understanding these clinical, pharmacological, and microbiological components and their underlying relationship can provide a scientific basic for proper antibiotic use and reduction of antibiotic resistance in neonates and infants. This highlights the necessity of a close multidisciplinary collaboration between physicians, pharmacists, clinical pharmacologists and microbiologist to assure the optimal utilization of antibiotics in neonates and young infants.

Keywords: antibiotics, empirical phase, exposure, neonates, targeted phase, sepsis

INTRODUCTION

Despite a decline in child mortality during the last decades, close to 6 million children died before the age of 5 years in 2015 with almost half of these patients dying during the neonatal period (1). Neonates are immunologically immature, have reduced skin barrier, reduced humoral response and a diminished microbial diversity in gut microbiota, all contributing to a higher risk of life-threatening bacterial infection, often presenting as sepsis (2–5). Sepsis is defined as a clinical condition resulting from a dysregulated immune response, triggered by an infection. The initiation of the pro-inflammatory cascade may cause widespread tissue injury (6–9). In 2015, infectious diseases were responsible for 9.5% of neonatal deaths worldwide, mainly focusing on lower and middle income countries where healthcare and appropriate antibiotics may be difficult to access (1). It should be noted that sepsis continues to impact not only neonates, but also affects a considerable proportion of young and older infants receiving intensive care. A recent study showed that global prevalence of severe sepsis in pediatric intensive care units is 8.2% (10).

The diagnosis of sepsis in neonates and infants is complex, and a complete discussion on clinical decision-making about initiations of antibiotics is beyond the scope of this review (11). Early antibiotic therapy for potential bacterial infection in sepsis is critical with antibiotics generally being started empirically, meaning before microbiological results are available. Antibiotic treatment is often started before sepsis is confirmed by microbiological diagnostics because of the lack of sensitive blood cultures together with the insufficient predictive performance of these analytics and as well as the possibility of sampling from the infection site. In settings with restricted availability of standard diagnostic tools or a high level of prior antibiotic exposure, for example because of availability of antibiotics over the counter, a definitive diagnosis may not be reached (12).

Neonatal sepsis can be divided into early and late onset neonatal sepsis (EONS and LONS), which reflects the timing of onset of symptoms, type and virulence of organism and associated pathogenesis (2). First, EONS is defined by a life-threatening infection during the 1 days of life. In developed countries Group B *Streptococcus* and *Escherichia coli* account for most episodes of EONS, whereas *Klebsiella* is the most common organism in low and middle income countries (13, 14). Risk factors for EONS are prematurity, premature and prolonged rupture of membranes, intrapartum maternal fever (>38°C) and maternal Group B *Streptococcus* colonization (3, 15, 16). As expected, neonates with a very low birth weight (VLBW, <1,500 g) are more susceptible to an infection (16, 17). Second, LONS is characterized by the onset of symptoms more than 72 h after birth. Among VLBW neonates, Gram-positive organisms are most commonly associated with LONS, although it has been shown that the mortality rate is 2–3 times higher in neonates with Gram-negative infections. Prolonged indwelling catheter use and other invasive procedures are potential risk factors (16). Third, invasive infections during infancy are mostly caused by *Streptococcus pneumoniae.* Because of vaccinations, infections caused by *Haemophilus influenzae* type b are less common in developed countries compared to resource limited settings (7). Currently, *Salmonella* spp. is one of the most common organisms causing sepsis in low and middle income countries (18).

In the first 2 years of life, maturational processes affect drug clearance and make antibiotic dosing more challenging, compared to older infants where dosing is mainly adjusted by body weight and renal function. Most of the current dosing guidelines for antibiotic treatment are simply extrapolated from adult studies and it has been reported that dosing recommendations across intensive care units and international guidelines are highly variable and inconsistent (19). We review and discuss key components and their underlying relationships relevant to antibiotic dose optimization in neonates and infants with suspected or confirmed sepsis (**Figure 1**).

OPTIMIZATION OF ANTIBIOTIC THERAPY IN SEPSIS: EMPIRICAL VS. TARGETED TREATMENT

In a clinical setting, there is generally no time to wait for the result from microbiologic samples when there is suspected sepsis. Antibiotic treatment can therefore be viewed as having two phases, namely an initial, empirical treatment phase followed by a targeted treatment phase once a causative pathogen is confirmed (**Figure 2**). Both phases are time-related, and antibiotic dose optimization may focus on either efficacy or safety, respectively.

Empirical Treatment Phase

In the 1 hours to days of treatment, the primary focus is to deliver effective treatment. During this earliest stage mortality is directly related to the effects of the life-threatening infection and managing toxicity is less central. As the causative organism generally remains unknown, selection of the antibiotic regimen needs to take into account the overall epidemiology of sepsis in the age group of the patient (19).

A key parameter describing susceptibility to antibiotics and used in dose-finding is the minimal inhibitory concentration, or MIC, which reflects the lowest antibiotic concentration needed to inhibit visible growth of the pathogen (20). MIC breakpoints for pathogens are established based on various *in vitro* tests and are applied to an entire population. Initial antibiotic doses should be targeting the "worst-case" minimal inhibitory concentrations, captured by the phrase "go hard and go home" (21). During the empirical treatment phase, the benefits (e.g., high probability that causative pathogens are killed) outweigh the risks (e.g., development of renal toxicity) and therefore a certain trade-off in dosing regimen to achieve relatively high exposures in relation to non-pathogen specific MIC may be acceptable.

Targeted Treatment Phase

After an initial empirical treatment there are two possible outcomes. Treatment may be discontinued because the clinical picture of sepsis cannot be microbiologically confirmed and an alternative diagnosis emerges. On the other hand, the microbiological cause confirming the diagnosis of sepsis may be identified. In the latter case treatment will be continued and toxicity issues become more important. During this

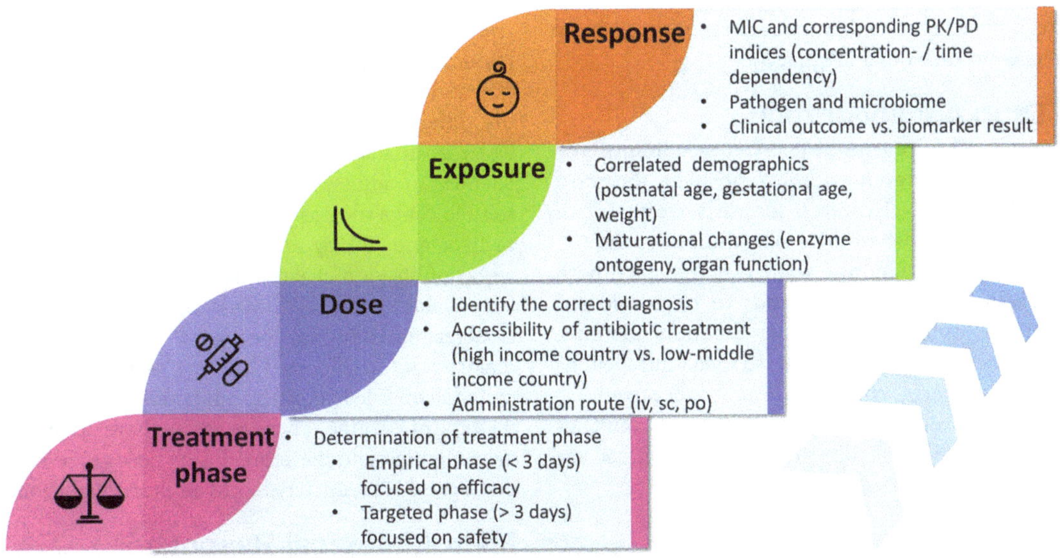

FIGURE 1 | Flowchart illustrating key components and factors influencing the concepts concerning antibiotic treatment in neonates and infants. MIC, minimal inhibitory concentration; PK, pharmacokinetics; PD, pharmacodynamics; iv, intravenous; sc, subcutaneous; po, oral.

targeted treatment phase, antibiotic dose optimization will be individualized to achieve an optimal efficacy-safety balance (**Figure 2**). When patients experience or are at high risk of toxicity (for example because of renal failure), three options are available: if susceptibility testing suggests a less toxic alternative, antibiotic treatment may be switched; depending on the exact infection and treatment response, only a short course is necessary and treatment may be stopped; or the antibiotic is question is considered the optimal therapeutic choice, in which case dose adjustments will be needed, possibly combined with therapeutic drug monitoring (TDM).

Antibiotic Drug Monitoring

The relationship between antibiotic dose and exposure is subject to high levels of inter- and intra-individual variability and to achieve effective antibiotic exposure, antibiotic drug monitoring is becoming crucial. This variability is known to be increased in patients with life-threatening infection, when rapid pathophysiological fluctuations even over the course of a few hours can impact the pharmacokinetics, and therefore the relationship between dose and antibiotic exposure. Reliable measurements are a prerequisite for effective TDM, accordingly turn-around times >24 h should be disregarded for critically ill patients (22). TDM is used to personalize the dosing strategies to ensure antimicrobial exposures which have therapeutic success and low probabilities of toxicity and generation of antimicrobial resistance (23). The percentage of patients with sub-therapeutic concentrations decreased from 58 to 40% after applying TDM for vancomycin in preterm and term neonates (24). Adequate antibiotic drug monitoring requires expertise in different fields and calls for the collaboration of physicians together with the lab technicians and clinical pharmacologists.

While the above is likely to be applicable to any antibiotic treatment, different antibiotics have different characteristics

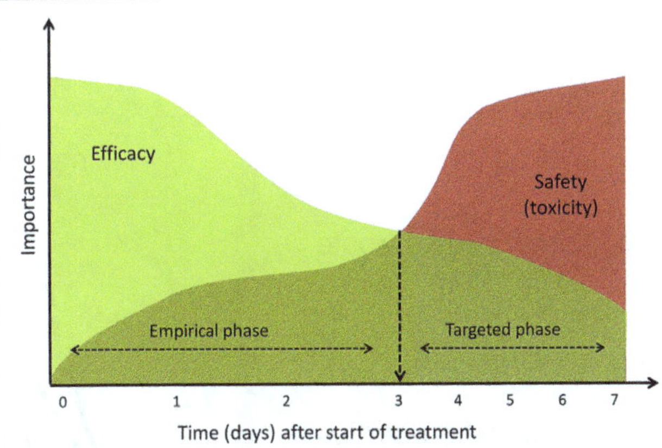

FIGURE 2 | Conceptual visualization of impact of efficacy and toxicity during antibiotic treatment. During the empirical phase, focus lies on an efficacious treatment and when sepsis is confirmed (~3 days) treatment can be individualized and focus should shift to the safety of treatment.

which are reflected in their pharmacological behavior. Most β-lactams have a wide therapeutic window, meaning that even high exposure is unlikely to be associated with toxicity. In contrast, aminoglycosides and glycopeptides have a narrow therapeutic window and require more attention to avoid toxicity.

UNDERSTANDING DOSE, DRUG ADMINISTRATION, EXPOSURE, AND RESPONSE

Clinical pharmacology aims to predict both efficacy and safety based on drug properties, population or individual pharmacokinetic behavior (PK) and pharmacodynamic, microbiological characteristics (PD). In order to understand optimal and individualized dosing of antibiotic treatment, one should be aware of the drug related processes in the human body and their influences on each other (**Figure 3**).

Dose and Drug Administration

A drug can have several formulations and can be administered through various routes, intravenous and oral being the most frequently used (**Figure 3A**). However, for early treatment of neonatal sepsis, oral administration is not clinically relevant. The route and method of administration can influence both PK and PD processes, and therefore needs to be considered when determining optimized dosing recommendations. Aminoglycosides are mostly administered via intravenous bolus dosage to achieve effective peak concentrations, due to concentration dependent properties. In countries where healthcare may be difficult to access, intramuscular administration is often applied.

Drug Exposure

The relationship between dose and drug exposure is governed by pharmacokinetics, defined by the kinetic processes abbreviated as ADME, which defines the absorption, distribution, metabolism, and excretion of a drug (**Figure 3B**). Due to dynamic maturation processes neonates and infants have marked differences compared to adults in terms of physiology affecting the different pharmacokinetic stages (25, 26). The total body water in infancy is decreasing over time (80–90% compared to 55–60% in adults), which influences the distribution of water soluble drugs such as gentamicin. Drug eliminating organs such as liver and kidney are immature at birth. During the first 2 weeks of life glomerular filtration rate increases rapidly reaching adult values within 1–2 years (27, 28). The metabolic capacity is determined by the ontogeny of metabolizing enzymes (a majority of them located in liver). Generally, the rate of hepatic metabolism is low at birth and increases over time, depending on the type of enzyme. These processes have an impact on exposure of antibiotics, and therefore dosing needs to be adjusted based on demographic characteristics of an individual neonate or infant.

Microbiological Response

Pharmacodynamic (PD) and microbiological aspects focus on the effects of a given drug on the pathogen and body (**Figure 3C**). In

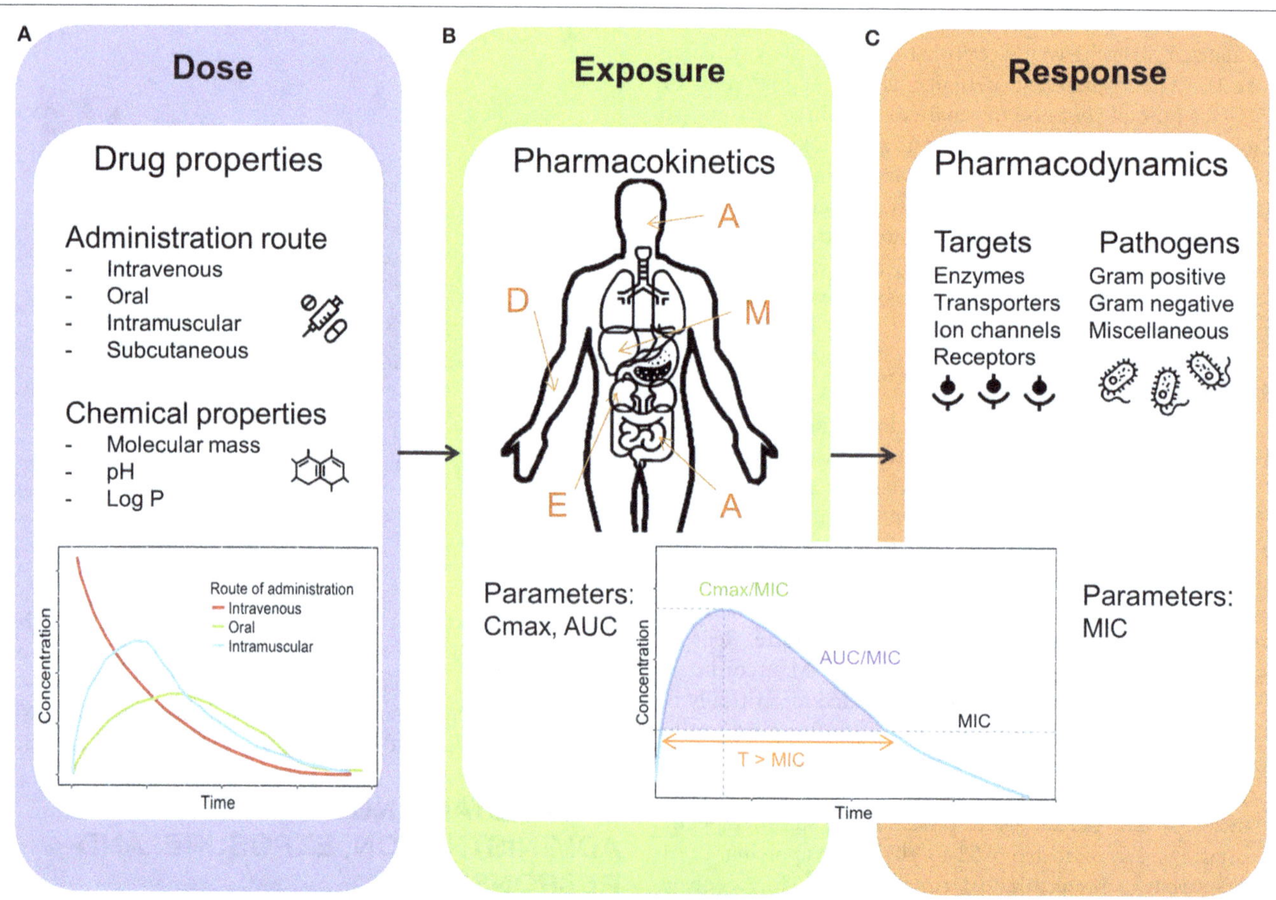

FIGURE 3 | General overview illustrating pharmacological key components. **(A)** Dose: drug properties and administration routes. **(B)** Exposure: Pharmacokinetic processes and parameters, A, Absorption (e.g., intestines); D, Distribution (e.g., blood circulation); M, Metabolism (e.g., liver); E, Excretion (e.g., kidneys); Cmax, peak concentration; AUC, area under the concentration-time curve. **(C)** Response: Pharmacodynamics, targets and pathogens, MIC, minimal inhibitory concentration; T > MIC, time above MIC.

order to elicit an effect, antibiotics need to reach certain exposure levels to kill causative pathogens of a sepsis. The exposure induced by the antibiotic dose will cause a response, but the main target being the pathogen. Currently, the MIC-based approach is most frequently applied to link drug exposure to microbiological response (**Figure 3C**).

Understanding the PK of antibiotics is necessary but not sufficient for optimizing and individualizing dosing strategies. It is essential to also understand characteristics and dynamics of the target (pathogen) as well (29). The growth of the pathogen needs to be inhibited or, even better, stopped entirely by the antibiotic agent depending on the MIC (**Table 1**). However the MIC may not be a fixed value, but rather changes over time, for example in the context of antibacterial resistance, and is also subject to measurement errors to the test system (variations in pH, incubation time, etc.) (38).

An increase in MICs, which is the result of decreasing susceptibility of a pathogen in a population, must in many cases be accompanied by dose adjustments to ensure effective exposure and maximize the effect. Recent changes to the interpretation of the so-called intermediate breakpoint as representing susceptibility for which successful treatment outcomes are likely with adjustments of the dosing regimen reflect this (10).

UNDERSTANDING THE LINK BETWEEN ANTIBIOTIC EXPOSURE AND MICROBIOLOGICAL RESPONSE

With a limited pipeline of new antibiotics, relying on proper use and understanding the link between antibiotic exposure (PK) and microbiological response (pharmacodynamics, PD) is a key issue concerning dosing optimization of the presently available antibiotics (29).

In order to describe relationships between drug exposure and microbiological effects, exposure-response parameters are used. A PK/PD index is defined as the quantitative relationship between an exposure-related parameter (e.g. plasma concentration) and a microbiological parameter (e.g. MIC) (39). Antibiotic classes can be characterized by different properties in terms of PK/PD indices. The optimal target index is frequently identified based on animal dose fractionation studies (37). Already in the early 1950s Eagle *et al.* noticed the time dependent properties of penicillin, and realized that penicillins are best administered as continuous infusions, whereas a concentration dependent agent is better given as an intravenous bolus to achieve high maximum concentrations (40, 41).

Concentration Dependent Microbiological Response

The bacterial killing rate of concentration dependent antibiotics increases at high levels of the antibiotic; this applies to aminoglycosides and fluoroquinolones. For aminoglycosides, the antibacterial effect is related to the peak concentration (C_{max}/MIC). Depending on the antibiotic class, different ratios apply (**Table 1**). The magnitude of the peak concentration is often associated with the bacterial killing efficiency (go hard and go home paradigm) (21, 40, 42). In addition, concentration dependent antibiotics frequently exhibit a post antibiotic effect (PAE). The PAE is defined as the suppression of bacterial growth after the exposure of bacteria to an antibiotic (even in absence of host defense mechanism) (43).

Shifts in MIC can lead to a situation where dosing recommendations need to be revised to achieve optimal treatment. For gentamicin, for example, an increase in MIC from 0.5 to 1.0 mg/L means that, in order to achieve similar efficacy (similar ratio of $Cmax/MIC$), the dose should be increased from 5 to 7.5 mg/kg in neonates (19).

Time Dependent Microbiological Response

The effect of time dependent antibiotics relies on the length of time that the antibiotic is in contact with causative pathogen. For β-lactams the antibacterial effect is considered to be time dependent and therefore the PK/PD index *Time/MIC* is used (**Figures 3B,C**). This index is generally transformed to $fT>MIC$; this reflects the percentage of time for which the free fraction of drug concentration remains above the MIC (**Table 1**). For β-lactams (penicillins, cephalosporins, carbapenems) it has been proposed that dosing schedules should maintain plasma concentrations above MIC for at least 50% of the dosing interval, but the efficacy of β-lactams is enhanced with longer exposure times. The post antibiotic effect is limited for β-lactams with an exception for carbapenems (40). Continuous infusions can potentially improve target attainment for $fT>MIC$, they may, however, be impractical in many settings (44). Decreased mortality has been associated with continuous infusion of β-lactam antibiotics in critically ill patients with severe sepsis (45).

Other Relevant Indices for Microbiological Response

Several studies have shown the importance of a third index, namely *AUC/MIC* (21, 38). AUC reflects the area under the concentration-time curve and represents the antibiotic exposure over time. This parameter is often used for concentration independent antibiotics with extended post antibiotic effects, such as vancomycin. Bacterial regrowth is inhibited, even when the concentration falls below MIC, but the effect is not dependent on the peak concentration (37). Few antibiotics, such as aminoglycosides and fluoroquinolones have been linked to multiple classes and multiple corresponding indices, leading to differences in dosing recommendations and guidelines.

CHALLENGES OF ANTIBIOTIC DOSE OPTIMIZATION IN NEONATES AND INFANTS

Currently, TDM of antibiotics is not widely used for antibiotic dose optimization in neonates and infants suffering from life-threatening infections. This is mainly related to practical barriers of implementing TDM for improving treatment effectiveness, such as the lack of rapid and reliable methods of analysis of the antibiotic or the possibility that the pharmacologic

TABLE 1 | Pharmacokinetic and pharmacodynamic indices for antimicrobial agents together with their target value and bactericidal characteristics.

PK/PD indices and their target values				
Antimicrobial agents	**PK/PD index**	**Target value for clinical antibacterial efficacy**	**PK/PD properties**	**References**
Aminoglycosides	Cmax/MIC		Concentration dependent killing (maximize drug concentration)	
Gentamicin		≥8		(22)
Amikacin		8–10		(30)
Tobramycin		8–12		(31)
β-lactams	fT > MIC	T>MIC > 40%	Time dependent killing (maximize exposure time)	(32)
Penicillins		T>MIC > 50–60%		(33)
Carbapenems		T>MIC > 40–50%		(33)
Cephalosporins		T>MIC > 60–70%		(33)
Glycopeptides			Time and concentration dependent killing (maximize daily amount of dose)	
Vancomycin	AUC24/MIC	400		(34)
Quinolones				
Levofloxacin	AUC/MIC	100		(35)
Ciprofloxacin	AUC/MIC	125		(36)
Fluoroquinolones	AUC24/MIC	100–125 (Gram-negatives) 25–35 (Gram-positives)		(37)

Cmax: maximum antibacterial concentration, MIC: minimal inhibitory concentration, AUC: area under the concentration-time-curve, AUC24: area under the concentration time curve over 24 hours, fT > MIC: percentage of time for which the free fraction of drug remains above MIC.

effect is not readily measurable (due to interactions with other drugs) (46) Beta-lactam antibiotics in particular would benefit from dose adaptations based on measured levels, as these are often the backbone of empiric treatment (47). Technical bottlenecks include long turn-around times for samples, lack of commercial assays and challenging pre-analytics, and in the pediatric population the need for relatively large samples volumes (**Table 2**). The required sampling volume, relative to the circulating blood volume is a crucial barrier, especially in preterm infants whose blood volume is limited. Furthermore, concentration measurements are often collected from plasma since these are relatively easy to obtain, although these levels appear to be a poor descriptor of the activities of the drug at site of action in individual patients.

Moreover, although the MIC-based approach is well-established as a measure of the potency of an antibiotic drug, it is determined in an *in vitro* setting, where the conditions are dissimilar from those at the site of infection in the *in vivo* situation. Better understanding of population-specific MICs is demanded to guide empiric antibiotic treatment (40, 48). Additionally, antibacterial activity is a dynamic process and since MIC is a one-point threshold value, the MIC can only provide an approximation on the antibacterial effect (38).

The key issue in optimizing antibiotic exposure in critically ill patients is to respond to expectedly variable PK in patients with life-threatening illness and at risk of infection caused by bacteria with potentially problematic antibiotic resistance. Critical illness leads to time-variation in multiple factors, potentially requiring frequent dose adjustments in the most vulnerable patients rather than simple *a priori* dose stratification. More knowledge is required concerning tissue penetration of antibiotics in critically ill neonates and infants (49). Furthermore, drug dosing is currently being adjusted for patients with impaired kidney function (risk for toxicity), whereas for patients with augmented renal clearance (elevated drug clearance) no dose adjustments are being recommended (50). Although the underlying physiological mechanisms of augmented renal clearance are not yet fully understood, augmented renal clearance has not only been observed in critically ill adults, but also in pediatric patients (50, 51). Consequently, there is a real need for reliable assessment and monitoring of kidney function in neonates and infants. Serum creatinine values are still widely used, although the accuracy and usefulness of this biomarker can be questioned in neonates as various parts of kidneys are maturing at different rates (52).

TABLE 2 | Challenges to overcome the burden of sepsis and the opportunities to improve diagnostic tools, measurement techniques and implementation of modeling and simulation techniques.

Challenges; what is missing?	Opportunities
• Uniform sepsis definitions for all age groups across the pediatric age range	• Identify of biomarkers (e.g., presepsin or cystatin C) with accurate thresholds
• Diagnostic tools to identify pathogens and infection	• Use microdialysis to measure drug concentrations at target site
• Adequate descriptors of drug concentration at target site	• Implement therapeutic antibiotic monitoring, especially in patients with life-threatening infections
• Understanding PK/PD relationships and parameters which can characterize the dynamic process of antibacterial activity	• Apply kill-curves approach to describe changing antibacterial activity
• Reliable measurements for GFR in the pediatric population (augmented renal clearance)	• Multidisciplinary collaboration and communication between research groups and physicians
• Straightforward applications of model-based approaches	• Implement modeling and simulation strategies in clinical settings (e.g., for individual dose optimization)
• Implementation of adjusted dosing guidelines in clinical practice	• Develop understandable time-saving software tools for individualized dosing

The application of pharmacometric modeling and simulation will be needed to truly support antibiotic dosing optimization based on the knowledge of the dose-concentration-effect relationship (53). The modeling and simulation strategy is still underutilized, although it has been shown that mechanistic modeling such as physiological-based pharmacokinetic (PBPK) models have good predictive value and enable extrapolation by using information about the drug and the physiology (54, 55). Despite modeling and simulation being frequently reported in the literature, the results and adjusted dosing recommendations are not yet implemented in daily clinical practice (56). Dose adjustment and individualization of antibiotics is crucial. For instance, administration of an inefficacious (too low) dose of antibiotics in patients with increased drug clearance can have a negative impact on patient outcome and antibiotic resistance.

OPPORTUNITIES: HOW TO CLOSE KNOWLEDGE GAPS

The search for a quantitative, scientific rationale to further enhance dosing regimens and drug combinations can benefit tremendously from modeling and simulation strategies when there is on-going communication and exchange between research groups and clinicians (**Table 2**) (57). In order to apply these quantitative methods directly in clinical practice, it is essential to communicate the strengths and applicability of the model to the users (mostly physicians). User-friendly decision support tools, which provide quantitative, scientific output without requiring additional time-consuming activities during routine clinical practice, would be valuable (54, 56). An example of these software tools is the model-supported TDM tool for precision dosing TDMx (http://www.tdmx.eu/). Since there are several population PK models published for antimicrobial agents, researchers should assess new data or use existing data to extend and improve existing population PK models (56, 58). Pharmacometric PK/PD models can help identify the optimal (effective and safe) therapeutic window necessary to successfully treat an infection (59).

In contrast to the MIC, which reflects the susceptibility of a pathogen at only one time point, bacterial kill-curves can offer more detailed information about the killing activity as a function over time and might even be used to identify the presence of resistant subpopulations (60, 61). Bacterial kill-curves are very labor intensive and until the method is automated and widely implementable, this approach might not be practical (61).

Furthermore, in recent decades novel non-invasive techniques have provided information about the process of target site distribution. Microdialysis provides direct measurement of concentrations of unbound antibiotics at the site of action when the site of infection is not the bloodstream (40, 62). Measurement of the free (unbound) drug concentration in the interstitial fluid is better correlated with the antimicrobial efficacy, compared to concentration measurements in plasma. Microdialysis offers a useful sampling tool which can quantify the unbound antibiotic at infection sites (29). Other non-invasive techniques such as dried blood spot analysis or TDM from sweat are considered as innovative and promising methods to tackle the known barriers (30, 31, 34).

CONCLUSIONS

There are still numerous challenges to overcome the burden of sepsis in neonates and infants, of which the lack of implementation of optimized, individualized dosing recommendations can be considered as remarkably important. Key components for optimal antibiotic treatment of sepsis in neonates and infants are indicated as treatment phase, dose, drug exposure and microbiological response. During the first days of treatment the focus lies on establishing an effective dose, thereafter the balance is shifting toward ensuring a safe and effective treatment. In neonates and young infants, drug exposure is affected by developmental changes such as maturation of organ function and metabolizing enzymes, which requires dosing adjustments. The response or treatment effect can be determined by the microbiological parameters (MIC) together with the pathogen characteristics (time- or concentration dependent). Understanding these clinical, pharmacological and microbiological components and their underlying relationship might provide a basis for proper antibiotic use and reduction of antibiotic resistance. This also illustrates the necessity of a close multidisciplinary collaboration between physicians, pharmacists, pharmacometricians, clinical pharmacologists and microbiologists to assure optimal utilization of antibiotics in neonates and infants.

AUTHOR CONTRIBUTIONS

TvD, JB, and MP drafted the concept of the review. TvD wrote the first draft of the manuscript and generated tables and figures. JB contributed to the sections considering infectious diseases. JvdA and MP contributed to the clinical pharmacology section. All authors critically revised the manuscript, and approved the final version before submission.

ACKNOWLEDGMENTS

TvD, JB, JvdA, and MP would like to thank the Eckenstein-Geigy Foundation in Basel, Switzerland for their financial support.

REFERENCES

1. Liu L, Oza S, Hogan D, Chu Y, Perin J, Zhu J, et al. Global, regional, and national causes of under-5 mortality in 2000–15: an updated systematic analysis with implications for the Sustainable Development Goals. *Lancet* (2016) 388:3027–35. doi: 10.1016/S0140-6736(16) 31593-8
2. Shane AL, Stoll BJ. Neonatal sepsis: progress towards improved outcomes. *J Infect.* (2014) 68:S24–S32. doi: 10.1016/j.jinf.2013.09.011
3. Simonsen KA, Anderson-Berry AL, Delair SF, Davies HD. Early-onset neonatal sepsis. *Clin Microbiol Rev.* (2014) 27:21–47. doi: 10.1128/CMR.00031-13
4. Malek A, Sager R, Kuhn P, Nicolaides KH, Schneider H. Evolution of maternofetal transport of immunoglobulins during

human pregnancy. *Am J Reproduct Immunol.* (1996) 36:248–55. doi: 10.1111/j.1600-0897.1996.tb00172.x
5. Gritz EC, Bhandari V. The Human Neonatal Gut Microbiome: a brief review. *Front Pediatr.* (2015) 3:17. doi: 10.3389/fped.2015.00017
6. Randolph AG, McCulloh RJ. Pediatric sepsis: important considerations for diagnosing and managing severe infections in infants, children, and adolescents. *Virulence* (2014) 5:179–89. doi: 10.4161/viru.27045
7. Plunkett A, Tong J. Sepsis in children. *BMJ.* (2015) 350:h3017. doi: 10.1136/bmj.h3017
8. Singer M, Deutschman CS, Seymour CW, Shankar-Hari M, Annane D, Bauer M, et al. The third international consensus definitions for sepsis and septic shock (Sepsis-3). *JAMA.* (2016) 315:801–10. doi: 10.1001/jama.2016.0287
9. Goldstein B, Giroir B, Randolph A. International pediatric sepsis consensus conference: definitions for sepsis and organ dysfunction in pediatrics. *Pediatr Crit Care Med.* (2005) 6:99. doi: 10.1097/00130478-200501000-00041
10. Kahlmeter G, Committee ES. EUCAST proposes to change the definition and usefulness of the susceptibility category 'Intermediate'. *Clin Microbiol Infect.* (2017) 23:894–5. doi: 10.1016/j.cmi.2017.08.015
11. Schlapbach LJ, Kissoon N. Defining pediatric sepsis. *JAMA Pediatr.* (2018) 172:312–4. doi: 10.1001/jamapediatrics.2017.5208.
12. Le Doare K, Barker CI, Irwin A, Sharland M. Improving antibiotic prescribing for children in the resource-poor setting. *Br J Clin Pharmacol.* (2015) 79:446–55. doi: 10.1111/bcp.12320
13. Stoll BJ, Hansen NI, Sánchez PJ, Faix RG, Poindexter BB, Van Meurs KP, et al. Early onset neonatal sepsis: the burden of group B Streptococcal and *E. coli* disease continues. *Pediatrics* (2011) 127:2010–217. doi: 10.1542/peds.2010-2217
14. Kuhn P, Dheu C, Bolender C, Chognot D, Keller L, Demil H, et al. Incidence and distribution of pathogens in early-onset neonatal sepsis in the era of antenatal antibiotics. *Paediatr Perinat Epidemiol.* (2010) 24:479–87. doi: 10.1111/j.1365-3016.2010.01132.x
15. Russell AB, Kumar R. Early onset neonatal sepsis: diagnostic dilemmas and practical management. *Arch Dis Childhood-Fetal Neonatal Ed.* (2015) 100:F350–F4. doi: 10.1136/archdischild-2014-306193
16. Camacho-Gonzalez A, Spearman PW, Stoll BJ. Neonatal infectious diseases: evaluation of neonatal sepsis. *Pediatr Clin North Am.* (2013) 60:367. doi: 10.1016/j.pcl.2012.12.003
17. Cohen-Wolkowiez M, Moran C, Benjamin DK, Cotten CM, Clark RH, Benjamin Jr DK, et al. Early and late onset sepsis in late preterm infants. *Pediatr Infect Dis J.* (2009) 28:1052. doi: 10.1097/INF.0b013e3181acf6bd
18. Becker JU, Theodosis C, Jacob ST, Wira CR, Groce NE. Surviving sepsis in low-income and middle-income countries: new directions for care and research. *Lancet Infect Dis.* (2009) 9:577–82. doi: 10.1016/S1473-3099(09)70135-5
19. van Donge T, Pfister M, Bielicki J, Csajka C, Rodieux F, van den Anker J, et al. Quantitative analysis of gentamicin exposure in neonates and infants calls into question its current dosing recommendations. *Antimicrobial Agents Chemother.* (2018) 62: 02004–17. doi: 10.1128/AAC.02004-17
20. Mueller M, de la Pe-a A, Derendorf H. Issues in pharmacokinetics and pharmacodynamics of anti-infective agents: kill curves versus MIC. *Antimicrobial Agents Chemother.* (2004) 48:369–77. doi: 10.1128/AAC.48.2.369-377.2004
21. Lipman J, Boots R. A new paradigm for treating infections: 'Go Hard and Go Home'. *Crit Care Resuscit.* (2009) 11:276. Available online at: https://cicm.org.au/CICM_Media/CICMSite/CICM-Website/Resources/Publications/CCR%20Journal/Previous%20Editions/December%202009/12_2009_Dec_Rev-A-new-paradigm.pdf
22. Muller AE, Huttner B, Huttner A. Therapeutic drug monitoring of beta-lactams and other antibiotics in the intensive care unit: which agents, which patients and which infections? *Drugs* (2018) 78:439–51. doi: 10.1007/s40265-018-0880-z
23. Roberts JA, Norris R, Paterson DL, Martin JH. Therapeutic drug monitoring of antimicrobials. *Br J Clin Pharmacol.* (2012) 73:27–36. doi: 10.1111/j.1365-2125.2011.04080.x
24. Sinkeler FS, de Haan TR, Hodiamont CJ, Bijleveld YA, Pajkrt D, Mathôt RAA. Inadequate vancomycin therapy in term and preterm neonates: a retrospective analysis of trough serum concentrations in relation to minimal inhibitory concentrations. *BMC Pediatr.* (2014) 14:193. doi: 10.1186/1471-2431-14-193
25. Allegaert K, Velde M, Anker J. Neonatal clinical pharmacology. *Pediatr Anesthesia* (2014) 24:30–8. doi: 10.1111/pan.12176
26. van den Anker JN, Schwab M, Kearns GL. Developmental pharmacokinetics. *Pediatr Clin Pharmacol.* (2011) 205:51–75. doi: 10.1007/978-3-642-20195-0_2
27. Wilbaux M, Fuchs A, Samardzic J, Rodieux F, Csajka C, Allegaert K, et al. Pharmacometric approaches to personalize use of primarily renally eliminated antibiotics in preterm and term neonates. *J Clin Pharmacol.* (2016) 56:909–35. doi: 10.1002/jcph.705
28. Rodieux F, Wilbaux M, van den Anker JN, Pfister M. Effect of kidney function on drug kinetics and dosing in neonates, infants, and children. *Clin Pharmacokinet.* (2015) 54:1183–204. doi: 10.1007/s40262-015-0298-7
29. Marchand S, Chauzy A, Dahyot-Fizelier C, Couet W. Microdialysis as a way to measure antibiotics concentration in tissues. *Pharmacol Res.* (2016) 111:201–7. doi: 10.1016/j.phrs.2016.06.001
30. Kiang TK, Ensom MH. A qualitative review on the pharmacokinetics of antibiotics in saliva: implications on clinical pharmacokinetic monitoring in humans. *Clin Pharmacokinet.* (2016) 55:313–58. doi: 10.1007/s40262-015-0321-z
31. Kiang TK, Ranamukhaarachchi SA, Ensom MH. Revolutionizing therapeutic drug monitoring with the use of interstitial fluid and microneedles technology. *Pharmaceutics* (2017) 9:43. doi: 10.3390/pharmaceutics9040043
32. Knippenberg B, Page-Sharp M, Salman S, Clark B, Dyer J, Batty KT, et al. Validation and application of a dried blood spot assay for biofilm-active antibiotics commonly used for treatment of prosthetic implant infections. *Antimicrobial Agents Chemother.* (2016) 60:4940–55. doi: 10.1128/AAC.00756-16
33. Drusano GL. Antimicrobial pharmacodynamics: critical interactions of 'bug and drug'. *Nat Rev Microbiol.* (2004) 2:289. doi: 10.1038/nrmicro862
34. Hawwa AF, AlBawab A, Rooney M, Wedderburn LR, Beresford MW, McElnay JC. A novel dried blood spot-LCMS method for the quantification of methotrexate polyglutamates as a potential marker for methotrexate use in children. *PLoS ONE* (2014) 9:e89908. doi: 10.1371/journal.pone.0089908
35. Zeitlinger MA, Dehghanyar P, Mayer BX, Schenk BS, Neckel U, Heinz G, et al. Relevance of soft-tissue penetration by levofloxacin for target site bacterial killing in patients with sepsis. *Antimicrobial Agents Chemother.* (2003) 47:3548–53. doi: 10.1128/AAC.47.11.3548-3553.2003
36. Forrest A, Nix DE, Ballow CH, Goss TF, Birmingham M, Schentag J. Pharmacodynamics of intravenous ciprofloxacin in seriously ill patients. *Antimicrobial Agents Chemother.* (1993) 37:1073–81. doi: 10.1128/AAC.37.5.1073
37. Schmidt S, Barbour A, Sahre M, Rand KH, Derendorf H. PK/PD: new insights for antibacterial and antiviral applications. *Curr Opin Pharmacol.* (2008) 8:549–56. doi: 10.1016/j.coph.2008.06.010
38. Mouton JW, Muller AE, Canton R, Giske CG, Kahlmeter G, Turnidge J. MIC-based dose adjustment: facts and fables. *J Antimicrob Chemother.* (2017) 73:564–8. doi: 10.1093/jac/dkx427
39. Mouton JW, Dudley MN, Cars O, Derendorf H, Drusano GL. Standardization of pharmacokinetic/pharmacodynamic (PK/PD) terminology for anti-infective drugs. *Int J Antimicrob Agents* (2002) 19:355–8. doi: 10.1016/S0924-8579(02)00031-6
40. Sherwin K, Zhuang L, Derendorf H. Pharmacokinetics and pharmacodynamics in antibiotic dose optimization. *Expert Opin Drug Metabol Toxicol.* (2016) 12:93–114. doi: 10.1517/17425255.2016.1123250
41. Eagle H, Fleischman R, Levy M. Continuous vs. discontinuous therapy with penicillin: the effect of the interval between injections on therapeutic efficacy. *N E J Med.* (1953) 248:481–8. doi: 10.1056/NEJM195303192481201
42. Ehrlich P. Address in Pathology, ON CHEMIOTHERAPY: delivered before the Seventeenth International Congress of Medicine. *Br Med J.* (1913) 2:353–9. doi: 10.1136/bmj.2.2746.353
43. Spivey J. The postantibiotic effect. *Clin Pharmacy* (1992) 11:865–75.
44. Zaidi AK, Tikmani SS, Warraich HJ, Darmstadt GL, Bhutta ZA, Sultana S, et al. Community-based treatment of serious bacterial infections in newborns and young infants: a randomized controlled trial assessing three antibiotic regimens. *Pediatr Infect Dis J.* (2012) 31:667–72. doi: 10.1097/INF.0b013e318256f86c
45. Roberts JA, Abdul-Aziz M-H, Davis JS, Dulhunty JM, Cotta MO, Myburgh J, et al. Continuous versus intermittent β-lactam infusion in severe sepsis. A

meta-analysis of individual patient data from randomized trials. *Am J Respirat Crit Care Med.* (2016) 194:681–91. doi: 10.1164/rccm.201601-0024OC

46. Soldin OP, Soldin SJ. Therapeutic drug monitoring in pediatrics. *Ther Drug Monit.* (2002) 24:1.
47. Versporten A, Bielicki J, Drapier N, Sharland M, Goossens H, Group AP, et al. The Worldwide Antibiotic Resistance and Prescribing in European Children (ARPEC) point prevalence survey: developing hospital-quality indicators of antibiotic prescribing for children. *J Antimicrob Chemother.* (2016) 71:1106–17. doi: 10.1093/jac/dkv418
48. Kent A, Kortsalioudaki C, Monahan IM, Bielicki J, Planche TD, Heath PT, et al. Neonatal gram-negative infections, antibiotic susceptibility and clinical outcome: an observational study. *Arch Dis Childhood-Fetal Neonatal Ed.* (2016) 101:F507–12. doi: 10.1136/archdischild-2015-309554
49. Smits A, De Cock PA. Antibiotic PK/PD research in critically ill neonates and children: how do we proceed? *Int J Pharmac.* (2018) 3:1–3. doi: 10.4155/ipk-2017-0019
50. van den Anker JN, Knibbe CA, Tibboel D. Augmented renal clearance in critically Ill pediatric patients: does it impact the outcome of pharmacotherapy? *Pediatr Crit Care Med.* (2017) 18:901–2. doi: 10.1097/PCC.0000000000001264
51. De Cock PA, Standing JF, Barker CI, de Jaeger A, Dhont E, Carlier M, et al. Augmented renal clearance implies a need for increased amoxicillin-clavulanic acid dosing in critically ill children. *Antimicrob Agents Chemother.* (2015) 59:7027–35. doi: 10.1128/AAC.01368-15
52. Finney H, Newman D, Thakkar H, Fell J, Price CJA. Reference ranges for plasma cystatin C and creatinine measurements in premature infants, neonates, and older children. *Arch Dis Child.* (2000) 82:71–5. doi: 10.1136/adc.82.1.71
53. Standing JF. Understanding and applying pharmacometric modelling and simulation in clinical practice and research. *Br J Clin Pharmacol.* (2017) 83:247–54. doi: 10.1111/bcp.13119
54. Germovsek E, Kent A, Metsvaht T, Lutsar I, Klein N, Turner MA, et al. Development and evaluation of a gentamicin pharmacokinetic model that facilitates opportunistic gentamicin therapeutic drug monitoring in neonates and infants. *Antimicrob Agents Chemother.* (2016) 60:4869–77. doi: 10.1128/AAC.00577-16
55. Edginton AN, Schmitt W, Willmann S. Development and evaluation of a generic physiologically based pharmacokinetic model for children. *Clin Pharmacokinet.* (2006) 45:1013–34. doi: 10.2165/00003088-200645100-00005
56. Darwich A, Ogungbenro K, Vinks A, Powell J, Reny JL, Marsousi N, et al. Why has model-informed precision dosing not yet become common clinical reality? Lessons from the past and a roadmap for the future. *Clin Pharmacol Therapeut.* (2017) 101:646–56. doi: 10.1002/cpt.659
57. Samardzic J, Allegaert K, Wilbaux M, Pfister M, van den Anker JN. Quantitative clinical pharmacology practice for optimal use of antibiotics during the neonatal period. *Expert Opin Drug Metabol Toxicol.* (2016) 12:367–75. doi: 10.1517/17425255.2016.1147559
58. Van Donge T, Mian P, Tibboel D, Van Den Anker J, Allegaert K. Drug metabolism in early infancy: opioids as an illustration. *Expert Opin Drug Metabol Toxicol.* (2018) 14:287–301. doi: 10.1080/17425255.2018.1432595
59. Trivedi A, Lee RE, Meibohm B. Applications of pharmacometrics in the clinical development and pharmacotherapy of anti-infectives. *Expert Rev Clin Pharmacol.* (2013) 6:159–70. doi: 10.1586/ecp.13.6
60. Liu P, Müller M, Derendorf H. Rational dosing of antibiotics: the use of plasma concentrations versus tissue concentrations. *Int J Antimicrobial Agents* (2002) 19:285–90. doi: 10.1016/S0924-8579(02)00024-9
61. Barbour AM, Schmidt S, Zhuang L, Rand K, Derendorf H. Application of pharmacokinetic/pharmacodynamic modelling and simulation for the prediction of target attainment of ceftobiprole against meticillin-resistant Staphylococcus aureus using minimum inhibitory concentration and time–kill curve based approaches. *Int J Antimicrobial Agents* (2014) 43:60–7. doi: 10.1016/j.ijantimicag.2013.08.016
62. Müller M, dela Pe-a A, Derendorf H. Issues in pharmacokinetics and pharmacodynamics of anti-infective agents: distribution in tissue. *Antimicrobial Agents Chemother.* (2004) 48:1441–53. doi: 10.1128/AAC.48.5.1441-1453.2004

Permissions

All chapters in this book were first published by Frontiers; hereby published with permission under the Creative Commons Attribution License or equivalent. Every chapter published in this book has been scrutinized by our experts. Their significance has been extensively debated. The topics covered herein carry significant findings which will fuel the growth of the discipline. They may even be implemented as practical applications or may be referred to as a beginning point for another development.

The contributors of this book come from diverse backgrounds, making this book a truly international effort. This book will bring forth new frontiers with its revolutionizing research information and detailed analysis of the nascent developments around the world.

We would like to thank all the contributing authors for lending their expertise to make the book truly unique. They have played a crucial role in the development of this book. Without their invaluable contributions this book wouldn't have been possible. They have made vital efforts to compile up to date information on the varied aspects of this subject to make this book a valuable addition to the collection of many professionals and students.

This book was conceptualized with the vision of imparting up-to-date information and advanced data in this field. To ensure the same, a matchless editorial board was set up. Every individual on the board went through rigorous rounds of assessment to prove their worth. After which they invested a large part of their time researching and compiling the most relevant data for our readers.

The editorial board has been involved in producing this book since its inception. They have spent rigorous hours researching and exploring the diverse topics which have resulted in the successful publishing of this book. They have passed on their knowledge of decades through this book. To expedite this challenging task, the publisher supported the team at every step. A small team of assistant editors was also appointed to further simplify the editing procedure and attain best results for the readers.

Apart from the editorial board, the designing team has also invested a significant amount of their time in understanding the subject and creating the most relevant covers. They scrutinized every image to scout for the most suitable representation of the subject and create an appropriate cover for the book.

The publishing team has been an ardent support to the editorial, designing and production team. Their endless efforts to recruit the best for this project, has resulted in the accomplishment of this book. They are a veteran in the field of academics and their pool of knowledge is as vast as their experience in printing. Their expertise and guidance has proved useful at every step. Their uncompromising quality standards have made this book an exceptional effort. Their encouragement from time to time has been an inspiration for everyone.

The publisher and the editorial board hope that this book will prove to be a valuable piece of knowledge for researchers, students, practitioners and scholars across the globe.

List of Contributors

Dominik Ochocinski
Department of Anesthesiology, University of Florida, Gainesville, FL, United States

Mansi Dalal and L. Vandy Black
Division of Pediatric Hematology/Oncology, University of Florida, Gainesville, FL, United States

Silvana Carr and Judy Lew
Division of Pediatric Infectious Disease, University of Florida, Gainesville, FL, United States

Kevin Sullivan
Department of Anesthesiology, University of Florida, Gainesville, FL, United States
Congenital Heart Center, University of Florida, Gainesville, FL, United States

Niranjan Kissoon
Department of Pediatrics, University of British Columbia and BC Children's Hospital, Vancouver, BC, Canada
Center for International Child Health, British Columbia Children's Hospital, Vancouver, BC, Canada

Etienne Javouhey
Pediatric Emergency and Critical Care Unit, Hospices Civils de Lyon, Hôpital Femme Mère Enfant, Bron, France
Faculté de Médecine Lyon Est, Université de Lyon, Domaine de la Buire, Lyon, France

Claire Jamen
Pediatric Emergency and Critical Care Unit, Hospices Civils de Lyon, Hôpital Femme Mère Enfant, Bron, France

Pierre-Adrien Bolze
Service de Gynécologie et Obstétrique, Hospices Civils de Lyon, Hôpital Femme Mère Enfant, Bron, France

Gerard Lina and Olivier Dauwalder
Centre National de Référence des Staphylocoques, Institut des Agents Infectieux, Centre de Biologie et de Pathologie Nord, Hospices Civils de Lyon, Lyon, France
Laboratoire de Bactériologie, Centre de Biologie et de Pathologie Nord, Institut des Agents Infectieux, Hospices Civils de Lyon, Lyon, France
Centre International de Recherche en Infectiologie (CIRI), Inserm U1111, Université Lyon 1, Ecole Normale Supérieure de Lyon, CNRS UMR5308, Lyon, France

Michèle Bes
Centre National de Référence des Staphylocoques, Institut des Agents Infectieux, Centre de Biologie et de Pathologie Nord, Hospices Civils de Lyon, Lyon, France
Centre International de Recherche en Infectiologie (CIRI), Inserm U1111, Université Lyon 1, Ecole Normale Supérieure de Lyon, CNRS UMR5308, Lyon, France

Yves Gilletand
Pediatric Emergency and Critical Care Unit, Hospices Civils de Lyon, Hôpital Femme Mère Enfant, Bron, France
Centre National de Référence des Staphylocoques, Institut des Agents Infectieux, Centre de Biologie et de Pathologie Nord, Hospices Civils de Lyon, Lyon, France
Centre International de Recherche en Infectiologie (CIRI), Inserm U1111, Université Lyon 1, Ecole Normale Supérieure de Lyon, CNRS UMR5308, Lyon, France

Cédric Badiou
Centre International de Recherche en Infectiologie (CIRI), Inserm U1111, Université Lyon 1, Ecole Normale Supérieure de Lyon, CNRS UMR5308, Lyon, France

Anne Tristan, Frédéric Laurent and François Vandenesch
Faculté de Médecine Lyon Est, Université de Lyon, Domaine de la Buire, Lyon, France
Centre National de Référence des Staphylocoques, Institut des Agents Infectieux, Centre de Biologie et de Pathologie Nord, Hospices Civils de Lyon, Lyon, France
Laboratoire de Bactériologie, Centre de Biologie et de Pathologie Nord, Institut des Agents Infectieux, Hospices Civils de Lyon, Lyon, France
Centre International de Recherche en Infectiologie (CIRI), Inserm U1111, Université Lyon 1, Ecole Normale Supérieure de Lyon, CNRS UMR5308, Lyon, France

Claire Poyart
Centre National de Références des Streptocoques – Groupe Hospitalier Paris Centre Cochin-Hôtel Dieu-Broca, Assistance Publique Hôpitaux de Paris, Paris, France
Institut Cochin Université Sorbonne Paris Descartes, Paris, France
INSERM 1016, Institut Cochin, Paris, France
CNRS, UMR8104, Institut Cochin, Paris, France

Aurelie Portefaix
Pediatric Emergency and Critical Care Unit, Hospices Civils de Lyon, Hôpital Femme Mère Enfant, Bron, France
EPICIME-CIC 1407 de Lyon, Inserm, Service de Pharmacotoxicologie, Hospices Civils de Lyon, Bron, France

Ben Gelbart
Paediatric Intensive Care Unit Royal Children's Hospital, Melbourne, VIC, Australia Murdoch Childrens Research Institute, Melbourne, VIC, Australia
The University of Melbourne, Melbourne, VIC, Australia

Claus Klingenberg
Pediatric Research Group, Faculty of Health Sciences, University of Tromsø-Arctic University of Norway, Tromsø, Norway
Department of Pediatrics and Adolescence Medicine, University Hospital of North Norway, Tromsø, Norway
Paediatric Research Group, Department of Clinical Medicine, UiT The Arctic University of Norway, Tromsø, Norway

René F. Kornelisse
Division of Neonatology, Department of Pediatrics, Erasmus MC-Sophia Children's Hospital, Erasmus University Medical Center, Rotterdam, Netherlands

Giuseppe Buonocore
Department of Molecular and Developmental Medicine, University of Siena, Siena, Italy

Rolf F. Maier
Children's Hospital, University Hospital, Philipps University of Marburg, Marburg, Germany

Martin Stocker
Department of Pediatrics, Children's Hospital Lucerne, Lucerne, Switzerland
Pediatric and Neonatal Intensive Care Unit, Children's Hospital Lucerne, Lucerne, Switzerland

Angelika Berger
Division of Neonatology, Pediatric Intensive Care & Neuropediatrics, Department of Pediatrics and Adolescent Medicine, Medical University of Vienna, Vienna, Austria

Simone S. Schüller
Division of Neonatology, Pediatric Intensive Care & Neuropediatrics, Department of Pediatrics and Adolescent Medicine, Medical University of Vienna, Vienna, Austria
Precision Vaccines Program, Division of Infectious Diseases, Department of Medicine, Boston Children's Hospital, Boston, MA, United States
Harvard Medical School, Boston, MA, United States

Boris W. Kramer and Eduardo Villamor
Department of Pediatrics, Maastricht University Medical Centre (MUMC+), Maastricht, Netherlands
School for Oncology and Developmental Biology (GROW), Maastricht University, Maastricht, Netherlands

Andreas Spittler
Department of Surgery, Research Labs & Core Facility Flow Cytometry, Medical University of Vienna, Vienna, Austria

Ofer Levy
Precision Vaccines Program, Division of Infectious Diseases, Department of Medicine, Boston Children's Hospital, Boston, MA, United States
Harvard Medical School, Boston, MA, United States
Broad Institute of MIT and Harvard, Boston, MA, United States

Min Xu, Liping Wang, Jintong Tan and Yongjun Zhang
Department of Neonatology, Xinhua Hospital, Shanghai Jiaotong University School of Medicine, Shanghai, China

Lan Hu and Chao Chen
Department of Neonatology, Children Hospital of Fudan University, Shanghai, China,

Heyu Huang and Lisu Huang
Department of Pediatric Infectious Diseases, Xinhua Hospital, Shanghai Jiaotong University School of Medicine, Shanghai, China

Xi Zhang
Clinical Research Unit, Xinhua Hospital, Shanghai Jiaotong University School of Medicine, Shanghai, China

Laurence Dillenseger, Claire Langlet, Dominique Astruc and Pierre Kuhn
Service de Pédiatrie II, Hôpital de Hautepierre, Strasbourg, France

Silvia Iacobelli and Jean Bernard Gouyon
Service de Réanimation Néonatale et Pédiatrique, Néonatologie, CHU La Réunion, Saint Pierre, France

Thomas Lavaux and Charline Ratomponirina
Laboratoire de Biochimie et de Biologie Moléculaire, Hôpital de Hautepierre, Strasbourg, France

Marc Labenne
Service de Réanimation Pédiatrique, Hôpital Timone 2, Marseille, France

François Severac
Service de Santé Publique, Nouvel Hôpital Civil, Strasbourg, France

Alexa Dierig and Ulrich Heininger
Infectious Diseases and Vaccinology, University of Basel Children's Hospital, Basel, Switzerland

Christoph Berger and Christa Relly
Division of Infectious Diseases and Hospital Epidemiology, Children's Research Center, University Children's Hospital Zurich, Zurich, Switzerland

Philipp K. A. Agyeman and Christoph Aebi
Department of Pediatrics, Inselspital, Bern University Hospital, University of Bern, Bern, Switzerland

Sara Bernhard-Stirnemann
Cantonal Hospital Aarau, Children's Hospital, Aarau, Switzerland

Eric Giannoni
Department Mother-Woman-Child, Service of Neonatology, Lausanne University Hospital, Lausanne, Switzerland
Infectious Diseases Service, Lausanne University Hospital, Lausanne, Switzerland

Alex Donas
Department of Pediatrics, Children's Hospital Lucerne, Lucerne, Switzerland

Klara M. Posfay-Barbe
Pediatric Infectious Diseases Unit, Children's Hospital of Geneva, University Hospitals of Geneva, Geneva, Switzerland

Anita Niederer-Loher and Christian R. Kahlert
Children's Hospital of Eastern Switzerland St. Gallen, St. Gallen, Switzerland

Paul Hasters
Department of Neonatology, University Hospital Zurich, Zurich, Switzerland

Thomas Riedel
Department of Pediatrics, Cantonal Hospital Graubuenden, Chur, Switzerland

Luregn J. Schlapbach
Department of Pediatrics, Inselspital, Bern University Hospital, University of Bern, Bern, Switzerland
Faculty of Medicine, The University of Queensland, Brisbane, QLD, Australia
Paediatric Critical Care Research Group, Mater Research Institute, University of Queensland, Brisbane, QLD, Australia
Paediatric Intensive Care Unit, Lady Cilento Children's Hospital, Children's Health Queensland, Brisbane, QLD, Australia
Paediatric Intensive Care Unit, Queensland Children's Hospital, Children's Health Queensland, Brisbane, QLD, Australia

Simon Nadel
Paediatric Intensive Care Unit, St. Mary's Hospital and Imperial College London, London, United Kingdom

Nelly Ninis
Paediatrics, St Mary's Hospital, London, United Kingdom

Julie E. Hibbert
Centre for Neonatal Research and Education, University of Western Australia, Perth, WA, Australia

Andrew Currie
Centre for Neonatal Research and Education, University of Western Australia, Perth, WA, Australia
School of Veterinary and Life Sciences, Murdoch University, Perth, WA, Australia

Tobias Strunk
Centre for Neonatal Research and Education, University of Western Australia, Perth, WA, Australia
Neonatal Directorate, King Edward Memorial Hospital for Women, Subiaco, WA, Australia

Li (Danny) Liang
Faculty of Medicine, University of Toronto, Toronto, ON, Canada

Naima Kotadia
Faculty of Medicine, University of British Columbia, Vancouver, BC, Canada

Lacey English
School of Medicine, University of North Carolina, Chapel Hill, NC, United States

J. Mark Ansermino
Center for International Child Health, British Columbia Children's Hospital, Vancouver, BC, Canada
Department of Anesthesiology, Pharmacology and Therapeutics, Faculty of Medicine, University of British Columbia, Vancouver, BC, Canada
Department of Anesthesia, British Columbia Children's Hospital and University of British Columbia, Vancouver, BC, Canada

Jerome Kabakyenga
Maternal Newborn and Child Health Institute, Mbarara University of Science and Technology, Mbarara, Uganda
Faculty of Medicine, Mbarara University of Science and Technology, Mbarara, Uganda

Matthew O. Wiens
Center for International Child Health, British Columbia Children's Hospital, Vancouver, BC, Canada
Department of Anesthesiology, Pharmacology and Therapeutics, Faculty of Medicine, University of British Columbia, Vancouver, BC, Canada
Faculty of Medicine, Mbarara University of Science and Technology, Mbarara, Uganda

Pascal M. Lavoie
Division of Neonatology, Department of Pediatrics, University of British Columbia, Vancouver, BC, Canada

Neha Gupta, Robert Richter and Michele Kong
Division of Pediatric Critical Care Medicine, Department of Pediatrics, University of Alabama at Birmingham, Birmingham, AL, United States

Stephen Robert
Division of Pediatric Critical Care Medicine, Cedars-Sinai Medical Center, Los Angeles, CA, United States

Robert J. Sepanski
Department of Quality Improvement, Children's Hospital of The King's Daughters, Norfolk, VA, United States

Sandip A. Godambe and Arno L. Zaritsky
Department of Pediatrics, Eastern Virginia Medical School, Children's Hospital of The King's Daughters, Norfolk, VA, United States

Colleen M. Badke and Lauren E. Marsillio
Division of Critical Care Medicine, Ann & Robert H. Lurie Children's Hospital of Chicago, Chicago, IL, United States
Department of Pediatrics, Northwestern University Feinberg School of Medicine, Chicago, IL, United States

L. Nelson Sanchez-Pinto
Division of Critical Care Medicine, Ann & Robert H. Lurie Children's Hospital of Chicago, Chicago, IL, United States
Department of Pediatrics, Northwestern University Feinberg School of Medicine, Chicago, IL, United States
Stanley Manne Children's Research Institute, Chicago, IL, United States

Debra E. Weese-Mayer
Department of Pediatrics, Northwestern University Feinberg School of Medicine, Chicago, IL, United States
Center for Autonomic Medicine in Pediatrics, Ann & Robert H. Lurie Children's Hospital of Chicago, Chicago, IL, United States
Stanley Manne Children's Research Institute, Chicago, IL, United States

Nchafatso Gikenyi Obonyo
Initiative to Develop African Research Leaders (IDeALDELTAS), Kilifi, Kenya
KEMRI-Wellcome Trust Research Programme, CGMRC, Kilifi, Kenya
Critical Care Research Group, The Prince Charles Hospital, Chermside, QLD, Australia
Wellcome Trust Centre for Global Health Research, Imperial College London, London, United Kingdom

Luregn Jan Schlapbach
Paediatric Critical Care Research Group, Child Health Research Centre, The University of Queensland, South Brisbane, QLD, Australia
Paediatric Intensive Care Unit, Queensland Children's Hospital, South Brisbane, QLD, Australia
Department of Pediatrics, Inselspital Universitätsspital Bern, Bern, Switzerland
Faculty of Medicine, The University of Queensland, Herston, QLD, Australia

John Francis Fraser
Critical Care Research Group, The Prince Charles Hospital, Chermside, QLD, Australia
Faculty of Medicine, The University of Queensland, Herston, QLD, Australia
School of Medicine, Griffith University, Gold Coast, QLD, Australia

Anouk Goerens and Thomas J. Neuhaus
Department of Pediatrics, Children's Hospital Lucerne, Lucerne, Switzerland

Dirk Lehnick
Clinical Trial Unit, University of Lucerne, Lucerne, Switzerland

Michael Büttcher
Department of Pediatrics, Children's Hospital Lucerne, Lucerne, Switzerland
Infectious Diseases Unit, Children's Hospital Lucerne, Lucerne, Switzerland

Karin Daetwyler, Matteo Fontana, Petra Genet, Davide Morgillo, Sina Pilgrim and Katharina Schwendener-Scholl
Department of Pediatrics, Children's Hospital Lucerne, Lucerne, Switzerland
Pediatric and Neonatal Intensive Care Unit, Children's Hospital Lucerne, Lucerne, Switzerland

Marco Lurà and Nicolas Regamey
Department of Pediatrics, Children's Hospital Lucerne, Lucerne, Switzerland
Pediatric Pulmonology Unit, Children's Hospital Lucerne, Lucerne, Switzerland

Amanda Harley
Paediatric Critical Care Research Group, Child Health Research Centre and Faculty of Medicine, The University of Queensland, Brisbane, QLD, Australia
Paediatric Intensive Care Unit, Queensland Children's Hospital, Children's Health Queensland, Brisbane, QLD, Australia
School of Nursing, The University of Queensland, Brisbane, QLD, Australia

Jos M. Latour
Faculty of Health and Human Sciences, School of Nursing and Midwifery, University of Plymouth, Plymouth, United Kingdom

Eirin Esaiassen and Jorunn Pauline Cavanagh
Paediatric Research Group, Department of Clinical Medicine, UiT The Arctic University of Norway, Tromsø, Norway
Department of Paediatrics, University Hospital of North Norway, Tromsø, Norway

Erik Hjerde and Nils P. Willassen
Department of Chemistry, Norstruct, UiT The Arctic University of Norway, Tromsø, Norway

Tanja Pedersen
Department of Paediatrics, Haukeland University Hospital, Bergen, Norway

Jannicke H. Andresen
Department of Neonatal Intensive Care, Oslo University Hospital, Oslo, Norway

Siren I. Rettedal
Department of Paediatrics, Stavanger University Hospital, Stavanger, Norway Ragnhild Støen
Department of Paediatrics, St. Olavs University Hospital, Trondheim, Norway
Department of Laboratory Medicine, Children's and Women's Health, University of Science and Technology, Trondheim, Norway

Britt Nakstad
Department of Paediatric and Adolescents Medicine, Akershus University Hospital, Nordbyhagen, Norway
Institute of Clinical Medicine, Faculty of Medicine, University of Oslo, Oslo, Norway

Manon Tauzin and Gilles Dassieu
Neonatal Intensive Care Unit, Centre Hospitalier Intercommunal de Créteil, Créteil, France

Robert Cohen
ACTIV, Association Clinique et Thérapeutique Infantile du Val de Marne, Saint-Maur des Fossés, France
Université Paris Est, IMRB- GRC GEMINI, Créteil, France
Clinical Research Center, Centre Hospitalier Intercommunal de Créteil, Créteil, France
Groupe de Pathologie Infectieuse Pédiatrique, Paris, France
Unité Court Séjour, Petits Nourrissons, Service de Néonatologie, Centre Hospitalier Intercommunal de Créteil, Créteil, France

Xavier Durrmeyer
Neonatal Intensive Care Unit, Centre Hospitalier Intercommunal de Créteil, Créteil, France
Université Paris Est, IMRB- GRC GEMINI, Créteil, France
Inserm, U1153, Obstetrical, Perinatal and Pediatric Epidemiology Team, Epidemiology and Biostatistics Sorbonne, Paris Descartes University, Paris, France

Jérôme Barre
Clinical Research Center, Centre Hospitalier Intercommunal de Créteil, Créteil, France
Department of Pharmacology, Centre Hospitalier Intercommunal de Créteil, Créteil, France

Laurence Caeymaex
Neonatal Intensive Care Unit, Centre Hospitalier Intercommunal de Créteil, Créteil, France
Clinical Research Center, Centre Hospitalier Intercommunal de Créteil, Créteil, France
Department of Research in Ethics EA1610 Studies on Science and Technics, Paris Est University, Créteil, France

Tamara van Donge
Paediatric Pharmacology and Pharmacometrics, University Children's Hospital Basel, University of Basel, Basel, Switzerland

Julia A. Bielicki
Paediatric Pharmacology and Pharmacometrics, University Children's Hospital Basel, University of Basel, Basel, Switzerland
Paediatric Infectious Diseases Research Group, Institute for Infection and Immunity, St George's, University of London, London, United Kingdom

John van den Anker
Paediatric Pharmacology and Pharmacometrics, University Children's Hospital Basel, University of Basel, Basel, Switzerland
Intensive Care and Department of Paediatric Surgery, Erasmus MC-Sophia Children's Hospital, Rotterdam, Netherlands
Division of Clinical Pharmacology, Children's National Health System, Washington, DC, United States

Marc Pfister
Paediatric Pharmacology and Pharmacometrics, University Children's Hospital Basel, University of Basel, Basel, Switzerland
Certara LP, Princeton, NJ, United States

Index

P

R

S

T

V

www.ingramcontent.com/pod-product-compliance
Lightning Source LLC
LaVergne TN
LVHW082137200926
848484LV00008B/2065
* 9 7 9 8 8 8 7 4 0 3 7 0 0 *